AF771529

Healthcare: Planning and Management

Healthcare: Planning and Management

Edited by Codie Horton

hayle medical
New York

Hayle Medical,
750 Third Avenue, 9th Floor,
New York, NY 10017, USA

Visit us on the World Wide Web at:
www.haylemedical.com

© Hayle Medical, 2018

This book contains information obtained from authentic and highly regarded sources. Copyright for all individual chapters remain with the respective authors as indicated. All chapters are published with permission under the Creative Commons Attribution License or equivalent. A wide variety of references are listed. Permission and sources are indicated; for detailed attributions, please refer to the permissions page and list of contributors. Reasonable efforts have been made to publish reliable data and information, but the authors, editors and publisher cannot assume any responsibility for the validity of all materials or the consequences of their use.

ISBN: 978-1-63241-499-1

The publisher's policy is to use permanent paper from mills that operate a sustainable forestry policy. Furthermore, the publisher ensures that the text paper and cover boards used have met acceptable environmental accreditation standards.

Trademark Notice: Registered trademark of products or corporate names are used only for explanation and identification without intent to infringe.

Printed in China.

Cataloging-in-Publication Data

Healthcare : planning and management / edited by Codie Horton.
p. cm.
Includes bibliographical references and index.
ISBN 978-1-63241-499-1
1. Medical care. 2. Health planning.
3. Health services administration. I. Horton, Codie.
RA427 .H43 2018
362.1--dc23

Table of Contents

Preface

Healthcare focuses on the diagnosis and treatment of illnesses found in human beings. It can be divided into three levels-primary care, secondary care and tertiary care. Pharmacy, nursing, psychology, medicine, etc. all fall under the umbrella of healthcare. This book unfolds the innovative aspects of healthcare management which will be crucial for the progress of this field in the future. It attempts to assist those with a goal of delving into the field of healthcare.

All of the data presented henceforth, was collaborated in the wake of recent advancements in the field. The aim of this book is to present the diversified developments from across the globe in a comprehensible manner. The opinions expressed in each chapter belong solely to the contributing authors. Their interpretations of the topics are the integral part of this book, which I have carefully compiled for a better understanding of the readers.

At the end, I would like to thank all those who dedicated their time and efforts for the successful completion of this book. I also wish to convey my gratitude towards my friends and family who supported me at every step.

Editor

1

Isolation Facilities for Highly Infectious Diseases in Europe – A Cross-Sectional Analysis in 16 Countries

Stefan Schilling[1]*, Francesco Maria Fusco[2], Giuseppina De Iaco[3], Barbara Bannister[4], Helena C. Maltezou[5], Gail Carson[6], Rene Gottschalk[7], Hans-Reinhard Brodt[8], Philippe Brouqui[9], Vincenzo Puro[2], Giuseppe Ippolito[2], for the European Network for Highly Infectious Diseases project members¶

1 Department for Internal Medicine, Staedtische Kliniken Moenchengladbach, Moenchengladbach, Germany, **2** Department for Infectious Diseases, National Institute for Infectious Diseases "Lazarro Spallanzani", Rome, Italy, **3** Department for Internal Medicine, Azienda Ospedaliero, Universitaria Ospedali Riuniti delle Marche, Torrette, Italy, **4** Department for Infectious Diseases, The Royal Free Hospital, London, United Kingdom, **5** Department for Interventions in Health-Care Facilities, Hellenic Center for Disease Control and Prevention, Athens, Greece, **6** Department of Rare and Imported Pathogens, Health Protection Agency, Porton, United Kingdom, **7** Department for Infectious Diseases, Port Health Authorities, Frankfurt am Main, Germany, **8** Department for Infectious Diseases, Goethe University Frankfurt, Frankfurt am Main, Germany, **9** Department for Infectious Diseases and Tropical Medicine, Marseilles University, Marseille, France

Abstract

Background: Highly Infectious Diseases (HIDs) are (i) easily transmissible form person to person; (ii) cause a life-threatening illness with no or few treatment options; and (iii) pose a threat for both personnel and the public. Hence, even suspected HID cases should be managed in specialised facilities minimizing infection risks but allowing state-of-the-art critical care. Consensus statements on the operational management of isolation facilities have been published recently. The study presented was set up to compare the operational management, resources, and technical equipment among European isolation facilities. Due to differences in geography, population density, and national response plans it was hypothesized that adherence to recommendations will vary.

Methods and Findings: Until mid of 2010 the European Network for Highly Infectious Diseases conducted a cross-sectional analysis of isolation facilities in Europe, recruiting 48 isolation facilities in 16 countries. Three checklists were disseminated, assessing 44 items and 148 specific questions. The median feedback rate for specific questions was 97.9% (n = 47/48) (range: n = 7/48 (14.6%) to n = 48/48 (100%). Although all facilities enrolled were nominated specialised facilities' serving countries or regions, their design, equipment and personnel management varied. Eighteen facilities fulfilled the definition of a High Level Isolation Unit'. In contrast, 24 facilities could not operate independently from their co-located hospital, and five could not ensure access to equipment essential for infection control. Data presented are not representative for the EU in general, as only 16/27 (59.3%) of all Member States agreed to participate. Another limitation of this study is the time elapsed between data collection and publication; e.g. in Germany one additional facility opened in the meantime.

Conclusion: There are disparities both within and between European countries regarding the design and equipment of isolation facilities. With regard to the International Health Regulations, terminology, capacities and equipment should be standardised.

Editor: Alex Friedrich, University Medical Center Groningen, Netherlands

Funding: The "European Network for Highly Infectious Diseases – EuroNHID" is co-funded by the European Commission/DG SANCO under the EU contract number 2006205. Neither the Commission nor DG SANCO had an influence on the study design, data collection, or interpretation of results. The funders had no role in study design, data collection and analysis, decision to publish, or preparation of the manuscript.

Competing Interests: The authors have declared that no competing interests exist.

* Email: stefan.schilling@kgu.de

¶ Membership of the European Network for Highly Infectious Diseases is provided in the Acknowledgments.

Introduction

The term highly infectious diseases (HID) defines mostly viral and bacterial infections that (i) are easily transmissible from person to person; (ii) cause a life-threatening clinical illness with no or few treatment options; and (iii) pose a threat for both health care workers and the public, thus requiring specific infection control measures and public health planning [1]. Included in this definition are viral haemorrhagic fevers (e.g. Filo-, Arena- or Bunyavirus infections); some respiratory syndromes (e.g. severe acute respiratory syndrome (SARS)-Coronavirus, or pneumonic plague); as well as any (re−) emerging infectious agent transmissible from person-to-person [2]. In Europe, HIDs have caused several events within the last decade: SARS affected eight European nations in 2003; Lassa virus has repeatedly been imported to Europe; and Crimean Congo Haemorrhagic Fever virus infections are increasing in several Mediterranean regions, and have also been imported to central Europe and the United

Kingdom (UK) [3–7]. Recently detected agents like the new human Middle East Respiratory Syndrome Coronavirus underline the continuous challenge faced [8].

Patients with suspected or proven HIDs should be cared for in a clinical environment that provides safe, secure, high-quality, and appropriate care with optimal infection containment, prevention and control procedures [1]. Consensus statements on the operational management and design of isolation facilities have been published in Europe and the United States of America [1;9]. In addition, the European Commission has funded projects to enhance early recognition of cases by training front-line health care workers (HCWs) and standardizing diagnostic methodology [10–12]. Despite such efforts, no pooled data on isolation facilities resources, such as infrastructure design, technical equipment, capacity and access to intensive care, do exist.

The study presented was performed by the European Network for Highly Infectious Diseases, EuroNHID, and set up to compare the operational management, resources, and technical equipment among isolation facilities with recommendations published. Due to differences in geography, population density, national response plans, and experience with HIDs in participating countries, it was hypothesized that the level of adherence to recommendations may vary. The objective of this article is to present data about infrastructure design and resources, technical equipment, available personnel, and access to intensive care.

Methods

Setting

EuroNHID consists of infectious disease clinicians and public health officers with expertise in the management of HIDs identified via their National Health Authorities. Administrative and scientific aspects are managed by an Italian Coordination Team, and a Steering Committee, including partners from France, Germany, Greece, and the UK. Both committees started their work in 2007, and reported all organizational and scientific developments to the project members. Names and countries of all project members are listed above.\

Study design

Three checklists were developed and based on project-member's experience, available literature, national preparedness plans, and guidelines of international authorities for the management of HIDs [13]. Each checklist contained questions addressing specific items of interest, and answers were structured as open-ended, closed, semi-open or free text options. Overall, the checklists included 44 items and 148 specific questions.

Checklist one contained three major sections: Infrastructure; technical equipment; and personnel management. A fourth section on Emergency Departments was not obligatory [14]. All checklists can be downloaded after free registration from: www.EUNID.eu.

The checklists underwent a pilot application to identify structural gaps and sources of misinterpretation [13]. The facilities of the Steering Committee members and one external facility applied the checklists and cross-checked all itmes for their applicability, but no external validation process was conducted. Following minor changes, the checklists were disseminated to all eligible facilities until December 2009 and expected to be re-submitted within three months. Data provided were cross-checked by personal on-site visits by a coordination team member in all but four centres enrolled. Investigator (the National Project Representative) and observer (the Coordination Team member) bias may be ruled out, as all data recorded were cross-checked on-site and agreed with the facilities operational manager or director.

Participants

Until November 2009, the Coordination Team collected data on eligible isolation facilities to be included into the survey. National Health Authorities of all European Union (EU) member states were contacted to identify their will to participate. Participating National Health Authorities were requested to identify clinical facilities responsible for the admission, assessment, and care of HID patients in their country, and to nominate a National Project Representative.

Role of the funding source

EuroNHID was co-funded by the European Commission/ Director General for Consumers and Health (DG SANCO) for an initial period of 36 months and extended to 42 months without additional funding. A technical and scientific report on all data collected during the project was delivered to the Commission in December 2010. For details please follow: http://ec.europa.eu/research/health/infectious-diseases/emerging-epidemics/projects/143_en.html.

Results

Participants

Until mid of 2010, 48 isolation facilities in 16 European countries were recruited into this survey (Table 1). Recruitment was closed by the end of 2009 with the exception of Norway, who received questionnaires by end of 2009 and submitted data by spring of 2010. Data collection and on-site visits were finalised in spring 2010. Except for Norway, all participating countries were EU member states. Data were collected from all existing facilities in participating countries except for Spain, where data were only collected in the Catalonia region. Overall, the median feedback rate for checklist 1 was 97.9% (n = 47/48), with a range from n = 7/48 (14.6%) to n = 48/48 (100%) of centres providing valid answers to specific questions. All data provided in this article represent a minimum feedback from 44 facilities (>90%).

Background data on facilities evaluated

The majority of facilities were constructed or underwent major re-construction in the year 2001 or later (n = 32/47; 66.7%) and are located on the same campus or in direct connection with a general hospital (n = 41/48; 85.4%). Most facilities have designated rooms (n = 23/48; 47.9%) or wards (n = 18/48; 37.5%) located within other hospital structures, and seven facilities are located within a separate building (n = 7/48; 14.6%). National guidelines for the construction of isolation facilities were available for 17 facilities whereas 29 were (re−) constructed in the absence of specific requirements (37% and 63%, respectively). Three facilities accept paediatric (6.3%), and 14 (29.2%) accept adult patients, only, whereas most facilities provide care for both (n = 31/48; 64.6%). The number of isolation beds per facility ranges from one to 56, with a median of 9.3 beds for adult and 7.2 for paediatric patients. With respect to the overall population, the number of beds ranges from 0.05 to 17.9 per one million inhabitants (median: 1.7) (Table 1). The majority of all facilities uses their beds on a daily basis for routine patients (n = 37/48; 77,1%), while the remainder provide bed capacities reserved for HID cases, only (n = 11/48, 22.9%).

Except for the United Kingdom, all countries (n = 46/48; 95.4%) use barrier nursing techniques with high level Personal Protective Equipment (hl-PPE) (21). 37 facilities (n = 37/46; 80.4%) have a response time of less than five hours after a case is notified, the remainder demand up to 10 hours to be fully operational (n = 9/46; 19.6%). Only eight (16.7%) of all facilities

Table 1. Number of isolation facilities, existence of High Level Isolation Units, and isolation beds for highly infectious patients per participating country.

Participating country	Overall number of facilities enrolled#	Overall number of isolation beds	Number of isolation beds/million of population*
Austria	1	24	2.87
Bulgaria	2	64	8.46
Denmark	1	56	10.12
Finland	2 (1)	57	10.65
France	12 (5)	112	1.73
Germany	8 (6)	44	0.54
Greece	6 (1)	20	1.77
Ireland	2 (1)	4	0.89
Italy	2 (2)	5	0.08
Luxembourg	1	15	29.87
Malta	1	3	7.26
Norway	1 (1)	4	0.82
Poland	1	2	0.05
Slovenia	1	2	0.97
Spain	5	38	0.58§
United Kingdom	2 (1)	3	0.05

(#): Numbers in brackets indicate the amount of High Level Isolation Units per country, if existing. (*): Total population calculated on the basis of Eurostat [30]. (§): Facilities enrolled are located in the Catalonia region, only.

evaluated lacked any experience in the management of suspected or proven HID cases. Among the remainder, most had experience with infections due to SARS (n = 13/48; 27.8%), and viral haemorrhagic fevers (n = 9/48; 18.8%).

Technical equipment

Essential technical requirements for isolation facilities includes: Negative pressure in the isolation room(s); an anteroom; aerosol-tight doors and windows; High Efficacy Particulate Air (HEPA) filtration of exhausted air; and a surface of walls, floors and ceiling withstanding disinfection procedures [1]. All but five facilities enrolled (n = 43/48; 89.6%) provide negative pressure in the isolation area, and the majority (n = 34/48; 70.8%) is also equipped with all other essential equipment investigated. In facilities with two or less additional items, most often HEPA filtration of exhausted air and anterooms were missing (n = 7 and 5/14 facilities, respectively) (Figure 1).

Additional technical requirements not considered essential, but benefitting infection control and HCW safety, includes: self-closing doors; audio and/or visual negative pressure indicators; an exclusive evacuation pathway; and an internal communication system (for HCW-HCW and HCW-patient communication) [1]. At least 3 additional technical requirements are found in the majority of facilities (n = 34/48; 70.8%). Most often, an internal communication system (n = 43/48; 89.6%) and negative pressure indicators (n = 40/48; 83.3%) were present, while an exclusive evacuation pathway was missing in half of all facilities enrolled (n = 27/48, 56.3%).

Access to Intensive Care

Thirty-three facilities (68.8%) provide intensive care, available for patients within the isolation facility. Twelve facilities (25%) rely on a designated isolation room within standard intensive care units, three (6.3%) have no access to intensive care capacities (Figure 2). Equipment for the monitoring of vital parameters and advanced life support is available in all 48 facilities. In contrast, mechanical ventilators are available either permanently in twelve (25%) or on call in thirty-two facilities (66.7%), but not accessible at all in four (8.3%). Forty-two facilities (87.5%) have either permanent or on-call access to blood gas analyzers, whereas six have not (12.5%). Hence, out of forty-five facilities reporting intensive care provision, one (2.2%) lacks a mechanical ventilator, and three (6.7%) have no ability to monitor their ventilation therapy.

Personnel

Almost all facilities (93.6%; n = 44/47) report permanent access to specifically trained infectious diseases doctors. 45/48 (93.75%) facilities report providing intensive care, but only 34 of those (75.5%) have access to specifically trained intensive care specialists. In addition, out of 34 facilities indicating to provide care for pediatric HID patients, only 11 (32.4%) report either permanent or on-call access to pediatricians. Compared with available doctors, even fewer facilities report access to specifically trained infectious diseases nurses (n = 41/48; 85.4%), but intensive care nurses are available in a comparable number of facilities (n = 32/45; 71.1%) (Figure 3).

All but two facilities indicate 24-hour access to specifically trained medical and non-medical staff (n = 45/47; 95.7%), although 72.9% (n = 35/48) only have specific protocols to contact staff responsible for the operation of the facility. A shift plan to limit the number of HCWs exposed to patients as well as the duration of working under hl-PPE exists in 70.8% of facilities (n = 34/48). Permanent access to technicians was lacking in eleven facilities (n = 11/48; 22.9%).

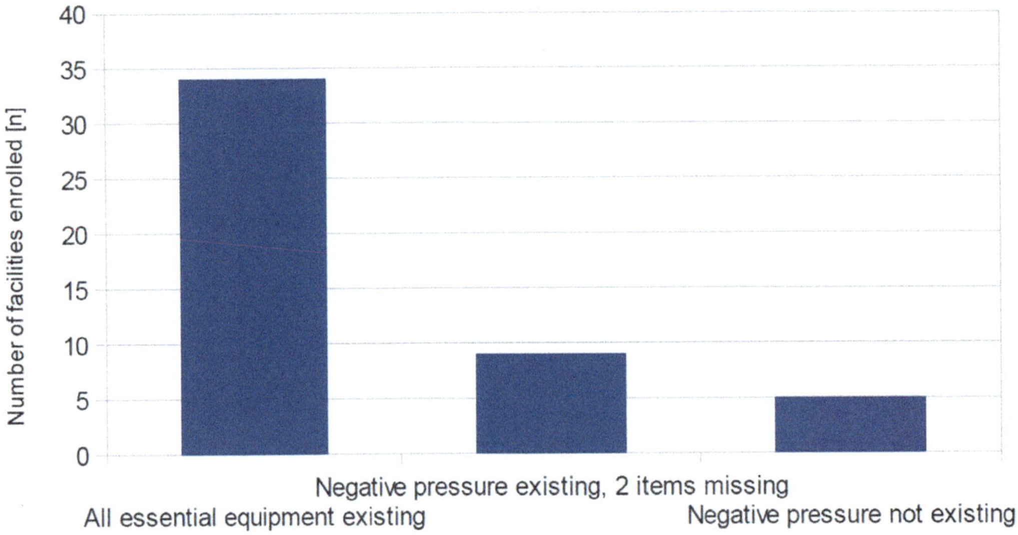

Figure 1. Existence of technical equipment essential for infection control and HCW's safety. Number of enrolled facilities and adherence to recommended equipment (overall response n = 48/48). Access to all essential equipment was reported from 34 facilities; negative pressure existing, but 2 other items missing in 9 facilities; and no negative pressure available in 5 facilities.

Conclusions

All participating facilities were evaluated for their adherence to recommendations for the operational management of isolation facilities published [1]. As hypothesized, the level of adherence to recommendations varied, both within and between participating countries.

Hence, three categories of isolation facilities representing different levels of adherence were defined:

(i) High Level Isolation Units (HLIU), defined as operating independently from other hospital resources and specifically equipped; (ii) Isolation Rooms, defined as specifically equipped but only partially independent from other hospital resources; and (iii) Referral Centers, neither specifically equipped nor functionally independent.

According to this classification, all facilities enrolled were categorized as shown in Figure 4. Few facilities completely fulfilled recommendations for HLIUs (n = 18/48; 37.5%). Six of those are located in Germany, five in France, two in Italy, and one each in the UK, Finland, Greece, Ireland, and Norway. Such HLIUs are constructed and equipped for the admission, assessment and long-term critical care of HID patients.

Most facilities assessed did partially meet the recommendations, but lacked infrastructural components, or preconditions for personnel management (n = 25/48; 52%). Such were labeled 'Isolation Rooms' considered effective to assess HID patients and provide short-term medical care until a patient can be transferred

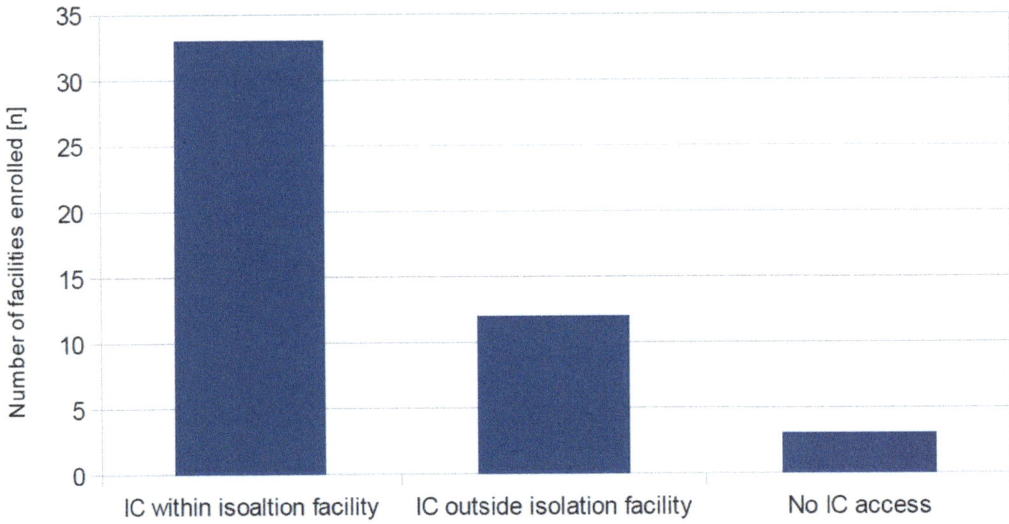

Figure 2. Access to and location of Intensive Care beds for HID patients. Number of facilities enrolled with Intensive Care (IC) capacity and location of IC beds (overall response n = 48/48). 33 facilities provide IC beds within the isolation area, and 12 in designated rooms on standard IC wards.

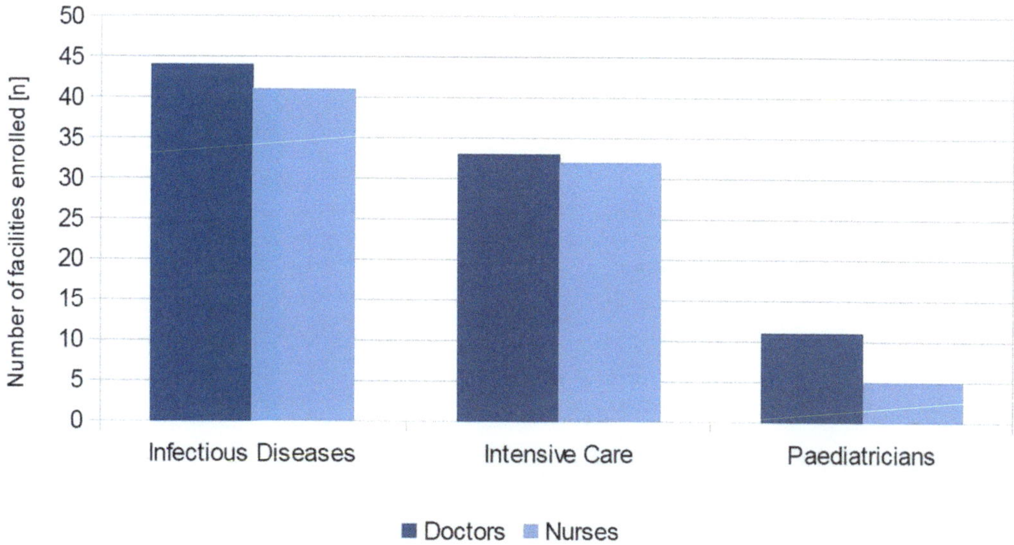

Figure 3. Access to specifically trained personnel. Number of facilities enrolled with access to specifically trained personnel (overall response n = 48/48). Access to Infectious Disease and Intensive Care doctors or nurses is provided in the majority of facilities, but specifically trained personnel for paediatric patients is rarely available.

to a HLIU. Of these, five each are located in France, Greece, and Spain; two in Germany; and one each in Denmark, Finland, Ireland, Luxembourg, Malta, Poland and Slovenia.

The remaining facilities (n = 5/48; 10.4%) are considered to function as 'Referral Centers' where suspected HID cases can be assessed within daily routine, but even short-term critical care cannot be provided without an increased risk of nosocomial infections. Two of such facilities are located in Bulgaria and France, each, and one in Austria.

Discussion

Within the last decades, autochthonous outbreaks or imported cases of HIDs have affected Europe with significant impact, and new pathogens are emerging. Most European countries have established national response plans including specialised clinical care facilities for the management of such scenarios [3–7,15–17]. This article presents the first standardised analysis on the operational management, infrastructure, and technical equipment of 48 isolation facilities in 16 European countries. Data provided may support national authorities to assess their level of preparedness but have to be adapted to single member states' needs and resources. With regard to the implementation of the International Health Regulations [18], terminology, capacities and equipment accessible in isolation facility should be documented and standardised on a European level.

Although all EU member states were invited to join the project by DGSANCO, only 16 agreed to participate, thus data presented

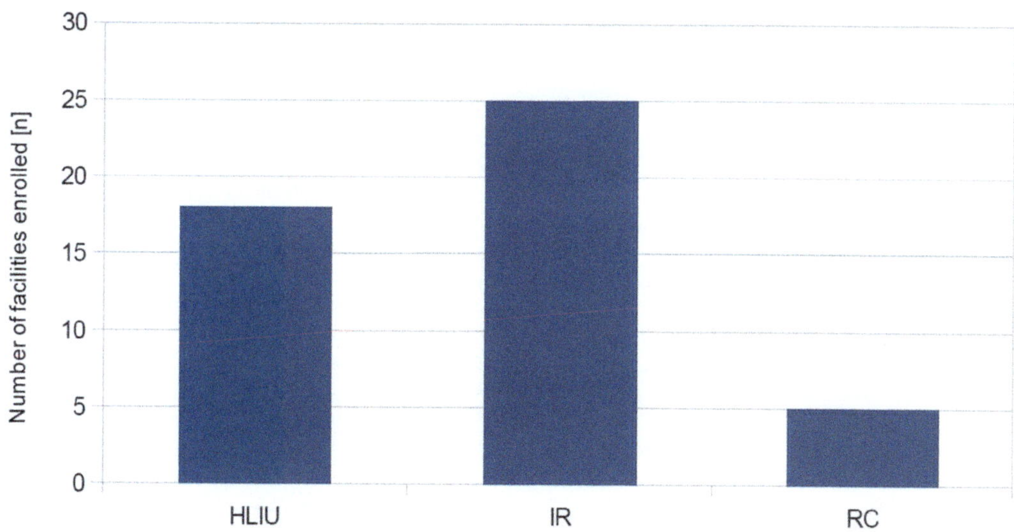

Figure 4. Classification of enrolled facilities by adherence to EUNID recommendations. Number of facilities classified by adherence to published recommendations: 18/48 facilities fulfilled the criteria of 'High Level Isolation Units' (HLIU); 25 met criteria for 'Isolation Rooms' and 5 for 'Referral Centres'.

are not representative for the EU in general. A major limitation of this study is the time elapsed between data collection and publication: e.g. in Germany one another facility has opened in the meantime. Hence, a periodical re-assessment of facilities and countries should be achieved, aiming for a permanently updated record of national preparedness. In addition, the checklists applied did not undergo an external validation process (e.g. a Delphi Cycle) due to limitations of funds and project duration, and present published guidelines, only. Hence, within the data collection process, misinterpretations occurred and items needed to be excluded from the data analysis presented here.

Half of all countries assessed have at least one HLIU according to the recommendations [1]. Compared to the definition, 18 facilities fulfilled the criteria applied, but the majority of all facilities enrolled could not operate independently from other facilities. The high rate of incompliance with the recommendations depicted here can be explained by the absence of legally binding documents by the time most facilities were constructed. After SARS and the US anthrax attacks in 2001, the political will was to enhance public preparedness, but no standard was agreed on. Only few countries (e.g. the UK) had specific guidelines at hand, but the vast majority of facilities were constructed using laboratory- or operational theatre guidelines adapted to local needs and infrastructure prerequisites. An earlier inventory of isolation rooms in Europe by our group faced this problem, when EU countries were asked to report on negative pressure rooms for HID patients [19]: The overall number of rooms exceeded most expectations, but both technical and infrastructural conditions were not well defined. Hence, an overreporting of any isolation room' with available led to the impression of a well prepared health system, although other aspects of equipment and personnel were not addressed. Given the definitions for different levels of isolation facilities proposed now, a reassessment of the EU's capacities could lead to more accurate data. Furthermore, the allocation of funds for hospital's biological event preparedness has decreased since the SARS pandemic, and is not harmonised within the EU. Hence, as our data show, the level of adherence to the recommendations mirrors the economical situation in the EU, with the highest level of adherence in the economical most stable countries. The situation in the United States of America is comparable: a consensus on the operational management of isolation units consistent with the European approach exists, but only three facilities fulfill those criteria, although hospital preparedness for biological events is mandatory [9,20]. The contrary can be found in Israel, where the capability to manage HID patients is mandatory for every public hospital, and dedicated HLIUs are absent [21].

As HLIUs are designed for single imported cases or small clusters in the beginning of an outbreak, only, they do not compensate for surge capacity planning in major biological events [1]. Besides infrastructure and equipment, additional features which support effective functioning of such specialised centres were addressed in this survey and recently published [22–25]. Access to a transportation system for HID patients plays an important role in distribution of isolation facilities and is reflected by the overall amount isolation facilities per country. Balancing the necessary access to a focus of expertise with available transport logistics leads to either a centralised or a de-centralised approach to the location of specific facilities, and ambulance dispatch recording can be of use in early warning systems for outbreak detection [26].

Most documented HID cases demanded supportive intensive care [16,17,27], and access to such is considered essential for HLIUs [1]. In order to allocate funds most effectively, a balance between infection control excellence and operational feasibility should be sought. Basic specifications for HLIU provision, including access to intensive care equipment and trained personnel, should be developed in order to facilitate a common standard of best clinical practice. Key issues are the composition of a permanently available multidisciplinary medical and non-medical team, the ability and physical fitness to work with PPE, and reliable timelines and shifts to prevent accidents or mistakes due to exhaustion [1,28]. Data depicted in this article do highlight available personnel as the most crucial pitfall in operating isolation facilities: Compared to the complicane with technical equipment recommendations, the lack of specifically trained staff is surprising, especially for HCWs trained in intensive and paediatric care. It should be mentioned that all facilities with experience in proven HIDs provide more sophisticated human resources management such as shift-and surge capacity planning as an outcome of their experience.

The overall investment for an isolation facility, and HLIUs in particular, is high, in terms of costs for construction and maintenance, medical and infection control equipment, human resources and training activities. Even in time of economical constraints, employers "are obliged to ensure the health and safety of workers", as defined by the European Commission [29]. Without adequate protection, HCWs may acquire and transmit infections, with potential dramatic impact on the health system, and the economic solidity of a country, as documented during the SARS epidemic in Canada. For these reasons, we believe that specialized isolation facilities, and HLIUs in particular, still represent a critical infrastructure to which each EU Member State should have access, within the country or through pre-defined agreements with neighbouring countries where such facilities are available. Whether such capacities should be reserved for HID cases, only, or also used on routine basis, is part of an ongoing discussion. Financial constraints within hospitals and the host country may benefit from a routine-use concept, although such facilities demand more frequent maintenence due to damage on technical equipment. In addition, access to routine use beds for training of HCWs is reduced, and patients need to be relocated to other rooms once the facility receives an HID case. In contrast, reserved bed capacities demand additional personnel and material for routine functional checks, thus considered cost- ineffective. The major benefit from reserved capacities is a full access for training and no delay in patients admission since no evacuation of others is needed.

The WHO IHRs define the need of preparedness for infectious diseases outbreaks, but a European, if not international, consensus on the funding and minimum number of isolation capacities is not in sight. Although HIDs are rare events, they cause dynamic and often rapidly evolving issues in need of comprehensive solutions and may challenge the capacity of healthcare systems. Leadership and funding at both national and European level are required to harmonize preparedness plans, terminology and communication to weaken the impact of future infectious disease outbreaks with cross-border potential. In order to achieve a balance between saving lives and protecting HCWs in hazardous environments, national and international collaboration should continue to share experiences, and provide standardized training and equipment.

Acknowledgments

The 'European Network for Highly Infectious Diseases – EuroNHID' is co-funded by the European Commission/DG SANCO under the EU contract number 2006205. Neither the Commission nor DG SANCO had an influence on the study design, data collection, or interpretation of results. Other members of the EuroNHID have supported the authors listed in providing data of their facilities (in alphabetical order of the country): Norbert Vetter (Austria), Mira Kojouharova (Bulgaria), Kremena Parmakova (Bulgaria), Peter Skinhoej (Denmark), Heli Siikamaki (Finland), Christian Perronne (France), all members of the "Ständige Arbeitsgemeinschaft der Kompetenz- und Behandlungszentren – StAKoB" (Germany), Olga Adrami (Greece), John Lambert (Republic of Ireland), Simone Lanini (Italy), Robert Hemmer (Luxembourg), Michael Borg (Malta), Anne Lise Fjellet (Norway), Arne Broch Brantsæter (Norway), Andrzej Horban (Poland), Franc Strle (Slovenia), Antoni Trilla (Spain). We also thank Ramona Iacovino for administrative assistance and all European centres for data contribution.

Author Contributions

Conceived and designed the experiments: SS FMF. Performed the experiments: SS FMF. Analyzed the data: SS FMF GDI. Wrote the paper: SS FMF. Reviewing of the questionnaire design and content: SS FMF GDI BB HM GC RG HRB PB VP GI. Data interpretation: SS FMF GDI BB HM GC RG HRB PB VP GI. Final approval of the manuscript: SS FMF GDI BB HM GC RG HRB PB VP GI.

References

1. Bannister B, Puro V, Fusco FM, Heptonstall J, Ippolito G, et al. (2009) Framework for the design and operation of high level isolation units: consensus of the European Network of Infectious Diseases. Lancet Infect Dis. Jan 9(1): 45–56.
2. Brouqui P, Puro V, Fusco FM, Bannister B, Schilling S, et al. (2009) Infection control in the management of highly pathogenic infectious diseases: consensus of the European Network of Infectious Disease. Lancet Infect Dis. May 9(5): 301–11.
3. Drosten C, Preiser W, Günther S, Schmitz H, Doerr HW (2003) Severe acute respiratory syndrome: identification of the etiological agent. Trends Mol Med. Aug 9(8): 325–7.
4. Kitching A, Addiman S, Cathcart S, Bischop L, Krahe D, et al. (2009) A fatal case of Lassa fever in London, January 2009. Euro Surveill 14: pii: 19117.
5. Atkin S, Anaraki S, Gothard P, Walsh A, Brown D, et al. (2009) The first case of Lassa fever imported from Mali to the United Kingdom, February 2009. Euro Surveill 14: pii: 19145.
6. Barr DA, Aitken C, Bell DJ, Brown CS, Cropley I, et al. (2013) First confirmed case of Crimean-Congo Haemorrhagic Fever in the UK. Lancet 382: 1458.
7. Ergönül O (2006) Crimean-Congo haemorrhagic fever. Lancet Infect Dis. Apr; 6(4): 203–14.
8. Zaki AM, van Boheemen S, Bestebroer TM, Osterhaus ADME, Fouchier RAM (2012) Isolation of a Novel Coronavirus from a Man with Pneumonia in Saudi Arabia N Engl J Med 367: 1814–20.
9. Smith PW, Anderson AO, Christopher GW, Cieslak TJ, Devreede GJ, et al. (2006) Designing a Biocontainment Unit to Care for Patients with Serious Communicable Diseases: A Consensus Statement. Biosec and Bioterr. 4(4): 351–65.
10. Baka A, Fusco FM, Puro V, Vetter N, Skinhoj P, et al. (2007) A curriculum for training healthcare workers in the management of highly infectious diseases. Euro Surveill. Jun 1; 12(6): E5–6.
11. Nisii C, Castilletti C, Di Caro A, Capobianchi MR, Brown D, et al. (2009) The European network of Biosafety-Level-4 laboratories: enhancing European preparedness for new health threats. Clin Microbiol Infect Aug 15(8): 720–6.
12. European Commission, Community Research and Development Service European Training and Research Centre for Imported and Highly Contagious Diseases. Available: http://epp.eurostat.ec.europa.eu/portal/page/portal/population/data/main_tables. Accessed 2012 Oct 1.
13. Fusco F, Schilling S, Puro V, Brodt HR, Follin P, et al. (2009) EuroNHID checklists for the assessment of highlevel isolation units and referral centres for highly infectious diseases: results from the pilot phase of a European survey. Clin Microbiol Infect. Aug 15(8): 711–9.
14. Fusco FM, Schilling S, De Iaco G, Brodt HR, Brouqui P, et al. (2012) Infection control management of patients with suspected highly infectious diseases in emergency departments: data from a survey in 41 facilities in 14 European countries. BMC Infect Dis. Jan 28; 12: 27.
15. Günther S, Feldmann H, Geisbert TW, Hensley LE, Rollin PE, et al. (2011) Management of accidental exposure to Ebola virus in the biosafety level 4 laboratory, Hamburg, Germany. J Infect Dis. Nov; 204 Suppl 3: S785–90.
16. van Paassen J, Bauer MP, Arbous MS, Visser LG, Schmidt-Chanasit J, et al. (2012) Acute liver failure, multiorgan failure, cerebral oedema, and activation of proangiogenic and antiangiogenic factors in a case of Marburg haemorrhagic fever. Lancet Infect Dis. Aug 12(8): 635–42.
17. Danielsson N, on behalf of the ECDC Internal Response Team, Catchpole M (2012) Novel coronavirus associated with severe respiratory disease: Case definition and public health measures. Euro Surveill 17(39): pii = 20282.
18. Rodier G, Hardiman M, Plotkin B, Ganter B (2006) Implementing the International Health Regulations (2005) in Europe. Euro Surveill11(12): pii = 664.
19. Fusco FM, Puro V, Baka A, Bannister B, Brodt HR, et al. (2009) Isolation rooms for highly infectious diseases: an inventory of capabilities in European countries. J Hosp Infect. Sep;73(1): 15–23.
20. U.S. Department of Health and Human Services (2005) National Bioterrorism Hospital Preparedness Program FY 2005 Continuation Guidance. Washington, DC: U.S. Department of Health and Human Services, Health Resources and Services Administration, Healthcare Systems Bureau.
21. World Health Organization, Regional Office for Europe (2012) Assessment of heath-system crisis preparedness: Israel. World Health Organisation.
22. De Iaco G, Puro V, Fusco FM, Schilling S, Maltezou HC, et al. (2012) Personal protective equipment management and policies: European network for highly infectious diseases data from 48 isolation facilities in 16 European countries. Infect Control Hosp Epidemiol. Oct;33(10): 1008–16.
23. Maltezou HC, Fusco FM, Schilling S, De Iaco G, Gottschalk R, et al. (2012) Infection control practices in facilities for highly infectious diseases across Europe J Hosp Infect. 81(3): 184–191.
24. Schilling S, Maltezou HC, Fusco FM, De Iaco G, Brodt HR, et al. (2013) Transportation capacity for patients with highly infectious diseases in Europe: A survey in 16 nations. Clin Microbiol Infect 19 (Suppl. 2): in press. doi: 10.1111/1469-0691.12290.
25. Thiberville SD, Schilling S, De Iaco G, Fusco FM, Thomson G, et al. (2012) Diagnostic issues and capabilities in 48 isolation facilities in 16 European countries: data from the EuroNHID surveys. BMC Research Notes, 5: 527.
26. Bork KH, Klein BM, Mølbak K, Trautner S, Pedersen UB, et al. (2006) Surveillance of ambulance dispatch data as a tool for early warning. Euro Surveill 11(12): pii = 669.
27. Menne J, Nitschke M, Stingele R, Abu-Tair M, Beneke J, et al. on behalf of the EHEC-HUS consortium (2012) Validation of treatment strategies for enterohaemorrhagic Escherichia coli O104:H4 induced haemolytic uraemic syndrome: case-control study. BMJ 345: e4565.
28. Kaji AH, Koenig KL, Lewis RJ (2007) Current Hospital Disaster Preparedness JAMA 298(18): 2188–2190.
29. European Commission (1989) Council Directive 89/391/EEC of 12 June 1989 on the introduction of measures to encourage improvements in the safety and health of workers at work. Official Journal 183, 29.6.89.
30. European Commission, Eurostat. Available: http://epp.eurostat.ec.europa.eu/portal/page/portal/population/data/main_tables. Database used: population on January 1st 2010. Accessed 2012 Oct 1.

2

Geographic Variation of Failure-to-Rescue in Public Acute Hospitals in New South Wales, Australia

Hassan Assareh[1,2]*, Lixin Ou[1], Jack Chen[1], Kenneth Hillman[1], Arthas Flabouris[3], Stephanie J Hollis[1]

1 Simpson Centre for Health Services Research, Australian Institute of Health Innovation & South Western Sydney Clinical School, University of New South Wales, Sydney, New South Wales, Australia, **2** Epidemiology, Western Sydney Local Health District, Sydney, New South Wales, Australia, **3** Intensive Care Unit, Royal Adelaide Hospital, Adelaide, South Australia, Australia

Abstract

Despite the wide acceptance of Failure-to-Rescue (FTR) as a patient safety indicator (defined as the deaths among surgical patients with treatable complications), no study has explored the geographic variation of FTR in a large health jurisdiction. Our study aimed to explore the spatiotemporal variations of FTR rates across New South Wales (NSW), Australia. We conducted a population-based study using all admitted surgical patients in public acute hospitals during 2002–2009 in NSW, Australia. We developed a spatiotemporal Poisson model using Integrated Nested Laplace Approximation (INLA) methods in a Bayesian framework to obtain area-specific adjusted relative risk. Local Government Area (LGA) was chosen as the areal unit. LGA-aggregated covariates included age, gender, socio-economic and remoteness index scores, distance between patient residential postcode and the treating hospital, and a quadratic time trend. We studied 4,285,494 elective surgical admissions in 82 acute public hospitals over eight years in NSW. Around 14% of patients who developed at least one of the six FTR-related complications (58,590) died during hospitalization. Of 153 LGAs, patients who lived in 31 LGAs, accommodating 48% of NSW patients at risk, were exposed to an excessive adjusted FTR risk (10% to 50%) compared to the state-average. They were mostly located in state's centre and western Sydney. Thirty LGAs with a lower adjusted FTR risk (10% to 30%), accommodating 8% of patients at risk, were mostly found in the southern parts of NSW and Sydney east and south. There were significant spatiotemporal variations of FTR rates across NSW over an eight-year span. Areas identified with significantly high and low FTR risks provide potential opportunities for policy-makers, clinicians and researchers to learn from the success or failure of adopting the best care for surgical patients and build a self-learning organisation and health system.

Editor: Eli Samuel Rosenberg, Emory University Rollins School of Public Health, United States of America

Funding: This work is supported by National Health And Medical Research Council Project grants-Australia (APP1009916 and APP1020660). The funders had no role in study design, data collection and analysis, decision to publish, or preparation of the manuscript.

Competing Interests: The authors have declared that no competing interests exist.

* Email: h.assareh@unsw.edu.au

Introduction

Adverse events during hospitalisation and complications after surgery can be quite common. In the U.S., approximately one-fifth of patients who underwent surgery in 1997 died due to treatable complications [1]. In Australia, between 15 to 20% of patients experienced at least one complication after the surgery; 5% to 7% of them died prior to discharge [2–4]. Timely recognition and effective treatment of the complication once it occurs can prevent patient death [5]. Silber and colleagues [6] proposed to measure Failure-to-Rescue (FTR), defined as the proportion of deaths among surgical in-patients with treatable complications, as a hospital quality indicator. Effective management of treatable post-operative complications reportedly made a larger contribution to patient survival than pre-operation patient characteristics or operation type [7]. Since the Agency for Healthcare Research and Quality (AHRQ) adopted FTR as one of its patient safety indices [8], the concept has gained wide acceptance and now used to evaluate and compare post-operative care across hospitals [9–14]. FTR was found to have the highest incidence rate (91.13 per 1000 cases) among all the patient safety indicators and accounted for 6.7% of the total number of preventable patient safety incidents in the U.S. between 2007–2009 [15]. Two studies reported a decreased FTR rate of 2.4% to 6% within one decade [16,17].

FTR rate varies across patients and hospitals with different characteristics. Older patients and those with higher pre-operative comorbidities have a higher risk of complication and risk of death after surgery [7,18,19]. Studies in both U.S. and European hospitals revealed that patients undergoing surgery in hospitals with a high mortality rate did not suffer from excessive complications compared to patients in lower mortality rate hospitals, but were less likely to survive due to lower quality of care [20–24]. Ghaferi and colleagues [25] also showed that patients in small hospitals which had only slightly higher complications rates (odds ratio 1.17), were exposed to substantially higher FTR rates compared to patients in large hospitals. They suggested that large hospitals were more capable of effectively rescuing patients from complications compared to their low volume counterparts.

The success of regional policy interventions and quality improvement programs varies, resulting in a different level of care quality across catchment areas. There are significant variations in post non-cardiac surgery mortality rates among 28

European nations [26] and in complication and mortality rates among U.S. hospitalised patients across different states during 2009–2011 [27], reflecting the potential different areal risk of FTR and other adverse outcomes. Furthermore, a better understanding of the spatial distributions of FTR may facilitate the design and prioritisation of regional quality improvement interventions [26].

Accordingly, we aimed to investigate the spatiotemporal pattern of post-surgery FTR rate for all public acute hospital patients in New South Wales (NSW), Australia during 2002–2009, in order to enhance our understanding of geographical variation of FTR across NSW.

Methods

Data source and study population

We used records from the NSW Admitted Patient Data Collection (APDC) database. The APDC is administrated by NSW Ministry of Health including all admitted patient services provided by NSW public and private healthcare facilities. The APDC includes information on patient demographics, medical conditions and procedures, hospital characteristics, and separations (discharges, transfers and deaths) from all public and private hospitals, as well as day procedure centres in NSW. The medical records for each episode of care in the APDC were assigned with codes based on the International Statistical Classification of Diseases and Related Health Problems, Tenth Revision, Australian Modification (ICD-10-AM) 4th edition [28]. Of all admissions at 497 healthcare facilities in NSW between 1st January 2002 to 31st December 2009, we included all 82 public acute hospitals in NSW (9,221,128 admissions; 57.4% of all admissions) in our study, excluding community and private facilities, multipurpose and non-acute centres, psychiatric and rehabilitation facilities, nursing home and hospices, and two children's hospitals and one other hospital (data was unavailable).

Measures and covariates

Following methodology by AHRQ, we defined FTR as mortality among surgical patients who developed at least one of six serious treatable complications during hospitalisation; including acute renal failure, deep vein thrombosis or pulmonary embolism, pneumonia, sepsis, shock or cardiac arrest, gastrointestinal haemorrhage or acute ulcer [8]. The six abovementioned complications were identified by secondary diagnostic codes (ICD-10-AM) that were translated from the AHRQ definition (ICD-9-CM) by Victorian Government Health Information [29]. Applying AHRQ inclusion criteria [8], patients who had elective surgery within two days of admission, aged between 18–90 years (inclusive) and who were transferred to an acute care facility were considered in the population study. 4,362,624 admissions in 82 acute hospitals were included (47.3% of all NSW public acute hospital admissions). Ethical approval was obtained from the University of NSW Human Research Ethics Committee (LNR/11/CIPHS/64).

We selected NSW Local Government Areas (LGA; 153 in total) as the spatial units through the aggregation of patient postcode (651 in total) using appropriate concordance references [30]. NSW is also divided into 15 Local Health Districts (LHDs) and three hospital networks which can be categorized into two classes: Metropolitan (eight LHDs and three networks), and Rural and Regional NSW (seven LHDs). Aggregated age and gender of patients and the distance between patient residential postcode and the treating hospital in each study year at LGA level were included in the adjustment. We also utilised a LGA-level advantage and disadvantage index of Socio-Economic Indices for Areas (SEIFA) as a covariate with lower values indicating more disadvantage in the area [31]. Similarly, using Accessibility/Remoteness Index Australia Plus (ARIA+), a remoteness score (varying between zero to fifteen with higher values indicating more remoteness) was obtained for each LGA and employed as a covariate [32]. Aggregated covariates was generated using mean for scale variables (age, SEIFA, ARIA+ and distance), and percentage of females (0–100) among all patients for gender. 77,130 admissions (%1.7 of 4,362,624 admissions) were excluded due to either missing items in covariates or patient's non-NSW residential location. We initially examined the Elixhauser and the Charlson Index comorbidities based on the ICD-10 coding scheme [33]. We did not include either of them in the adjustment given the recent reports that these indices may introduce misleading results possibly due to geographical variations and biases in the coding [34–36].

Statistical analysis

To test the presence of any geographical variations of FTR across NSW LGAs over the study period (2002–2009), we examined spatial autocorrelation of the outcome across LGAs. We applied an empirical Bayes index modification of Moran's I [37] to evaluate the global association. Local spatial association measures (LISA) were also used to identify clusters. A cluster of neighbouring LGAs with high (or low) FTR rates and significant local indicators was regarded as a hot (or cold) spot [38,39]. The neighbourhood effect for each LGA was limited to the first order of neighbours, LGAs with a shared common boundary, which implies that the neighbour LGAs are more related than distant LGAs. We then utilised spatiotemporal modelling techniques to investigate spatial and temporal patterns of adjusted FTR rates across LGAs during the study period. We derived areal adjusted relative risk (compared to overall FTR rate) using a geo-additive mixed effect model where a Poisson distribution underlies the observed FTR count, y_{it}, for i^{th} LGA, $i: 1, \ldots, n$, at t^{th} year, $t: 1, \ldots, T$ [40]. A Bayesian hierarchical model was defined to incorporate effects of covariates and spatial and temporal structure through random and fixed components. We followed the model specification proposed for spatiotemporal models in Gaussian Markov Random Field framework [41,42]. For spatial patterns, we used two latent random effects components: a spatially structured random effect, u_i, which was modelled as a so-called intrinsic Conditionally Autoregressive (iCAR); and a spatially unstructured effect, v_i, which was modelled as an independent normal distribution [41,43]. The former accounts for any spatial autocorrelation, whilst the latter captures unexplained variation across LGAs and over dispersion. p_i is the known LGA-specific offset parameter, the number of patients who developed complications. To model temporal patterns, we extended the parametric formulation proposed by Bernardinelli and colleagues [44]. In a semi-parametric approach, we included two time trends, linear and quadratic, as the fixed effect in the model (a linear, δ_1, and a quadratic, δ_2), and then added a random effect term, φ_t, to account for any departure from the parametric fixed effects. We set time at the centre of study period (2005.5); therefore time varies between -3.5 and 3.5 for the linear term, and between 0.25 and 12.25 for the quadratic term. To incorporate interaction between space (LGAs) and time (linear and quadratic), two additional random effect terms, γ_{1i} and γ_{2i}, were incorporated into the model. These terms are analogous to the random slope formulation capturing model differential trends of the ith LGA, since they can be interpreted as the amount by which the time trends of ith LGA differ from the overall linear and quadratic time trends [44,45]. Five year×LGA-specific covariates, x_{itj}, comprising average age, proportion of females in the population at risk, square root of average distance between patients residential postcode and treating hospital, SEIFA and ARIA+ were added into the model. Covariates were set as continues variables and assumed to have fixed effects.

$$y_{it} Poisson(\mu_{it})$$

$$\log(\mu_{it}) = \log(p_{it}) + \alpha + \sum_{j=1}^{k} \beta_j x_{itj} + u_i + v_i$$
$$+ \delta_1 t + \delta_2 t^2 + \varphi_t + \gamma_{1i} t + \gamma_{2i} t^2$$

In prior specification, we let fixed effects, α, β_j, δ_1 and δ_2, follow a zero-mean normal distribution with a very large variance of 10^3. The unstructured random spatial term v_i, and all random effect terms, φ_t, γ_{1i} and γ_{2i}, were set as a zero-mean normal distribution with an unknown precision following a Gamma distribution with shape and scale parameters of $a=1$ and $b=2000$, respectively. A similar Gamma prior was also used for the precision parameter of the structured spatial term, u_i, in iCAR. This setting led to non-informative priors with large variances imposing no pattern [46,47]. To test if spatial effect is evident, we applied a recommended posterior-based probability, $p(exp(u_i+v_i)>1)$, criterion with a 10% threshold [44,48,49]. To be consistent, a similar significance level was applied for other effects and analyses.

We employed non-informative zero-mean normal priors using the default and recommended settings for the precision [49]. Although prior specification in Bayesian setting is arbitrary and may lead to a different conclusion, this full Bayesian geo-additive model was reported to be relatively insensitive to the choice of prior [46]. In our sensitivity analysis, no deviation in results was seen when less defuse priors including a normal distribution with a variance of $\sigma^2=5,10,100$ and a Gamma with a smaller scale parameter of $b=10,100,100$ were employed. The robustness of the results was not unexpected due to the small effect sizes which were obtained for all components including intercept, $-3.12<\alpha,\beta_j,u_i,v_i,\delta_1,\delta_2,\varphi<0.032$. Moreover, use of a highly informative prior which may affect likelihood and lead to different results is not justifiable in the absence of any prior evidence. We limited the neighbouring effect to the LGAs with shared borders; other settings such as distance based configuration may be of interest for further investigation. The model without LGA-specific temporal patterns was preferred over the model with random space-time interaction terms, γ_{1i} and γ_{2i}, according to the smaller Deviance Information Criterion [50], 3064.8 vs. 3068.5, respectively. We only presented results from the superior model.

The spatiotemporal model was computed using Integrated Nested Laplace Approximation (INLA) methods. This is a computation technique for Bayesian latent Gaussian models which outperforms traditional Markov chain Monte Carlo (MCMC) methods while providing very precise estimates [42,45,51]. Data preparation was conducted in Stata 12.0 [52]. Statistical analyses and modelling were performed using INLA package [49,53], built on 26 May 2013 (www.rinla.org) within R environment version 3.0.0 [54].

Results

Of 4,285,494 elective surgical admissions for NSW residents during 2002–2009, across 82 NSW public acute hospitals, 58,590 (1.3%) patients residing in NSW developed at least one of the six complications of interest. Approximately 14% of them died prior to discharge, equivalent to an incidence rate of 1.88 per 1000 surgical patients. Males and older patients tended to have a higher risk of death compared to their counterparts (Table 1). Crude FTR rate slightly varied across years. There were large variations among LHDs (SD = 2.58%) and LGAs (SD = 4.28%). Patients who resided in metropolitan areas had lower crude FTR rates compared to those patients residing in non-metropolitan areas. Patients residing in regions with the highest SEIFA score (4th quartile) had the lowest FTR rate. The remoteness of patients' residential locations and the distance between the residential postcode and the treating hospital were associated with different crude FTR rates. Patients residing in very remote areas had the highest FTR rate.

Figure 1 shows the overall crude rate of FTR for all LGAs in NSW within the study period (2002–2009). The most densely populated LGAs in NSW, located within Sydney Metropolitan LHDs are shown on the right panel of Figure 1. Wentworth LGA, the far south west region of NSW within Far West LHD, had no patients with a post-operative complication and, therefore, no FTR was observed. The rate varied from less than 1% in Bombala and Murrumbidgee LGAs both located in the two southern LHDs of NSW, to 26.6% in Gilgandra in the centre of the state within Western NSW LHD. A non-zero Moran I index of 0.325 (p-value = 0.001) obtained in the preliminary spatial analysis revealed a significant spatial autocorrelation. This positive value suggests neighbouring LGAs tended to have similar levels of FTR. Five main clusters each comprising of at least three highly correlated LGAs were identified based on LISA statistics. Two clusters with high FTR rates, H1 and H2 (hot spots), were located in the state's centre towards the northern part of NSW, largely within Western NSW LHD (H1), and in the eastern coastline of NSW within Hunter New England LHD (H2), with rate averages of 18.4% and 18.0%, respectively. Of three cold spots, clusters of LGAs with low rates, two were found in the southern part of NSW within Murrumbidgee (C1) and Southern NSW (C2) LHDs, and one in South Eastern Sydney LHD (C3), with average rates of 3.3%, 6.9%, and 6.7%, respectively. Clusters are presented in Figure 1.

Smoothed relative risks of FTR after adjustment for age, gender, time trend, distance, SEIFA and ARIA+ scores were obtained using a spatiotemporal model. Posterior estimates of rates are shown in Figure 2. Overall FTR rate in NSW was the reference level in the calculation of relative risks. LGAs with significant deviation from the state average are illustrated in Figure 2 by light or dark grey shading.

Of the 153 LGAs, nine regions had a significantly higher risk of FTR, with an excessive risk ranging from 30% to 50%, compared to the state average. These regions were mostly located in the mid-eastern coastline of NSW within Hunter New England, and Sydney Western and South Western LHDs, accommodating 24% of all patients at risk across NSW. Of 31 LGAs with a lower level of excessive risk (10% to 30%), 22 LGAs significantly deviated from the state average. They were found within Western NSW and Sydney Metropolitan LHDs. Overall, 48% of all NSW patients at risk resided within 31 LGAs with higher FTR rates; see Table S1 for more details. Eight LGAs had significantly lower FTR rate (RR ranged from 0.7 to 0.8), three in Sydney South Eastern LHD and five in the southern NSW. We also found 18 low FTR LGAs with a smaller deviation from the state average

Table 1. Distribution and proportion of patients who developed at least one post-surgery complication (population at risk) and died (failure-to-rescue) across patients' and incidences' characteristics.

Characteristics	Patients at risk		Patients died		FTR rate
Age*					
>=18 yr&<35 yr	3602	(6.15%)	167	(2.03%)	4.64%
>=35 yr&<55 yr	9989	(17.05%)	719	(8.73%)	7.20%
>=55 yr&<75 yr	22564	(38.51%)	2974	(36.11%)	13.18%
>=75 yr<90	22435	(38.29%)	4376	(53.13%)	19.51%
Mean ± SD†	66.23±16.61		72.22±13.44		-
Median ± IQ†	70.00±23.18		75.84±17.01		-
Gender*					
Female	27020	(46.12%)	3490	(42.37%)	12.92%
Male	31570	(53.88%)	4746	(57.63%)	15.03%
Mean ± SD (%Female)†	44.51%±6.86%		41.46%±13.60%		-
Median ± IQ (%Female)†	45.42%±6.41%		42.22%±14.07%		-
Quartiles of distance travelled*					
1st quartile (<17.6 km)	32690	(55.79%)	4551	(55.25%)	13.92%
2nd quartile (>=17.6 km & <71.1 km)	16418	(28.02%)	2458	(29.85%)	14.97%
3rd quartile (>=71.1 km & <121.7 km)	6933	(11.83%)	858	(10.42%)	12.38%
4th quartile (>=121.7 km)	2549	(4.36%)	369	(4.48%)	14.46%
Mean ± SD†	88.22±88.42		97.76±97.44		-
Median ± IQ†	71.11±104.04		83.10±118.83		-
Year*					
2002	5402	(9.23%)	680	(8.25%)	12.59%
2003	5116	(8.73%)	691	(8.39%)	13.51%
2004	6371	(10.87%)	923	(11.21%)	14.49%
2005	7085	(12.09%)	1023	(12.42%)	14.44%
2006	7447	(12.71%)	1146	(13.91%)	15.39%
2007	8560	(14.61%)	1222	(14.84%)	14.28%
2008	9090	(15.51%)	1330	(16.15%)	14.63%
2009	9519	(16.25%)	1221	(14.83%)	12.83%
Mean ± SD§	7323.75±1648.05		1029.50±246.73		13.95%±0.95%
Median ± IQ§	7226.00±2564.00		1085.00±355.80		14.30%±1.19%
Quartiles of SEIFA*					
1st quartile (most disadvantaged)	7883	(13.45%)	1215	(14.82%)	15.41%
2nd quartile	13911	(23.74%)	1877	(22.90%)	13.49%
3rd quartile	20857	(35.61%)	3219	(39.26%)	15.43%
4th quartile (most advantaged)	15939	(27.20%)	1887	(23.02%)	11.84%
Categories of ARIA+*					
Highly Accessible (<=0.2)	37194	(63.48%)	5345	(64.90%)	14.37%
Accessible (>0.2 & <=2.4)	13685	(23.36%)	1864	(22.63%)	13.62%
Moderately Accessible (>2.4 & <=5.92)	6862	(11.71%)	904	(10.97%)	13.17%
Remote (>5.92 & <=10.53)	607	(1.04%)	82	(1.00%)	13.53%
Very Remote (>10.53 & <=15)	242	(0.41%)	41	(0.50%)	16.83%
Local health district*					
Metropolitan	35998	(61.44%)	4949	(60.09%)	13.75%
Rural & Regional NSW	22592	(38.56%)	3287	(39.91%)	14.55%
Mean ± SD‡	3661.85±2967.23		514.77±482.91		13.41%±2.58%
Median ± IQ‡	2724.00±2395.00		410.20±280.20		12.54%±4.02%
Local government areas					
Mean ± SD†	383.90±545.70		53.83±90.91		12.59%±4.28%
Median ± IQ†	167.80±390.65		19.91±47.57		12.38%±5.21%

Table 1. Cont.

Characteristics	Patients at risk	Patients died	FTR rate
Total	58590	8236	14.06%

* Significant at 0.01 using $\chi2$ test.
Note: 1502 FTR cases were excluded due to non-NSW postcodes. Summary statistics were calculated over (†) LGAs, (§) years 2002–2009, and (‡) LHDs.

(RR ranged from 0.8 to 0.9), mostly within Murrumbidgee, Sydney and Sydney South Eastern LHDs. Areas with a lower risk of FTR accommodated 8% of NSW patients at risk; see Table S2 for more details.

We found a significant linear and quadratic time effect in the spatiotemporal model (Table 2), where the risk of FTR peaked between 2005 and 2006, and then declined afterwards (Figure 3). As summarised in Table 2, LGAs accommodating a greater proportion of older patients had a higher risk of FTR compared to regions with younger patients (RR = 1.03). LGAs with a higher percentage of female patients had a significantly lower FTR risk (RR = 0.97). Socio-economically advantaged LGAs exhibited a lower risk of FTR (RR = 0.99). Remoteness of patients' residence area was not associated with FTR. Patients who underwent surgery in farther hospitals experienced a higher risk of FTR (RR = 1.021).

Discussion

We simultaneously studied spatial and temporal variation of post-operative failure-to-rescue in 82 public acute hospitals across NSW between 2002 and 2009. We found 8236 (14%) deaths among patients who developed at least one complication after surgery. Patients residing in 31 LGAs mostly located in the centre and mid-eastern coast line of NSW were exposed to a higher risk of FTR (varying from 10% to 50%) compared to the state average. In contrast, within 26 LGAs, located in the southern part of NSW and Sydney eastern regions, levels of FTR risk were 10% to 30% lower. The yearly FTR rate was in the highest level in 2005.

Timely recognition and management of post-operative complications has been considered as a patient safety indicator [8,29,55]. Hospitals responding differently to such complications results in the inequality of care provided and varying post-complication death rate at the hospital level and different geographic regions. [15,21,26,27]. Our study demonstrated such a variation across LGAs of NSW. It showed that despite the close proximity of some areas, in particular within Sydney LHDs where several hospitals are accessible, patients residing in some LGAs were exposed to a higher level of FTR risk than those residing in neighbouring regions. Variation in the practice of quality initiatives aiming at the effective recognition and response to surgical complications at hospital and regional levels, as well as differences in the hospital characteristics, may have contributed to the observed discrepancies. For example, one study showed that the implementation of a Medical Emergency Team (MET) system was associated with a significant decrease in complication and post-operative death rates [56,57]. It has also been shown that large hospitals have a lower FTR rate compared to small hospitals [25]. However, our study found that the LGAs comprising of highly populated areas within metropolitan LHDs with large hospitals had excessive FTR risks. Blacktown (in the western Sydney area) and Newcastle (North of Sydney) areas, which accommodated over 10% of all patients at risk, exhibited excessive FTR risks above 43%. Conversely, patients from areas with a lower population density such as in western parts of NSW, who predominantly underwent surgery in small centres, did not experience a higher FTR rate. Further hospital-level investigation is required to address and verify the effect of volume, staffing and other centre-based characteristics [14,58].

The overall FTR rate of 14% in NSW was close to the national rates seen in the U.S.; 15.3% to 10.3% between 1998 and 2007 [16]. During 2002–2009 in NSW, the current study confirmed the significant quadratic trend of FTR found in our previous study using individual patient data [59]. In contrast with the consistently

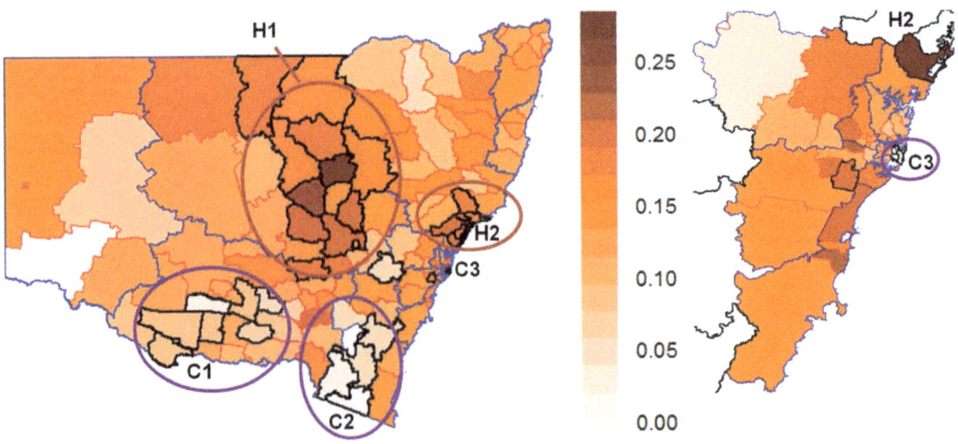

Figure 1. Crude FTR rate for each LGA (separated by red borders) in NSW over the study period (2002–2009). LGAs with significant LISA index (p-value<0.1), indication of clusters, are highlighted with black borders and labelled (H: hot spot, C: cold spot). LHDs are separated by blue borders. LGAs within Sydney metropolitan LHDs are enlarged in the right panel.

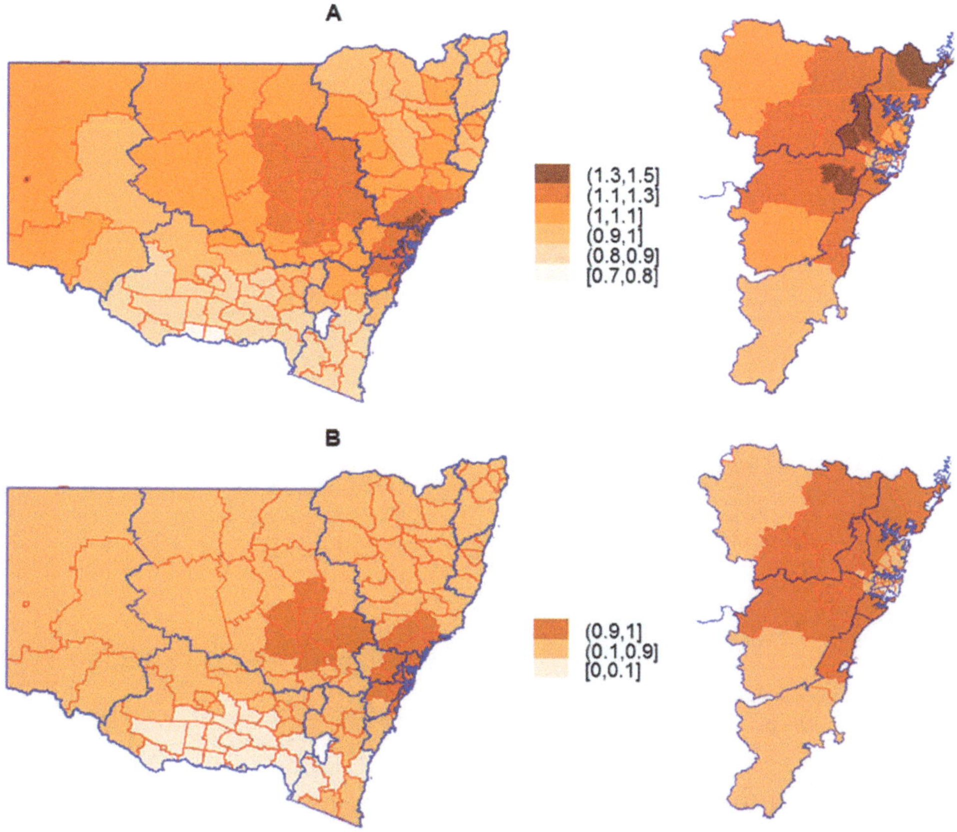

Figure 2. Smoothed relative risk of FTR for each LGA (separated by red borders) in NSW over the study period (2002-2009), adjusted for age, gender, distance, SEIFA and ARIA+ scores: (a) Relative risk posterior estimates (reference level is state average), $exp(u_i+v_i)$; (b) Posterior probability of relative risk greater than 1 (state average), $p(exp(u_i+v_i)>1)$. LHDs are separated by blue borders. LGAs within Sydney metropolitan LHDs are enlarged in the right panel.

decreasing trend in the U.S. [16], NSW demonstrated an increasing trend until 2005–2006, followed by a decreasing trend to 2009. More importantly, our study showed that such a recent decreasing FTR trend was uniform across all different LGAs. Such trajectory in the FTR rate may be due to national and state-wide quality and safety programs advocated by Australian Commission on Safety and Quality in Healthcare (ACQSHC) [60] and Clinical Excellence Commission (CEC) of NSW [61] founded in 2006 and late 2004, respectively. CEC and ACQSHC had launched and sustained specific programs in targeting specific complications such as deep vein thrombosis and sepsis.

Our finding that older patients experienced a higher risk of FTR is consistent with previous study findings [7,18]. However, our findings that male patients had a higher rate of FTR was in line with one study [18] but not others which reported no gender effect on post-operative mortality [3,62,63]. Further analysis on

Table 2. Relative risk posterior estimates and 90% credible intervals for temporal effect and covariates in the spatiotemporal model of FTR across LGAs of NSW over the study period (2002–2009).

Covariates	RR	90% CI
Year	0.986	0.976–0.996
Year^2	0.987	0.982–0.991
Age	1.033	1.026–1.040
Gender (% female)	0.967	0.941–0.995
Distance travelled	1.021	1.000–1.042
SEIFA score	0.989	0.983–0.996
ARIA+ score	0.978	0.939–1.018

Note: Effects of year (linear and quadratic) were obtained where time was centred on the middle of study period (2005.5). Effect of SEIFA score was obtained for 10 unit increments in the raw scores varying from 816 to 1155 in NSW. Effect of distance travelled was obtained for square root of the raw values. Effect of gender was obtained for 10 unit increments in the percentage of females among all patients.

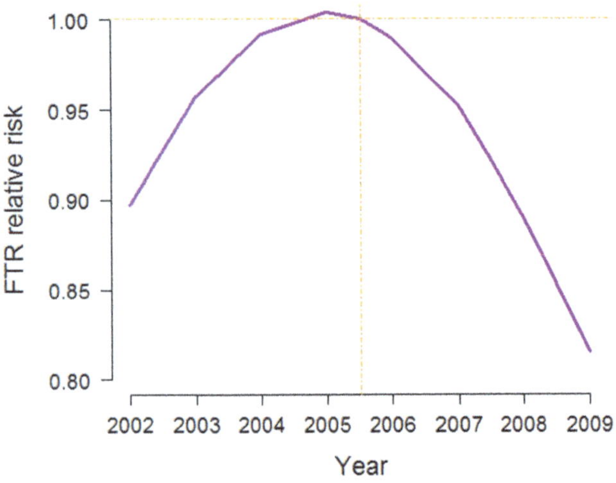

Figure 3. Temporal pattern of FTR in NSW over the study period (2002–2009). Relative risk posterior estimates were obtained from the spatiotemporal model, $exp(\varphi+\delta_1 t+\delta_2 t^2)$, in which time was centred on mid-2005 and adjusted for age, gender, distance, SEIFA and ARIA+ scores.

patient characteristics at an individual level, not LGA-aggregated, is required for verification of gender effect or other potentially contributing factors.

Patient safety indicators have been introduced in the U.S. and Australia [8,29] and currently the routine measurement and reporting of indicators have been broadly adopted [15,20,27]. To our knowledge, the current study was the first to investigate the geographical variation of FTR in a large health jurisdiction in Australia. Our findings provide policy-makers with FTR risk distribution that is not just patient or hospital based. It presents results on a large geographical scale that may reflect the impact of multi-factorial determinants such as local area health policy, quality improvement initiatives, hospital culture and compliance with best practice. It may also be related to complex patients-level factors (i.e. age, gender, case mix, severity and comorbidity). Moreover, other environmental factors such as transportation, local referral system and accessibility of different health facilities may also play a role in patient outcomes. We examined the effects of remoteness of patients' residence locations and distance between patient residential address and treating hospital. We found that the proximity to the treating hospital was associated with the reduced FTR rate. Despite that hospital location was reported as a contributing factor [17,64], no study directly investigated the impact of the distance between patients residential location and the treating hospital. Our identified hot spots provide local health authorities and hospital networks with pre-targeted areas for in-depth case studies on how and why this was the case and what lessons could be learnt and shared. Equally, cold spots may provide decision-makers, clinicians and researchers with valuable insights into how post-surgical care could be better delivered and avoidable deaths prevented. Although this study did not primarily aim to directly identify and compare the best or worst performers, it illustrates areas in which preferred practices and outcomes are delivered. The presence of geographical variation across LGAs and LHDs also reinforces the importance of continual monitoring and public reporting of health system performances in order to create a self-learning health system with a focus on patient-centred care [65].

Finally, the current study utilised the most recent development in computation techniques from Bayesian hierarchical modelling framework for spatiotemporal modelling. This approach allowed us a stable and fast estimation of the most complex spatial regression model in comparison to the conventional MCMC approach [42,45,51]. Our study included all NSW public acute hospital patients spanning an eight–year period and was based on an accepted AHRQ definition which makes cross-country comparison possible. Our study however, had some limitations. Firstly, our model was constructed on a LGA level which may suffer from ecological fallacy. As a result, our model only included limited covariates in the adjustment. We did not specifically examine the relationship between hospital level outcome and geo-spatial distributions. Future studies, however, should investigate other extended models to explore the impact of patient and hospital characteristics on the outcome. These results would help to identify high risk patients prior to their operation and evaluate the effects of post-operative quality improvement policies and initiatives [20,57].

Conclusions

There were significant spatial-temporal variations of FTR across NSW over an eight-year span. Such variations demonstrate a significant ecological effect that cannot be explained purely by hospital differences. Both the hot spots and cold spots identified provide potential opportunities for policy-makers, clinicians and researchers to learn from the success or failure of adopting the best care for surgical patients in building a self-learning organisation and health system.

Supporting Information

Table S1 List of LGAs with a significantly higher adjusted relative risk of FTR.

Table S2 List of LGAs with a significantly lower adjusted relative risk of FTR.

Author Contributions

N/A. Conceived and designed the experiments: HA JC AF KH. Performed the experiments: HA LO JC. Analyzed the data: HA LO JC. Contributed reagents/materials/analysis tools: HA JC AF SH. Wrote the paper: HA JC AF KH SH.

References

1. Needleman J, Buerhaus P, Mattke S, Stewart M, Zelevinsky K (2002) Nurse-staffing levels and the quality of care in hospitals. New England Journal of Medicine 346: 1715–1722.
2. Bellomo R, Goldsmith D, Russell S, Uchino S (2002) Postoperative serious adverse events in a teaching hospital: a prospective study. Medical Journal of Australia 176: 216–218.
3. Kable A, Gibberd R, Spigelman A (2002) Adverse events in surgical patients in Australia. International Journal for Quality in Health Care 14: 269–276.
4. Moje C, Jackson TJ, McNair P (2006) Adverse events in Victorian admissions for elective surgery. Australian Health Review 30: 333–343.
5. Silber JH, Romano PS, Rosen AK, Wang Y, Even-Shoshan O, et al. (2007) Failure-to-Rescue: Comparing Definitions to Measure Quality of Care. Medical Care 45: 918–925 910.1097/MLR.1090b1013e31812e31801cc.
6. Silber JH, Williams SV, Krakauer H, Schwartz JS (1992) Hospital and patient characteristics associated with death after surgery. A study of adverse occurrence and failure to rescue. Medical Care 30: 615–629.

7. Khuri SF, Henderson WG, DePalma RG, Mosca C, Healey NA, et al. (2005) Determinants of long-term survival after major surgery and the adverse effect of postoperative complications. Annals of surgery 242: 326–341.
8. Agency for Healthcare Research and Quality (2009) AHRQ quality indicators: patient safety indicators: technical specifications (Version 4.1). Agency for Healthcare Research and Quality.
9. Scarborough JE, Pappas TN, Bennett KM, Lagoo-Deenadayalan S (2012) Failure-to-Pursue Rescue: Explaining Excess Mortality in Elderly Emergency General Surgical Patients with Preexisting "Do-Not-Resuscitate" Orders. Annals of Surgery 256: 453–461.
10. Schmid A, Hoffman L, Happ MB, Wolf GA, DeVita M (2007) Failure to rescue: a literature review. Journal of nursing administration 37: 188–198.
11. Sermeus W, Aiken L, Van den Heede K, Rafferty A, Griffiths P, et al. (2011) Nurse forecasting in Europe (RN4CAST): Rationale, design and methodology. BMC Nursing 10: 6.
12. Simpson KR (2006) Measuring perinatal patient safety: review of current methods. Journal of Obstetric, Gynecologic, & Neonatal Nursing 35: 432–442.
13. Talsma A, Jones K, Liu G, Campbell DA (2010) Failure to rescue measure: validation of community-and hospital-acquired complications. Journal of Nursing Administration 40: 417–423.
14. Unruh LY, Zhang NJ (2012) Nurse staffing and patient safety in hospitals: New variable and longitudinal approaches. Nursing Research 61: 3–12.
15. HealthGrades (2013) Variation in patient safety outcomes and the importance of being informed. U.S.: HealthGrades.
16. Downey JR, Hernandez-Boussard T, Banka G, Morton JM (2012) Is patient safety improving? National trends in patient safety indicators: 1998–2007. Health services research 47: 414–430.
17. Semel ME, Lipsitz SR, Funk LM, Bader AM, Weiser TG, et al. (2012) Rates and patterns of death after surgery in the United States, 1996 and 2006. Surgery 151: 171–182.
18. Story DA, Leslie K, Myles PS, Fink M, Poustie SJ, et al. (2010) Complications and mortality in older surgical patients in Australia and New Zealand (the REASON study): a multicentre, prospective, observational study. Anaesthesia 65: 1022–1030.
19. Sheetz KH, Waits SA, Krell RW, Campbell DAJ, Englesbe MJ, et al. (2013) Improving Mortality Following Emergent Surgery in Older Patients Requires Focus on Complication Rescue. Annals of Surgery 258: 614–617.
20. Ghaferi AA, Birkmeyer JD, Dimick JB (2009) Complications, failure to rescue, and mortality with major inpatient surgery in Medicare patients. Annals of surgery 250: 1029–1034.
21. Ghaferi AA, Birkmeyer JD, Dimick JB (2009) Variation in hospital mortality associated with inpatient surgery. New England Journal of Medicine 361: 1368–1375.
22. Glance LG, Dick AW, Meredith JW, Mukamel DB (2011) Variation in hospital complication rates and failure-to-rescue for trauma patients. Annals of surgery 253: 811–816.
23. Almoudaris AM, Mamidanna R, Bottle A, Aylin P, Vincent C, et al. (2013) Failure to rescue patients after reintervention in gastroesophageal cancer surgery in england. JAMA Surgery 148: 272–276.
24. Henneman D, Snijders HS, Fiocco M, Leersum NJ, Kolfschoten NE, et al. (2013) Hospital Variation in Failure to Rescue after Colorectal Cancer Surgery: Results of the Dutch Surgical Colorectal Audit. Annals of Surgical Oncology 20: 2117–2123.
25. Ghaferi AA, Birkmeyer JD, Dimick JB (2011) Hospital volume and failure to rescue with high-risk surgery. Medical Care 49: 1076–1081.
26. Pearse RM, Moreno RP, Bauer P, Pelosi P, Metnitz P, et al. (2012) Mortality after surgery in Europe: a 7 day cohort study. The Lancet 380: 1059–1065.
27. HealthGrades (2013) American Hospital Quality Outcomes: Healthgrades Report to the Nation.
28. National Centre for Classification in Health N (2004) The International Statistical Classification of Diseases and Related Health Problems, Tenth Revision, Australian Modification (ICD-10-AM). Sydney: NCCH, Faculty of Health Sciences, The University of Sydney.
29. Victorian Government Health Information (2006) Patient Safety Indicators-Translated Technical Specifications. Melbourne: Victorian State Government, Department of Health.
30. Australian Bureau of Statistics (2006) Local Government Area from Postal Area 2006 Concordance. Canberra: Australian Bureau of Statistics.
31. Australian Bureau of Statistics (2011) Census of population and housing: socio-economic indexes for areas (SEIFA), Australia. Canberra: Australian Bureau of Statistics.
32. Glover JD, Tennant SK (2003) Remote areas statistical geography in Australia: notes on the accessibility/remoteness index for Australia (ARIA+ version): Public Health Information Development Unit, The University of Adelaide.
33. Quan H, Sundararajan V, Halfon P, Fong A, Burnand B, et al. (2005) Coding algorithms for defining comorbidities in ICD-9-CM and ICD-10 administrative data. Medical care 43: 1130–1139.
34. Song Y, Skinner J, Bynum J, Sutherland J, Wennberg JE, et al. (2010) Regional variations in diagnostic practices. New England Journal of Medicine 363: 45–53.
35. Welch HG, Sharp SM, Gottlieb DJ, Skinner JS, Wennberg JE (2011) Geographic variation in diagnosis frequency and risk of death among Medicare beneficiaries. JAMA 305: 1113–1118.
36. Wennberg JE, Staiger DO, Sharp SM, Gottlieb DJ, Bevan G, et al. (2013) Observational intensity bias associated with illness adjustment: cross sectional analysis of insurance claims. BMJ 346: f549.
37. Assuncao RM, Reis EA (1999) A new proposal to adjust Moran's I for population density. Statistics in medicine 18: 2147–2162.
38. Anselin L (1995) Local indicators of spatial association—LISA. Geographical analysis 27: 93–115.
39. Ord JK, Getis A (1995) Local spatial autocorrelation statistics: distributional issues and an application. Geographical analysis 27: 286–306.
40. Kammann E, Wand MP (2003) Geoadditive models. Journal of the Royal Statistical Society: Series C (Applied Statistics) 52: 1–18.
41. Rue H, Held L (2005) Gaussian Markov random fields: theory and applications: CRC Press.
42. Rue H, Martino S, Chopin N (2009) Approximate Bayesian inference for latent Gaussian models by using integrated nested Laplace approximations. Journal of the royal statistical society: Series b (statistical methodology) 71: 319–392.
43. Besag J, York J, Mollié A (1991) Bayesian image restoration, with two applications in spatial statistics. Annals of the Institute of Statistical Mathematics 43: 1–20.
44. Bernardinelli L, Clayton D, Pascutto C, Montomoli C, Ghislandi M, et al. (1995) Bayesian analysis of space—time variation in disease risk. Statistics in Medicine 14: 2433–2443.
45. Schrödle B, Held L (2011) Spatio-temporal disease mapping using INLA. Environmetrics 22: 725–734.
46. Bernardinelli L, Clayton D, Montomoli C (1995) Bayesian estimates of disease maps: how important are priors? Statistics in Medicine 14: 2411–2431.
47. Schrödle B, Held L (2011) A primer on disease mapping and ecological regression using INLA. Computational statistics 26: 241–258.
48. Meng CYK, Dempster AP (1987) A Bayesian Approach to the Multiplicity Problem for Significance Testing with Binomial Data. Biometrics 43: 301–311.
49. Blangiardo M, Cameletti M, Baio G, Rue H (2013) Spatial and Spatio-Temporal models with R-INLA. Spatial and spatio-temporal epidemiology 4: 33–49.
50. Spiegelhalter DJ, Best NG, Carlin BP, Van Der Linde A (2002) Bayesian measures of model complexity and fit. Journal of the Royal Statistical Society: Series B (Statistical Methodology) 64: 583–639.
51. Schrödle B, Held L, Riebler A, Danuser J (2011) Using integrated nested Laplace approximations for the evaluation of veterinary surveillance data from Switzerland: a case-study. Journal of the Royal Statistical Society: Series C (Applied Statistics) 60: 261–279.
52. StataCorp (2011) Stata Statistical Software: Release 12. College Station, TX: StataCorp LP. 12 ed. College Station, TX: StataCorp LP.
53. Martino S, Rue H (2009) Implementing approximate Bayesian inference using Integrated Nested Laplace Approximation: A manual for the inla program. Department of Mathematical Sciences, NTNU, Norway.
54. RDC Team (2013) R: A language and environment for statistical computing. R Foundation Statistical Computing.
55. Silber JH, Williams SV, Krakauer H, Schwartz JS (1992) Hospital and patient characteristics associated with death after surgery: a study of adverse occurrence and failure to rescue. Medical care: 615–629.
56. Bellomo R, Goldsmith D, Uchino S, Buckmaster J, Hart G, et al. (2004) Prospective controlled trial of effect of medical emergency team on postoperative morbidity and mortality rates. Critical care medicine 32: 916–921.
57. Shelton A, Jones D, Story DA, Heland M, Bellomo R (2013) Survey of attitudes of nurses and junior doctors to co-management of high risk surgical patients. Contemporary nurse: 2253–2276.
58. Pasquali SK, Li JS, Burstein DS, Sheng S, O'Brien SM, et al. (2012) Association of Center Volume With Mortality and Complications in Pediatric Heart Surgery. Pediatrics 129: e370–e376.
59. Ou L, Chen J, Assareh H, Hollis SJ, Hillman K, et al. (2013) Trends in the rates of complications, failure-to-rescue and 30-day mortality among surgical patients in New South Wales, Australia (2002 to 2009).
60. Department of Health (2006) Australian Commission on Safety and Quality in Health Care. Australia.
61. NSW Health (2004) NSW Clinical Excellence Commision Directions Statement. Sydney.
62. McNicol L, Story DA, Leslie K, Myles PS, Fink M, et al. (2007) Postoperative complications and mortality in older patients having non-cardiac surgery at three Melbourne teaching hospitals. Medical journal of Australia 186: 447–452.
63. Davis P, Lay-Yee R, Briant R, Ali W, Scott A, et al. (2002) Adverse events in New Zealand public hospitals I: occurrence and impact.
64. Griffiths P, Jones S, Bottle A (2013) Is "failure to rescue" derived from administrative data in England a nurse sensitive patient safety indicator for surgical care? Observational study. International Journal of Nursing Studies 50: 292–300.
65. Chen J (2010) Public reporting of health system performance: a rapid review of evidence on impact on patients, providers and healthcare organisations. Sydney: Sax Institute.

3

Execution of Diagnostic Testing Has a Stronger Effect on Emergency Department Crowding than Other Common Factors

Takahisa Kawano[1]*, Kei Nishiyama[2], Hiroyuki Hayashi[3]

1 Department of Emergency Medicine, University of Fukui Hospital, Fukui, Japan, **2** Department of Primary Care and Emergency Medicine, Kyoto University Graduate School of Medicine, Kyoto city, Japan, **3** Department of General Medicine, University of Fukui Hospital, Fukui, Japan

Abstract

Study Objective: We compared the effects of execution of diagnostic tests in the emergency department (ED) and other common factors on the length of ED stay to identify those with the greatest impacts on ED crowding.

Methods: Between February 2010 and January 2012, we conducted a cross-sectional, single-center study in the ED of a large, urban, teaching hospital in Japan. Patients who visited the ED during the study period were enrolled. We excluded (1) patients scheduled for admission or pharmaceutical prescription, and (2) neonates requiring intensive care transferred from other hospitals. Multivariate linear regression was performed on log-transformed length of ED stay in admitted and discharged patients to compare influence of diagnostic tests and other common predictors. To quantify the range of change in length of ED stay given a unit change of the predictor, a generalized linear model was used for each group.

Results: During the study period, 55,285 patients were enrolled. In discharged patients, laboratory blood tests had the highest standardized β coefficient (0.44) among common predictors, and increased length of ED stay by 72.5 minutes (95% CI, 72.8–76.1 minutes). In admitted patients, computed tomography (CT) had the highest standardized β coefficient (0.17), and increased length of ED stay by 32.7 minutes (95% CI, 40.0–49.9 minutes). Although other common input and output factors were significant contributors, they had smaller standardized β coefficients in both groups.

Conclusions: Execution of laboratory blood tests and CT had a stronger influence on length of ED stay than other common input and output factors.

Editor: Robert Lane Schmidt, University of Utah School of Medicine, United States of America

Funding: Financial incentives were provided to the authors by the Emergency Promotion Foundation (http://www.fasd.or.jp/). This foundation has no role in study design, data collection and analysis, decision to publish, or preparation of the manuscript.

Competing Interests: The authors have declared that no competing interests exist.

* Email: maketenakunarakattenake@hotmail.com

Introduction

Background

Emergency department (ED) crowding represents a serious problem in emergency medicine. In Japan, 13,000 patients needing critical care experienced ambulance diversion at least four times during one emergency transport; nearly one-quarter of this ambulance diversion was caused by ED crowding. [1] Further, ED crowding does not only cause this ambulance diversion, but also delays treatment in the ED, which adversely affects patient outcomes. Indeed, increased mortality has been observed in patients admitted from the ED when ED crowding is severe. [2].

Recently, diagnostic tests in ED were recognized as one of major contributors to ED crowding. [3] For example, when laboratory tests are ordered for ED patients, an additional 80 minutes are reportedly added to the length of ED stay. [4] However, other contributors to ED crowding have been identified. For example, entry overload contributed to ED crowding in Australia. [5] High hospital bed occupancy can block admissions from the ED and prolong patient stay in the ED. [6] Additionally, patient age is an independent contributor to ED crowding, with older patients staying longer than young patients. [7] The glut of factors contributing to ED crowding has precluded an effective prioritization of interventions to reduce the problem. To establish effective interventions, identifying contributing factors and understanding the extent of their contributions to ED crowding is necessary.

We hypothesized that execution of diagnostic tests in ED has a close relation to ED crowding both in admitted and discharged patients. Here, we assessed the influence of diagnostic tests and other common contributors on the length of ED stay in each group toward the identification of factors whose negative impact on ED stay can be mitigated through appropriate policies and procedures.

Methods

Study design and setting

We conducted a cross-sectional, single-center study in the ED of the Fukui Prefectural Hospital in Fukui, Japan. The Fukui Prefectural Hospital, a large teaching hospital in an urban setting, has the largest ED in the mid-Fukui Prefecture area, where approximately 380,000 residents live. Another large academic hospital with an ED is located in this area. These hospitals serve both urban and rural communities in an area of 830 km^2 with a population density of 450 persons per km^2. The area has 7 fire departments and 7 emergency dispatch centers. Fukui Prefectural Hospital has 1,082 beds and 14 intensive care unit beds. The main treatment location at the ED has four beds for serious cases or patients being resuscitated. There are also four examination rooms for low-acuity patients and four beds for observation. Almost all patients who visited this ED were self-referred. The ED accepts all patients regardless of their age, including pediatric patients. The ED performs simple radiologic studies, laboratory blood tests, urinalysis, CT, MRI, and electrocardiography. Laboratory blood tests are analyzed in a central laboratory; a point-of-care test for blood gas analysis, cardiac troponin level, and β-human chorionic gonadotropin is available, and for admitted patients, laboratory blood tests were conducted routinely. General staffing comprises six residents, one attending physician, and three nurses per shift. Residents are responsible for the first encounter with almost all patients who come to the ED. However, the attending physician begins evaluation of high-acuity patients without awaiting evaluation by residents. All other specialist consultants are available when necessary.

Selection of participants

Patients who visited the ED at Fukui Prefectural Hospital from February 1, 2010 to January 31, 2012 were enrolled in our study. We excluded (1) patients who were scheduled for admission or pharmaceutical prescription, and (2) neonates requiring intensive care who were transferred from other hospitals. The regular reception desks at our hospital are closed on weekends. Patients arriving for scheduled admission or pharmaceutical prescription visit the reception desk at the ED. Patients needing pharmaceutical prescription mainly receive daily intravenous antibiotic administration at outpatient clinics. These patients quickly depart the ED without any evaluation or treatment, so the length of ED stay of these patients is small. Neonates requiring intensive care who are transferred from another hospital typically stay in the ED during registration only, so their length of ED stay is also small. Because these patients rarely consume any ED resources beyond registration, we excluded them. We classified participants into admitted and discharged patient groups to consider patient acuity in this study.

Outcomes

Study outcome was the length of ED stay, one of the most common proxy measures of overcrowding. [8] The length of ED stay was defined as the time, in minutes, from registration in the ED to ED departure.

Definitions

We chose 14 variables for assessment in this study following review of the literature. To understand the causes of ED crowding, the input-throughput-output conceptual model has been accepted. [9] According to the model, the 14 variables in this study were classified into four categories; input factors, or those relating to patient entry to the ED; throughput factors, or those relating to ED care processes; output factors, or those relating to the disposition of patients from the ED by discharge or hospital admission; and other factors. Input factors in this study included mode of arrival, number of walk-in, and the number of ambulance arrivals. Throughput factors in this study included diagnostic tests (laboratory blood tests, radiography, CT, MRI, ultrasonography, and electrocardiography). Output factors in this study included hospital bed occupancy and ED boarding. Patient age, arrival time and percentage of hospital admissions were included as other factors.

Mode of arrival represented the method of patient entry to the ED, by ambulance or walk-in. [10] Number of walk-ins was defined as the number of walk-in patients arriving in the ED each hour. The number of ambulance arrivals at the ED was calculated hourly. Laboratory blood tests were defined as those blood tests analyzed in the central laboratory; point-of-care blood tests were excluded. Hospital bed occupancy was defined as the percentage of hospital beds occupied daily. [6] ED boarding was defined as the number of patients at each hour who stayed in the ED for more than 1 hour after admission by an ED physician. [6] Arrival time was classified into 3 shifts (08:00–15:59, 16:00–23:59, and 00:00–07:59) to assess the effect of staffing on the length of ED stay. The percentage of admissions represented the percentage of hospital admissions originating from the ED per day. [11].

Measurement

We obtained data from the electronic medical record (EMR) system and the electronic hospital administrative data system of our hospital. Patient age, arrival time, time of decision to admit, departure time, disposition of patient, mode of arrival, and execution of any diagnostic tests were obtained from the EMR of each patient. This record is considered to be accurate because every patient account is generated from it. When a patient needs to be admitted, the physician orders admission through EMR. Nurses follow the necessary procedures after this order and transfer patients to hospital wards. If patients have to wait in the ED for the arrangement of a hospital bed, nurses record these patients and provide care to them appropriately. We obtained this nursing record to calculate ED boarding. ED clerks obtained the number of available hospital beds at 09:00 each day from the electronic hospital administrative data system and calculated hospital bed occupancy. We could not obtain hourly hospital bed occupancy information.

Statistical analysis

To compare influence of diagnostic tests and other predictors on length of ED stay of admitted and discharged patients, multivariate linear regression was performed in each group (see database in Appendix S1). Length of ED stay in this study was not normally distributed, which corresponded to findings of previous studies (Absolute skew value 2.24, absolute kurtosis 9.54). [6] Therefore, we applied the natural log transform to length of ED stay. For sample sizes greater than 300, the distribution is considered normal if the absolute skew value was less than 2 and the absolute kurtosis less than 7. [12] Thus, the log-transformed length of ED stay in this study was considered as normally distributed (absolute skew value 0.42, absolute kurtosis 1.02). We subsequently obtained the standardized partial regression coefficient (standardized β coefficient) of each predictor to compare their influences on length of ED stay. Each predictor was measured in different units of measurement and had a different variance, so we could not compare each regression coefficient in original units in this model. Therefore, to make their variance equal, the model was applied to standardized predictors, and we accessed the contribution of predictors to LOS using their standardized β coefficients. We tested this model for multicolinearity by measuring the variance inflation factor. The inflation factor of laboratory blood tests in admitted patients was more than 10 and considered to have multicolinearity. Thus, laboratory blood tests were excluded from the analysis of admitted patients.

To quantify the range of change in length of ED stay of each group given a unit change in the value of the predictor, a generalized linear model (GLM) with a log-link function and gamma distribution was conducted. GLM is commonly used to analyze length of ED stay because of its skewedness. [3,6] Laboratory blood tests in admitted patients also demonstrated multicolinearity in this model by measurement of the variance inflation factor, and were excluded from the analysis of admitted patients.

Descriptive analyses were conducted with the use of frequency tabulations. We described the medians and interquartile ranges (IQR) for all variables. All analyses were conducted with STATA version 12.1 (STATA Corp LP, College Station, TX). The authors had full access to the data and take responsibility for its integrity. All authors have read and agreed to the content of the manuscript.

Ethical Statement

The study protocol accorded with the guidelines for epidemiologic studies issued by the Ministry of Health, Labor and Welfare of Japan. [13] The ethics committees in Fukui Prefectural Hospital approved the research protocol. According to the guidelines, the requirement of written informed consent was allowed to be waived by the ethics committees, because our study didn't include any personally identifiable information. [13,14] We posted the poster about our study protocol on the bulletin board in the ED instead of written informed consent.

Results

Patient characteristics

During the study period, 56,296 patients visited the ED. Of these, 979 patients who were scheduled to visit the ED for admission or pharmaceutical prescription, as well as 32 newborn babies who were transferred from other hospitals, were excluded. The study therefore included 55,285 (98.2%) of the total patients who visited the ED. Of the included patients, 7,883 (14.3%) were admitted to the hospital, and 47,402 (85.7%) were discharged (Figure 1).

The median (quartiles) age of included patients was 35 years [interquartile range (IQR), 14–62 years]. Of the included patients, 14.0% were transported to the ED by ambulance (Table 1). The median length of ED stay for all patients was 91 minutes (IQR, 54–154 minutes). The median lengths of ED stay for the discharged and admitted patients were 83 minutes (IQR, 51–137 minutes) and 162 minutes (IQR, 113–234 minutes), respectively.

Laboratory blood tests were the most frequent examination ordered in the ED; 20,125 patients (36.4%) received these tests, and all admitted patients had laboratory blood tests in the ED (Table 2). Of other diagnostic tests available, radiographies, CTs, ultrasonographies, electrocardiograms, and MRIs were conducted on 16,820 (30.4%), 11,696 (21.2%), 10,794 (19.5%), 10,663 (19.3%), and 1,360 patients (2.5%), respectively (Table 2). Admitted patients underwent these diagnostic tests in ED more frequently than discharged patients.

Discharged patients

We compared the influence of input, throughput, and output factors on length of stay in the ED through multivariate regression in discharged patients (Table 3). The cross correlation of included variables in this analysis was described in table 4. In discharged patients, laboratory blood testing, a throughput factor, had the highest standardized β coefficient (0.44) among possible predictors and increased length of ED stay by 74.5 minutes. CT and radiography-throughput factors-also had high standardized β coefficients (0.17 and 0.16) and increased length of ED stay by 32.7 and 27.0 minutes respectively. Number of walk-ins (common input factor) and hospital bed occupancy (common output factor) were statistically significant contributors in log-transformed regression analysis. However, these factors had smaller absolute standardized β coefficients than the diagnostic tests (0.09 and 0.01). Number of walk-ins increased length of ED stay by only 1.8 minutes per increase of the number of hourly walk-in patients.

Admitted patients

In admitted patients, laboratory blood tests were omitted due to multicolinearity in both log-transformed regression analysis and GLM. The cross correlation of included variables for the admitted patient analysis was also described in table 6. CT had the highest standardized β coefficient (0.25) among possible predictors and increased length of ED stay by 44.9 minutes (Table 5). Number of walk-ins and ED boarding (common output factors) were also statistically significant contributors in log-transformed regression analysis. However, these factors had smaller standardized β coefficients than CT (0.07 and 0.02). Number of walk-ins also increased length of ED stay by only 2.3 minutes per increase in the number of hourly walk-in patients.

Limitations

Several limitations existed in this study. First, we did not classify participants in this study according to severity and complexity of their medical condition, because we could not obtain triage results. The severity and complexity likely affected physicians' decisions regarding diagnostic testing in the ED. This is the most important limitation in this study. Second, the findings were obtained from a single institution over two years, which might reduce the generalizability of the conclusions. However, our approach corresponds to that of previous studies of ED crowding in a single site; [8] therefore, our findings may be generalizable, especially to other teaching hospitals. Third, our institution is a teaching facility, requiring emergency physicians to evaluate and treat patients after initial evaluation by resident physicians. This additional step might extend the ED stay. [15] Fourth, although ambulance diversion and patients leaving before evaluation are important measures in ED crowding, we did not include them in this study because we did not measure them. Fifth, staffing in ED and the number of consultations were also not measured. [11] We cannot exclude possible bias from these unmeasured factors. Sixth, we could not obtain hourly hospital bed occupancy due to insufficiency of our electronic hospital administrative data system. Ideally, data analysis would be performed according to the precise hospital bed occupancy at particular times because hospital bed occupancy changes every hour. However, previous studies have also used daily hospital bed occupancy and found an association with length of ED stay. [11,16] Finally, we could not distinguish necessary diagnostic tests from unnecessary tests in our study. These unnecessary diagnostic tests might contribute to extended patient stay in the ED.

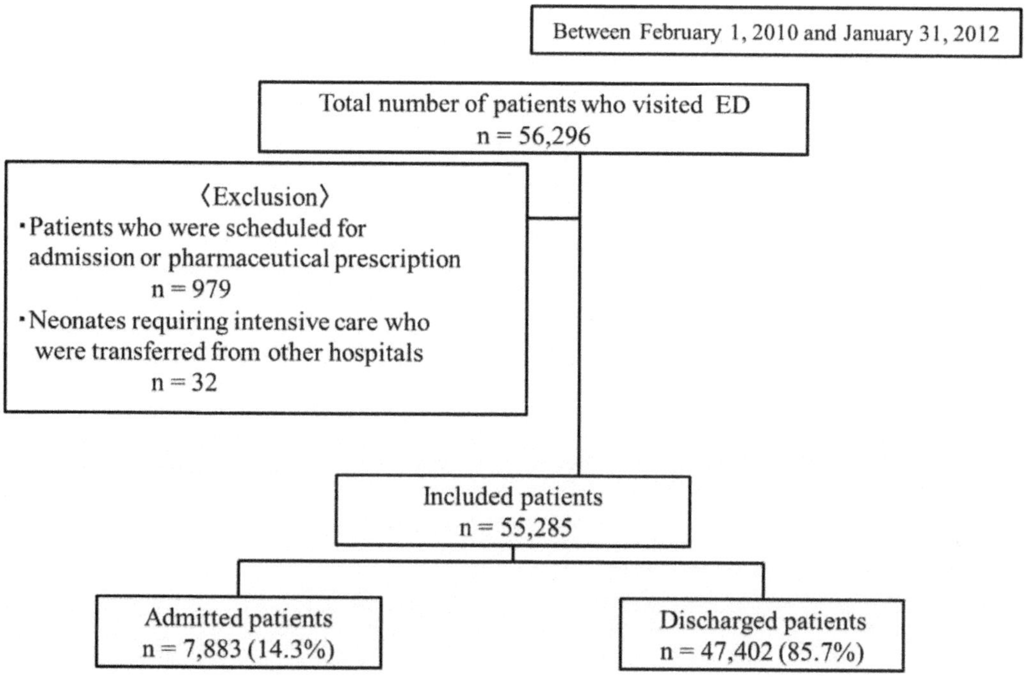

Figure 1. Patient flow diagram. ED, emergency department.

Table 1. Patient demographics and primary outcome.

	Total (n = 55,285)
Median patients age, y (IQR)	35 (14–62)
Walk-in patients, n	48,558
per day, n (IQR)	55 (46–80)
08:00 to 15:59, n (IQR)	15 (12–32)
16:00 to 23:59, n (IQR)	32 (27–39)
0:00 to 07:59, n (IQR)	9 (6–12)
Ambulance, n	6760
per day, n (IQR)	9 (7–1)
08:00 to 15:59, n (IQR)	4 (2–5)
16:00 to 23:59, n (IQR)	3 (2–5)
0:00 to 07:59, n (IQR)	1 (1–3)
Admissions, n	7,843
per day, n (IQR)	10 (8–13)
Percentage of admission, % (IQR)	15.4 (11.5–19.1)
Hospital bed occupancy	
per day, % (IQR)	74.1 (70.6–75.8)
ED boarding	
per day, n (IQR)	2 (1–3)
Deaths, n (%)	185 (1.6)
Median Length of ED stay	
Total patients, min (IQR)	92 (55–154)
Discharged patients, min (IQR)	83 (51–137)
Admitted patients, min (IQR)	162 (113–234)

IQR, interquartile range; ED, emergency department.

Table 2. The number of diagnostic tests in ED.

Number of diagnostic examination in ED	Total patients (n = 55,285)	Admitted patients (n = 7,843)	Discharged patients (n = 47442)	P value
X-ray, n	16,820	6778	9905	
proportion of examined patients per day, % (IQR)	31 (26−36)	88 (80−100)	20.9 (17.3−25.5)	<0.01
Computed tomography, n	11,696	4357	7326	
proportion of examined patients per day, % (IQR)	22 (17−26)	55.6 (44.4−6.7)	16.1 (11.9−20.6)	<0.01
Magnetic resonance imaging, n	1,360	653	706	
proportion of examined patients per day, % (IQR)	2 (1−4)	7.7 (0−13.3)	1.4 (0−2.4)	<0.01
Blood examination, n	20,125	7843	12016	
proportion of examined patients per day, % (IQR)	37 (31−43)	100 (100−100)	26.4 (21.1−31.4)	-
Ultrasonography, n	10,794	2693	7998	
proportion of examined patients per day, % (IQR)	20 (15−25)	33.3 (25−4.4)	17.2 (13.6−2.0)	<0.01
Electrocardiogram, n	10,663	5523	5143	
proportion of examined patients per day, % (IQR)	20 (15−25)	71.4 (60.8−81.3)	11.2 (7.8−15.1)	<0.01

IQR, interquartile range.

Table 3. Comparison of the effects of input, throughput, and output factors on the length of ED stay for discharged patients.

	Discharged patients (n = 47442)			
Characteristic	standardized β coefficient	95% CI	Additional length of stay, minutes	95% CI
Input factors				
Mode of arrival				
Walk-in	Reference			
Ambulance	−0.02*	−0.03−−0.01	2.4	<−0.5−4.9
Number of walk-in patients	0.09*	0.08−0.97	1.8*	1.6−2.0
Number of ambulance arrivals	0.02*	0.02−0.03	2.6*	1.7−3.4
Throughput factors				
No diagnostic test	Reference			
Radiography	0.17*	0.16−0.17	27.0*	25.6−28.6
Computed tomography	0.16*	0.16−0.17	32.7*	31.0−34.5
Magnetic resonance imaging	0.06*	0.05−0.07	38.3*	33.4−43.2
Ultrasonography	0.08*	0.08−0.09	13.6*	12.0−15.2
Laboratory blood tests	0.44*	0.44−0.45	74.5*	72.8−76.1
Electrocardiogram	<0.01	<−0.01−0.01	1.6	−0.5−3.7
Output factors				
Bed occupancy	−0.01*	−0.02−−0.01	−0.1	−0.2−0.7
ED boarding	0.01	<−0.01−0.01	0.7	−0.5−2.0
Other factors				
Patient age	0.04*	0.03−0.05	0.2*	0.2−0.2
Arrival				
08:00–15:59	Reference			
16:00–23:59	<−0.01	−0.01−<0.01	−3.0*	−4.4−−1.8
0:00–07:59	<0.01	<−0.01−0.01	− 0.1	−1.9−1.9
Percentage of admissions	<0.01	<−0.01−<0.01	0.2*	0.1−0.3

*,P<0.05; 95% CI, 95% confidence intervals; ED, emergency department.

Table 4. Cross correlation of input, throughput, and output factors on the length of ED stay for discharged patients.

Characteristic	Ambulance arrival	Number of walk-in patients	Number of ambulance arrivals	Radiography	Computed tomography	Magnetic resonance imaging	Ultrasonography	Laboratory blood tests
Ambulance arrival	1							
Number of walk-in patients	−0.0901	1						
Number of ambulance arrivals	0.3521	0.195	1					
Radiography	0.1971	−0.0441	0.0757	1				
Computed tomography	0.2536	−0.0885	0.0764	0.1627	1			
Magnetic resonance imaging	0.0833	−0.048	0.0295	0.0444	0.1961	1		
Ultrasonography	0.1654	−0.114	0.0283	0.0989	0.1905	−0.0144	1	
Laboratory blood tests	0.2803	−0.0999	0.0893	0.2218	0.3084	0.1246	0.267	1
Electrocardiogram	0.2605	−0.0996	0.0741	0.2649	0.2411	0.1291	0.1978	0.4087
Bed occupancy	0.0227	−0.2207	−0.0302	0.01	0.0462	0.0276	0.0413	0.0358
ED boarding	−0.0127	0.0506	0.0056	−0.0087	−0.0083	−0.0103	−0.0157	−0.0156
Patient age	0.1659	−0.0644	0.0476	0.1883	0.2812	0.1332	0.1321	0.2912
Arrival 16:00–23:59	−0.0644	0.1643	0.0188	−0.034	−0.0665	−0.0466	−0.0478	−0.059
Arrival 0:00–07:59	0.0479	−0.3665	−0.0926	−0.0026	0.0455	0.0126	0.1082	0.0499
Percentage of admissions	0.0542	−0.2895	0.0557	0.031	0.0568	0.029	0.0499	0.057
	Electrocardiogram	Bed occupancy	ED boarding	Patient age	Arrival 16:00–23:59	Arrival 0:00–07:59	Percentage of admissions	
Electrocardiogram	1							
Bed occupancy	0.0399	1						
ED boarding	−0.0091	−0.0069	1					
Patient age	0.3324	−0.0127	−0.0049	1				
Arrival 16:00–23:59	−0.0646	0.1164	0.0122	−0.1337	1			
Arrival 0:00–07:59	0.0482	0.0063	−0.095	0.0385	−0.4229	1		
Percentage of admissions	0.0569	0.2707	0.0683	0.0352	0.0986	0.024	1	

ED, emergency department.

Table 5. Comparison of the effects of input, throughput, and output factors on the length of ED stay for admitted patients.

	Admitted patients (n = 7,843)			
Characteristic	**standardized β coefficient**	**95% CI**	**Additional length of stay, minutes**	**95% CI**
Input factors				
Mode of arrival				
Walk-in	Reference			
Ambulance	−0.20*	−0.22−−0.17	−38.6*	−44.1−−3.1
Number of walk-in patients	0.06*	0.04−0.09	2.3*	1.4−3.1
Number of ambulance arrivals	0.01	−0.01−0.04	1.2	−2.0−4.3
Throughput factors				
No diagnostic test	Reference			
Radiography	0.06*	0.03−0.08	2.5	−4.7−9.7
Computed tomography	0.25*	0.23−0.27	44.9*	40.0−49.9
Magnetic resonance imaging	0.14*	0.12−0.16	53.9*	45.6−62.3
Ultrasonography	0.07*	0.04−0.09	12.5*	7.6−17.4
Laboratory blood tests	omitted			
Electrocardiogram	0.01	<−0.01−0.04	−0.4	−0.7−0.5
Output factors				
Bed occupancy	−0.01	−0.03−0.01	−0.1	−0.7−0.5
ED boarding	0.02*	<0.01−0.04	2.2	−2.5−6.8
Other factors				
Patient age	0.01	<−0.02−0.03	0.1*	<0.1−0.2
Arrival				
08:00–15:59	Reference			
16:00–23:59	−0.05*	−0.08−−0.03	−12.9*	−17.8−−8.0
0:00–07:59	0.08*	0.06−0.11	36.5*	29.2−43.7
Percentage of admissions	0.02	<−0.01−0.04	0.3	−0.1−0.8

*, P<0.05; 95% CI, 95% confidence intervals; ED, emergency department.

Discussion

In this analysis of input, output, and throughput factors contributing to length of ED stay, laboratory blood testing had the strongest influence on length of ED stay in discharged patients, increasing it by 74.5 minutes compared to those discharged patients who did not have blood tests. CT testing had a strong influence on length of ED stay in admitted patients, increasing it by 44.9 minutes compared to that of admitted patients who did not undergo CT. Input and output factors also had significant influences on length of ED stay. However, their contributions did not have as great an impact as these diagnostic tests. Our findings will enable ED physicians to prioritize the contribution of input, throughput, and output factors to ED crowding and identify diagnostic tests that have a close relationship with length of ED stay both in discharged and admitted patients.

While many input, throughput, and output factors contributed to ED crowding, hospital bed insufficiency has been considered a major contributor to ED crowding. [17] However, the strength of contribution of this hospital bed insufficiency to ED crowding was not compared with those of other factors in any study. Indeed, ED physicians could not effectively set priorities of countermeasures against ED crowding because a lot of recommendations about solutions for input, throughput, and output factors were treated equally. [17] In our study, comparing the effect of input, throughput, and output factors on length of ED stay revealed that diagnostic tests, especially laboratory blood tests and CT, have a stronger effect on ED stay than other factors. Our findings suggest that interventions aimed at improving efficacy of diagnostic tests, especially laboratory blood tests and CT, should be explored.

The finding of the association between diagnostic testing and ED stay may result from two phenomena: the complex process of these diagnostic tests, and the use of unnecessary testing. First, the process of acquiring diagnostic tests takes many steps. For example, laboratory blood tests require placing the order, sampling patient blood, transporting it to the laboratory, analyzing it, and reporting of the results to the physician. This process, namely turnaround time of diagnostic tests, is considered as an important determinant of length of ED stay. [18] Thus, turnaround time of diagnostic tests might contribute to extended stay in ED of patients who had these tests in our study. Second, in general, physicians select diagnostic tests for patients who were considered to be high acuity or of complex medical condition. [19,20] However, these tests do not always yield additional value to management of these patients. [21] For example, one study reported that physicians established and used guidelines to select diagnostic tests for patients with an acute limp. This practice reduced the number of unnecessary tests, and the length of ED stay of these patients decreased. [22] Our study implies the improvement of turnaround time of laboratory blood tests and CT

Table 6. Cross correlation of input, throughput, and output factors on the length of ED stay for admitted patients.

Characteristic	Ambulance arrival	Number of walk-in patients	Number of ambulance arrivals	Radiography	Computed tomography	Magnetic resonance imaging	Ultrasonography	Electrocardiogram
Ambulance arrival	1							
Number of walk-in patients	−0.1181	1						
Number of ambulance arrivals	0.501	0.1558	1					
Radiography	0.1261	−0.0527	0.0753	1				
Computed tomography	0.1214	−0.0469	0.0505	0.2432	1			
Magnetic resonance imaging	0.0679	−0.0302	0.0221	0.0534	0.1934	1		
Ultrasonography	0.1107	−0.0884	0.0352	0.1471	0.2145	−0.0848	1	
Electrocardiogram	0.1731	−0.0906	0.0821	0.4485	0.2731	0.1073	0.2004	1
Bed occupancy	0.0496	−0.2389	−0.0038	0.0211	0.0146	0.0153	0.0725	0.0162
ED boarding	−0.0326	0.0525	−0.01	−0.0146	−0.0135	−0.0007	−0.028	−0.0271
Patient age	0.2223	−0.0771	0.1286	0.3038	0.2484	0.1231	0.1417	0.4673
Arrival 16:00–23:59	−0.0437	0.2523	−0.0013	−0.1196	−0.0502	−0.0541	−0.0341	−0.1117
Arrival 0:00–07:59	0.076	−0.3022	−0.0553	0.0336	0.0607	0.0393	0.1084	0.0719
Percentage of admissions	0.071	−0.2799	0.108	0.0001	0.0172	0.016	0.0244	0.0183
	Bed occupancy	ED boarding	Patient age	Arrival 16:00–23:59	Arrival 0:00–07:59	Percentage of admissions		
Bed occupancy	1							
ED boarding	0.0019	1						
Patient age	0.0295	−0.0161	1					
Arrival 16:00–23:59	0.0364	0.0197	−0.119	1				
Arrival 0:00–07:59	−0.0058	−0.0889	0.011	−0.3228	1			
Percentage of admissions	0.2564	0.0562	0.0611	0.0268	−0.0246	1		

ED, emergency department.

and the reduction of unnecessary testing might be effective solutions for ED crowding.

Numerous countermeasures on ED crowding have been investigated. Redirection of low-acuity patients to alternative facilities and ambulance diversion were studied as countermeasures controlling ED volume. [23,24] However, our findings suggest that restrictions on input factors may not be most effective to reduce the length of ED stay. An increase of one in the number of walk-in patients and ambulance arrivals prolonged patient stay in ED by only 1.8 and 2.6 minutes respectively; however, the execution of laboratory blood tests added another 74 minutes to stay of discharged patients. Another proposed countermeasure against ED crowding is the use of observation units to improve admission flow from the ED. [25] Once again, however, output factors may not have as strong an influence on length of ED stay as throughput factors. Our findings suggest that countermeasures on input and output factors might not be as effective as countermeasures on diagnostic tests.

Our study has some weaknesses. First, input factors in this study may have a smaller effect on the length of ED stay than they would in large EDs. However, large EDs with annual patients volumes of over 60,000 account for only 11% of total EDs in U.S. [26] Annual patient volume of our ED matches that of mid-sized EDs in the U.S., where annual patient volumes are 20,000–40,000; these EDs comprise 25% of total EDs in the U.S. [26] Indeed, the effect of input factors on the length of ED stay increases with increased patient volume, but this trend is observed at both large and small EDs. [26] This, the findings of our study may be most generalizable to mid- and small-sized EDs. Second, the hospital bed occupancy in this study was not as high as that of previous studies. [6,27] However, an effect of bed occupancy on the length of ED stay was observed in EDs where median hospital bed occupancy was around 70%. [11,16] The effect of hospital bed occupancy seems to be limited in this study and our findings should be validated in the EDs with higher hospital bed occupancy.

Conclusion

In our study, performance of diagnostic tests had a stronger relationship to increased length of ED stay than other common input and output factors both in discharged and admitted patients. In addition to other known factors that can contribute to ED crowding, emergency providers should develop an improved sensitivity to the time costs associated with the diagnostic testing they order and how these can detrimentally affect patient length of stay.

Acknowledgments

The authors would like to thank Miho Tamamura and Kyoko Kawano for research assistance.

Author Contributions

Conceived and designed the experiments: TK KN. Analyzed the data: TK KN HH. Contributed reagents/materials/analysis tools: TK KN HH. Contributed to the writing of the manuscript: TK.

References

1. Ministry of Internal Affairs and Communications (2010) Reserch of the acceptance of ambulance in the medical institution in 2009 (Japanese). Available: http://www.fdma.go.jp/neuter/topics/houdou/h22/2203/220318_6houdou.pdf. Accessed July 13 2013.
2. Sun BC, Hsia RY, Weiss RE, Zingmond D, Liang LJ, et al. (2013) Effect of emergency department crowding on outcomes of admitted patients. Ann Emerg Med 61: 605–611 e606.
3. Kocher KE, Meurer WJ, Desmond JS and Nallamothu BK (2012) Effect of testing and treatment on emergency department length of stay using a national database. Acad Emerg Med 19: 525–534.
4. Oredsson S, Jonsson H, Rognes J, Lind L, Goransson KE, et al. (2011) A systematic review of triage-related interventions to improve patient flow in emergency departments. Scand J Trauma Resusc Emerg Med 19: 43.
5. Fatovich DM, Hirsch RL (2003) Entry overload, emergency department overcrowding, and ambulance bypass. Emerg Med J 20: 406–409.
6. Hillier DF, Parry GJ, Shannon MW, Stack AM (2009) The effect of hospital bed occupancy on throughput in the pediatric emergency department. Ann Emerg Med 53: 767–776 e763.
7. Kawano T, Nishiyama K, Anan H, Tujimura Y (2014) Direct relationship between aging and overcrowding in the ED, and a calculation formula for demand projection: a cross-sectional study. Emerg Med J 31: 19–23.
8. Timm NL, Ho ML, Luria JW (2008) Pediatric emergency department overcrowding and impact on patient flow outcomes. Acad Emerg Med 15: 832–837.
9. Asplin BR, Magid DJ, Rhodes KV, Solberg LI, Lurie N, et al. (2003) A conceptual model of emergency department crowding. Ann Emerg Med 42: 173–180.
10. McCarthy ML, Zeger SL, Ding R, Levin SR, Desmond JS, et al. (2009) Crowding delays treatment and lengthens emergency department length of stay, even among high-acuity patients. Ann Emerg Med 54: 492–503 e494.
11. Asaro PV, Lewis LM and Boxerman SB (2007) The impact of input and output factors on emergency department throughput. Acad Emerg Med 14: 235–242.
12. Kim HY (2013) Statistical notes for clinical researchers: assessing normal distribution (2) using skewness and kurtosis. Restor Dent Endod 38: 52–54.
13. Nakayama T, Sakai M, Slingsby BT (2005) Japan's ethical guidelines for epidemiologic research: a history of their development. J Epidemiol 15: 107–112.
14. Halperin H, Paradis N, Mosesso V Jr, Nichol G, Sayre M, et al. (2007) Recommendations for implementation of community consultation and public disclosure under the Food and Drug Administration's "Exception from informed consent requirements for emergency research": a special report from the American Heart Association Emergency Cardiovascular Care Committee and Council on Cardiopulmonary, Perioperative and Critical Care: endorsed by the American College of Emergency Physicians and the Society for Academic Emergency Medicine. Circulation 116: 1855–1863.
15. Chin L, Fleisher G (1998) Planning model of resource utilization in an academic pediatric emergency department. Pediatr Emerg Care 14: 4–9.
16. Asaro PV, Lewis LM, Boxerman SB (2007) Emergency department overcrowding: analysis of the factors of renege rate. Acad Emerg Med 14: 157–162.
17. Affleck A, Parks P, Drummond A, Rowe BH, Ovens HJ (2013) Emergency department overcrowding and access block. CJEM 15: 359–370.
18. Chan L, Reilly KM, Salluzzo RF (1997) Variables that affect patient throughput times in an academic emergency department. Am J Med Qual 12: 183–186.
19. Simon AE, Lukacs SL, Mendola P (2011) Emergency department laboratory evaluations of fever without source in children aged 3 to 36 months. Pediatrics 128: e1368–1375.
20. Singal BM, Hedges JR, Rousseau EW, Sanders AB, Berstein E, et al. (1992) Geriatric patient emergency visits. Part I: Comparison of visits by geriatric and younger patients. Ann Emerg Med 21: 802–807.
21. Reed L, Baskett A, Watkins N (2009) Managing children with acute non-traumatic limp: the utility of clinical findings, laboratory inflammatory markers and X-rays. Emerg Med Australas 21: 136–142.
22. McCanny PJ, McCoy S, Grant T, Walsh S, O'Sullivan R (2013) Implementation of an evidence based guideline reduces blood tests and length of stay for the limping child in a paediatric emergency department. Emerg Med J 30: 19–23.
23. Washington DL, Stevens CD, Shekelle PG, Henneman PL, Brook RH (2002) Next-day care for emergency department users with nonacute conditions. A randomized, controlled trial. Ann Intern Med 137: 707–714.
24. Lagoe RJ, Jastremski MS (1990) Relieving overcrowded emergency departments through ambulance diversion. Hosp Top 68: 23–27.
25. Gomez-Vaquero C, Soler AS, Pastor AJ, Mas JR, Rodriguez JJ, et al. (2009) Efficacy of a holding unit to reduce access block and attendance pressure in the emergency department. Emerg Med J 26: 571–572.
26. Pines JM, Decker SL, Hu T (2012) Exogenous predictors of national performance measures for emergency department crowding. Ann Emerg Med 60: 293–298.
27. Forster AJ, Stiell I, Wells G, Lee AJ, van Walraven C (2003) The effect of hospital occupancy on emergency department length of stay and patient disposition. Acad Emerg Med 10: 127–133.

Data-Driven Decisions for Reducing Readmissions for Heart Failure: General Methodology and Case Study

Mohsen Bayati[1], Mark Braverman[2], Michael Gillam[3], Karen M. Mack[3], George Ruiz[3], Mark S. Smith[3], Eric Horvitz[4]*

1 Stanford University, Stanford, California, United States of America, **2** Princeton University, Princeton, New Jersey, United States of America, **3** MedStar Health and Washington Hospital Center, Washington, D. C., United States of America, **4** Microsoft Research and University of Washington School of Medicine, Redmond, Washington, United States of America

Abstract

Background: Several studies have focused on stratifying patients according to their level of readmission risk, fueled in part by incentive programs in the U.S. that link readmission rates to the annual payment update by Medicare. Patient-specific predictions about readmission have not seen widespread use because of their limited accuracy and questions about the efficacy of using measures of risk to guide clinical decisions. We construct a predictive model for readmissions for congestive heart failure (CHF) and study how its predictions can be used to perform patient-specific interventions. We assess the cost-effectiveness of a methodology that combines prediction and decision making to allocate interventions. The results highlight the importance of combining predictions with decision analysis.

Methods: We construct a statistical classifier from a retrospective database of 793 hospital visits for heart failure that predicts the likelihood that patients will be rehospitalized within 30 days of discharge. We introduce a decision analysis that uses the predictions to guide decisions about post-discharge interventions. We perform a cost-effectiveness analysis of 379 additional hospital visits that were not included in either the formulation of the classifiers or the decision analysis. We report the performance of the methodology and show the overall expected value of employing a real-time decision system.

Findings: For the cohort studied, readmissions are associated with a mean cost of $13,679 with a standard error of $1,214. Given a post-discharge plan that costs $1,300 and that reduces 30-day rehospitalizations by 35%, use of the proposed methods would provide an 18.2% reduction in rehospitalizations and save 3.8% of costs.

Conclusions: Classifiers learned automatically from patient data can be joined with decision analysis to guide the allocation of post-discharge support to CHF patients. Such analyses are especially valuable in the common situation where it is not economically feasible to provide programs to all patients.

Editor: Harry Zhang, Old Dominion University, United States of America

Funding: The research was supported as a project at Microsoft Research (http://research.microsoft.com/en-us/), a basic science research unit of Microsoft. Microsoft Research is an open research laboratory (with no publication controls) exploring curiosity-driven research with multiple concentrations in basic and applied computer science. MBa was also a postdoctoral researcher in Microsoft Research during 2007–2009 and received research support from Microsoft Research during 2010–12. MBa also received support by National Science Foundation award number 1216011. MBr was a postdoctoral researcher in Microsoft Research during 2008–2010 and received research support from Microsoft Research during 2010–11. MBr was also supported by a Natural Science and Engineering Research Council of Canada through its Discovery Grant program. MBr was supported by Microsoft Research (http://research.microsoft.com/en-us/) and also by the Natural Science and Engineering Research Council of Canada through its Discovery Grant program, by the Alfred P. Sloan Fellowship and by the National Science Foundation. The funders had no role in study design, data collection and analysis, decision to publish, or preparation of the manuscript.

Competing Interests: The authors declare that no competing interests exist. The authors know of no conflicts with the independent scholarship of the collaborations of researchers at Microsoft Research, Stanford, Princeton, and MedStar Health on this study.

* Email: horvitz@microsoft.com

Introduction

The increasing availability of large quantities of clinical data being captured by electronic health record systems frames opportunities for generating predictive models from that data to enhance healthcare. We first describe the construction of a predictive model that forecasts the likelihood that heart failure patients will be rehospitalized within 30 days of their discharge. Then, we show how the predictive model can be coupled with an automated decision analysis, which uses patient-specific predictions about readmissions within a cost-benefit model, to provide guidance on the patient-specific allocation of readmission reduction programs. We discuss how such a coupling creates a valuable *data to prediction to action* pipeline that can be implemented within a decision-support system to guide interventions. We describe methods for employing a cohort of test patients, held out from the development of the predictive models, to characterize the overall value of using a real-time decision system given uncertainty in costs and efficacies. This approach provides a foundation for understanding the relationship between interventions that promise to reduce readmission rates at some cost and predictive models that provide forecasts about individual patients' readmission risk.

High rates of rehospitalization within 30 days of discharge reported at multiple health centers have motivated studies of the use of predictive models to identify patients at the highest risk for readmission and the feasibility of using these inferred likelihoods to guide clinical decision making. In a 2007 report to the U.S. Congress, the Medicare Payment Advisory Commission (MedPAC) indicated that as much as $12B is spent annually by Medicare on potentially preventable readmissions within 30 days of patient discharge [1]. Beyond monetary costs, readmission within a short time horizon may be an indicator of poor quality of care with implications for the quality and length of patient lives. Incentives that would encourage hospitals to reduce the rates of unnecessary readmissions have been proposed and are being implemented [2].

Numerous programs for reducing readmissions have been implemented and tested over the past twenty years [3–11]. These programs have sought reductions in readmissions via investments in post-discharge care coordination, patient education and self-management support, scheduled outpatient visits, and telemedicine. A recent survey of readmission reduction programs can be found in [12].

Post-discharge intervention studies described in the literature often report some reduction in readmission rates associated with the intervention being studied. Reported reductions in rates of readmission vary from a few percentage points to 50% or more. Reported per-patient intervention costs vary from a low of $180 [13–14] to $1,200 [15]. Results span savings of thousands of dollars per patient to reported net losses. [16].

Even when an intensive post-discharge program is found effective in preventing readmissions, it may be prohibitively expensive to provide such an intervention to an entire patient cohort. However, net savings may be achieved when the same interventions are applied in a selective manner to patients identified as being at high risk for readmission.

Some readmission reduction programs have been implemented as patient-specific, with enrollment of patients into the prevention program determined by risk scores [17–20]. Detailed surveys of such scores are provided in [21–22]. A notable example is LACE [17]. LACE and related scores are designed to be simple enough to be calculated manually at time of discharge.

We give an end-to-end demonstration of the methodology of per-patient cost-benefit analysis based on a risk score that is automatically inferred from EHR data. We perform a sensitivity analysis of the overall effectiveness of readmission reduction programs over reported ranges of efficacies and costs of interventions and probe the expected value of embedding a real-time system providing these automated inferences in the clinical workflow. Finally, we compare the utility of our score for the end-to-end process to that of LACE and show that even relatively modest improvements in prediction quality can make a substantial difference in the utility of an intervention.

The advances introduced include: (1) a means for harnessing data available in the local EHR to build the best possible predictive model based on the locally available data; (2) the ability to embed computational guidance on risk rather than relying on heuristic policies or manual calculations of risk scores; (3) the ability to use local financial data to perform a calibrated cost-benefit analysis that recommends an intervention based on the optimal expected payoff; and (4) the ability to perform offline analyses to probe the value of embedding real-time guidance on interventions in a clinical setting via exploring implications of different combinations of costs and benefits of the interventions. The results highlight the importance of combining predictions with decision analysis.

Materials and Methods

We performed the studies on de-identified patient data drawn from the EHR system for a large tertiary urban hospital serving the Metropolitan Washington DC area. Approval for data access and analysis was granted by hospital's institutional review board.

The patient cohort consists of all Medicare patients who were admitted as inpatients to the hospital during July 1, 2007–June 30, 2010 and were discharged alive with heart failure as their primary diagnosis (ICD9 codes 402.01, 402.11, 402.91, 404.01, 404.03, 404.11, 404.13, 404.91, 404.93, and 428.x).

For each visit we defined a target binary variable to describe the patient's 30-day bounce-back status (bb_{30}). We defined all-cause rehospitalizations occurring within 30 days as $bb_{30}=1$ and no rehospitalization as $bb_{30}=0$. The correct value of bb_{30} was obtained using data files provided by the U.S. Centers for Medicare & Medicaid Services (CMS) to the hospital in April 2011. Our goal was to estimate the probability of $bb_{30}=1$ for patients where the value of bb_{30} is unknown.

We divided the cohort into a derivation cohort, consisting of all visits that started between July 1, 2007–June 30, 2009, and a validation set of all visits that started between August 1, 2009–June 30, 2010. In order to build a predictive model, the following information was extracted from the EHR database for each patient:

- *Patient information*: age, gender, marital status, family support.
- *Visit information*: date, time, duration, type (inpatient, emergency, or outpatient), source (emergency, transfer, etc.).
- *Medical information*: history of diagnoses, lab results, medications, medical history, chief complaint, attending and admitting doctors.

For the analysis of costs, we gathered cost information for these visits from the hospital's administrative database. To be consistent with CMS definitions, we excluded the following visits that did not meet criteria for calculation of hospital readmission rates according to CMS 30-day mortality and readmission patient-level data files sent to the hospital.

- Patient was not enrolled in fee for service (FFS) Parts A and B (the standard U.S. Federal-funded health coverage for those over 65) during the 12 consecutive months prior to the index admission or in the 30 days after discharge.
- Patient died during the index hospitalizations.
- Patent left against medical advice (AMA).
- Patient was transferred to another acute care facility.

- Additional admission within 30 days of discharge from an index admission (an admission cannot be considered both an index admission and a readmission).

Our eligible cohort was reduced to 1,172 hospital visits including 793 visits in the derivation cohort and 379 visits in the validation group. Further refinement of the cohort to account for readmissions of patients to other medical facilities is presented in accompanied Text S1.

Model-building and variable selection

We encoded the information about each visit as a vector of binary variables of size 3,388. The variables were extracted automatically from the patient visit data. We used logistic regression to compute probabilities of rehospitalization for cases in the validation set. Since our model contains a large set of variables relative to the cohort size, we use the LASSO technique to select the most predictive variables and avoid overfitting [23–24]. Overfitting is a challenge in statistics and machine learning that can specialize the predictive model to the training cases and provide predictors that do not ideally generalize to future, previously unseen cases. The optimal parameters of LASSO were selected based on a cross-validation analysis. The details of this analysis are described in the accompanied Text S1.

We also implemented LACE [17] in our cohort and compared its predictive accuracy with the statistical classifier using area under receiver-operator characteristic (ROC) curve and reclassification analysis. Details of this implementation and calibration of both LACE and the classifier is provided in the accompanied Text S1.

From Predictions to Decisions

We coupled the predictive classifier for readmission with a decision model to perform patient-specific decision analyses for guiding post-discharge interventions. The decision model takes into account the predicted probability of readmission, cost and efficacy of applying the intervention, and average cost of readmission and allocates the interventions. We made the following simplifying assumptions:

- The cost of applying an intervention is on a per-patient basis and is the same for all patients. Most prior studies make this assumption. Interventions include assuring an outpatient visit within a specified time frame, rendering additional patient education, performing follow-up phone calls, and providing a fixed number of home visits.
- The expected cost $C_{readmit}$ of readmission is *a priori* the same for all patients. $C_{readmit}$ may include not just the monetary cost of a readmission, but also a penalty for the reduced quality of care associated with presentations warranting avoidable hospital readmissions. $C_{readmit}$ may be set by the hospital using a variety of considerations or just be calculated from past financial data. We obtained $C_{readmit}$ using the latter option by calculating the empirical average readmission costs for patients in the derivation cohort.
- The efficacy of the intervention is *a priori* the same $P_{success}$ for the entire cohort of patients. For example, an intervention that reduces the readmission rate by 25% reduces the readmission risk of each patient to whom it is applied by 25%.

Without the intervention, the expected cost of readmission for a patient whose probability of being readmitted within 30 days is p is

$$C_0(p) = p \times C_{readmit},$$

which is the full cost of a readmission, weighted by the likelihood of the readmission. The intervention adds $C_{intervene}$ to the cost of treatment but promises to reduce the readmission probability to $p(1 - P_{success})$, thus bringing the total expected cost to

$$C_1(p) = C_{intervene} + p(1 - P_{success})C_{readmit}.$$

The expected cost of the outcomes associated with the cases of intervention and nonintervention as functions of p are plotted in **Figure 1**. The expected utility of the intervention is the difference of these expected values, $U(p) = C_0(p) - C_1(p)$. For low values of p, the intervention is not warranted, as $C_0(p) < C_1(p)$ and $U(p) < 0$. For high values of p, $U(p)$ becomes positive and the intervention becomes beneficial. Note that the expected utilities associated with the intervention and default post-discharge programs cross at a threshold probability, which we denote by p^*. At this probability of readmission, the expected utility for the intervention and default programs are equal. We seek to maximize the overall benefit of the program for all patients by taking patient-specific actions that maximize the net expected benefit for each patient. The ideal policy for maximizing utility is to apply the intervention to patients for whom $U(p) > 0$, or equivalently

$$p \geq p^* = \frac{C_{intervene}}{P_{success} \times C_{readmit}}$$

The predictive model provides patient-specific estimates of the readmission probability p based on the available data, and we use the model to predict for each patient whether $p \geq p^*$.

Finally, to explore the importance of the accuracy of the classifier in this analysis, we repeated the study using the LACE score instead of the output of the learned classifier and compared the results of the two analyses.

Software packages

All statistical analysis including construction of the classifier, cross-validation analysis, model calibration, and decision optimization was performed using R and Matlab.

Results

Model validation

The optimal classifier achieved an overall area under the curve (AUC) of 0.66 on the validation cohort. This is 10% improvement over the predictive model presented in [20], which obtained an AUC equal to 0.60, and an 11% improvement over LACE [17], which had an AUC of 0.59 in the validation cohort. The cross-validation AUC for the classifier and LACE for the derivation cohort is 0.69±0.0198 ($p_{value} < 0.05$) and 0.59±0.0093 ($p_{value} < 0.05$), respectively. The difference is statistically significant ($p_{value} < 0.001$). The fractions of readmissions to outside hospitals in the derivation and validation cohorts are 35.2% and 47.9%, respectively. This significant increase in outside readmissions highlights a major challenge of predicting readmissions in our data as the patient population and patterns of engagements with the hospital has significantly changed. If we remove from the

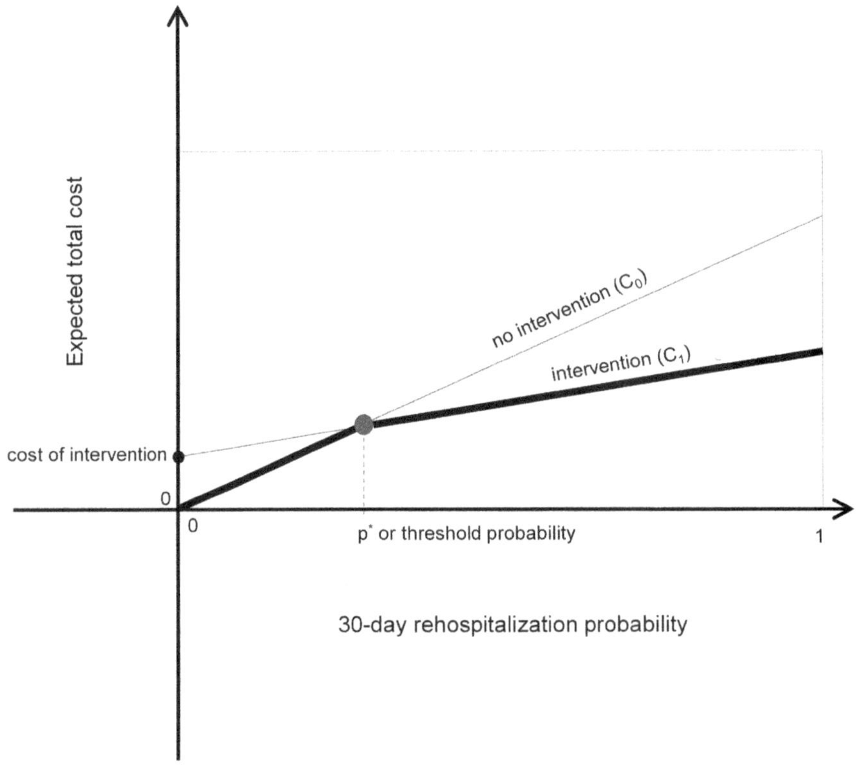

Figure 1. Plots of utility of outcomes for the intervention and no-intervention cases, showing relationship of potential expected utilities of outcomes achieved with a postdischarge program that reduces the rate of readmission versus the default of making no special intervention. Darker lines highlight ideal policy for any predicted likelihood of rehospitalization.

validation cohort all patients who were readmitted to outside hospitals, the AUC of the classifier on the validation cohort is 0.71.

The observed and predicted probabilities of rehospitalization provided by the predictive model for both derivation and validation cohorts are shown in **Figure 2**. The reclassification of patients from the three risk groups obtained by LACE to the three risk groups obtained by the learned classifier is shown in **Table 1**.

Predictive variables

The optimal model automatically selects a subset of 253 variables from 3,388 available variables to avoid overfitting to the derivation data. **Tables 2** and **3** show lists of the variables identified as most influential in predicting rehospitalization within 30 days. The variables are separated into lists of findings that provide the most evidential support for (**Table 2**) and against (**Table 3**) a patient being rehospitalized and are clustered within each list into diagnosed diseases, medications, lab results, and patterns of engagement with the healthcare system. Observations on engagement include such statistics as time since the last hospitalization and the number of hospitalizations in the last year.

Exploring the value of a real-time decision system

The patient-specific decision analyses applied to each of the CHF patients in the validation cohort using the utility model described in the Materials and Methods section identifies patients in the validation cohort who would have received the post-discharge intervention according to a policy of minimizing expected care costs. We compared the efficacy of using such patient-specific decision analyses to the use of a simpler *uniform policy*, where interventions are allocated homogeneously to either all or none of the patients, based on an analysis of which of the two possible uniform policies (*apply to all* versus *apply to none*) has the highest net expected value.

Table 4 compares the percentage of total readmission costs ($1,291,300) that would be saved, as predicted by the model, through using a patient-specific decision analysis as opposed to offering interventions to all patients in a uniform manner for efficacies (reduction in readmission rate) assumed to be 25%, 35% and for costs of intervention set to $800, $1,300, and $1,800. **Table 4** also shows the percentage of total expected readmissions prevented with the patient-specific analysis versus the best uniform policy. **Table 4** also displays the cost savings achieved by the patient-specific decision analysis when LACE is used in place of the statistical classifier. Using the poorer-performing LACE score for identifying patients at risk for readmissions translates into lower savings and narrower bands of usefulness across regimes defined by the costs and efficacies of programs.

We note that information in **Table 4**, representing details about the value and appropriateness of using patient-specific versus uniform policies depends on the costs, efficacies, and the predictive power of the classifier derived from data. Improvements in the accuracy of classifiers lead to greater selectivity in the application of programs and greater overall benefits to patients and hospitals. For example, by using the patient-specific decision analysis in the application of an intervention that costs $1,300 and that is 35% effective, 3.8% of rehospitalization costs can be saved and 18.2% of readmissions can be prevented. However, applying the intervention to all patients does not save dollars. Rather, providing the program to all patients adds 3.2% to the total costs.

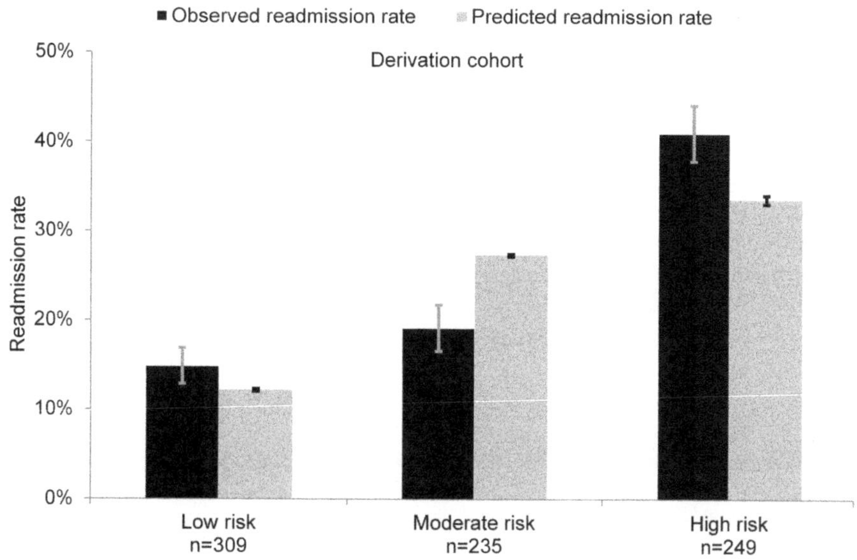

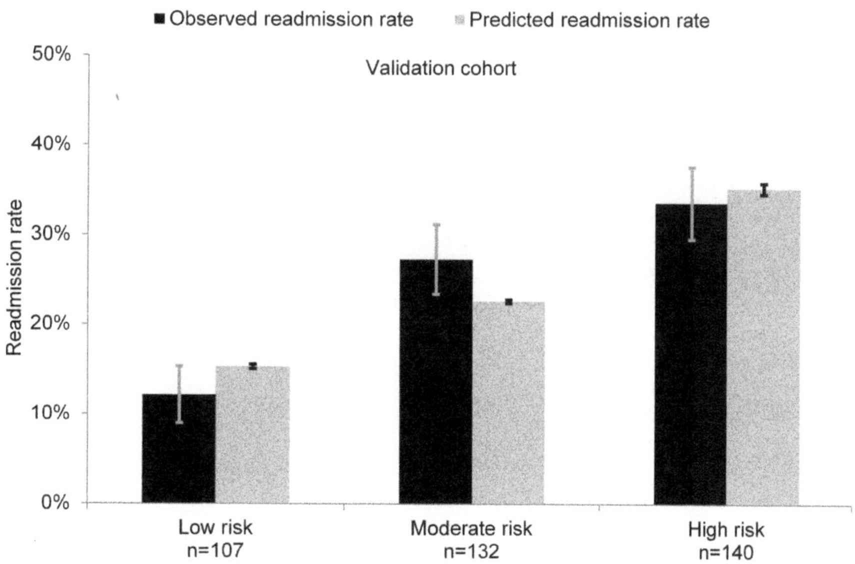

Figure 2. Study of calibration of likelihoods generated by predictive model. Figures show number of patients in each of three risk groups of derivation cohort (top) and validation cohort (bottom) with observed and predicted readmission rates within a margin of error with $p_{value}<0.05$.

Table 1. Reclassification of patients from the three risk groups obtained by LACE to revised risk groups obtained by the classifier.

Reclassification matrix

		Classifier			
		Low risk	**Moderate risk**	**High risk**	**Total reclassified (%)**
LACE	**Low risk (%)**	35.8	36.2	28.0	**64.2**
	Moderate risk (%)	16.8	33.6	49.6	**66.4**
	High risk (%)	0.0	23.5	76.5	**23.5**

Table 2. Top variables selected by machine learning procedure that increase risk of readmission within 30 days.

Top supportive evidence			
Variable class	**Variable description**	**Log Odds Ratio**	**Log Odds Ratio Standard Error[1]**
Lab Results	Lymphocyte % is low	0.0128	0.0027
Patterns of Engagement	Patient was admitted in past 6 months	0.0112	0.0031
Lab Results	BUN is high	0.0038	0.0012
Lab Results	Glucose level random is elevated	0.003	0.0012
Lab Results	Monocyte absolute is low	0.0028	0.0012
Other Diagnoses	History of nondependent abuse of drugs (ICD9 305.x)	0.0018	0.001
Other Diagnoses	History of chronic airway obstruction, not elsewhere classified (ICD9 496.x)	0.0017	0.0008
Other Diagnoses	History of gastrointestinal hemorrhage (ICD9 578.x)	0.0014	0.0007
Lab Results	AST is elevated	0.0013	0.0006
Other Diagnoses	History of cardiomyopathy (ICD9 425.x)	0.001	0.0006
Lab Results	Magnesium is low	0.001	0.0006
Lab Results	INR is elevated	0.0009	0.0004
Patterns of Engagement	Patient has been in isolated room in hospital	0.0009	0.0006
Lab Results	BNP is high	0.0007	0.0005

These are variables that receive positive log-odds ratio with the largest magnitude.
1. Obtained from sample standard error for cross-validation odds ratios

Intervention decisions obtained using LACE in lieu of the learned classifier would achieve only 0.5% savings and prevented only 2.6% of readmissions.

Given the ranges of costs and efficacies of post-discharge programs reported in the literature, the efficacy of a specific new program may not be known at the time that a new program is formulated. To build insights about the value of employing a real-time decision system in light of such uncertainty, we introduce an automated analysis of the *net expected value of a decision system* in a clinical environment. For each of a large number of different pairs of assumed efficacy and cost of intervention, we apply the data to prediction to action pipeline for all patients in the validation cohort, using the hospital-specific classifier that we have generated from local data. This sensitivity analysis provides the overall reduction in readmissions or savings for each pair of independently varied cost and efficacy. We performed this analysis and combined the multiple studies into a contour map visualization of the expected savings across the spectrum of cost and efficacy of the intervention. The contour map in **Figure 3**(a) represents the expected reductions in costs achieved with the use of a real-time decision system that performs guidance on patient-specific enrollment versus performing no special intervention for different combinations of cost and efficacies of programs. **Figure 3**(b) considers the boost in savings achieved by using the

Table 3. Top variables selected by machine learning procedure that decrease risk of readmission within 30 days.

Top disconfirming evidence			
Variable class	**Variable description**	**Log Odds Ratio**	**Log Odds Ratio Standard Error[1]**
Patterns of Engagement	Number of emergency room visits during past 6 months <2	−0.0607	0.0035
Lab results	Hematocrit % is normal	−0.0442	0.0043
Lab results	BNP is normal	−0.044	0.0049
Lab results	Alkaline phosphatase is normal	−0.0428	0.0033
Lab results	Chloride is normal	−0.0428	0.0042
Cardiac medications	Patient is not on digoxin therapy	−0.0396	0.0039
Lab results	MCHC % is low	−0.0387	0.0039
Changes in lab results	TSH variation during current visit is low	−0.0343	0.003
Changes in lab results	CO2 variation during current visit is low	−0.0318	0.0039
Changes in lab results	RDW variation during current visit is low	−0.0308	0.0038
Changes in lab results	MCV variation during current visit is low	−0.0306	0.0036

These are variables that receive negative log-odds ratio with largest magnitude.
1. Obtained from sample standard error for cross-validation odds ratios

Table 4. Comparison of savings achieved and readmissions prevented for post-discharge programs with different costs and efficacies.

Comparison of savings

		Savings or losses				Readmissions prevented		
Cost of intervention	**Efficacy**	**Patient-specific analysis and classifier**	**Patient-specific analysis and LACE**	**Intervention applied to all patients**	**Best uniform policy**	**Patient-specific analysis and classifier**	**Patient-specific analysis and LACE**	**Best uniform policy**
$300	25%	16.2%	15.9%	16.2%	16.2%	25.0%	24.5%	25.0%
	35%	26.2%	26.2%	26.2%	26.2%	35.0%	35.0%	35.0%
$800	25%	5.4%	1.3%	1.5%	1.5%	17.4%	2.9%	25.0%
	35%	13.2%	9.1%	11.5%	11.5%	31.4%	22.2%	35.0%
$1,300	25%	0.7%	0.0%	−13.2%	0.0%	5.2%	0.0%	0.0%
	35%	3.8%	0.5%	−3.2%	0.0%	18.2%	2.6%	0.0%
$1,800	25%	0.3%	0.0%	−27.8%	0.0%	0.8%	0.0%	0.0%
	35%	0.8%	0.0%	−17.8%	0.0%	7.3%	0.0%	0.0%

Three policies are compared: patient specific analysis using the classifier, patient-specific analysis using LACE, best uniform policy. For comparison of savings an additional column demonstrates the policy that applies intervention to every patient may lead to loss (or savings).

patient-specific decision guidance over the best uniform policy. The best uniform policy refers to the intervention being performed for all patients or none of the patients, depending on which outcome is better. The contour map demonstrates that the use of a real-time decision-analytic system for guidance would not yield net savings when the intervention is inexpensive and efficient, as it is best in that situation to apply the intervention to the entire population. Likewise, decision-analytic guidance would not be useful when the intervention is very expensive and inefficient, as such a program would not be cost-effective for any patients. However, for interventions with more intermediate costs and efficacies, relative savings of nearly 10% can be realized for the population we have studied, given predictions available from the classifier. **Figure 3**(c) considers the same boost in cost savings achieved by the patient-specific decision analysis over the use of the LACE score. The use of the poorer-performing LACE score for identifying patients at risk for readmissions translates to significantly lower savings and narrower regimes of applicability across regimes defined by the costs and efficacies of programs.

Discussion and Conclusions

Implications for readmission reduction

As demonstrated by the results displayed in **Table 4** and **Figure 3**, selective patient enrollment based on automatic risk stratification, could be applied effectively to take advantage of interventional programs that are too expensive to be applied to the entire population of heart failure patients.

The value of performing patient-specific decision analyses will generally increase with increases in classification accuracy, which can be achieved with larger training sets as well as more complete medical information about individual patients. A readmission prediction study [25] conducted in a Veterans Health Administration (VA) Hospital considered a heart failure patient cohort of $n = 198{,}460$, including data from a cross-hospital EHR containing the long-term medical histories of patients. Using this more extensive data, a statistical classifier was created with an AUC of 0.82. We found that 47% of the readmission patients in our cohort were readmitted to outside medical facilities within 30 days of their initial hospitalization for heart failure. We found that we had sparse EHR data on this substantial proportion of patients and that this may have detracted from the predictive power of our model. The results of the VA study highlight the value of implementing a shared patient database among the different hospitals that patients visit over time.

Analysis and insights enabled by the electronic capture of clinical data

We see the construction and use of predictive models that are custom tailored to populations as having the ability to deliver predictions of higher accuracy than those produced by simpler clinical rules designed for application across all hospitals. We envision that the *data to prediction to action* pipeline will become more widely used as EHR systems become more prevalent. We now outline several benefits of using local patient data to construct classifiers to predict outcomes, as compared to relying on simpler rules such as LACE.

Automated risk calculation

The classifier for predictions is constructed entirely from data available within the EHR. In real-time clinical use, findings on specific patients can be drawn automatically from the EHR, requiring no additional time from the practitioners. The computed risk scores can in turn be used to recommend enrollment into

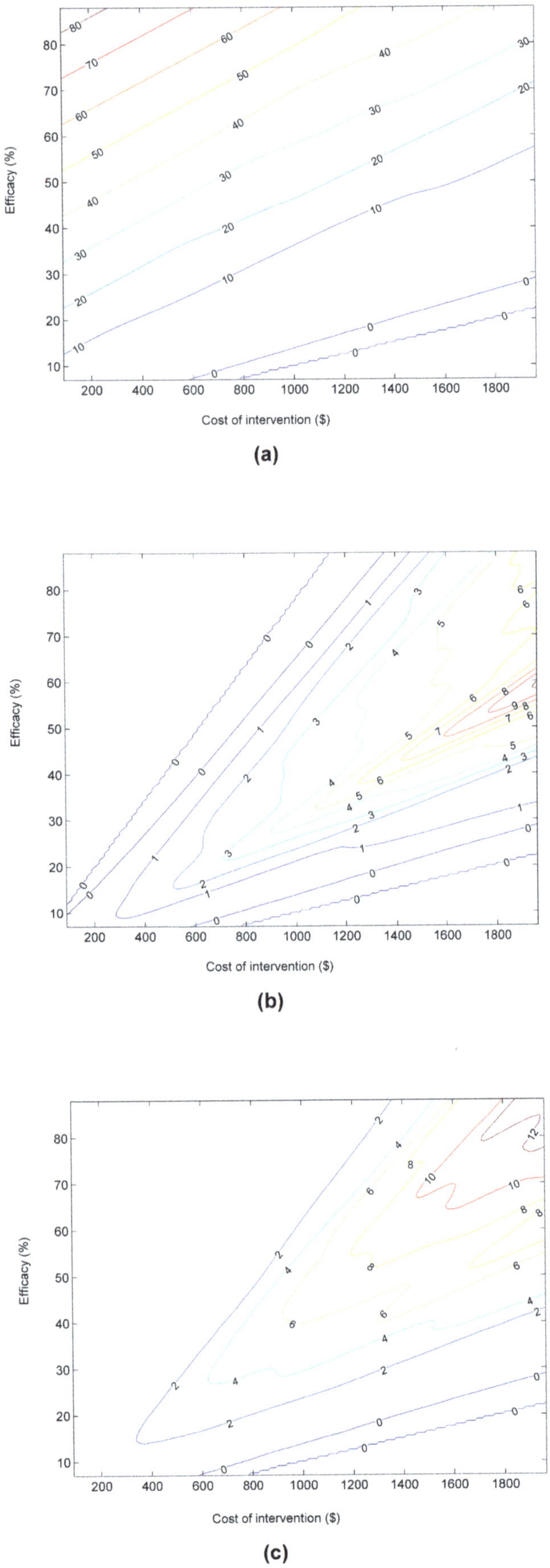

Figure 3. Contour maps capturing cost savings for ranges of program costs and efficacies: (a) savings with decision analysis over no intervention; (b) savings achieved with automated decision analysis over that of applying best uniform policy; (c) savings achieved with automated decision analysis over the use of LACE score, highlighting value of using more accurate predictive model. The labels on contour maps show percentage savings.

prevention programs as part of the workflow. Currently, such enrollment is performed typically using a pencil-and-paper form, or an application specifically designed for this purpose, and observations about patients and their health are manually entered or checked, making it difficult to consider multiple influencing factors. The risk estimation methods we describe do not place additional demands on practitioners and enable large numbers of patients to be screened for multiple intervention and prevention programs. Such automation also enables valuable data on the efficacy of interventions to be collected and harnessed. Moreover, when data on outcomes associated with interventions is accrued in the EHR, we can extend the methodology described in this paper to estimate both the readmission risk and the likelihood of the intervention succeeding at the level of an individual patient or patient subpopulation, further amplifying the effect of the intervention program.

Emphasis on local data

The predictive model is constructed entirely using local data. If our aim is to make the best possible predictions, taking local populations, data collection, and practice patterns into account will almost always be important in achieving the highest predictive performance. This raises the question of how a model trained within one hospital would perform when validated at a different hospital. As readmission patterns and prevalence vary by hospital and by region [26], a risk-stratification model that is not constructed locally will not be able to take into account the location-specific trends, details of care activities, and patient population. Unlike a generic risk rule, a locally trained classifier will be able to adjust as changes in the hospital's patterns of care occur over time.

Clinical face validity of observations

In reviewing the most predictive variables found by the classifier, we found that low lymphocyte percentage (top variable in **Table 2**) has previously been linked to poor outcomes in early postdischarge period of hospitalized HF patients [27] and low hematocrit (second top variable in **Table 3**) has been related to lower risk of heart failure [28]. However, a benefit of the data-driven approach is that we make use of all available data in constructing a predictive model. This means that we do not restrict the analysis solely to variables that have been found valid in previous studies. This characteristic is important because a learning algorithm may derive significant predictive power from variables that have poor face validity and appear arbitrary. This predictive power can stem from correlations among seemingly irrelevant variables available in the EHR and other, more interpretable variables that are not captured in the patient record. Variables identified as discriminatory may serve as proxies for other variables that would be more understandable, but are not available in the system. For example, in one of our studies on predicting general readmissions to the hospital, we discovered that "cocaine test: negative" raises the likelihood that the patient will be readmitted. A subsequent inquiry revealed that clinicians would be unlikely to administer a cocaine screening unless they had reason to suspect that a patient may be a drug abuser. Thus, the observation that the test was administered at all is linked to a higher-level assessment by the physician that the patient belongs to a vulnerable population—an assessment that is not recorded directly in the health database. Classifiers derived from all of the data available in the EHR will generally perform as well or better than models restricted only to those variables that have widely recognized clinical significance or that mesh with intuition as understandable or obvious indicators of risk with respect to a specific target ailment. We note that great care must be taken in interpreting the clinical relevance of variables flagged by such models as discriminating. Such observations are not necessarily involved in a *causal* manner nor suggest new paths to intervention. Observations identified as useful by the learning procedure may reflect local care patterns and not necessarily correspond to a generalizable risk factor. At the same time, variables identified as discriminating for a given predictive task may unearth new clinical insights and frame directions for study and intervention.

On limitations of local predictive tools

A potential drawback of the analytical pipeline that we have presented versus traditional risk-stratification scores is that its implementation would require some amount of computing resources. As the approach is data driven and relies only on data within the EHR, it can be implemented by the hospital, by the EHR vendor, or by an independent third party, further lowering the cost of implementing such a predictive system.

Another limitation of this study is the fact that it is based on retrospective data. A more rigorous validation would entail performing a randomized controlled experiment. However, the results provide a first step to demonstrate the applicability of risk stratification for guiding allocation of post-discharge interventions in a cost-effective manner.

Acknowledgments

We thank Paul Koch, Dobroslav Kolev, and Hank Rappaport for assistance with data access and interpretation.

Author Contributions

Conceived and designed the experiments: M. Bayati M. Braverman MG KMM GR MSS EH. Performed the experiments: M. Bayati M. Braverman EH. Analyzed the data: M. Bayati M. Braverman KMM EH. Contributed reagents/materials/analysis tools: M. Bayati M. Braverman MG KMM MSS EH. Wrote the paper: M. Bayati M. Braverman KMM MSS EH.

References

1. Medicare Payment Advisory Commission (2013) Promoting greater efficiency in Medicare, report to Congress. Medicare Payment Advisory Commission. Available at: http://www.medpac.gov/documents/jun07_entirereport.pdf.
2. Center for Medicare and Medicaid Services (2009) Proposed changes to the hospital inpatient prospective payment system for acute care hospitals. Federal Register. May 22;74(98): 24166. Available at: http://edocket.access.gpo.gov/2009/pdf/E9-10458.pdf.
3. Gonseth J, Guallar-Castillon P, Banegas JR, Rodriguez-Artalejo F (2004) The effectiveness of disease management programmes in reducing hospital re-admission in older patients with heart failure: a systematic review and meta-analysis of published reports. Eur Heart J. 25: 1570–1595.
4. Gwadry-Sridhar F, Flintoft V, Lee DS, Lee H, Guyatt GH (2004) A systematic review and meta-analysis of studies comparing readmission rates and mortality rates in patients with heart failure. Arch Intern Med.164: 2315–2320.
5. Jovicic A, Holroyd-Leduc JM, Straus SE (2006) Effects of self-management intervention on health outcomes of patients with heart failure: A systematic review of randomized controlled trials. BMC Cardiovasc Disord. 6: 43.
6. Koelling T (2005) Multifaceted outpatient support can improve outcomes for people with heart failure: commentary. Evid Based Cardiovasc Med.; 9: 138–141.
7. Krumholz HM, Amatruda J, Smith GL, Mattera JA, Roumanis SA, et al. (2002) Randomized trial of an education and support intervention to prevent readmission of patients with heart failure. J Am Coll Cardiol.39: 83–89.
8. McAlister FA, Lawson FM, Teo KK, Armstrong PW (2001) A systematic review of randomized trials of disease management programs in heart failure. Am J Med. 110: 378–384.
9. Phillips CO, Wright SM, Kern DE, Singa RM, Shepperd S, et al. (2004) Comprehensive discharge planning with postdischarge support for older patients with congestive heart failure: a meta-analysis. JAMA. 291: 1358–1367.
10. Rich M, Beckham V, Wittenberg C, Leven CL, Freedland K., et al. (1995) A multidisciplinary intervention to prevent the readmission of elderly patients with congestive heart failure. N. Engl J Med. 333: 1190–1195.
11. Hernandez AF, Greiner MA, Fonarow GC, Hammill BG, Heidenreich PA, et al. (2010) Relationship between early physician follow-up and 30-day readmission among Medicare beneficiaries hospitalized for heart failure. JAMA. 303: 1716–1722.
12. Boutwell A, Griffin F, Hwu S (2009) Effective interventions to reduce rehospitalizations: a compendium of 15 promising interventions. Cambridge, MA: Institute for Healthcare Improvement;. Available at http://ah.cms-plus.com/files/STAAR_A_Compendium_of_Promising_Interventions.pdf.
13. Anderson C, Deepak B, Amoateng-Adjepong Y, Zarich S (2005) Benefits of comprehensive inpatient education and discharge planning combined with outpatient support in elderly patients with congestive heart failure. Congestive Heart Failure. 11: 315–321.
14. Coleman EA, Parry C, Chalmers S, Min SJ (2006) The care transitions intervention: Results of a randomized controlled trial. JAMA. 166: 1822–1828.
15. Kasper EK, Gerstenblith G, Hefter G, Van Anden E, Brinker JA, et al. (2002) A randomized trial of the efficacy of multidisciplinary care in heart failure outpatients at high risk of hospital readmission. J Am Coll of Cardiol. 39: 471–480.
16. Peikes D, Chen A, Schore J, Brown R (2002) Effects of care coordination on hospitalization, quality of care, and health care expenditures among Medicare beneficiaries: 15 randomized trials. JAMA. 301: 603–618.
17. Van Walraven C, Dhalla IA, Bell Ch, Etchells E, Stiell IG (2010) Derivaiton and validation of an index to predict early death or unplanned readmission after discharge from hospital to the community. CMAJ. 6: 51–557.
18. Amarasingham R, Moore BJ, Tabak YP, Drazner MH, Clark CA, et al. (2010) An automated model to identify heart failure patients at risk for 30-day readmission or death using electronic medical record data. Med Care. 48(11):981–8.
19. Wang L, Porter B, Maynard C, Bryson C, Sun H, et al. (2012) Predicting Risk of Hospitalization or Death Among Patients With Heart Failure in the Veterans Health Administration. Am J Cardiol. 110(9):1342–9.
20. Keenan PS, Normand ST, Lin Z, Drye EE, Bhat KR, et al. (2008) An administrative claims measure suitable for profiling hospital performance on the basis of 30-day all-cause readmission rates among patients with heart failure. Circulation.1: 29–37.
21. Kansagara D, Englander H, Salanitro A, Kagen D, Theobald C, et al. (2011) Risk prediction models for hospital readmission: a systematic review. JAMA. 306(15):1688–1698.
22. Giamouzis G, Kalogeropoulos A, Georgiopoulou V, Smith LS, Dunbar S, et al. (2011) Hospitalization epidemic in patients with heart failure: risk factors, risk prediction, knowledge gaps, and future directions. J Card Fail. 17(1):54–75.
23. Chen S, Donoho D (1994) Basis pursuit, Signals, Systems and Computers, (1):41–44.
24. Tibshirani R (1996) Regression shrinkage and selection via the lasso. J Royal Statistics Society Series B. 58: 267–288.
25. Wang L, Porter B, Maynard C, Bryson C, Sun H, et al. (2012) Predicting risk of hospitalization or death among patients with heart failure in the veterans health administration. Am J Cardiol. 110(9):1342–9.
26. Jencks SF, Williams MV, Coleman EA (2009) Rehospitalizations among patients in the Medicare fee-for-service program. New Engl J Med. 360: 1418–1428
27. Vaduganathan M, Ambrosy A, Greene S, Mentz R, Subacius H, et al. (2012) Predictive value of low relative lymphocyte count in patients hospitalized for heart failure with reduced ejection fraction: insights from the EVEREST trial, Circ Heart Fail. 5(6):750–8.
28. Coglianese E, Qureshi M, Vasan R,Wang Th, Moore L (2012) Usefulness of the Blood Hematocrit Level to Predict Development of Heart Failure in a Community, Am J Cardiol. 109(2): 241–245.

5

Acute Kidney Injury Enhances Outcome Prediction Ability of Sequential Organ Failure Assessment Score in Critically Ill Patients

Chih-Hsiang Chang[1,2], Pei-Chun Fan[1,2], Ming-Yang Chang[1,2], Ya-Chung Tian[1,2], Cheng-Chieh Hung[1,2], Ji-Tseng Fang[1,2], Chih-Wei Yang[1,2], Yung-Chang Chen[1,2]*

1 Kidney Research Center, Department of Nephrology, Chang Gung Memorial Hospital, Taipei, Taiwan Chang Gung University College of Medicine, Taoyuan, Taiwan, **2** Chang Gung University College of Medicine, Taoyuan, Taiwan

Abstract

Introduction: Acute kidney injury (AKI) is a common and serious complication in intensive care unit (ICU) patients and also often part of a multiple organ failure syndrome. The sequential organ failure assessment (SOFA) score is an excellent tool for assessing the extent of organ dysfunction in critically ill patients. This study aimed to evaluate the outcome prediction ability of SOFA and Acute Physiology and Chronic Health Evaluation (APACHE) III score in ICU patients with AKI.

Methods: A total of 543 critically ill patients were admitted to the medical ICU of a tertiary-care hospital from July 2007 to June 2008. Demographic, clinical and laboratory variables were prospectively recorded for post hoc analysis as predictors of survival on the first day of ICU admission.

Results: One hundred and eighty-seven (34.4%) patients presented with AKI on the first day of ICU admission based on the risk of renal failure, injury to kidney, failure of kidney function, loss of kidney function, and end-stage renal failure (RIFLE) classification. Major causes of the ICU admissions involved respiratory failure (58%). Overall in-ICU mortality was 37.9% and the hospital mortality was 44.7%. The predictive accuracy for ICU mortality of SOFA (areas under the receiver operating characteristic curves: 0.815 ± 0.032) was as good as APACHE III in the AKI group. However, cumulative survival rates at 6-month follow-up following hospital discharge differed significantly ($p < 0.001$) for SOFA score ≤ 10 *vs.* ≥ 11 in these ICU patients with AKI.

Conclusions: For patients coexisting with AKI admitted to ICU, this work recommends application of SOFA by physicians to assess ICU mortality because of its practicality and low cost. A SOFA score of ≥ "11" on ICU day 1 should be considered an indicator of negative short-term outcome.

Editor: Giovanni Camussi, University of Torino, Italy

Funding: The authors have no support or funding to report.

Competing Interests: The authors have declared that no competing interests exist.

* Email: cyc2356@adm.cgmh.org.tw

Introduction

Although there are currently numerous co-existing clinical scores for critically ill patients [sequential organ failure assessment (SOFA) [1], Simplified Acute Physiology *Score (SAPS)* [2,3], Acute Physiology and Chronic Health Evaluation (APACHE) [4–6]], none of them has sufficient accuracy to predict outcome. Raising the sensitivity and specificity and increasing the number of parameters in order to enhance statistical power reduce the simplicity and cost effectiveness for clinical use. Given the aging population and numerous cases of co-morbidity in intensive care unit (ICU) setting today, acute kidney injury (AKI) remains a common and serious complication [7–9]. Pathophysiological factors associated with AKI are also incriminated in the failure of other organs, indicating that AKI is often part of a multiple organ failure syndrome. The occurrence of individual organ system failures varies among patients admitted to the ICU with AKI, with different degrees of association existing between individual organ system failures and ICU mortality. From this viewpoint, the SOFA score is an excellent tool for assessing the extent of organ dysfunction in critically ill patients with AKI [10,11]. However, there is no extant literature comparing these scoring systems in the setting of AKI defined by the risk of renal failure, injury to kidney, failure of kidney function, loss of kidney function, and end-stage renal failure (RIFLE) classification in critically ill patients [12].

We hypothesized that the discriminative power of the SOFA score in predicting ICU mortality is further enhanced for patients with AKI compared to those without. Therefore, we undertook a post hoc analysis of a prospectively accumulated database, to explore 3 ICU mortality scoring systems (SOFA and APACHE II & III) in critically ill patients with/without AKI and to compare

Table 1. Demographic data and clinical characteristics according to total v.s. AKI v.s. non-AKI.

	Total (n = 543)	AKI (n = 187)	Non-AKI (n = 356)	*p*-value
Age (years)	62.2±0.7	64.1±1.1	61.6±0.9	NS (0.09)
Male/Female	390/153	130/57	260/96	NS (0.359)
Length of ICU stay (days)	11.7±0.5	13.7±1.0	10.7±0.7	0.009
Length of hospital stay (days)	21.5±0.9	22.1±1.6	21.2±1.0	NS (0.60)
Body weight on ICU admission (kg)	62.3±0.6	61.4±1.0	62.8±0.8	NS (0.27)
GCS, ICU first day (points)	11±0.2	10±0.3	12±0.2	<0.001
MAP, ICU admission (mmHg)	77.1±1.7	73.8±1.5	79.7±2.7	NS (0.083)
Serum creatinine, ICU first day (mg/dl)	2.1±0.1	3.5±0.2	1.3±0.1	<0.001
Arterial HCO_3^-, ICU first day	21.7±0.3	19.3±0.5	22.9±0.3	<0.001
Serum sodium, ICU first day (mg/dl)	138.3±0.3	138.0±0.7	138.5±0.4	NS (0.545)
Bilirubin, ICU first day (mg/dl)	4.3±0.4	6.6±0.8	3.1±0.3	<0.001
Albumin, ICU first day (g/l)	2.8±0.1	2.5±0.1	3.0±0.1	<0.001
Blood Sugar, ICU first day (mg/dl)	168.4±4.8	182.1±10.3	161±5.0	NS (0.073)
Hemoglobin, ICU first day (g/dl)	10.4±0.1	9.7±0.2	10.8±0.1	<0.001
Platelets, ICU first day ($x10^3/\mu L$)	166.4±4.8	143.4±8.0	178.5±5.9	<0.001
Leukocytes, ICU first day ($x10^3/\mu L$)	10.9±0.3	11.9±0.7	9.7±0.4	0.005
PaO_2/FiO_2, ICU first day (mmHg)	279.6±6.6	260.2±10.4	289.9±8.3	0.031
ICU mortality (%)	220 (40.5)	116 (62.0)	104 (29.2)	<0.001
Hospital mortality (%)	243 (44.8)	131 (70.1)	112 (31.5)	<0.001
Need for renal replacement therapy (%)	34 (6.2)	34 (18.1)	–	–
Underlying diseases				
Diabetes mellitus (%)	164 (30.2)	67 (35.8)	97 (27.2)	0.044
Hypertension (%)	188 (34.6)	57 (30.4)	131 (36.7)	NS (0.135)
Cardiovascular disease (%)	148 (27.3)	47 (25.1)	101 (28.4)	NS (0.421)
Chronic kidney disease (%)	113 (20.8)	62 (33.1)	51 (14.3)	<0.001
Liver disease (%)	191 (35.2)	74 (39.6)	117 (32.9)	NS (0.120)
Malignancy (%)	105 (19.3)	35 (18.7)	70 (19.7)	NS (0.791)
Score systems				
APACHE II, ICU first day (mean ± SE)	18.0±0.4	23.2±0.6	15.2±0.4	<0.001
APACHE III, ICU first day (mean ± SE)	72.4±1.5	94.3±2.3	60.2±1.6	<0.001
SOFA, ICU first day (mean ± SE)	7.4±0.2	10.5±0.3	5.8±0.2	<0.001
RIFLE, ICU first day (mean ± SE)	0.8±0.1	2.0±0.1	–	–
RIFLE-R (%)	66 (12.2)	66 (35.3)	–	–
RIFLE-I (%)	54 (9.9)	54 (28.9)	–	–
RIFLE-F (%)	67 (12.3)	67 (35.8)	–	–

Abbreviation: AKI, acute kidney injury; NS, not significant; ICU, intensive care unit; SE, standard error; GCS, Glasgow coma scale; MAP, mean arterial pressure; PaO2, arterial partial pressure of oxygen; FiO2, fraction of inspired oxygen; APACHE, Acute Physiology and Chronic Health Evaluation; SOFA, sequential organ failure assessment; RIFLE, risk of renal failure, injury to the kidney, failure of kidney function, loss of kidney function, and end-stage renal failure.

the scores in these heterogeneous groups in three ICU admission settings.

Materials and Methods

Study participants and data collection

This investigation was carried out at three ICUs of one tertiary-care referral center between July 2007 and June 2008. These ICUs included two medical ICUs and one coronary care unit (CCU). The Chang Gung Memorial Hospital Institutional Review Board approved the study and waived the need of informed consent because there was no breach of privacy and the study did not interfere with clinical decisions related to patient care (approval No. 101-3059B). The patient information was anonymized and de-identified prior to analysis. There were 885 admissions during this period; final diagnosis and admission duration were reviewed first. Patients were excluded if they stayed in the ICU for less than 1 day (n = 89) or had repeated ICU admission (n = 56). Patients under 18 years of age, with organ transplant and end-stage renal disease (ESRD) with long-term dialysis were excluded (n = 154). To determine the ICU outcomes, we also excluded patients admitted to the ICU for observation after invasive procedures (n = 43).

Finally, a total of 543 cases were enrolled in this study. Post hoc analysis of a prospectively accumulated database examined the

Table 2. Demographic data and clinical characteristics of total population, non-AKI and AKI groups according to ICU mortality.

	Total			Non-AKI group			AKI group		
	Survival (n = 337)	**Non-survival (n = 206)**	***p*-value**	**Survival (n = 266)**	**Non-survival (n = 90)**	***p*-value**	**Survival (n = 71)**	**Non-survival (n = 116)**	***p*-value**
Age (years)	62.8±0.9	62.1±1.0	NS (0.616)	60.4±1.7	62.1±1.0	NS (0.396)	65.8±1.8	62.9±1.4	NS (0.223)
Male/Female	218/82	172/71	NS (0.802)	194/72	66/24	NS (0.981)	52/19	78/38	NS (0.387)
Length of ICU stay (days)	8.4±0.6	15.8±0.9	<0.001	8.7±0.7	16.7±1.6	<0.001	12.3±1.3	14.6±1.3	NS (0.241)
Length of hospital stay (days)	23.4±1.2	19.2±1.2	0.016	22.5±1.3	17.3±1.6	0.012	34.3±2.9	14.7±1.3	<0.001
Body weight on ICU admission (kg)	63.3±0.8	61.0±0.9	NS (0.055)	63.9±0.9	59.5±1.4	0.011	60.8±1.5	61.7±1.3	NS (0.666)
GCS, ICU first day (points)	12.7±0.2	9.9±0.3	<0.001	12.7±0.3	10.8±0.5	0.001	11.9±0.5	8.9±0.5	<0.001
MAP, ICU admission (mmHg)	80.1±3.8	75.1±1.4	NS (0.170)	81.7±4.3	76.1±2.4	NS (0.370)	80.5±2.7	71.3±1.8	0.008
Serum creatinine, ICU first day (mg/dl)	1.7±0.1	2.5±0.1	<0.001	1.7±0.1	1.8±0.2	NS (0.444)	2.9±0.6	2.7±0.4	NS (0.765)
Arterial HCO_3^-, ICU first day	22.8±0.4	20.2±0.4	<0.001	23.1±0.4	22.1±0.7	NS (0.220)	20.6±0.8	18.5±0.6	0.021
Bilirubin, ICU first day (mg/dl)	1.8±0.2	7.4±0.7	<0.001	2.3±0.3	5.2±0.8	0.001	2.1±0.6	9.3±1.1	<0.001
Albumin, ICU first day (g/l)	3.1±0.1	2.5±0.1	<0.001	3.2±0.1	2.5±0.1	<0.001	2.6±0.6	2.4±0.4	0.014
Hemoglobin, ICU first day (g/dl)	11.1±0.2	9.6±0.1	<0.001	11.2±0.2	9.7±0.3	<0.001	10.2±0.3	9.4±0.2	0.022
Platelets, ICU first day ($x10^3/\mu L$)	186.8±6.1	141.7±7.4	<0.001	185.8±6.2	157.6±16.7	NS (0.077)	178.1±13.5	122.1±9.4	0.001
PaO_2/FiO_2, ICU first day (mmHg)	301.5±8.6	252.4±9.9	<0.001	308.2±9.3	233.9±16.7	<0.001	283.5±16.7	246.5±13.2	NS (0.086)
Score systems									
APACHE II, ICU first day (mean ± SE)	14.5±0.4	23.8±0.5	<0.001	13.0±0.4	21.0±0.7	<0.001	19.1±0.8	25.9±0.7	<0.001
APACHE III, ICU first day (mean ± SE)	54.3±1.5	94.1±1.9	<0.001	54.5±1.6	82.2±2.9	<0.001	75.5±2.6	106.6±2.8	<0.001
SOFA, ICU first day (mean ± SE)	5.3±0.2	10.1±0.3	<0.001	5.0±0.2	8.2±0.4	<0.001	7.7±0.4	12.2±0.3	<0.001
RIFLE, ICU first day (mean ± SE)	0.5±0.1	1.4±0.1	<0.001	–	–	–	1.5±0.1	2.3±0.1	<0.001

Abbreviation: AKI, acute kidney injury; NS, not significant; ICU, intensive care unit; SE, standard error; GCS, Glasgow coma scale; MAP, mean arterial pressure; PaO2, arterial partial pressure of oxygen; FiO2, fraction of inspired oxygen; APACHE, Acute Physiology and Chronic Health Evaluation; SOFA, sequential organ failure assessment.

Table 3. Causes of ICU admission.

	All patients n (%)	Survivors n (%)	Non-survivors n (%)	*p*
Respiratory failure	315 (58.0)	152 (45.1)	163 (79.1)	<0.001
Cirrhosis with severe UGI bleeding	118 (21.7)	57 (16.9)	61 (29.6)	<0.001
CHF functional class IV	113 (20.8)	94 (27.9)	19 (9.2)	<0.001
Hepatic encephalopathy	108 (19.9)	42 (12.5)	66 (32.0)	<0.001
Shock	103 (19.0)	48 (14.72)	55 (26.7)	<0.001
Severe sepsis	103 (19.0)	33 (9.8)	70 (34.0)	<0.001
AMI	102 (18.8)	93 (27.6)	9 (4.4)	<0.001
ARDS	91 (16.8)	41 (12.2)	50 (24.3)	<0.001
HCC rupture	26 (4.8)	13 (3.9)	13 (6.3)	NS (0.194)
Arrhythmia	22 (4.1)	22 (6.5)	0 (0)	<0.001
Others[a]	22 (4.1)	14 (4.2)	8 (3.9)	NS (0.877)

Abbreviation: ICU, intensive care unit; UGI, upper gastrointestinal; CHF, congestive heart failure; AMI, acute myocardial infarction; ARDS, acute respiratory distress syndrome; HCC, hepatocellular carcinoma; NS, not significant;
[a]Acute pancreatitis severe form, cardiac tamponade, status epilepticus, pulmonary embolism, renal infraction.

demographics and clinical characteristics recorded on the first day of ICU admission.

Definitions

Pertinent medical history included respiratory failure (need for mechanical ventilation), AKI (based on the RIFLE classification), severe upper gastrointestinal (GI) bleeding (defined as massive GI bleeding combined with shock or need of ventilator assistance for procedure), congestive heart failure (CHF, based on Framingham criteria and defined as New York Heart Association functional class IV), hepatic encephalopathy grade II (according to World Congresses of Gastroenterology), shock (defined as hypotension with systolic arterial blood pressure of 90 mm Hg despite adequate fluid resuscitation), severe sepsis (defined as presence of 2 or more systemic inflammatory response syndrome criteria, proven or suspected infection) and associated organ dysfunction (according to modified American College of Chest Physicians and Society of Critical Care Medicine consensus criteria), acute myocardial infarction (AMI, defined according to the 2007 Expert Consensus Document of Circulation from the European Heart Journal), acute respiratory distress syndrome (based on the American-European Consensus Conference), hepatic carcinoma rupture (diagnosed by image and ascites puncture), arrhythmia (defined as ventricular tachycardia, ventricular filtrations, 2- or 3-degree AV block) [12–16]. The worst physiological and biochemical values on the first day of ICU admission were recorded. Neurological scoring was not performed in patients who were paralyzed or sedated since their conditions were not classified as neurological failure. The best verbal response for in-patients who had been intubated but not sedated was determined according to clinical judgment. Illness severity was assessed by the following scoring systems: APACHE II, III and SOFA [1,4,5,17]. The RIFLE was also evaluated at the time of ICU admission. Baseline serum creatinine (SCr) was the first value measured during hospitalization. The modification of diet in renal disease (MDRD) formula was used to estimate the baseline SCr levels in 45 patients because these patients had been admitted directly to the ICU and their previous SCr levels were unknown [12].

Table 4. Causes of AKI.

	All AKI patients (n = 187)	AKI Survivors (n = 71)	AKI Non-survivors (n = 116)	*p*
Sepsis without shock	37 (19.8)	13 (18.3)	24 (20.7)	NS (0.692)
Sepsis with shock	27 (14.4)	6 (8.5)	21 (18.1)	NS (0.068)
Hypovolemic shock(UGI bleeding, HCC rupture)	24 (12.8)	12 (16.9)	12 (10.3)	NS (0.193)
Decompensated heart failure	12 (6.4)	9 (12.7)	3 (2.6)	0.011
AMI	15 (8.0)	11 (15.5)	4 (3.4)	0.005
ARDS	32 (17.1)	10 (14.1)	22 (19.0)	NS (0.390)
Hepatorenal syndrome	22 (11.8)	2 (2.8)	20 (17.2)	0.002
Contrast induced nephropathy	9 (4.8)	5 (7.0)	4 (3.4)	NS (0.304)
Others[a]	9 (4.8)	3 (4.2)	6 (5.2)	NS (1.000)

Abbreviation: AKI, acute kidney injury; NS, not significant; UGI, upper gastrointestinal; HCC, hepatocellular carcinoma; AMI, acute myocardial infarction; ARDS, acute respiratory distress syndrome.
[a]Acute pancreatitis severe form, cardiac tamponade, status epilepticus, pulmonary embolism, renal infraction.

Table 5. Calibration and discrimination for the scoring methods in predicting ICU mortality.

	Calibration			Discrimination		
	goodness-of-fit (χ^2)	df	*p*	AUROC ± SE	95% CI	*P*
Total						
APACHE II	15.362	8	0.052	0.802±0.019	0.764–0.839	<0.001
APACHE III	10.041	8	0.262	0.829±0.018	0.793–0.865	<0.001
SOFA	9.870	8	0.274	0.817±0.019	0.780–0.854	<0.001
RIFLE	5.690	2	0.058	0.703±0.025	0.655–0.752	<0.001
AKI group						
AKI total						
APACHE II	17.254	8	0.028	0.745±0.037	0.672–0.818	<0.001
APACHE III	4.800	8	0.779	0.815±0.032	0.752–0.877	<0.001
SOFA	7.263	8	0.508	0.815±0.032	0.751–0.878	<0.001
RIFLE	3.540	1	0.060	0.772±0.035	0.704–0.893	<0.001
RIFLE-R						
APACHE II	3.556	8	0.829	0.737±0.068	0.604–0.870	0.010
APACHE III	7.806	8	0.350	0.830±0.052	0.727–0.933	<0.001
SOFA	8.683	8	0.370	0.833±0.050	0.735–0.930	<0.001
RIFLE-I						
APACHE II	6.799	8	0.450	0.754±0.068	0.621–0.888	0.002
APACHE III	8.987	8	0.343	0.776±0.070	0.638–0.914	0.005
SOFA	8.944	8	0.347	0.787±0.069	0.651–0.923	0.003
RIFLE-F						
APACHE II	5.564	8	0.591	0.704±0.112	0.485–0.923	NS (0.121)
APACHE III	7.952	8	0.438	0.803±0.125	0.558–0.998	0.043
SOFA	3.602	8	0.824	0.832±0.064	0.707–0.956	0.008
Non-AKI group						
APACHE II	9.280	8	0.319	0.771±0.027	0.719–0.823	<0.001
APACHE III	8.080	8	0.426	0.791±0.027	0.739–0.843	<0.001
SOFA	11.725	8	0.164	0.756±0.028	0.702–0.810	<0.001

Abbreviation: ICU, intensive care unit; df, degree of freedom; AUROC, areas under the receiver operating characteristic curve; SE, standard error; CI, confidence interval; APACHE, Acute Physiology and Chronic Health Evaluation; SOFA, sequential organ failure assessment; AKI, acute kidney injury; RIFLE, risk of renal failure, injury to the kidney, failure of kidney function, loss of kidney function, and end-stage renal failure.

Statistical analysis

Continuous variables were summarized by mean and standard error unless otherwise stated. The Kolmogorov-Smirnov test was used to determine the normal distribution for each variable. Student's *t*-test was used to compare the means of continuous variables and normally distributed data; otherwise, the Mann-Whitney U test was used. Categorical data were tested using the Chi-square test or Fisher's exact test. Furthermore, the Hosmer-Lemeshow goodness-of-fit test was used for calibration when evaluating the number of observed and predicted deaths in risk groups for the entire range of death probabilities. Discrimination was assessed using the area under a receiver operating characteristic curve (AUROC), which was compared by a nonparametric approach. The AUROC analysis calculated cutoff values, sensitivity, specificity, and overall correctness. Finally, cutoff points were calculated with acquiring the best Youden index. The index is defined as sensitivity+specificity -1, where sensitivity and specificity are calculated as proportions. Youden index has minimum and maximum values of -1 and $+1$, respectively, with a value of $+1$ representing the optimal value for an algorithm. Cumulative survival curves as a function of time were generated by the Kaplan-Meier approach and compared with a log rank test. All statistical tests were two-tailed; a value of $p<0.05$ was considered statistically significant.

Results

Subject characteristics

Five hundred and forty-three critically ill patients admitted to medical ICUs were enrolled. Table 1 shows demographic data, clinical characteristics and illness severity of patients with AKI and non-AKI. The median patient age was 62 years. Three hundred and ninety (71.8%) patients were males and 153 (28.2%) were females. Among these patients, one hundred and eighty-seven (34.4%) patients had AKI at ICU admission as determined by the RIFLE classification. Compared to non-AKI patients, the AKI group had a longer ICU stay, low hemoglobin (Hb) ($p<0.001$), less serum albumin ($p<0.001$), as well as more hospital and ICU mortality.

Table 2 shows the demographic data and scoring systems of ICU survivors and non-survivors. In the non-survival group of the total population, these patients had longer ICU stays but fewer hospital days. In addition, low Hb ($p<0.001$) and serum albumin

Table 6. Subsequent ICU mortality predicted after ICU admission.

Predictive Factors	Cutoff Point	Youden Index	Sensitivity (%)	Specificity (%)	Overall Correctness (%)
Total					
APACHE II	20[a]	0.46	88	56	72
APACHE III	80[a]	0.51	70	80	75
SOFA	7[a]	0.48	85	64	74
RIFLE	R[a]	0.34	93	34	64
AKI group					
APACHE II	21[a]	0.41	75	67	71
APACHE III	93[a]	0.49	68	82	75
SOFA	10[a]	0.47	75	73	74
RIFLE	I[a]	0.36	78	58	68
RIFLE-R					
APACHE II	24[a]	0.36	53	83	68
APACHE III	83[a]	0.56	90	67	79
SOFA	11[a]	0.45	74	67	71
RIFLE-I					
APACHE II	19[a]	0.46	75	71	73
APACHE III	99[a]	0.39	43	96	69
SOFA	10[a]	0.44	63	79	72
RIFLE-F					
APACHE II	24[a]	0.36	53	83	68
APACHE III	83[a]	0.56	90	67	79
SOFA	12[a]	0.61	67	100	81
Non-AKI group					
APACHE II	16[a]	0.44	85	57	71
APACHE III	52[a]	0.45	95	49	72
SOFA	7[a]	0.39	69	70	70

Abbreviation: ICU, intensive care unit; APACHE, Acute Physiology and Chronic Health Evaluation; SOFA, sequential organ failure assessment; AKI, acute kidney injury.
[a]Value giving the best Youden index.

($p<0.001$) were also noted in these patients. Moreover, the non-AKI ICU non-survival patients still had a significantly longer ICU stay but fewer hospital days. They also had very significantly lower Hb ($p<0.001$) and serum albumin ($p<0.001$) on ICU day 1. After adjusting the SOFA score in the multivariate analysis, the Hb and serum albumin still reached a significant difference ($p<0.05$) for those non-AKI patients. Furthermore, the AKI ICU non-survival patients had significantly fewer hospital days but not significantly shorter ICU stay. They also tended to have low Hb ($p = 0.022$) and serum albumin ($p = 0.014$) on the first day of ICU admission. However, the Hb and serum albumin were not found to be significantly different for these AKI patients after adjusting the SOFA score in the multiple logistic regression.

The reasons for admission to the ICU are listed in Table 3. The major causes of ICU admission were respiratory failure (58%) and severe UGI bleeding (21.7%). The causes of AKI are listed in Table 4. The major causes of AKI are sepsis (34.2%), acute respiratory distress syndrome (ARDS) (17.1%) and hypovolemic shock (12.8%).

Hospital mortality, short-term prognosis and results of the scoring systems

Overall ICU mortality was 37.9% and the hospital mortality was 44.7%. As for the assessment of calibration, Table 5 lists goodness-of-fit, as measured by the Hosmer-Lemeshow analysis of predicted ICU mortality risk and the predictive accuracy of the APACHE III and SOFA scores in the different groups. In predicting the ICU mortality, the accuracy of SOFA was as good as that of APACHE III in the AKI group (AUROC: 0.815 ± 0.032). In the non-AKI group, APACHE III was superior to SOFA (AUROC: 0.791 ± 0.027 *vs.* 0.756 ± 0.028). To assess the values of selected cutoff points for predicting ICU mortality, the sensitivity, specificity and overall correctness of prediction were determined (Table 6). The APACHE III scores revealed the best Youden index and highest overall correctness of prediction in both groups. In the AKI group, ICU mortality rates differed significantly ($p<0.001$) below and above cutoffs for 93 APACHE III points and 10 SOFA points. Cumulative survival rates at 6-month follow-up following hospital discharge differed significantly ($p<0.001$) for non-AKI vs. AKI groups (Fig. 1). Figure 2 shows the cumulative rates of survival for patients with coexisting AKI admitted to ICU were dichotomized at 10 SOFA points or less, and more than 11 SOFA points ($p<0.001$). To evaluate the correlation among APACHE II, APACHE III, SOFA score and various severity of AKI, we compared the means between groups according to the RIFLE classification by using ANOVA. The chi-square for trends revealed that the APACHE II, APACHE III,

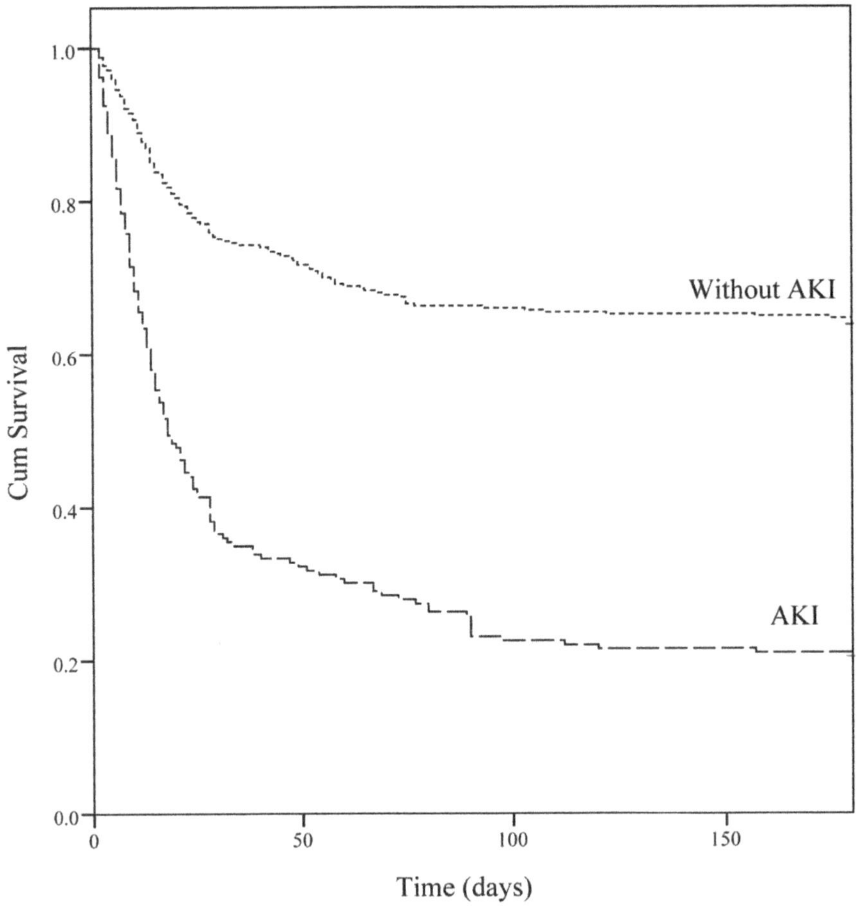

Figure 1. Comparison of cumulative survival between patients with and without acute kidney injury (AKI) (p<0.001).

SOFA score were all significantly different between non-AKI and AKI groups with varying severity ($P<0.001$) (Figure 3).

Discussion

This post hoc analysis of a prospectively accumulated database study included 543 heterogeneous patients with critical illnesses. The overall in-hospital mortality rate was 44.7%, which is consistent with figures obtained by previous studies indicating poor prognosis of ICU patients with septic shock, ARDS, AKI or hepatic cirrhosis. The occurrence of AKI in this work was 34.4% (187/543) and is in agreement with previous report indicating that the incidence was 35.8% of AKI (defined by the RIFLE classification) in a mixed ICU. The overall AKI group ICU mortality rate observed in this study was 62% (116/187), which was high compared to other studies [7–10,18]. The high mortality may have been attributed to the inclusion of two hundred and fifty-two patients (46.4%) with underlying cirrhosis and ninety-one patients (16.8%) with ARDS, both of which are positively associated with mortality in AKI patients [19–23]. In this study, we demonstrated that SOFA score at ICU day 1 has a comparable predictive ability for ICU mortality to APACHE III in the AKI group (AUROC 0.815 vs. 0.815). On the other hand, the APACHE III was superior to the SOFA score in the non-AKI group (AUROC 0.791 vs.0.756).

Renal failure is common in critically ill patients, and its occurrence is associated with an extremely high mortality rate [10,12,24,25]. Therefore, outcome prediction for short-term prognosis is needed to identify patients with high mortality risk from AKI. Since ICU patients with AKI is a syndrome and often is precipitated by and co-existing with other organ failure, the SOFA scores performance in evaluating the function of multi-organ systems was found to be as good as those of APACHE III in this work. Beyond the AKI, the mortality in an ICU setting is often related to age and co-existing co-morbidity, thus making the APACHE III score more accurate. When facing AKI patients, assessing the function of other organs is important [10]. We can simply use the six parameters to predict the outcomes and apply this score to help clinicians to focus their attention on more severe patients. Given that the SOFA score ignores diagnosis, age and co-morbid conditions, this score probably reflects the unique characteristics of the present patient group, whose prognosis can be predicted without considering the factors of age and diagnosis. The influence of age on outcome has been demonstrated to decrease with an increase in disease severity [26,27]. This can, at least partially, explain why age did not substantially influence the probability of mortality. The mortality rates greatly increased when SOFA scores of 11 or above were recorded in our study, which means that integrating the RIFLE classification and SOFA score, where ≥4 failed/dysfunction organs (including AKI), has fairly poor prognosis. Furthermore, researchers have come a long way in the study of the factors contributing to outcome in AKI patients. At present, the measure of AKI severity can be done using both ICU and specific AKI scores [11,28–31]. Among the current general ICU scores, APACHE III and SOFA scores

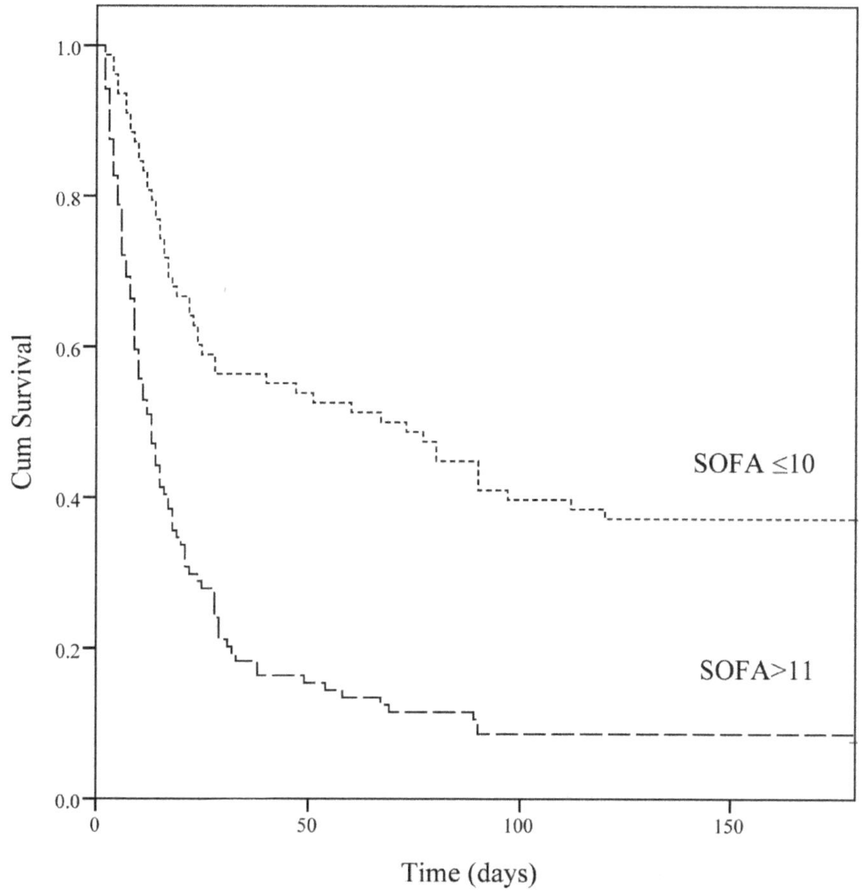

Figure 2. Cumulative survival for patients with coexisting AKI admitted to intensive care units were dichotomized at 10 SOFA points or less, and more than 11 SOFA points (p<0.001).

promise to be very useful. However, because the number and categorization of the variables considered in the APACHE III score is greater, it gains in statistical power but loses in simplicity, and thus the use of APACHE III entails extra cost [32].

In the non-AKI critically ill patients group, the discriminatory power of the APACHE III for predicting ICU mortality is superior to that of SOFA score. The non-AKI population in this study admitted to ICU was composed of a high proportion of subjects with AMI, CHF and cirrhosis. Anemia at baseline in patients with AMI undergoing primary percutaneous coronary intervention is common, and is strongly associated with adverse outcomes and increased mortality [33–35]. In CHF patients, low Hb values directly relate to poor peak oxygen consumption, disabling symptoms, and impaired survival [36,37]. Das *et al.* retrospectively evaluated the outcomes of 138 ICU cirrhotic patients and identified the independent risk factors for in hospital mortality as age, albuminemia, international normalized ratio and the SOFA score computed after discarding points for hematologic failure [38]. As responses to chronic disease, causes cachexia and malnutrition (low Hb and albumin) as well as a systemic inflammation. A lack of Hb and serum albumin prognostic factors in the SOFA score may account for its discriminative inferiority to APACHE III.

Despite the promising analytical results of this study, several important limitations should be recognized. First, this study was conducted at a single institution; consequently, the results may not be directly extrapolated to other patient populations. Second, scoring was performed only on the first day of ICU admission. Sequential application of these scoring systems (for example, daily or weekly) may reflect the dynamic aspects of clinical diseases and thus provide more complete data for mortality risk. Third, the patient population was heterogeneous and contained a high proportion of AMI, CHF, ARDS and cirrhotic patients, and may be viewed as a special subgroup of critically ill patients. Further validation in other cohorts with a multicenter study may be required in the future research. Finally, use of the prognostic instruments in patients already admitted to ICUs rather than as a preadmission screening tool may have skewed measurement results.

Various novel biomarkers such as NGAL (Neutrophil gelatinase-associated lipocalin), KIM-1 (Kidney Injury Molecule-1), interleukin-18 and cystatin C have been developed to assist early diagnosis, differential diagnosis and prognostic prediction in patients with AKI [39,40]. Combination of biomarkers and traditional scoring systems may further improve the sensitivity, specificity of clinical diagnosis and prognostic prediction, and remained to be clarified in the future.

Conclusions

In conclusion, this investigation demonstrated that the prognosis for AKI patients admitted to ICU is poor. The analytic data also highlighted the good discriminative power of the SOFA score in predicting ICU mortality of critically ill patients with AKI defined

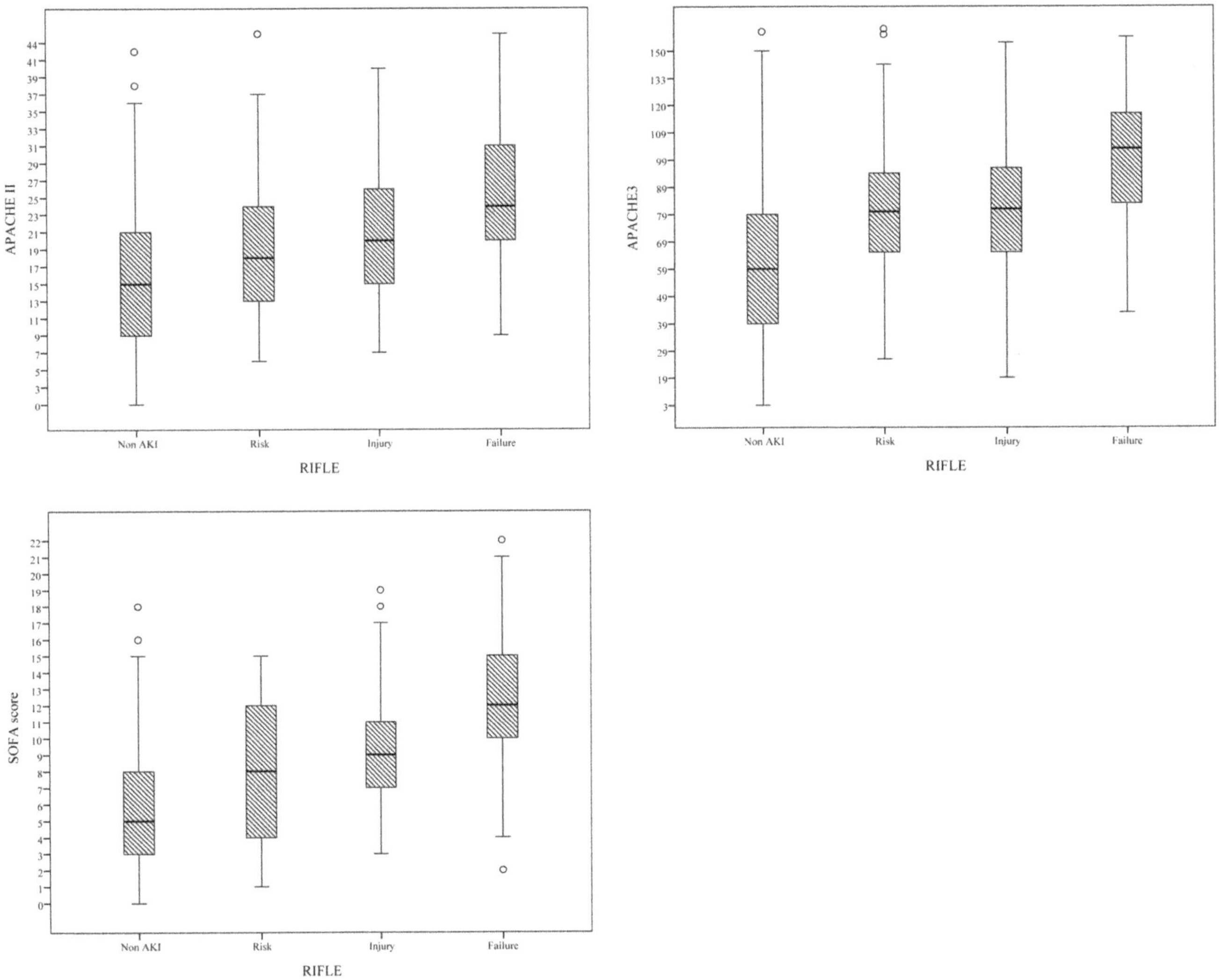

Figure 3. Box plot graph of APACHE II, APACHE III and SOFA score categorized by different AKI severity based on RIFLE classification. *P*<0.001 between groups by one-way analysis of variance (ANOVA).

by RIFLE classification. Considering the economy and ease of implementation, we suggest that SOFA score can increase the accuracy of short-term prognosis in this heterogeneous group of patients.

Acknowledgments

We thank all participants of the Kidney Research Center of Chang Gung Memorial Hospital, Linkou, Taiwan.

Author Contributions

Conceived and designed the experiments: CHC YCC. Performed the experiments: PCF MYC. Analyzed the data: YCT CCH. Contributed reagents/materials/analysis tools: JTF CWY. Contributed to the writing of the manuscript: CHC.

References

1. Vincent JL, Moreno R, Takala J, Willatts S, De Mendonca A, et al. (1996) The SOFA (Sepsis-related Organ Failure Assessment) score to describe organ dysfunction/failure. On behalf of the Working Group on Sepsis-Related Problems of the European Society of Intensive Care Medicine. Intensive Care Med 22: 707–710.
2. Le Gall JR, Lemeshow S, Saulnier F (1993) A new Simplified Acute Physiology Score (SAPS II) based on a European/North American multicenter study. Jama 270: 2957–2963.
3. Le Gall JR, Loirat P, Alperovitch A, Glaser P, Granthil C, et al. (1984) A simplified acute physiology score for ICU patients. Crit Care Med 12: 975–977.
4. Knaus WA, Zimmerman JE, Wagner DP, Draper EA, Lawrence DE (1981) APACHE-acute physiology and chronic health evaluation: a physiologically based classification system. Crit Care Med 9: 591–597.
5. Knaus WA, Wagner DP, Draper EA, Zimmerman JE, Bergner M, et al. (1991) The APACHE III prognostic system. Risk prediction of hospital mortality for critically ill hospitalized adults. Chest 100: 1619–1636.
6. Keegan MT, Gajic O, Afessa B (2011) Severity of illness scoring systems in the intensive care unit. Crit Care Med 39: 163–169.
7. Hoste EA, Clermont G, Kersten A, Venkataraman R, Angus DC, et al. (2006) RIFLE criteria for acute kidney injury are associated with hospital mortality in critically ill patients: a cohort analysis. Crit Care 10: R73.
8. Barrantes F, Tian J, Vazquez R, Amoateng-Adjepong Y, Manthous CA (2008) Acute kidney injury criteria predict outcomes of critically ill patients. Crit Care Med 36: 1397–1403.

9. Hsu RK, McCulloch CE, Ku E, Dudley RA, Hsu CY (2013) Regional variation in the incidence of dialysis-requiring AKI in the United States. Clin J Am Soc Nephrol 8: 1476–1481.
10. de Mendonca A, Vincent JL, Suter PM, Moreno R, Dearden NM, et al. (2000) Acute renal failure in the ICU: risk factors and outcome evaluated by the SOFA score. Intensive Care Med 26: 915–921.
11. Lin YF, Ko WJ, Wu VC, Chen YS, Chen YM, et al. (2008) A modified sequential organ failure assessment score to predict hospital mortality of postoperative acute renal failure patients requiring renal replacement therapy. Blood Purif 26: 547–554.
12. Bellomo R, Ronco C, Kellum JA, Mehta RL, Palevsky P (2004) Acute renal failure - definition, outcome measures, animal models, fluid therapy and information technology needs: the Second International Consensus Conference of the Acute Dialysis Quality Initiative (ADQI) Group. Crit Care 8: R204–212.
13. Thygesen K, Alpert JS, White HD, Jaffe AS, Apple FS, et al. (2007) Universal definition of myocardial infarction. Circulation 116: 2634–2653.
14. Ho KK, Anderson KM, Kannel WB, Grossman W, Levy D (1993) Survival after the onset of congestive heart failure in Framingham Heart Study subjects. Circulation 88: 107–115.
15. (1992) American College of Chest Physicians/Society of Critical Care Medicine Consensus Conference: definitions for sepsis and organ failure and guidelines for the use of innovative therapies in sepsis. Crit Care Med 20: 864–874.
16. Bernard GR, Artigas A, Brigham KL, Carlet J, Falke K, et al. (1994) The American-European Consensus Conference on ARDS. Definitions, mechanisms, relevant outcomes, and clinical trial coordination. Am J Respir Crit Care Med 149: 818–824.
17. Knaus WA, Draper EA, Wagner DP, Zimmerman JE (1985) APACHE II: a severity of disease classification system. Crit Care Med 13: 818–829.
18. Liu KD, Altmann C, Smits G, Krawczeski CD, Edelstein CL, et al. (2009) Serum interleukin-6 and interleukin-8 are early biomarkers of acute kidney injury and predict prolonged mechanical ventilation in children undergoing cardiac surgery: a case-control study. Crit Care 13: R104.
19. du Cheyron D, Bouchet B, Parienti JJ, Ramakers M, Charbonneau P (2005) The attributable mortality of acute renal failure in critically ill patients with liver cirrhosis. Intensive Care Med 31: 1693–1699.
20. Jenq CC, Tsai MH, Tian YC, Lin CY, Yang C, et al. (2007) RIFLE classification can predict short-term prognosis in critically ill cirrhotic patients. Intensive Care Med 33: 1921–1930.
21. Scott RA, Austin AS, Kolhe NV, McIntyre CW, Selby NM (2013) Acute kidney injury is independently associated with death in patients with cirrhosis. Frontline Gastroenterol 4: 191–197.
22. Cooke CR, Kahn JM, Caldwell E, Okamoto VN, Heckbert SR, et al. (2008) Predictors of hospital mortality in a population-based cohort of patients with acute lung injury. Crit Care Med 36: 1412–1420.
23. Lin CY, Kao KC, Tian YC, Jenq CC, Chang MY, et al. (2010) Outcome scoring systems for acute respiratory distress syndrome. Shock 34: 352–357.
24. Liu KD, Matthay MA (2008) Advances in critical care for the nephrologist: acute lung injury/ARDS. Clin J Am Soc Nephrol 3: 578–586.
25. Hsu CY, Chertow GM, McCulloch CE, Fan D, Ordonez JD, et al. (2009) Nonrecovery of kidney function and death after acute on chronic renal failure. Clin J Am Soc Nephrol 4: 891–898.
26. Rockwood K, Noseworthy TW, Gibney RT, Konopad E, Shustack A, et al. (1993) One-year outcome of elderly and young patients admitted to intensive care units. Crit Care Med 21: 687–691.
27. Van Den Noortgate N, Mouton V, Lamot C, Van Nooten G, Dhondt A, et al. (2003) Outcome in a post-cardiac surgery population with acute renal failure requiring dialysis: does age make a difference? Nephrol Dial Transplant 18: 732–736.
28. Abosaif NY, Tolba YA, Heap M, Russell J, El Nahas AM (2005) The outcome of acute renal failure in the intensive care unit according to RIFLE: model application, sensitivity, and predictability. Am J Kidney Dis 46: 1038–1048.
29. Ahlstrom A, Kuitunen A, Peltonen S, Hynninen M, Tallgren M, et al. (2006) Comparison of 2 acute renal failure severity scores to general scoring systems in the critically ill. Am J Kidney Dis 48: 262–268.
30. Mehta RL (2003) Outcomes research in acute renal failure. Semin Nephrol 23: 283–294.
31. Chertow GM, Soroko SH, Paganini EP, Cho KC, Himmelfarb J, et al. (2006) Mortality after acute renal failure: models for prognostic stratification and risk adjustment. Kidney Int 70: 1120–1126.
32. Chen YC, Tian YC, Liu NJ, Ho YP, Yang C, et al. (2006) Prospective cohort study comparing sequential organ failure assessment and acute physiology, age, chronic health evaluation III scoring systems for hospital mortality prediction in critically ill cirrhotic patients. Int J Clin Pract 60: 160–166.
33. Anker SD, Voors A, Okonko D, Clark AL, James MK, et al. (2009) Prevalence, incidence, and prognostic value of anaemia in patients after an acute myocardial infarction: data from the OPTIMAAL trial. Eur Heart J 30: 1331–1339.
34. Aronson D, Suleiman M, Agmon Y, Suleiman A, Blich M, et al. (2007) Changes in haemoglobin levels during hospital course and long-term outcome after acute myocardial infarction. Eur Heart J 28: 1289–1296.
35. Hsu CY, Ordonez JD, Chertow GM, Fan D, McCulloch CE, et al. (2008) The risk of acute renal failure in patients with chronic kidney disease. Kidney Int 74: 101–107.
36. Maraldi C, Volpato S, Cesari M, Onder G, Pedone C, et al. (2006) Anemia, physical disability, and survival in older patients with heart failure. J Card Fail 12: 533–539.
37. Groenveld HF, Januzzi JL, Damman K, van Wijngaarden J, Hillege HL, et al. (2008) Anemia and mortality in heart failure patients a systematic review and meta-analysis. J Am Coll Cardiol 52: 818–827.
38. Das V, Boelle PY, Galbois A, Guidet B, Maury E, et al. (2010) Cirrhotic patients in the medical intensive care unit: early prognosis and long-term survival. Crit Care Med 38: 2108–2116.
39. Chen TH, Chang CH, Lin CY, Jenq CC, Chang MY, et al. (2012) Acute kidney injury biomarkers for patients in a coronary care unit: a prospective cohort study. PLoS One 7: e32328.
40. Han WK, Bailly V, Abichandani R, Thadhani R, Bonventre JV (2002) Kidney Injury Molecule-1 (KIM-1): a novel biomarker for human renal proximal tubule injury. Kidney Int 62: 237–244.

6

Prediction of Cardiovascular Risk Using Framingham, ASSIGN and QRISK2: How Well Do They Predict Individual Rather than Population Risk?

Tjeerd-Pieter van Staa[1,2,3]*, Martin Gulliford[4], Edmond S.-W. Ng[2], Ben Goldacre[2], Liam Smeeth[2]

1 Health eResearch Centre, Farr Institute for Health Informatics Research, University of Manchester, Manchester, United Kingdom, **2** Department of non-communicable diseases, London School of Hygiene & Tropical Medicine, London, United Kingdom, **3** Utrecht Institute for Pharmaceutical Sciences, Utrecht University, Utrecht, the Netherlands, **4** Primary Care and Public Health Sciences, King's College, London, United Kingdom

Abstract

Background: The objective of this study was to evaluate the performance of risk scores (Framingham, Assign and QRISK2) in predicting high cardiovascular disease (CVD) risk in individuals rather than populations.

Methods and findings: This study included 1.8 million persons without CVD and prior statin prescribing using the Clinical Practice Research Datalink. This contains electronic medical records of the general population registered with a UK general practice. Individual CVD risks were estimated using competing risk regression models. Individual differences in the 10-year CVD risks as predicted by risk scores and competing risk models were estimated; the population was divided into 20 subgroups based on predicted risk. CVD outcomes occurred in 69,870 persons. In the subgroup with lowest risks, risk predictions by QRISK2 were similar to individual risks predicted using our competing risk model (99.9% of people had differences of less than 2%); in the subgroup with highest risks, risk predictions varied greatly (only 13.3% of people had differences of less than 2%). Larger deviations between QRISK2 and our individual predicted risks occurred with calendar year, different ethnicities, diabetes mellitus and number of records for medical events in the electronic health records in the year before the index date. A QRISK2 estimate of low 10-year CVD risk (<15%) was confirmed by Framingham, ASSIGN and our individual predicted risks in 89.8% while an estimate of high 10-year CVD risk (≥20%) was confirmed in only 48.6% of people. The majority of cases occurred in people who had predicted 10-year CVD risk of less than 20%.

Conclusions: Application of existing CVD risk scores may result in considerable misclassification of high risk status. Current practice to use a constant threshold level for intervention for all patients, together with the use of different scoring methods, may inadvertently create an arbitrary classification of high CVD risk.

Editor: Adrian V Hernandez, Universidad Peruana de Ciencias Aplicadas (UPC), Peru

Funding: This study was supported by the Wellcome Trust as part of a programme to evaluate the feasibility of conducting pragmatic randomised trials within CPRD; this work was done as part of the assessment of eligibility for a trial comparing simvastatin and atorvastatin. LS is supported by a Senior Clinical Fellowship from the Wellcome Trust. MG was supported by the National Institute for Health Research (NIHR) Biomedical Research Centre at Guy's and St Thomas' NHS Foundation Trust and King's College London. The funders had no role in study design, data collection and analysis, decision to publish, or preparation of the manuscript. CPRD is owned by the UK Department of Health and operates within the Medicines and Healthcare products Regulatory Agency (MHRA). CPRD has received funding from the MHRA, Wellcome Trust, Medical Research Council, NIHR Health Technology Assessment programme, Innovative Medicine Initiative, UK Department of Health, Technology Strategy Board, Seventh Framework Programme EU, various universities, contract research organisations and pharmaceutical companies. The department of Pharmacoepidemiology & Pharmacotherapy, Utrecht Institute for Pharmaceutical Sciences has received unrestricted funding for pharmacoepidemiological research from GlaxoSmithKline, Novo Nordisk, the private-public funded Top Institute Pharma (www.tipharma.nl, includes co-funding from universities, government, and industry), the Dutch Medicines Evaluation Board, and the Dutch Ministry of Health. The funders had no role in study design, data collection and analysis, decision to publish, or preparation of the manuscript.

Competing Interests: The authors have the following interests: Utrecht Institute for Pharmaceutical Sciences has received unrestricted funding for pharmacoepidemiological research from GlaxoSmithKline and Novo Nordisk. There are no patents, products in development or marketed products to declare. Two authors (TvS and EN) were previously employed by the Clinical Practice Research Datalink (CPRD). CPRD provides data and trial services on a commercial basis for both academic and pharmaceutical industry researchers. CPRD did not have any role in writing the report, or any input into the content of the report.

* Email: tjeerd.vanstaa@manchester.ac.uk

Introduction

Cardiovascular disease (CVD) is a major cause of mortality and morbidity worldwide. It causes impaired quality of life and accounts for a large share of health services utilization [1]. Statins are widely used medications in the prevention of CVD. A recent Cochrane review reported that statins reduce the risk of mortality by 16% and CVD outcomes by 26% in people without a history of CVD [1]. Most guidelines recommend that statins should only be used in primary prevention in people with a high absolute CVD risk [2,3]. As an example, the National Collaborating Centre for Primary Care and Royal College of General Practitioners and the National Institute of Clinical Excellence (NICE) recommended in 2007 to use statins "…as part of the management strategy for the primary prevention of CVD for adults who have a 20% or greater 10-year CVD risk of developing CVD…" [2].

A large number of risk assessment tools have been developed to support clinicians in determining the long-term risks of CVD [4]. The Framingham, ASSIGN and QRISK2 risk scores are widely used to predict 10-year CVD risk for primary prevention. The Framingham risk score is based on a US cohort recruited several decades ago [5]. The ASSIGN risk score was derived from the Scottish Heart Health Extended Cohort [6] and the QRISK risk score from a large primary care database in England and Wales [7,8]. These scores were based on risk factors that can easily be measured in the general population. The Framingham, ASSIGN and QRISK2 risk scores have been validated by comparing observed to predicted risks in the overall population [9]. There is no consensus about what risk score to use for CVD risk assessment and guidelines for primary CVD prevention propose to use any risk score [10]. These three risk scores are currently being used in the UK to determine CVD risk.

A recent review of CVD risk prediction models recommended that claims of improved performance of new models over established models should be documented in several studies carried out by independent investigators [9]. There is little evidence about how accurately these risk scores predict high CVD risk in individuals. A risk score could perform well in the overall population if it consistently predicts low rather than high risks as those at high risks are typically only a minority [11]. The objective of this study was to evaluate the validity and reliability of the Framingham, ASSIGN and QRISK2 scores in predicting individual CVD risk.

Material and Methods

Data source

This study used data from the General Practice Research Database in the United Kingdom which is part of the Clinical Practice Research Datalink (CPRD), previously known as the General Practice Research Database. CPRD comprises the computerised medical records maintained by general practitioners (GPs). Almost all people in the UK are registered with a general practice. GPs play a key role in the UK health care system, as they are responsible for primary health care and specialist referrals. The GPs are typically informed by hospitals of diagnoses made during outpatient consultations and hospitalisations. The data recorded in the CPRD since 1987 include demographic information, prescription details, clinical events, preventive care provided, specialist referrals, hospital admissions and their major outcomes [12]. A recent review of validation studies found that medical data in the CPRD were generally of high quality [13]. Fifty-five studies of the CPRD recording of diseases of the circulatory system reported a median percentage of cases confirmed of 85.3% [13]. People in CPRD have now been linked individually and anonymously to the national registry of hospital admission (Hospital Episode Statistics [HES]) and death certificates. The linkages are performed using the patient's unique NHS number, date of birth, sex and postcode of residence. HES collect the dates of hospital admission and discharge and main diagnoses, as extracted from the medical records by coding staff in England. The death certificates list the date and causes of death. Linked data were available for 50% of the CPRD population as, at the time of the study, this only included practices in England willing to provide unique patient identifiers to the Trusted Third Party. The protocol of this study was approved by the CPRD Independent Scientific Advisory Committee.

Study populations

The main study population consisted of people aged 35–74 years, using the November 2011 version of CPRD and drawn from CPRD practices that participated in the linkages. The start of follow-up was one year after start of the patient's CPRD data collection or 1 January 1998, whichever date came last. HES and death certificates data were available from 1998 onwards. The end of follow-up was the patient's end of CPRD data collection or death. The index date at which the CVD risk assessment was conducted, was a randomly selected date during this period of follow-up. This approach was different from that used in the QRISK2 analysis, which set the index date to 1-1-1998 unless the patient's data collection started later (e.g. due to patient newly registering). The use of a random index date was preferred in order to investigate changes in data recording (a newly registered patient may have different levels of e.g. missing data). The following persons were excluded: (i) those with CVD prior to the index date or with missing dates, (ii) those prescribed a statin prior to the index date or with missing dates, (iii) those temporarily registered with the practice. Follow-up was censored at the date of a first statin prescription.

Outcomes

The following incident CVD outcomes were included:

(i) CVD as recorded by the GPs (myocardial infarction, angina, coronary heart disease, stroke and transient ischemic attack).
(ii) hospitalisation due to CVD as recorded by the hospital in HES (either primary or secondary admission diagnostic ICD10 codes): angina pectoris (I20); acute myocardial infarction (I21); complications following acute myocardial infarction (I23); other acute ischaemic heart disease (I24); chronic ischaemic heart disease (I25); cerebral infarction (I63); and stroke, not specified as haemorrhage or infarction (I64), as used for QRISK2 [8]. Additional codes included intracerebral haemorrhage (I61) and other nontraumatic intracranial haemorrhage (I62).
(iii) Death due to CVD as reported on a death certificate (primary or secondary cause). The ICD-10 codes were similar to those used for hospitalisations.

Death due to causes other than CVD was also measured.

Imputation for missing variables

Missing values for smoking status, systolic blood pressure, ratio of total serum cholesterol and high density lipoprotein (HDL) cholesterol and BMI were imputed (using MI and MIANALYZE imputation procedures in SAS). The imputation regression models included the risk factors as listed in supplementary Table 1, CVD occurrence, death due to causes other than CVD, duration of follow-up and interactions between CVD occurrence and death and duration of follow-up. Five imputation datasets were created and the effect estimates were based on the combination of point and variance estimates from these five datasets [14]. The same imputed values for each patient were used across the different risk scores.

CVD risk scores

Three risk scores were analysed including Framingham, ASSIGN and QRISK2. We did not analyse the Joint British Society 2 risk score [3] given the similarity to the Framingham risk score. The 10-year CVD risks at the index date as predicted by Framingham and ASSIGN were estimated using the publicly available risk equations [7,8]. The risks predicted by QRISK2

Table 1. Baseline characteristics of the study population.

Risk factor		Men (N = 924233)	Women (N = 927953)
Age at index date	Mean (sd)	49.5 (11.3)	50.5 (11.8)
Duration of follow-up after index date	Mean (sd)	3.2 (3.0)	3.4 (3.2)
	≥5 years	221588 (24.0%)	248012 (26.7%)
	≥10 years	37741 (4.1%)	47159 (5.1%)
Ethnicity	White	444617 (48.1%)	538979 (58.1%)
	Black	11699 (1.3%)	14820 (1.6%)
	Indian	8627 (0.9%)	9805 (1.1%)
	Other	17231 (1.9%)	22210 (2.4%)
	Unknown	442059 (47.8%)	342139 (36.9%)
Index of deprivation quintiles	1 (most deprived)	230269 (24.9%)	237408 (25.6%)
	2	221536 (24.0%)	227396 (24.5%)
	3	180771 (19.6%)	182010 (19.6%)
	4	170552 (18.5%)	167548 (18.1%)
	5 (least deprived)	121105 (13.1%)	113591 (12.2%)
Body mass index	Low (<20)	12661 (1.4%)	40105 (4.3%)
	Normal (≥20 - <26)	181156 (19.6%)	273038 (29.4%)
	Overweight (≥26)	249981 (27.0%)	273694 (29.5%)
	Unknown	480435 (52.0%)	341116 (36.8%)
Smoking status	No	264612 (28.6%)	388477 (41.9%)
	Past	120610 (13.0%)	115259 (12.4%)
	Current	193165 (20.9%)	171328 (18.5%)
	Unknown	345846 (37.4%)	252889 (27.3%)
Systolic blood pressure	Recorded	596319 (64.5%)	771566 (83.1%)
	Mean (sd)	133.1 (16.3)	128 (18.0)
Cholesterol HDL ratio	Recorded	158927 (17.2%)	168611 (18.2%)
	Mean (sd)	4.5 (1.4)	3.8 (1.2)
Number of records for medical events in the electronic health records in the year before	Mean (sd)	10 (14.5)	16.5 (17.6)
Treated hypertension		72459 (7.8%)	91125 (9.8%)
Diabetes mellitus		20144 (2.2%)	15778 (1.7%)
Atrial fibrillation		7247 (0.8%)	4351 (0.5%)
Chronic renal disease		4830 (0.5%)	6998 (0.8%)
Rheumatoid arthritis		4280 (0.5%)	10721 (1.2%)
Left ventricular hypertrophy		2297 (0.2%)	1361 (0.1%)

were calculated using the commercial software program as provided by CLINRISK Limited on a fee-paying licence using the 2012 version [http://qrisk.org/index.php]. The CVD risks as predicted by the risk scores were based on the risk factors measured at the index date. A previous study reported that lifestyle variables as recorded in CPRD (such as obesity and smoking) were important predictors for myocardial infarction [15].

CVD risks based on a competing risk regression model

We also estimated for each patient the individual long-term CVD risks as modelled by a competing risk Cox proportional hazards regression model [16]. This was done to estimate as accurately as possible the actual CVD risks for each patient in the study population, which could then be compared to the risks as predicted by the risk scores. Competing risk regression was used as standard Cox regression model has been reported to overestimate 10-year CVD risk of coronary heart disease [17]. Accounting for the risks of competing events (such as death due to non-CVD causes) may be important in the frail and older populations as CVD occurrence may be precluded by the development of other diseases. Fractional polynomials were used to model non-linear risk relations with the continuous variables [18]. The regression models were conducted separately by gender and three age groups.

The validation of risk scores involves the measurement of calibration and discrimination. Calibration is the comparison of observed and predicted event rates and discrimination the ability of the risk score to distinguish between people who do and do not experience the event of interest [19]. We assessed calibration by comparing observed (using competing risk life tables) and predicted event rates in subgroups as defined by the vigintiles of predicted risk (vigintiles are the values that divides the distribution of individuals into twenty groups of equal frequency). Discrimination is the extend a risk score is able to differentiate between those who develop the outcome and those who do not. Discrimination is typically assessed by estimating the c index [19]. Rather than estimating this c index which is a global measure and population average, we evaluated the predicted risks at the index date for those people who developed CVD during follow-up. Good discrimination would have occurred if CVD cases mostly developed in those with high predicted risks. External validation is typically recommended for models that need to be generalised to other populations [19]. Our competing risk regression model was not intended to be generalised but only to estimate as best as possible the individual risks in our study population. We also assessed reclassification by evaluating the consistency in prediction between the different risk scores.

Descriptive analyses

The main analysis consisted of a comparison of the predictions of CVD risk at the index date with the four risk scores for each individual patient. The intraclass correlation coefficients (ICCs) in individual risk prediction between the four risk scores were estimated [20]. We report the ICCs rather than Pearson correlation coefficients because the former provides a measure of agreement between scores while the latter shows how well one score predicts the other. This distinction is important when a threshold (such as 20%) is recommended for deciding the course of clinical intervention.

Two different analyses were conducted in order to evaluate bias with the risk scores. The first analysis concerned secular trend in CVD incidence. CVD incidence has decreased over several decades [21]. Thus, the risk scores may overestimate CVD risks in current practice. In order to estimate the potential effects of this secular trend, incidence rates were measured in each calendar year. The second bias analysis concerned multiple imputations as used in the QRISK2 estimation. This method assumes that the occurrence of missing data is random conditional on other observed patient characteristics. In UK general practice, risk factors are typically not recorded unless the patient visits the practice. People with certain conditions may also be more likely to be screened for risk factors which incur extra payments (Quality Outcome Framework). In order to evaluate the effects of imputation, Cox regression was used to compare the CVD incidence in people with imputed values (for BMI, systolic blood pressure, cholesterol and smoking status) and those with measured values. If the assumption behind multiple imputations is correct, it can be expected that the CVD rate is similar between those with recorded and imputed values (conditional on the other risk factors in the model). SAS version 9.2 was used for the analyses.

Results

The study population included 1.8 million persons with an average follow-up of 3.3 years (Table 1). Ethnicity was not recorded for about half of the men and one-third of the women. About one-quarter of the study population had a follow-up after the random date of at least 5 years. Women were more likely to have information on smoking status, BMI and systolic blood pressure. The extent of missing data decreased sharply over calendar time. In 1998, BMI was missing in 47.3% of people, smoking status in 47.3%, systolic blood pressure in 33.4% and cholesterol/HDL ratio in 97.8%; in 2010, these figures were 32.7%, 14.3%, 22.3% and 72.2%, respectively.

CVD outcomes occurred in 69,870 persons. Major risk factors for CVD included number of cigarettes smoked per day of 21+ (relative rate [RR] = 2.77 [95% CI 2.54–3.03] in women and RR = 2.45 [95% CI 2.32–2.59] in men), unknown ethnicity (RR = 0.46 [95% CI 0.45–0.48] and RR = 0.42 [95% CI 0.42–0.43]) and 50+ records in CPRD in the year before (RR = 5.75 [95% CI 5.33–6.20] and RR = 4.31 [95% CI 4.02–4.62]).

The CVD incidence decreased over calendar time. The age- and sex-adjusted RR of CVD was 0.61 (95% CI 0.59–0.63) in 2010 compared to 1998. This RR was 0.94 (95% CI 0.89–1.00) for hospitalisations due to CVD (as recorded in HES) and 0.52 (95% CI 0.49–0.54) for GP-recorded CVD. Death due to CVD (as recorded on death certificates) also decreased over calendar time (RR of 0.58 [95% CI 0.52–0.64]).

The calibration of the competing risk model showed small differences on average with observed risks across vigintiles of risk. The largest difference between predicted and observed CVD risk occurred in the vigintile with highest risk (predicted 10-year risk of 35.9% compared to an observed risk of 34.9%). The differences between observed and predicted 10-year risks were on average less than 0.2% in 16 vigintiles with lowest risk.

Table 2 shows the distribution of 10-year CVD risks as estimated by competing risk regression. In people aged 50 years or older, 22.9% had a 10-year CVD risk of ≥20% and 51.5% of risk of ≥10%. The risks varied considerably in this age group: the 5th percentile of 10-year CVD risk was 1.4% and 95th percentile 34.6%.

The level of agreement in CVD risk prediction was best between ASSIGN and QRISK (intraclass correlation coefficient of 0.93) and lowest between Framingham and estimated risks in CPRD (0.77). The correlation was 0.91 between Framingham and ASSIGN, 0.87 between Framingham and QRISK2, 0.80 between ASSIGN and estimated risks in CPRD and 0.84 between QRISK2 and estimated risks in CPRD. As shown in Table 3, the difference in the predicted 10-year CVD risks between QRISK2 and the risks predicted based a competing risk model was on average 0.4%, while the predicted 10-year CVD risk with Framingham was on average 2.3% higher and ASSIGN 1.4% higher compared to that predicted by the competing risk model. When analysing the concordance in estimates for individual persons, only 55.6% of persons had a small difference in the risks predicted by QRISK2 and the risks based on the competing risk model.

Table 4 shows the differences between Framingham, ASSIGN and QRISK2 compared to the estimated risks in CPRD stratified by the risk factors. The mean differences between QRISK2 predicted risks and estimated risks in CPRD increased by age. QRISK2 overestimated 10-year CVD risk by 2.2% in people aged ≥65 years compared to the risks estimated in CPRD while QRISK2 predicted and CPRD estimated risks were, on average, similar in younger people. The concordance between QRISK2 predicted risks and the estimated risks in CPRD changed over calendar time; QRISK2 underestimated 10-year CVD risk by 3.2% in 1998–2001 and overestimated risk by 2.2% in 2006–2010 compared to the estimated risks in CPRD. Larger deviations between the risks predicted by QRISK2 and risks estimated in CPRD occurred with different ethnicities, diabetes mellitus, left ventricular hypertrophy and number of records for medical events in the electronic health records in the year before the index date.

The differences in individual risk prediction between the risk scores were largest among people with higher CVD risks (Figure 1). In the lowest vigintile of risk, the risk predictions by QRISK2 were similar to the individual risks estimated in CPRD (absolute difference of less than 2%) for 99.9% of people; in the highest vigintile of risk, this was only 13.3%.

The risk scores predicted low 10-year CVD risk fairly consistently (Table 5). A QRISK2 estimate of low 10-year CVD

Table 2. Distribution of 10-year CVD risk as estimated for individual persons in the study population using competing risk regression stratified by age and gender.

Risk factor		Number of persons (%) in categories of 10-year CVD risk				10-year CVD risk			
		Risk of <10%	Risk of 10-15%	Risk of 15–20%	Risk of ≥20%	Mean	Median	5th percentile	95th percentile
All		1373431 (74.2%)	165004 (8.9%)	111837 (6.0%)	201914 (10.9%)	7.4	3.3	0.2	27.9
Age at index	35–49	959377 (96.0%)	24718 (2.5%)	8981 (0.9%)	6196 (0.6%)	2.4	1.2	0.2	8.9
	50+	414054 (48.5%)	140286 (16.4%)	102857 (12.1%)	195718 (22.9%)	13.2	10.4	1.4	34.6
Gender	Men	629258 (68.1%)	91544 (9.9%)	65487 (7.1%)	137944 (14.9%)	9.1	4.7	0.3	31.7
	Women	744173 (80.2%)	73460 (7.9%)	46351 (5.0%)	63970 (6.9%)	5.7	2.2	0.2	22.8

risk (<15%) was confirmed by Framingham, ASSIGN and the CPRD estimated risks in 89.8% of people. An estimate of high 10-year CVD risk (≥20%) by QRISK2 was confirmed in 48.6% of people.

The majority of CVD cases occurred in people who had a predicted 10-year CVD risk of less than 20% (Table 6). Only 41.1% of the cases were predicted by QRISK2 to have a 10-year CVD risk of ≥20% and 27.5% of the cases a 10-year CVD risk of less <10%.

Discussion

We found that all three risk scores (Framingham, ASSIGN and QRISK2) predicted the presence of low CVD risk consistently in individual persons. However, predictions of high CVD risk for individuals varied substantively between the risk scores and treatment strategies could be different depending on which risk score is being used. Most CVD cases occurred in people deemed to be at low CVD risk.

Population averages can hide substantial variability in prediction among individual persons and poor prediction of 'high risk' status as these estimates are often determined by the large majority of low risk individuals. As succinctly stated by Rose, the ability to estimate the average risk for a group may not be matched by any corresponding ability to predict which individuals are going to fall ill soon [11]. The present study confirmed Rose's observations for CVD prediction, with a considerable variability between risk scores in the prediction of high CVD risk and with most CVD cases occurring in people classified to have lower CVD risk.

The QRISK2 score was developed in a similar setting as the present study and the statistical methods were also broadly similar. As expected, we found that the averages of QRISK2 estimates and our competing risk predictions were reasonably consistent. Two validation studies of QRISK2 reported that the predicted and observed risks were on average similar and they concluded that QRISK2 was accurate in identifying a high risk population [22,23]. Our analyses of averages support these studies. But we also conducted analyses of individual risk predictions and reached opposite conclusions. We found substantial deviations between the QRISK2 estimates and our competing risk predictions. This was related to the inclusion into the competing risk models of several risk factors, as pre-defined in the protocol, which were found to be strong predictors of risk (such as calendar year, number of GP visits, region and indicators of missing data including ethnicity). Our approach, although not commonly used, allows for an examination of the performance of risk scores in individual persons rather than testing averages across populations. This regression approach should provide, as long as the model is specified correctly, a close representation of the observed risks across multiple risk factors. The regression models also included risk factors not used by the published risk scores, such as number of GP visits (e.g. there was a five-fold difference in CVD risk between women with frequent and no GP attendance). If the risk scores are to be used for individual risk prediction, the evaluation of performance should go beyond population averages.

A recent meta-analysis reported that statins reduced CVD risk mortality in people with low CVD risk. It concluded that the threshold for statin treatment should be reduced to a 10-year CVD risk of 10% [24]. A commentary of this study proposed that statins should be used by all by the age of 50 years as most people aged 50 years or older have higher risks. It stated, incorrectly, that 83% of the men older than 50 years and 56% of women older than 60 years have a 10-year CVD risk of ≥10% [25]. It is questionable whether whole populations should be treated if individual risks

Table 3. Concordance between the risks predicted by the different risk scores and those estimated by competing risk regression in CPRD.

					Difference in individual risk predictions						
					≤ −10%	Between −5 and −10%	Between −5 and −2%	Between −2 and +2%	Between +2 and +5%	Between +5 and +10%	≥ +10%
Comparator risk method	**Reference risk method**	**Mean predicted risk by comparator risk method**	**Mean predicted risk by reference risk method**	**Mean difference between the two methods**	**% of persons**	**% of persons**	**% of persons**	**% of persons**	**% of persons**	**% of persons**	**% of persons**
Framingham risk score	ASSIGN risk score	9.7	8.8	0.9	0.8	3.4	4.4	65.4	16.5	7.3	2.2
	QRISK2 risk score	9.7	7.8	1.9	1.4	3.7	5.2	46.3	25.8	14.1	3.5
	Individual risks estimated in CPRD using competing risk regression	9.7	7.4	2.3	2.9	4.9	6.2	39.1	22.8	16	8.1
ASSIGN risk score	Framingham risk score	8.8	9.7	−0.9	2.2	7.3	16.5	65.4	4.4	3.4	0.8
	QRISK2 risk score	8.8	7.8	1	1	2.5	6	61.5	24.1	3.7	1
	Individual risks estimated in CPRD using competing risk regression	8.8	7.4	1.4	3.6	5.5	6.8	41.7	27	11.3	4.2
QRISK2 risk score	Framingham risk score	7.8	9.7	−1.9	3.5	14.1	25.8	46.3	5.2	3.7	1.4
	ASSIGN risk score	7.8	8.8	−1	1	3.7	24.1	61.5	6	2.5	1
	Individual risks estimated in CPRD using competing risk regression	7.8	7.4	0.4	3.7	6.3	8.8	55.6	14.3	7.9	3.5

Table 4. Differences in individual risk predictions between risk scores and risks estimated using competing risk regression stratified by risk factors (selected results for larger differences).

		Framingham risk score		ASSIGN risk score		QRISK2 risk score	
Risk factor		**Mean difference with risks estimated using competing risk regression**	**Percentage of persons with difference between −2 and +2%**	**Mean difference with risks estimated using competing risk regression**	**Percentage of persons with difference between −2 and +2%**	**Mean difference with risks estimated using competing risk regression**	**Percentage of persons with difference between −2 and +2%**
Gender	Men	3.7	24.0	1.7	24.8	0.4	47.5
	Women	0.8	54.2	1.0	58.5	0.4	63.6
Age at index	35–44	2.0	58.9	1.5	59.9	0	84.4
	45–54	3.2	31.8	1.2	39.6	0	53.3
	55–64	2.8	22.2	0.5	24.1	0.3	26.5
	65–74	0.7	19.6	2.4	18.2	2.2	18.5
Calendar year index	1998–2000	−0.7	32.0	−1.7	34.6	−3.2	42.3
	2001–2003	1.6	38.0	0.6	39.8	−0.5	49.8
	2004–2006	2.8	41.2	1.9	44.3	1.0	57.5
	2007–2009	3.6	41.6	2.8	44.7	2.1	62.4
	2010–2011	3.8	42.3	3.1	44.0	2.2	66.1
Ethnicity	White	0	46.9	−0.7	51.1	−1.5	53.3
	Black	2.6	52.0	2.0	56.1	0	77.6
	Indian	2.5	46.2	−0.7	62.7	−0.2	64.7
	Unknown	5.1	27.9	4.1	27.9	2.8	56.8
Diabetes mellitus	no	2.2	39.6	1.2	42.2	0.3	56.3
	yes	3.3	17.6	7.7	13.3	3.6	18.7
Left ventricular hypertrophy	no	2.3	39.2	1.4	41.7	0.4	55.7
	yes	1.1	12.1	−15.2	11.4	−11.9	13.3
Number of records for medical events in the electronic health records in the year before	0	4.9	26.7	3.4	26.3	1.6	58.0
	1–3	3.9	34.8	2.7	36.3	1.1	60.2
	4–8	2.8	42.3	1.8	45.6	0.5	60.8
	9–18	1.7	43.6	0.9	47.4	0.1	55.3
	19–4	0.1	43.5	−0.3	46.9	−0.5	48.7
	50+	−2.6	37.3	−2.7	38.7	−1.9	37.6

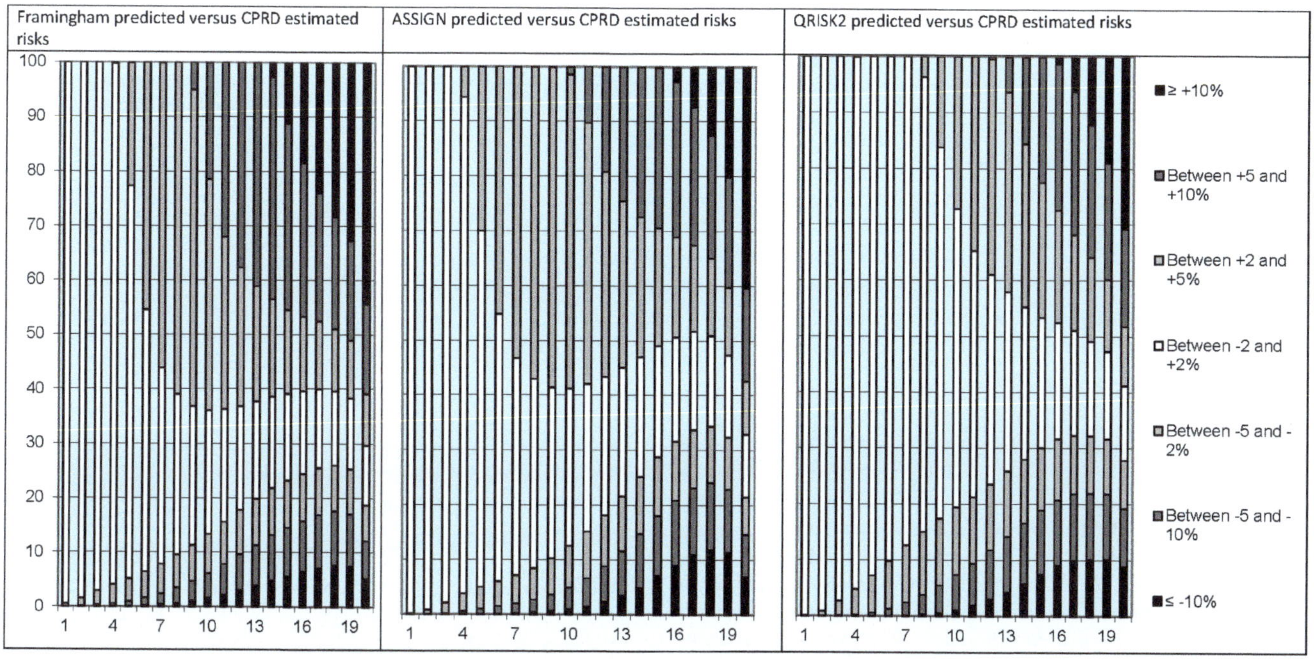

Figure 1. Absolute differences in individual 10-year CVD risk prediction between the Framingham, ASSIGN and QRISK2 risk scores and the individual risks estimated in CPRD using competing risk regression stratified by vigintiles of predicted risk. X-axis: Vigintiles of predicted risk. Y-axis: Percentage of persons.

vary greatly, as with CVD. Another question is how to deal with individuals who were not eligible for the trials (e.g. a 50-year old with normal LDL and C-reactive protein). There is no guarantee that the treatment effects as observed in trials can be generalised to populations different from those in the trials [26].

The strength of this study was the large size and representativeness of the study population, the well-documented data quality of CPRD [13] and the availability of linked hospital and death certificate data. There are several important limitations. Information on laboratory and physical measurements was missing for a large number of people. The extent of missing data decreased substantially over time. Reasons for this decrease include the availability of electronic communication between practices and laboratories and the incentivisation of practices in measuring and recording of data. We applied imputation techniques but found that people with imputed values had different CVD risks

Table 5. Consistency in risk predictions with risk scores or competing risk regression in predicting high and low CVD risk.

		Number of other risk scores with 10-year CVD risk of ≥20%			
		0	**1**	**2**	**3**
Reference risk method	**≥20%**	**% of persons**	**% of persons**	**% of persons**	**% of persons**
Framingham risk score		18.2	15.7	24.2	41.9
ASSIGN risk score		4.6	14.2	30.1	51.1
QRISK2 risk score		7.6	15.1	28.6	48.6
Individual risks estimated using competing risk regression		21.6	15.2	14.5	48.7
		Number of other risk scores with 10-year CVD risk of <15%			
		0	1	2	3
	<15%	% of persons	% of persons	% of persons	% of persons
Framingham risk score		0.6	2.3	3.5	93.5
ASSIGN risk score		0.4	2.2	8.2	89.2
QRISK2 risk score		0.4	2.6	7.3	89.8
Individual risks estimated using competing risk regression		3.8	3.1	5.9	87.2

Table 6. 10-year CVD risk at index date for persons who developed CVD after the index date (cases).

	10-year CVD risk at the index date#			
	<10%	10–15%	15–20%	≥20%
Risk method	N cases (%)	N cases (%)	N cases (%)	N cases (%)
Framingham risk score	15336 (21.9%)	13087 (18.7%)	11544 (16.5%)	29903 (42.8%)
ASSIGN risk score	18100 (25.9%)	12633 (18.1%)	11516 (16.5%)	27621 (39.5%)
QRISK2 risk score	19212 (27.5%)	10604 (15.2%)	11348 (16.2%)	28705 (41.1%)
Individual risks estimated using competing risk regression	14361 (20.6%)	9662 (13.8%)	10517 (15.1%)	35330 (50.6%)

#Rounded averages across the five imputation datasets.

compared to those without missing data. This is not unexpected as healthy people are less likely to visit their practice. Another limitation of this study concerned the use of socioeconomic status in the evaluation of the ASSIGN score. This score used the Scottish IMD and their values cannot be generalised to other regions in the UK. Our approach of standardising English to Scottish IMD may have introduced bias but the direction of bias is likely to have underestimated differences as socioeconomic status is, on average, higher in England. The recording of ethnicity in CPRD also has limitations as there was a substantive discrepancy in ethnicity between CPRD and HES in the recording of ethnicity. Another limitation is that the coding by practices of CVD has changed over calendar time [27] which may explain part of the trend of lower CVD rates over time. However, a secular trend was also observed with hospitalisations recorded in HES and death certificates. The main analyses in this study concerned comparisons of predictions by the different risk scores which are not affected by changes in CVD recording. Another consideration in this study was the use of a random index date rather than one based on the start of data collection. This approach reduced statistical power. However, our rationale for this was the objective to emulate the performance of risk scores in actual clinical practice, with assessments being done at arbitrary dates rather than at the start of data collection. There have also been major changes in the completeness of data recording over time: an imputation model that used an index date of 1-1-1998 did not converge due to high levels of missing cholesterol levels. The number of people with a follow-up exceeding 10 years was also larger than that in the studies for ASSIGN, Framingham and QRISK1 [5,6,8].

In conclusion, the Framingham, ASSIGN and QRISK2 risk scores do not predict the presence of high CVD risk well and consistently. Current practice to use any risk score in conjunction with a constant threshold level has inadvertently created an arbitrary classification of high CVD risk. Risk prediction strategies should be based on statistical models that are transparent, derived from a similar population, with data collected recently and updated regularly.

Author Contributions

Conceived and designed the experiments: TvS MG LS. Performed the experiments: TvS EN. Analyzed the data: TvS EN. Contributed reagents/materials/analysis tools: TvS EN. Wrote the paper: TvS MG LS BG.

References

1. Taylor F, Ward K, Moore TH, Burke M, Davey Smith G, et al. (2011) Statins for the primary prevention of cardiovascular disease. Cochrane database Syst Rev: CD004816. Available: http://www.ncbi.nlm.nih.gov/pubmed/21249663. Accessed 2013 December 26.
2. Cooper A, Nherera L, Calvert N, O'Flynn N, Turnbull N, et al. (2007) Clinical Guidelines and Evidence Review for Lipid Modification: cardiovascular risk assessment and the primary and secondary prevention of cardiovascular disease. Available: http://www.nice.org.uk/nicemedia/pdf/CG67fullguideline.pdf.
3. JBS 2: Joint British Societies' guidelines on prevention of cardiovascular disease in clinical practice (2005) Heart 91 Suppl 5: v1–52. Available: http://www.pubmedcentral.nih.gov/articlerender.fcgi?artid=1876394&tool=pmcentrez&rendertype=abstract. Accessed 2013 December 16.
4. Matheny M, McPheeters ML, Glasser A, Mercaldo N, Weaver RB, et al. (2011) Systematic review of cardiovascular disease risk assessment tools [Internet]. Rep No 11-05155-EF-1. Available: http://www.ncbi.nlm.nih.gov/entrez/query.fcgi?cmd=Retrieve&db=PubMed&dopt=Citation&list_uids=21796824.
5. Anderson KM, Odell PM, Wilson PWF, Kannel WB, Framingham MPH (n.d.) Cardiovascular disease risk profiles P (T > t) = p (log (;' -F > u }.
6. Woodward M, Brindle P, Tunstall-Pedoe H (2007) Adding social deprivation and family history to cardiovascular risk assessment: the ASSIGN score from the Scottish Heart Health Extended Cohort (SHHEC). Heart 93: 172–176. Available: http://www.pubmedcentral.nih.gov/articlerender.fcgi?artid=1861393&tool=pmcentrez&rendertype=abstract. Accessed 2013 August 22.
7. Hippisley-Cox J, Coupland C, Vinogradova Y, Robson J, May M, et al. (2007) Derivation and validation of QRISK, a new cardiovascular disease risk score for the United Kingdom: prospective open cohort study. BMJ 335: 136. Available: http://www.pubmedcentral.nih.gov/articlerender.fcgi?artid=1925200&tool=pmcentrez&rendertype=abstract. Accessed 2013 August 19.
8. Hippisley-Cox J, Coupland C, Vinogradova Y, Robson J, Minhas R, et al. (2008) Predicting cardiovascular risk in England and Wales: prospective derivation and validation of QRISK2. BMJ 336: 1475–1482. Available: http://www.pubmedcentral.nih.gov/articlerender.fcgi?artid=2440904&tool=pmcentrez&rendertype=abstract. Accessed 2013 September 1.
9. Siontis GCM, Tzoulaki I, Ioannidis JPA (2012) Comparisons of established risk prediction models for cardiovascular disease: systematic review. 3318: 1–11. doi:10.1136/bmj.e3318
10. Davies M, Khunti K, Webb D, Mostafa S, Gholap N, et al. (2012) Updated. The handbook for vascular risk assessment, risk reduction and risk management. Leicester.
11. Rose G (2008) Rose's strategy of preventive medicine. New York: Oxford University Press.
12. Williams T, van Staa TP, Puri S, Eaton S (2012) Recent advances in the utility and use of the General Practice Research Database as an example of a UK Primary Care Data resource. Ther Adv Drug Saf 3: 89–99.
13. Herrett E, Thomas SL, Schoonen WM, Smeeth L, Hall AJ (2010) Validation and validity of diagnoses in the General Practice Research Database: a systematic review. Br J Clin Pharmacol 69: 4–14. Available: http://www.pubmedcentral.nih.gov/articlerender.fcgi?artid=2805870&tool=pmcentrez&rendertype=abstract. Accessed 2013 September 2.
14. Rubin DB (1987) Multiple imputation for nonresponse in surveys. New York: John Wiley.
15. Delaney JAC, Daskalopoulou SS, Brophy JM, Steele RJ, Opatrny L, et al. (2007) Lifestyle variables and the risk of myocardial infarction in the general practice research database. BMC Cardiovasc Disord 7: 38. Available: http://www.pubmedcentral.nih.gov/articlerender.fcgi?artid=2241637&tool=pmcentrez&rendertype=abstract. Accessed 2014 June 20.
16. Cheng SC, Fine JP, Wei LJ (1998) Prediction of cumulative incidence function under the proportional hazards model. Biometrics 54: 219–228. Available: http://www.ncbi.nlm.nih.gov/pubmed/9544517.
17. Wolbers M, Koller MT, Witteman JCM, Steyerberg EW (2009) Prognostic models with competing risks: methods and application to coronary risk

prediction. Epidemiology 20: 555–561. Available: http://www.ncbi.nlm.nih.gov/pubmed/19367167. Accessed 2013 August 12.
18. Royston P, Sauerbrei W (2008) Multivariable model-building: A pragmatic approach to regression analysis based on fractional polynomials for modelling continuous variables. Chichester: John Wiley & Sons, Ltd.
19. Altman DG, Vergouwe Y, Royston P, Moons KGM (2009) Prognosis and prognostic research: validating a prognostic model. BMJ 338: b605. Available: http://www.ncbi.nlm.nih.gov/pubmed/19477892. Accessed 2013 December 26.
20. McGraw K, Wong S (1996) Forming inferences about some intraclass correlation coefficients. Psychol Methods 1: 30–46.
21. Smolina K, Wright FL, Rayner M, Goldacre MJ (2012) Determinants of the decline in mortality from acute myocardial infarction in England between 2002 and 2010: linked national database study. BMJ 344: d8059. Available: http://www.pubmedcentral.nih.gov/articlerender.fcgi?artid=3266430&tool=pmcentrez&rendertype=abstract. Accessed 26 December 2013.
22. Collins GS, Altman DG (2012) Predicting the 10 year risk of cardiovascular disease in the United Kingdom: independent and external validation of an updated version of QRISK2. 4181: 1–12. doi:10.1136/bmj.e4181
23. Collins GS, Altman DG (2010) An independent and external validation of QRISK2 cardiovascular disease risk score: a prospective open cohort study. BMJ 340: c2442. Available: http://www.pubmedcentral.nih.gov/articlerender.fcgi?artid=2869403&tool=pmcentrez&rendertype=abstract. Accessed 2013 December 26.
24. Mihaylova B, Emberson J, Blackwell L, Keech a, Simes J, et al. (2012) The effects of lowering LDL cholesterol with statin therapy in people at low risk of vascular disease: meta-analysis of individual data from 27 randomised trials. Lancet 380: 581–590. Available: http://www.pubmedcentral.nih.gov/articlerender.fcgi?artid=3437972&tool=pmcentrez&rendertype=abstract. Accessed 2013 August 9.
25. Ebrahim S, Casas JP (2012) Statins for all by the age of 50 years? Lancet 380: 545–547. Available: http://www.ncbi.nlm.nih.gov/pubmed/22607823. Accessed 2013 September 2.
26. Djulbegovic B, Paul A (2011) From efficacy to effectiveness in the face of uncertainty: indication creep and prevention creep. JAMA 305: 2005–2006. Available: http://www.ncbi.nlm.nih.gov/pubmed/21586716. Accessed 2013 December 26.
27. Gulliford MC, Charlton J, Ashworth M, Rudd AG, Toschke AM (2009) Selection of medical diagnostic codes for analysis of electronic patient records. Application to stroke in a primary care database. PLoS One 4: e7168. Available: http://www.pubmedcentral.nih.gov/articlerender.fcgi?artid=2744876&tool=pmcentrez&rendertype=abstract. Accessed 2013 September 2.

7

Activity-Based Funding of Hospitals and Its Impact on Mortality, Readmission, Discharge Destination, Severity of Illness, and Volume of Care

Karen S. Palmer[1]*, Thomas Agoritsas[2,3], Danielle Martin[4], Taryn Scott[2], Sohail M. Mulla[2], Ashley P. Miller[5], Arnav Agarwal[2], Andrew Bresnahan[6], Afeez Abiola Hazzan[2], Rebecca A. Jeffery[7], Arnaud Merglen[8], Ahmed Negm[9], Reed A. Siemieniuk[10], Neera Bhatnagar[11], Irfan A. Dhalla[12], John N. Lavis[2,13], John J. You[2], Stephen J. Duckett[14], Gordon H. Guyatt[2]

1 Faculty of Science Simon Fraser University, Burnaby, British Columbia, Canada, **2** Department of Clinical Epidemiology and Biostatistics, Faculty of Health Sciences, McMaster University, Hamilton, Ontario, Canada, **3** Divisions of General Internal Medicine and Clinical Epidemiology, University Hospitals of Geneva and Faculty of Medicine, University of Geneva, Geneva, Switzerland, **4** Department of Family and Community Medicine, Department of Health Policy Management and Evaluation, University of Toronto and Medical Affairs and Health Systems Solutions at Women's College Hospital, Toronto, Ontario, Canada, **5** Memorial University of Newfoundland, St. John's, Newfoundland, Canada, **6** Michael G. DeGroote School of Medicine, McMaster University, Hamilton, Ontario, Canada, **7** Faculty of Medicine, Dalhousie University, Halifax, Nova Scotia, Canada, **8** Paediatric Outcome Research Team, The Hospital for Sick Children, Toronto, Ontario, Canada and Division of General Pediatrics, University Hospitals of Geneva and Faculty of Medicine, University of Geneva, Geneva, Switzerland, **9** Rehabilitation School, McMaster University, Hamilton, Ontario, Canada, **10** Department of General Internal Medicine, Sunnybrook Health Sciences Centre, Toronto, Ontario, Canada, **11** Health Sciences Library, McMaster University, Hamilton, Ontario, Canada, **12** St. Michael's Hospital, Department of Medicine and Institute of Health Policy Management and Evaluation, University of Toronto, Toronto, Ontario, Canada, **13** McMaster Health Forum, Centre for Health Economics and Policy Analysis, Department of Political Science, McMaster University, Hamilton, Ontario, Canada and Department of Global Health and Population, Harvard School of Public Health, Boston, Massachusetts, United States of America, **14** Grattan Institute, Carlton, Victoria, Australia

Abstract

Background: Activity-based funding (ABF) of hospitals is a policy intervention intended to re-shape incentives across health systems through the use of diagnosis-related groups. Many countries are adopting or actively promoting ABF. We assessed the effect of ABF on key measures potentially affecting patients and health care systems: mortality (acute and post-acute care); readmission rates; discharge rate to post-acute care following hospitalization; severity of illness; volume of care.

Methods: We undertook a systematic review and meta-analysis of the worldwide evidence produced since 1980. We included all studies reporting original quantitative data comparing the impact of ABF versus alternative funding systems in acute care settings, regardless of language. We searched 9 electronic databases (OVID MEDLINE, EMBASE, OVID Healthstar, CINAHL, Cochrane CENTRAL, Health Technology Assessment, NHS Economic Evaluation Database, Cochrane Database of Systematic Reviews, and Business Source), hand-searched reference lists, and consulted with experts. Paired reviewers independently screened for eligibility, abstracted data, and assessed study credibility according to a pre-defined scoring system, resolving conflicts by discussion or adjudication.

Results: Of 16,565 unique citations, 50 US studies and 15 studies from 9 other countries proved eligible (i.e. Australia, Austria, England, Germany, Israel, Italy, Scotland, Sweden, Switzerland). We found consistent and robust differences between ABF and no-ABF in discharge to post-acute care, showing a 24% increase with ABF (pooled relative risk = 1.24, 95% CI 1.18–1.31). Results also suggested a possible increase in readmission with ABF, and an apparent increase in severity of illness, perhaps reflecting differences in diagnostic coding. Although we found no consistent, systematic differences in mortality rates and volume of care, results varied widely across studies, some suggesting appreciable benefits from ABF, and others suggesting deleterious consequences.

Conclusions: Transitioning to ABF is associated with important policy- and clinically-relevant changes. Evidence suggests substantial increases in admissions to post-acute care following hospitalization, with implications for system capacity and equitable access to care. High variability in results of other outcomes leaves the impact in particular settings uncertain, and may not allow a jurisdiction to predict if ABF would be harmless. Decision-makers considering ABF should plan for likely increases in post-acute care admissions, and be aware of the large uncertainty around impacts on other critical outcomes.

Editor: Eliana Jimenez-Soto, School of Population Health, The University of Queensland, Australia

Funding: KSP, DM, IAD, GHG received funds from the Canadian Institute for Health Research through a Knowledge Synthesis Grant, Priority Area: Evidence Informed Healthcare Renewal (http://www.cihr-irsc.gc.ca/e/193.html). The research was independent of any involvement from the sponsors of the study. The funders had no role in study design, data collection and analysis, decision to publish, or preparation of the manuscript.

Competing Interests: All authors have completed the ICMJE uniform disclosure form at www.icmje.org/coi_disclosure.pdf (available on request from the corresponding author) and declare as follows: (1) KSP, DM, IAD, GHG have non-salary support from the Canadian Institute for Health Research for the submitted work; (2) JL, JJY report that their institution received reimbursement from Canadian Institute for Health Research for the submitted work; (3) TS reports salary from Canadian Institute for Health Research for the submitted work; (4) TA and AM each report grants from the Swiss National Science Foundation during the period the study was conducted; (5) No financial relationships in the previous 3 years with companies that might have an interest in the submitted work; (6) No non-financial interests that influenced the submitted work.

* Email: kpalmer@sfu.ca

Introduction

As health care systems evolve, policymakers strive to design approaches to hospital funding that simultaneously boost efficiency, increase budget transparency to promote accountability [1], and expand volume of activity [2], all while maintaining quality of care [3], and assuring equitable access to hospital services [4].

Activity-based funding (ABF) is an alternative to other hospital funding mechanisms, such as negotiated funding through global budgets or block grants, per diem payments, or retrospective cost-based reimbursement. Increasingly popular, ABF is a significant policy intervention intended to re-shape incentives across health care systems [5].

Under ABF, hospitals receive a fixed amount for each episode of care delivered to each patient, regardless of length of stay or actual resources used (sometimes with refinements for outliers). The funding schedule is prospectively determined based on clinically meaningful diagnosis-based "bundles" of services within which patients can be expected to consume similar amounts of resources. The funding allocation for these bundles is intended to account for the anticipated complexity, type, volume, and intensity of care ordinarily provided to patients admitted with particular diagnoses. A variety of cost accounting systems underpin the processes used to set a prospective price for each bundle of services [6]. The price of each bundle coupled with the volume of bundles provided determines all or part of the facility's budget.

ABF was first developed in the United States (US) in response to rising health care costs coupled with economic stagnation, which together stimulated a radical restructuring of Medicare funding [7]. Beginning in 1983, the US implemented ABF based on Diagnosis-Related Groups (DRGs) to fund acute hospital care for Medicare beneficiaries [8]. Since then, other countries have adopted variants of this episode- or service-related bundling approach as the basis for their hospital funding.

Internationally, ABF is known by a variety of terms — often confused in translation leading to a lack of clarity in the literature — including Prospective Payment System (PPS in the US); Payment-by-Results (PbR in the English National Health Service); Fallpauschalen system/vergütung (in Germany); Innsatsstyrt finansiering (ISF in Norway); Forfaits par cas/leistungsbezogene Fallpauschale (in Switzerland); case-mix funding; volume-based funding; and service-based funding [9]. In this paper, we use the term ABF. All ABF funding systems are based on DRG-like grouping algorithms (such as AR-DRGs "Australian-refined"; case mix groups (CMG+) in Canada; health-resource groups (HRGs in England); Groupe Homogène des Malades (GHM) in France; G-DRGS in Germany; Diagnose Behandeling Combinatie (DBC in the Netherlands); Nord-DRGs in the Nordic countries; SwissDRG in Switzerland) [9–11]. ABF implementation differs in each jurisdiction where it is adopted, with many choices inherent in the precise design and accompanying rules.

Possible benefits of ABF may include reduced hospital costs [12,13], greater funding and spending transparency [4,9], improved efficiency [3,14]; reduced length of stay [15]; and shorter wait times [6]. Enthusiasts also claim that a culture change — by which patients are seen not as cost drivers but as "revenue generators" [3,5] — is a natural result of ABF. Possible detrimental consequences of ABF include increased mortality [16], increased readmission to hospital [17], rapid discharge of sick patients into ill-prepared community settings [18], an incentive to "upcode" diagnoses and thus "game" the system [19,20], focus on "profitable" over "unprofitable" patients and procedures compromising equitable access to care [21,22], and increased administrative and/or overall costs to the health care system [23,24].

Because it is natural for advocates and opponents to selectively cite evidence supporting their positions, to better inform decision-makers we undertook a systematic review of the worldwide evidence bearing on how ABF affects quality of care, access to care, equity, hospital and total health care system costs, length of stay, and efficiency. For this report, we focus on how ABF affects six key measures, each with the potential to affect patients and health care system capacity: acute care mortality (AC mortality); and post-acute care mortality (PAC mortality); readmission rates; discharge destination measured by discharge to post-acute care (PAC) following hospitalization; severity of illness; and volume of care. We also explored whether the impact of ABF on these six key measures varied according to either contextual factors of the health care systems, or the research methods used to assess the impact of ABF, by examining six pre-specified sub-groups: study location; study design; time elapsed after ABF implementation; adjustment for confounders; credibility of the methods; time of outcome assessment.

Methods

Our protocol (available upon request) provides a full description of our methods; a summary follows.

Eligibility Criteria

We included all studies providing original analyses of quantitative data that compared the impact of ABF versus alternative funding systems implemented in acute care settings (hospitals and non-hospital medical or surgical facilities) published in any language. We included before-after studies in single jurisdictions (before ABF vs. after ABF implementation), parallel group studies in multiple jurisdictions (jurisdictions without ABF vs. jurisdiction with ABF), or a combination of both designs (e.g. difference-in-difference analyses, time-series). We excluded editorials, letters, news, and notes as defined by the databases. For this report, we included only studies reporting data on at least one of our primary outcomes: AC mortality, PAC mortality, readmission rates, and discharge destination. For eligible studies that reported at least one of these primary outcomes, we also abstracted data on severity of illness and volume of care.

We excluded studies that did not include a comparator group in which ABF was not implemented. We further excluded studies that focused only on activity-based cost accounting systems; on differences in capital costs/acquisitions; on the intervention of pay-for-performance (a financial incentive for attaining targeted service goals [25]); and on systems based on a flat rate per diem or for another period of time, such as the Japanese Diagnosis Procedure Combination system, Chinese Hainan system, and Medicare Resource Utilization Groups.

Outcomes

Acute Care Mortality (AC Mortality) was defined as death rate per population per common time period in the ABF and no ABF comparator, starting at admission to acute care or at surgery. We excluded mortality measured only in-hospital or only from discharge since the potential influence of ABF may have been confounded by differences in length of stay in ABF and no ABF periods.

Post-Acute Care Mortality (PAC Mortality) was defined similarly to acute care mortality, except that mortality was measured starting from admission to PAC following a stay in acute care.

Hospital Readmission was defined as readmission rates per population per common time period (preferentially at 30 days) in the ABF and no ABF comparator.

Discharge Destination was defined as the proportion of patients discharged alive from acute care to PAC, rather than to home. PAC included: intermediate care facilities, nursing homes, PAC facilities designated under the US Centers for Medicare and Medicaid (i.e. skilled nursing facilities; in-patient rehabilitation facilities; long-term care hospitals; home health agencies), and similar facilities in other countries. If data were reported for different PAC destinations, we aggregated them for our analysis.

Changes in the distributions of reported severity of illness included differences in measures such as case mix, diagnostic codes, DRG points, or number of patients with comorbidities.

Changes in volume of care included differences in measures such as the number of patients treated or admitted or number of procedures or tests performed.

Search Strategy

Our search was limited to articles published from 1980 through 2012. We worked with a health information specialist to develop search terms; identified subject headings, terms, and keywords from key articles; and designed search strategies for ABF and related terms, such as DRGs and PPS, in combination with terms related to hospital and facility costs, and patient care. Studies were identified through bibliographic database searches of OVID MEDLINE, EMBASE, OVID Healthstar, CINAHL, Cochrane Central Register of Controlled Trials (CENTRAL), Health Technology Assessment, NHS Economic Evaluation Database, Cochrane Database of Systematic Reviews, and Business Source Complete. In each database, we undertook an iterative process to customize and refine search strategies. Appendix 1 (see File S1) presents a sample of our electronic search strategies.

In addition to electronic databases, we hand-searched reference lists of eligible studies and those of previously published reviews, books, websites, policy papers, personal files, and consulted with experts.

Study Selection

Using web-based systematic review software (DistillerSR) paired reviewers independently conducted screening; first title and abstracts, and then full texts of articles in which titles and abstracts appeared potentially eligible. We pre-defined screening rules, and reviewers completed calibration exercises prior to reviewing full texts.

Data Abstraction

Adhering to pre-defined abstraction rules, paired reviewers independently abstracted the following data from each article using standardized data abstraction forms custom built in DistillerSR and adapted to each study design: country and year of ABF implementation, data source, sampling methods, study population (type and number of patients and institutions), outcomes assessed, and results.

When studies reported data for several time periods before and after ABF implementation, we abstracted data from three time periods: 1) *no ABF*, defined as the first data point prior to ABF implementation within three years of implementation; 2) *early ABF*, defined as the first data point after ABF implementation irrespective of the proportion of ABF; 3) *late ABF*, defined as the data point farthest from ABF implementation up to 5 years following implementation, irrespective of the proportion of funding under ABF.

Whenever possible, we abstracted data to enable a meta-analysis for our primary outcomes. When data were not poolable, two abstractors independently abstracted narrative summaries including outcome direction, magnitude, and statistical significance.

Credibility Assessment

Pairs of reviewers independently assessed the credibility of individual studies according to a pre-defined scoring system documenting three criteria: 1) quality of data sources; 2) number of eligible outcomes simultaneously examined in the study; and 3) comprehensiveness and appropriateness of the adjustment for potential confounders. The maximum credibility score was 6 and the minimum 0, and higher credibility was *a priori* categorized as a score of 4 or more.

Eligibility, data abstraction, and credibility assessment conflicts between the two independent reviewers in each pair were resolved by discussion or if necessary with adjudication by a senior team member.

Heterogeneity and Hypothesized Sub-Group Effects

We hypothesized *a priori* that variability in results across studies might be due to the following: study location (US vs. international); study design (before-after vs. parallel-controlled study); time after ABF implementation (2 years or less = early ABF vs. more than 2 years = late ABF); adjustment for confounders (adjusted vs. unadjusted); credibility (higher vs. lower); and time of assessment of mortality or readmission (within 30 days vs. more than 30 days).

The comparison US vs. International may also be considered as an indirect comparison of: i) older studies (US) vs. more recent studies (International); ii) mainly cost-based reimbursement before ABF (US) vs. non-cost-based funding before ABF (International).

Data analysis

We pre-specified a set of conditions necessary to pool reported data in a meta-analysis. Data had to be either detailed unadjusted frequencies in the ABF and no ABF group, or effect estimates with: 1) a measure of variation (e.g. standard deviation, variance); or 2) sufficient statistical information (e.g. standard error, confidence intervals, exact p-values) along with exact number of patients at risk (Appendix 2, see File S1).

For studies that reported poolable data, we conducted a quantitative meta-analysis of 4 dichotomous outcomes – AC mortality, PAC mortality, hospital readmission, discharge to PAC – using random effects models. When both adjusted and unadjusted data were reported, we used adjusted data. The adjusted estimates determined the type of measure used in the pooling: risk ratios (RR) for discharge destination and readmission, and odds ratios (OR) for mortality data. When only hazard ratios (HR) or incidence rate ratios were reported we converted them to RR.

We assessed heterogeneity in results using the Cochrane's Q test [26] and calculated the I^2 [27]. We conducted all pre-specified sub-group analyses performing tests for interaction, with a p value <0.05 considered as statistically significant. When seven or more studies were available we addressed publication bias graphically using funnel plots.

For non-poolable data we recorded direction of outcome with ABF vs. no ABF (increase, decrease, mixed, no difference); magnitude (relative difference ≥5%, ≥1% to <5%, <1%, indeterminate or mixed); and statistical significance (p>.05, p≤ .05–.02, p≤.01–.002, p≤.001, p-value not reported), and considered possible differences in effect of study location (US vs. international) and study credibility (higher vs. lower).

Results

Figure 1 presents the flow of acquisition of eligible studies. Of 16,565 unique citations, 227 reported data from 64 countries addressing the impact of ABF on quality or access to care, equity, cost, or efficiency. Of these, 65 studies [16–18,28–89] reporting data from 10 countries — 50 US studies and 15 studies from other countries (i.e. Australia, Austria, England, Germany, Israel, Italy, Scotland, Sweden, Switzerland)— provided data on at least one of our primary outcomes. The weighted kappa coefficient for overall agreement across reviewer pairs screening full texts ranged from 0.72 to 0.86.

Table 1 presents the location, design, and sampling of the eligible studies, of which 36 provided data that contributed to the pooled analysis for at least one variable. The median number of outcomes reported per study was 3.0 (inter-quartile range 2.0 to 3.0).

Credibility of study results

Overall credibility of included studies was generally low, but varied across outcomes (Appendix 3, see File S1). The number of higher credibility studies ranged between 27% to 63% across studies with poolable outcomes and from 0% to 58% across studies with non-poolable outcomes.

The majority of studies did not provide satisfactory documentation of the quality of their data sources. From 64% to 80%

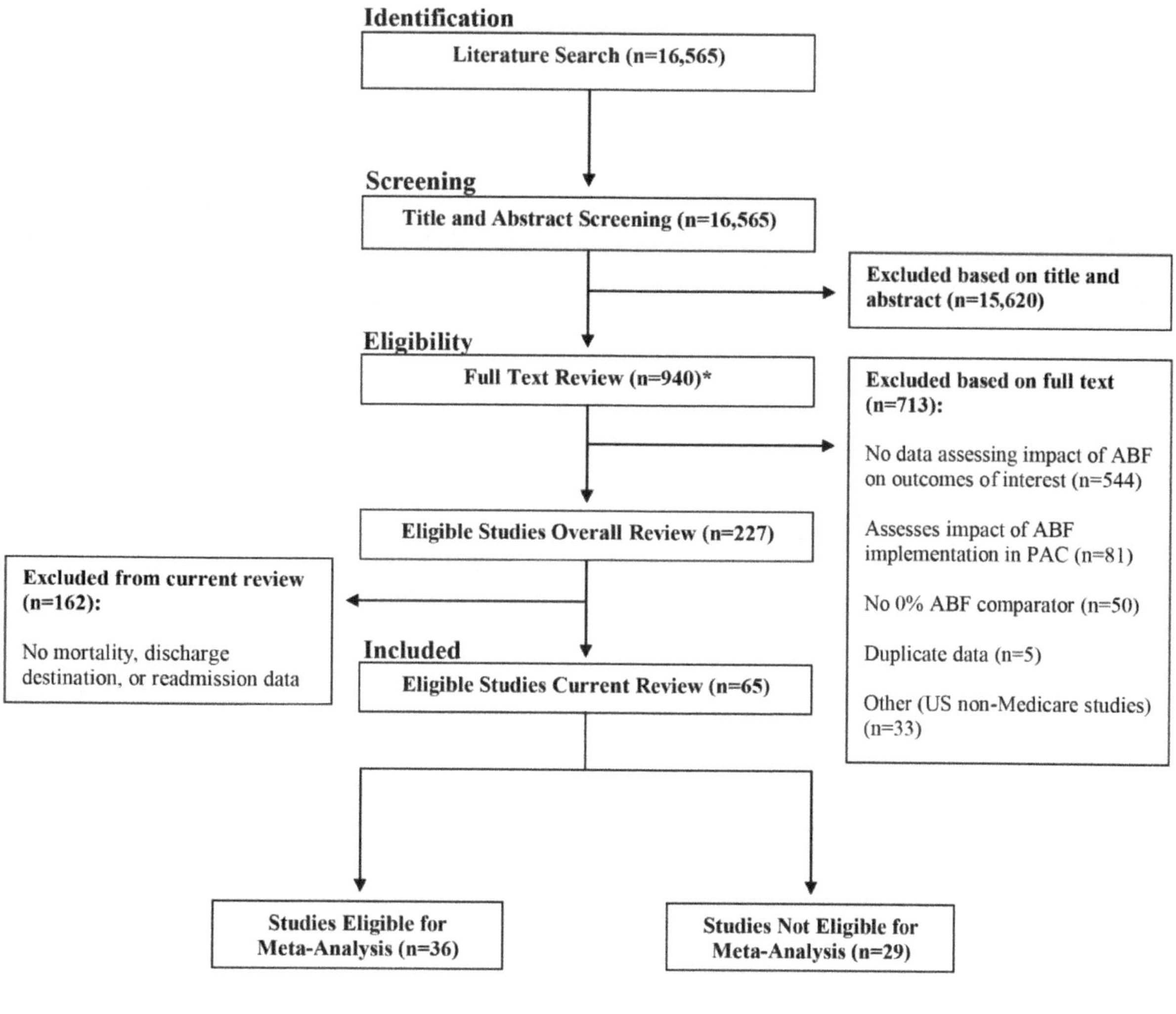

Figure 1. Prisma flow diagram.

**Full text articles for 5 references could not be retrieved.*

Table 1. Study Characteristics (Pooled and Non-Pooled).

Variable	Frequency N = 65		
	Pooled studies (n = 36)	**Non-Pooled studies (n = 29)**	**Total (N = 65)**
Study Demographics			
Type of Publication:			
Full-text journal article	35	29	64
Government report	1	0	1
Non-government report	0	0	0
Geographic Location of Study:			
USA	28	22	50
Australia	2	1	3
Austria	0	1	1
England	0	1	1
Germany	1	1	2
Israel	0	1	1
Italy	3	1	4
Scotland	0	1	1
Sweden	1	0	1
Switzerland	1	1	2
Methods			
Study Design			
Before vs. After ABF (single jurisdiction)	34	25	59
Parallel groups (multiple jurisdictions)	2	1	3
Parallel groups & before/after	0	3	3
Sampling Method			
Random	6	5	11
Convenience	20	16	36
All eligible institutions in a jurisdiction	10	9	19
Number of Patients Evaluated			
Less than 1,000	14	1	15
1,000 to 10,000	9	3	12
Greater than 10,000	7	7	14
Number of Institutions evaluated			
Less than 5	13	3	16
5 to 50	8	3	11
Greater than 50	6	15	21

Note: frequencies may not add to 65 as not all categories are mutually exclusive.

performed only minimal or no adjustment of their results, and 14% to 20% performed a comprehensive adjustment.

Main Findings

Table 2 summarizes the key results for pooled and non-pooled analyses across outcomes. Consistent and credible differences between ABF and no ABF were found only in discharge to PAC, which was greater with ABF (RR 1.24, 95% CI 1.18 to 1.31). Results also suggested an apparent increase in severity of illness with ABF, and possibly in readmission (with early ABF in the US and late ABF in other countries). In general, results were consistent between US studies and international studies, as well as between early and late implementation of ABF. Additional details of results by outcome follow.

AC Mortality

AC Mortality pooled results. Eight studies (six US; Switzerland; Germany) reporting poolable data demonstrated no difference in AC mortality between ABF and no ABF (OR = 1.03, 95% CI 0.93 to 1.15, p = 0.54, $I^2 = 57\%$) (Figure 2). Although the I^2 was relatively large, the results of the large studies were very consistent in showing no difference in AC mortality. None of our pre-specified sub-group analyses explained heterogeneity in findings (Appendix 4, see File S1). The funnel plot did not suggest publication bias (Appendix 5, see File S1). Appendix 6 (see File S1) presents details of study descriptions.

AC Mortality non-pooled results (Early ABF and Late ABF). Two studies (US; Scotland/England) reported that, early after ABF was implemented, mortality increased with small or indeterminate magnitude and without reporting p-values. One

Table 2. Summary of Findings of the Impact of ABF (Pooled and Non-Pooled).

	Pooled Analysis*	Non-Pooled Analysis*
AC Mortality	**No difference** (modest variability)	**Early ABF: Increase** (2 studies consistent)
		Late ABF: No difference (2 studies mixed)
PAC Mortality	**No difference** (modest variability)	**No difference** (1 study)
Readmission	**No difference** (high variability)	**Early ABF: Increase** (modest variability)
		Late ABF: US studies: No difference (high variability) **International: Increase** (2 studies mixed)
Discharge to PAC	**Overall increase** (modest variability) Possible subgroup effect: increase in US, no increase in international	**Increase** (modest variability)
Severity of illness	N/A	**Increase** (high variability)
Volume of Care	N/A	**No difference** (high variability)

**Note: In general, results were consistent between US studies and international studies, as well as between early and late implementation of ABF. We have specified occurrences where results credibly differed.*

study (Scotland/England) reported no difference in mortality late after ABF was implemented. A second study (US) reported that mortality increased in some sub-groups and decreased in others without reporting p-values. Appendices 7, 8, 9 (see File S1) present study descriptions, main findings, and analyses.

AC Mortality Summary. The pooled analysis showed no impact of ABF on mortality; non-pooled results show a possible increase in mortality in the early stages of ABF implementation, and mixed results later.

PAC Mortality

PAC Mortality results (pooled and non-pooled). Three US studies reported poolable data with very wide confidence intervals including both substantial decrease and appreciable increase in PAC mortality with ABF (RR = 0.80, 95% CI 0.52 to1.24, $p = 0.32$, $I^2 = 34\%$). The single additional US study reporting non-poolable data, suggested no difference in mortality with ABF. Appendices 10, 11, 12, 13 (see File S1) present the forest plot, study descriptions, main findings, and analyses.

Hospital Readmission

Readmission Pooled results. Twelve studies (eight US; two Australia; two Italy) reporting poolable data suggested no overall difference in readmissions (RR = 1.04, 95% CI 0.93 to 1.16, $p = 0.48$, $I^2 = 73\%$) (Figure 3). None of our pre-specified sub-group analyses explained the high variability in findings across studies, with some studies showing a significant increase [17,32] and others a significant decrease [78,83] in readmission rates with ABF

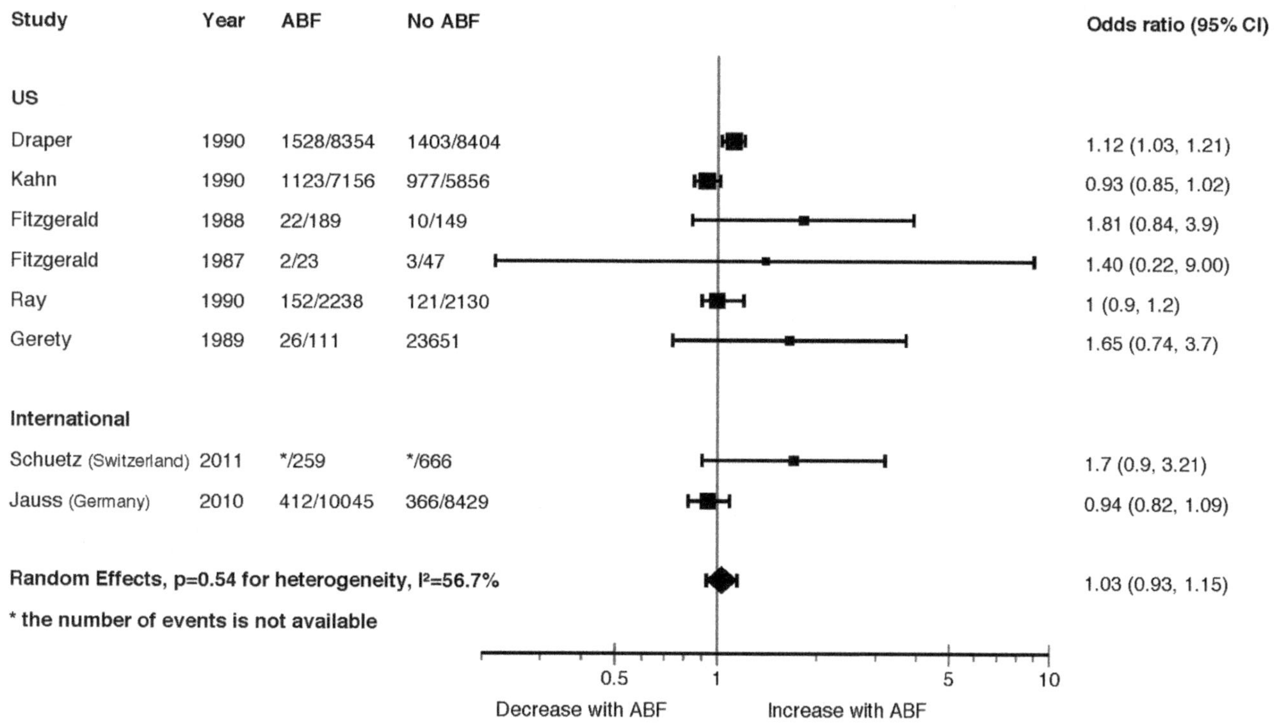

Figure 2. Acute Care Mortality Forest Plot.

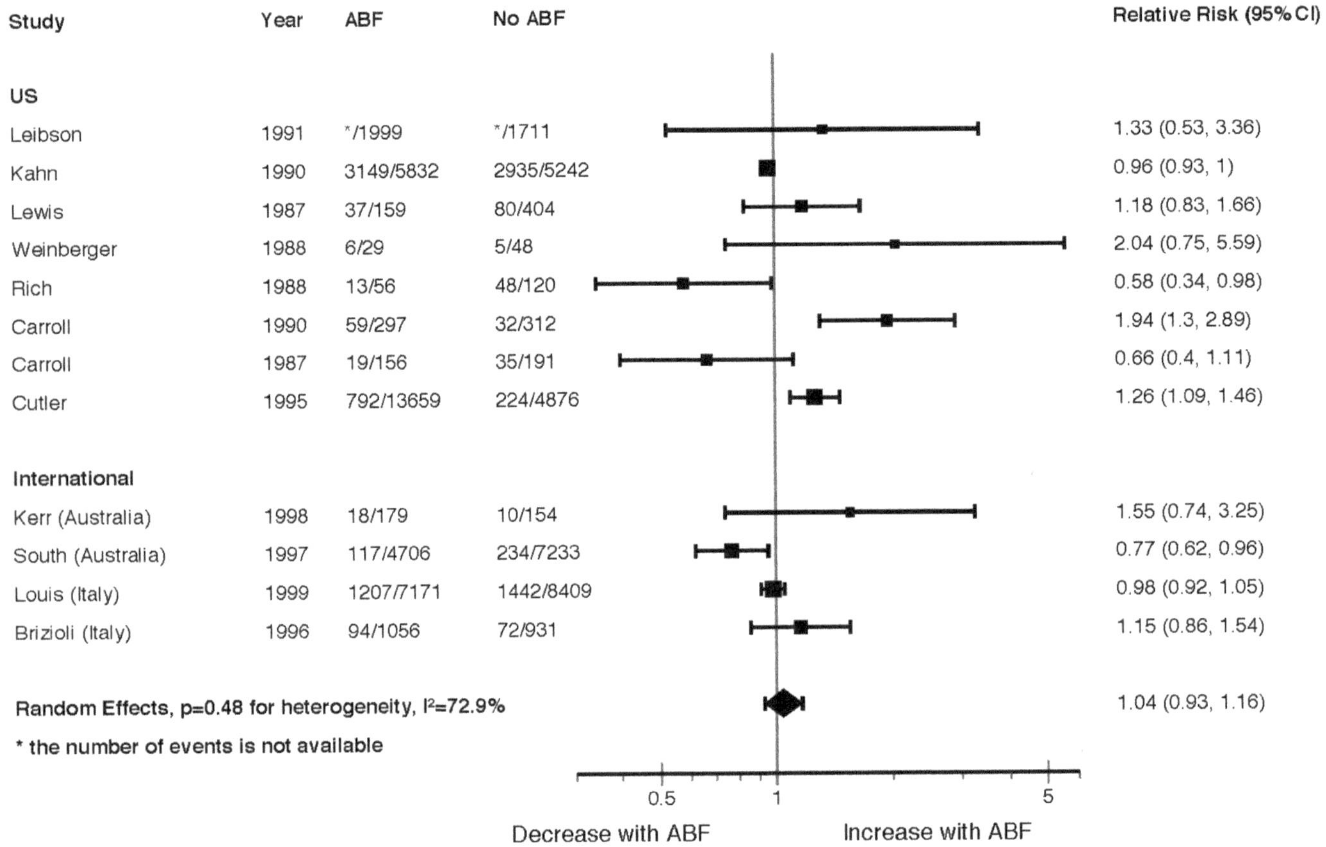

Figure 3. Readmission Forest Plot.

(Appendix 14, see File S1). We found no suggestion of publication bias (Appendix 15, see File S1). Appendix 16 (see File S1) presents study descriptions.

Even though it presented data amenable to statistical analysis, we excluded one US study [49] with a RR of readmission greater than 20 from our primary analysis. We attributed the results, which we found not credible, to "unbundling" cataract surgeries. Whereas prior to ABF, patients requiring bilateral cataract surgery would have both cataracts done in a single admission, under ABF they were discharged after the first cataract procedure and readmitted for the second eye. A sensitivity analysis in which we included this study showed a marked increase in heterogeneity, and thus a considerably widened confidence interval in our random effects model (RR = 1.40, 95% CI 0.66 to 2.94, $p = 0.38$, $I^2 = 100\%$).

Readmission Non-poolable results (Early ABF and Late ABF). Six studies (three US; Italy; Israel; England/Scotland) reported that early after ABF, readmissions increased, of which three reported a large increase. One US study reported a large decrease in readmissions. None of these studies reported p-values. Three studies (one US; Australia; Austria) reported no difference.

Three studies (one US; Switzerland; Germany) reported that late after ABF, readmissions increased, two of which reported a large increase. None of these studies reported p-values. Four studies (three US; England/Scotland) reported a decrease in readmissions of which two reported a large and, at least for some sub-groups, statistically significant difference. Three studies (all US) reported no difference. Appendices 17, 18, 19 (see file S1) present study descriptions, main findings, and analyses.

Readmission Summary. The pooled analysis showed no difference in readmissions after ABF, but some studies showed a significant increase and others a significant decrease. In the non-pooled analysis, most studies showed an increase in readmissions early in ABF. In the later ABF period, results were mixed.

Discharge Destination

Discharge to PAC Pooled results. Pooled data from twenty-two studies (19 US; Sweden; Germany; Italy) showed an increase in discharge to PAC with ABF (pooled RR = 1.24, 95% CI 1.18 to 1.31, $I^2 = 100\%$) (Figure 4). In a sub-group analysis, there was a 28% relative increase in discharge to PAC in the 19 US studies (RR = 1.28, 95% CI 1.22 to 1.36, $I^2 = 100\%$), but no difference in the 3 international studies (RR = 1.01, 95% CI 0.94 to1.09, $I^2 = 86\%$) (test for interaction $p = 0.04$) (Appendix 20, see File S1). Only one US study of lowest credibility showed a decrease in discharges to PAC with ABF [76]. Despite the very high I^2, the U.S. studies were consistent in showing an increase in discharge to PAC. None of our other pre-specified sub-groups explained the residual heterogeneity. The funnel plot did not suggest publication bias (Appendix 21, see File S1). Appendix 22 (see File S1) presents study descriptions.

Discharge to PAC Non-Pooled Results (Early ABF and Late ABF). Seven studies (all US) reported that early after ABF implementation there was a large increase in discharge to PAC; one reported $p < 0.01$, the others did not report p-values. One US study reported a large decrease in discharge to PAC without reporting an associated p-value. One US study reported mixed results.

Study	Year	ABF	No ABF	Relative Risk (95%CI)
US				
Leibson	1990	*/2093	*/1783	1.11 (0.93, 1.33)
Hing	1989	1202000/10508000	882000/10697000	1.39 (1.38, 1.39)
Fitzgerald	1988	113/189	56/149	1.58 (1.25, 2)
Qian	2011	***	***	2.03 (1.46, 2.81)
Fitzgerald	1987	11/23	10/47	2.25 (1.12, 4.51)
Kanda	1991	3.64**/454	3.31**/402	1.1 (0.25, 4.87)
Kahn	1990	783/815	709/746	1.01 (0.99, 1.03)
DesHarnais	1987	4818/34663	3460/34663	1.39 (1.34, 1.45)
Schmidt	2002	721/1992	421/1665	1.43 (1.29, 1.58)
Rich	1988	15/56	19/120	1.69 (0.93, 3.08)
Manton	1990	1208190/8785702	1101632/9785343	1.22 (1.22, 1.22)
Gay	1990	12535/116702	6749/108169	1.72 (1.67, 1.77)
Manton	1990	211/1039	243/1365	1.14 (0.97, 1.35)
Palmer	1989	105/196	100/190	1.02 (0.84, 1.23)
Kane	1987	36/279	27/237	1.13 (0.71, 1.81)
Mayer-Oakes	1988	31/79	18/74	1.61 (0.99, 2.62)
Long	1987	61987/416023	204027/1752356	1.28 (1.27, 1.29)
DesHarnais	1988	6209/28289	4176/28471	1.5 (1.44, 1.55)
Pfeiffer	1987	316/2758	1027/7729	0.86 (0.77, 0.97)
Random Effects, p < 0.0001 for heterogeneity, I²=99.7%				1.28 (1.22, 1.36)
International				
Stromberg (Sweden)	1997	1143/1178	975/1060	1.05 (1.03, 1.08)
Jauss (Germany)	2010	3694/10045	3187/8429	0.97 (0.94, 1.01)
Onder (Italy)	2001	32/378	53/584	0.93 (0.61, 1.42)
Random Effects, p =0.76 for heterogeneity, I²=85.8%				1.01 (0.94, 1.09)
Total				
Random Effects, p < 0.0001 for heterogeneity, I²=99.7%				1.24 (1.18, 1.31)

*** the number of events is not available**

**** mean rate (per 100 beds)**

***** total number of event=1160 and number of total population=12543**

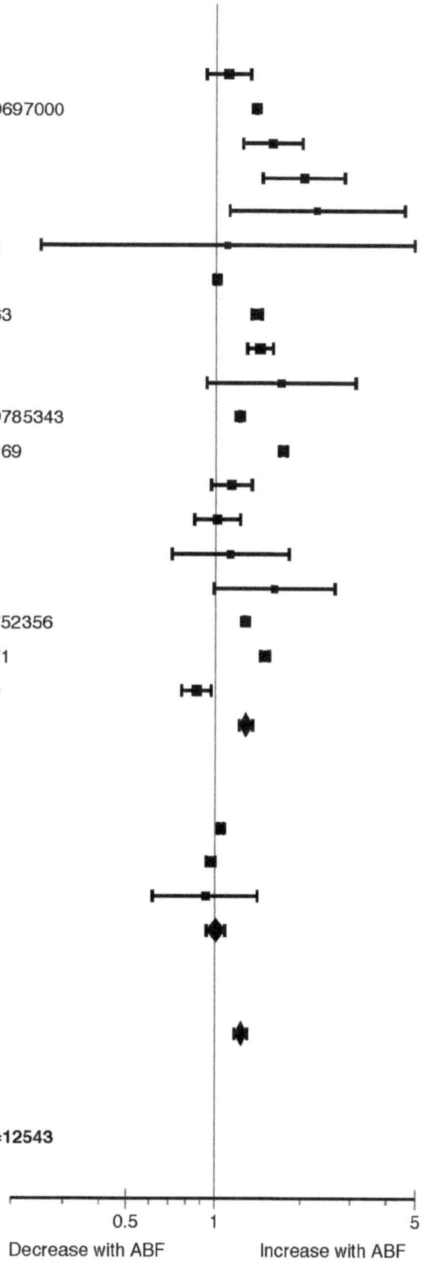

Figure 4. Discharge Destination Forest Plot.

Five studies (all US) reported that late after ABF, discharge to PAC increased; in four the increases were large. None of these studies reported p-values. One US study reported a large decrease in admissions to PAC ($p<0.05$). One US study reported an increase to some types of PAC and a decrease to others, and one an increase in two sub-groups and a decrease in one other. Study descriptions, main findings, and analyses are found in Appendices 23, 24, 25 (see File S1).

Discharge to PAC Summary. The pooled analysis showed a 24% increased risk of discharge to some form of PAC, a result consistent with the non-pooled data. The pooled analysis also showed a possible sub-group effect with a 28% increased risk of discharge to PAC in the 19 US studies, but the effect was not observed in the three international studies.

Severity of Illness

Severity of Illness Non-pooled results (Early ABF and Late ABF). Nine studies (six US; two Italy; Australia) reported that early after ABF implementation there was an increase in severity of illness of which seven reported a large effect (five US; Italy; Australia); of these, five reported some significant p-values. In two studies, the magnitude of the increase was not reported; of these, one reported a p-value of <0.01. Three studies (two US; Germany) reported that early after ABF there was a decrease in severity of illness. Three studies (two US; Australia) reported no difference and three studies (two US; Italy) reported mixed results.

Nine studies (eight US; Germany) reported that late after ABF there was an increase in severity of illness, large in five studies, moderate in two, and mixed in two; none reported p-values. Three studies (two US; Germany) reported a large decrease in severity of illness, two without reporting p-values and one reporting $p<0.01$. One study (US) reported no difference and four reported mixed results (three US; Switzerland). Study descriptions, main findings, and analyses tables are found in Appendices 26, 27, 28 (see File S1).

Severity of Illness Summary. Reported severity of illness increased both early and late after ABF in the majority of studies, though results varied across studies. There was no difference between US and international.

Volume of Care

Volume of Care Non-pooled results (Early ABF and Late ABF). Six studies (two US; Italy; Australia; Sweden; England/Scotland) reported that early after ABF implementation volume of care increased, of which five reported a large increase, but without reporting p-values. One study reported a significant increase in volume ($p<0.01$) but without reporting the magnitude. Eight studies (five US; two Italy; Switzerland) reported a decrease in volume of care of which six reported a large and one a moderate decrease; seven of these studies did not report p-values and one a large decrease with a p-value of <0.001. Three studies (two US; Austria) reported no difference and two (US; Australia) mixed results.

Six studies (five US; England/Scotland) reported that late after ABF volume of care increased, large in four studies and moderate in one (but without reporting p-values) and significant in one ($p<0.01$, but without reporting magnitude). Four studies (three US; Australia) reported a decrease in volume of care, of which three reported a large decrease but no p-values, and one reported $p<0.05$. One US study reported no difference and one mixed results. Study descriptions, main findings, and analyses tables are found in Appendices 29, 30, 31 (see File S1).

Volume of Care Summary. Results regarding the impact of ABF on volume of care showed high variability, with approximately the same number of studies showing an increase as decrease both early and late after ABF was implemented. There was no difference between US and international studies.

Discussion

Principal Findings

Our study is the first systematic review of the international literature addressing the impact of activity-based funding of hospitals. The evidence suggests no consistent impact of ABF on mortality in either acute or post-acute care. There was no impact on rates of readmission to hospital in the pooled analysis, but a suggestion of an increase in readmission early after ABF from the studies without poolable data. We found an apparent though highly variable increase in reported severity of illness, and no difference in volume of care, though this, too, was highly variable. Our most notable finding was a large increase in admissions to PAC after a hospital stay, though this appeared restricted to US and not international settings.

Strengths and Limitations

Strengths of this review included: explicit eligibility criteria; a comprehensive search that yielded a large number of eligible studies; assessment of the credibility of each eligible study; a rigorous approach to data abstraction and summarization of studies, both those that provided data amenable to statistical analysis and those that did not; tests of *a priori* hypotheses of possible explanations for heterogeneity; and duplicate assessment of eligibility, credibility, and data abstraction with third party adjudication when necessary.

The main limitation of our review lies in the deficiencies of the primary studies. The majority of eligible studies were before-after studies; thus, when differences are evident, they may be the result of temporal trends independent of ABF. This is of particular concern because hospital funding reform is rarely implemented as a solitary intervention. For instance, adoption of ABF in the English NHS was accompanied by a wave of competitive internal market reforms [90–92]. ABF introduction in the United States was followed by a restructuring of peer review organizations to externally audit physicians and hospitals for quality indicators [93]. Other secular trends that may confound attribution of outcome differences to ABF include changes in technology and related shifts from inpatient to outpatient care, and changes in other funding policies (for instance, funding for post-acute care).

Low credibility of many studies also limits strong inferences from the evidence. Credibility problems included lack of documentation of quality control and error rates in the administrative databases that provided data for the analyses; lack of statistical adjustment and, when present, lack of comprehensive and appropriate adjustment. However, we assessed whether the higher quality studies yielded different results than the lower quality studies. This was not the case, suggesting that inferences can be drawn from the whole body of evidence. In addition, many studies did not provide information necessary for inclusion in the pooled statistical analysis, nor did they report on the magnitude of effects, their statistical significance, or both. Inconsistency in study results, and the failure of our *a priori* hypotheses to explain the inconsistency, also decreases the strength of inferences from the results. There may be concomitantly implemented policies (e.g. quality improvement incentives) that may make it more likely that jurisdictions will see the potential benefits and not the potential harms of ABF; if this is so, our review provides no insight into what these strategies may be.

Finally, another limitation is the danger that upcoding in ABF settings led to differences in the recorded classification of severity after ABF was implemented [19]. Generally, in observational studies such as these, adjustment for key variables is crucial for making causal inferences. In this case, to the extent that upcoding exists, all adjusted analyses will be biased in favor of ABF. This concern is somewhat ameliorated by the similarity of effects in the adjusted and unadjusted analyses.

Relation to prior work

Prior reviews of ABF have shown variable results [2,4,24,94–98]. This is not surprising since none was systematic or comprehensive, and thus may be susceptible to study selection bias.

Prior studies have consistently established that the transition to ABF for hospitals initially decreased the length of hospital stay in the US and internationally, though it appeared to stabilize after the initial decrease [42,57,99]. Although we did not review this evidence systematically, prior non-systematic reviews have been highly consistent in their findings and conclusions. Accepting this finding as definitive, we did not include length of hospital stay as one of our outcomes.

Implications of our Findings

Our results represent the best available evidence, and thus the best guide for current decision-making regarding ABF. The results demonstrate that strong claims of either benefits or harms of ABF in the outcomes we studied are unwarranted. The appreciable inconsistency of results across studies in most outcomes suggests that there may be contexts in which ABF has substantial positive or negative consequences. For example, it may be the case that specific attributes of how ABF is implemented, such as with activity limits, or policies of non-payment for readmissions, could affect the outcomes we studied. We were not, however, able to abstract and analyze data for contextual factors that clearly explained differences in effect, and thus to determine the circumstances in which ABF is likely to produce positive or negative outcomes.

Reducing hospital length of stay is a worthwhile policy objective. Unless there are clear and substantial negative consequences to ABF, this alone might provide a rationale for its implementation. Our review failed to identify compelling evidence for such negative consequences, at least in terms of mortality or hospital readmissions, although some studies raise the possibility of detrimental effects on these outcomes under some circumstances. Again, however, the evidence does not allow us to identify the circumstances in which this is more likely to be the case.

ABF models have provided, in theory, a disincentive for hospitals to re-admit patients quickly [8,100–102]. Our data, however, provide low credibility evidence for a possible increase in readmission early after the implementation of ABF. Results, however, are highly variable and also consistent with no impact whatsoever of ABF on readmission.

The evidence may be obscuring a true increase in readmissions. For instance, patients may have been readmitted with a different admission diagnosis to avoid financial penalties for excess readmissions (even though this may attract charges of fraud) [103–105]; others may have been held in hospital under "out-patient observation status" but never technically readmitted [106,107]. This interpretation speaks to the literature on the opportunities for "gaming" under ABF systems [4,108], such as the cataract unbundling we have described in the results [49]. It is also possible that in response to earlier discharge, physicians intensified their follow-up care, thereby preventing readmissions [78]. The increased rate of discharge to post-acute care suggests that more intensive or more frequent use of post-hospital care may indeed have prevented an increase in readmission to acute care hospitals.

Our robust finding that, at least in the US, ABF is associated with increased discharge from hospital to PAC settings including rehabilitation facilities, home health agencies, and other forms of intermediate non-hospital health care suggests that introducing ABF may come at a price for patients recently discharged from acute care hospitals, but still needing care outside the hospital sector before returning home. The finding is not unanticipated: a funding model designed to reduce length of hospital stay provides a powerful incentive to discharge patients not yet medically stable enough to leave the health care system entirely.

Earlier discharge from hospital to PAC is not necessarily undesirable: assuming there is sufficient post-acute care capacity to meet demand it may be preferable for patients to enter a PAC facility, or to return home earlier with professional home care, rather than spend extra time in hospital. The danger, however, is that if health care systems are not equipped to deal with the additional burden of a potential 24% increase in patients requiring some form of post-acute care following their earlier discharge, then patients and their family caregivers at home will suffer [109]. Such a large increase in PAC admissions might also offset potential savings from any improved efficiency in acute care settings.

Further evidence supporting the increase in PAC discharges in the US following introduction of ABF includes the associated proliferation of cost-based post-acute facilities and programs that were initially exempt from ABF [110]. Between 1988 and 1997, expenditures on PAC increased at an average annual rate of 25 percent [111]. The increase in patients discharged to PAC, even in the US, may have been a temporary phenomenon. In 1997, the passage of legislation dramatically altered Medicare's PAC payment policies, shifting payment to PAC providers from a cost-basis to prospective payment. This change decreased the financial incentive for PAC facilities to admit from hospital those patients needing a relatively high intensity of care [112]. In an effort to ensure that care is provided in the most appropriate setting with shared resources, some health care systems are now considering other forms of bundled payment, beyond ABF of hospital-specific care, to cover the entire scope of services, across settings and providers —before, during, and after hospitalization — for a particular episode of care [113–115].

The evidence suggests that the rate of discharge to PAC may be a phenomenon restricted to the US. The credibility of this sub-group finding is, however, only moderate: although one of a relatively small number of *a priori* hypotheses and unlikely to be explained by chance (interaction p-value 0.04), the finding is based on only three studies outside of the US and is not consistent (one study conducted in Stockholm, Sweden showed a small but statistically significant increase in discharge to PAC with ABF [84]).

In countries like the US, where a post-acute care sector was highly developed as a policy response to the implementation of ABF in hospitals in 1983, the patient route to PAC was well-travelled. But in countries in which ABF is a more recent innovation, such as Sweden [84], Italy [74], and Germany [56], the apparent absence of increased PAC discharges suggests that underlying system and cultural differences may influence the impact of ABF. It may be, for instance, that having witnessed the substantial PAC sector that developed to accommodate the transformative effect of ABF in the US, European social service support systems developed primarily outside the institutional health care sector, meeting the post-acute care needs of patients at home, through community caregivers, or by families' shouldering the care burden. It may also be that patients in some countries are moved to PAC settings within the same hospital, thereby not being counted as discharged to PAC. Funding design outside the US may also have incorporated volume capping or volume growth moderation strategies (e.g. tapering payment for additional volume) which would have reduced the benefit to hospitals of earlier discharge to PAC – but also would make it less likely to shorten hospital stay [9].

Perhaps the most optimistic interpretation of the sub-group difference between international and US studies in PAC settings would be one of policy learning. Europe implemented ABF 20 years or more after the US. The US studies report data mostly from the 1980s, and their relevance may be somewhat limited given the refinements in ABF over time, such as the addition to the DRG classification system of a severity measure that may have, for example, increased the European LOS sufficiently that patients require less PAC. Alternatively, perhaps we have yet to see the full effect of ABF on Europe's health care systems, especially in the PAC sector. Published evidence about the development of Europe's PAC sector in the post-ABF era is scant [4]. That we have only three international studies in our review further limits the strength of any inferences about how ABF impacts discharges to PAC outside the US.

The policy implications of our results are uncertain. Should health systems now implementing ABF increase their capacity in the PAC setting to accommodate anticipated PAC discharges? Or can they anticipate that, as we found in the three international studies, discharges to PAC may not increase? In jurisdictions with limited informal networks of care providers or where community-based services are generally less well-developed, the risk of increased need for PAC facilities may be particularly high. If funding changes give rise to new demands for PAC, and if social protection systems are slow to adapt, hardship will follow. In countries in which hospital funding is almost exclusively provided by governments, but in which funding and delivery of post-acute care is a mixed public-private enterprise with families frequently paying out-of-pocket for long term care or home care services, any shift of care out of hospital and into the community sector has the potential to threaten equitable access to care.

The shortened LOS that appears to be associated with ABF should, in theory, pave the way for increasing volume of care, particularly number of admissions. Improving access to care by reducing waiting times is one potential policy objective of ABF and faster patient turnover could enable this. We found, however, no difference in volume of care, particularly number of acute admissions, with ABF, though the results were highly variable.

One concern, expressed by critics of ABF, is the potential to threaten equity of access by creating "profitable" and "unprofitable" diagnoses, or procedures, or programs — and thus patients — with resulting avoidance of unprofitable services [95,116,117]. For instance, one study found that following ABF implementation in South Carolina, the provision of TURP surgery declined by 25% for the "old-old" who tended to require longer hospital stays and have more complications, but increased 100% for the "young-old" [49]. To the extent that sicker patients are liable to be less profitable, our analysis does not support this concern: we did not find a decrease in severity of illness across populations admitted to hospital before and after ABF. Rather, we found an overall apparent increase, albeit highly variable, in the severity of illness.

This finding may be explained by differences in coding. Since ABF models tend to adjust hospital compensation for acuity, there is a financial incentive to code patients so they appear as sick as possible, thus maximizing reimbursement. Upcoding may be appropriate (if it represents legitimately better coding), questionable, or inappropriate. In Germany, for example, the introduction of ABF led to a very large increase in low birth weight babies and a decrease in normal birth weight babies over a 5-year period, with no biological or epidemiological explanation for this effect [118]. In the US, one study showed a decrease in overall case-fatality rate with ABF, coupled with a large increase in volume of septicaemia diagnoses, a combination highly suggestive of inappropriate upcoding [54]. To the extent that inappropriate upcoding occurs, it is likely to undermine at least one ABF policy objective: controlling costs to payer.

Conclusions

Inferences regarding the impact of ABF are limited both by inevitable study design constraints (randomized trails of ABF are unlikely to be feasible) and by avoidable weaknesses in methodology of many studies. Further, the variation in results across studies suggests that the impact of ABF may vary across settings, though the evidence does not provide strong clues of the determinants of differential effects. The ABF story thus provides testimony to how modifications in health policy without adequate evaluation leave their impact open to great uncertainty.

The most compelling evidence of any impact on ABF is on an initial, but likely not sustained, decrease in hospital length of stay following introduction of ABF, a possible increase in readmissions, and an increase in discharges to post-acute care. The latter impact may be restricted to the introduction of ABF in the US. Other effects are likely absent, or restricted to specific settings, and possibly manifest in different directions depending on the setting. Thus, the evidence on the variables we studied does not support either strong advocacy for, or strong rejection of, a change to ABF from other hospital funding methods.

Those considering adoption of ABF should be aware of the probable increase in admissions to post-acute care and other possible unintended adverse consequences that may arise. A paucity of consistent and conclusive evidence on the outcomes we studied, however, does not allow a jurisdiction to predict if ABF would be harmless. To this extent, despite the long and extensive experience, changing to an ABF system represents a leap of faith.

Supporting Information

File S1 Appendices 1–31.

Checklist S1 PRISMA Checklist.

Protocol S1

Acknowledgments

Lisa Buckingham (data abstraction form programmer); Qi Zhou (performed meta-analysis in consultation with research team); Lehana Thabane (statistical consultation); Linn Brandt, Alonso Carrasco, Wout de Boer, Markus Faulhaber, Toshi Furukawa, Alfonso Iorio, Annette Kristiansen, Ingmarie Skoglund, Jong Soue You, Per Olav Vandvik, Yuying Zhang (language translation); Canadian Doctors for Medicare, Health Quality Ontario (knowledge translation partners).

Author Contributions

Conceived of project: KSP DM IAD. Secured funds: KSP DM IAD GHG. Directed research project: KSP DM GHG. Served as PI: KSP. Directed methodology: GHG. Gave extensive input on methodology: TA. Research Coordinator and managed database: TS. Developed literature search terms: NB. Consultation on literature search terms development: KSP DM. Conducted literature search: NB. Screened titles/abstracts and full texts: KSP TA DM TS SMM APM. Abstracted data: TA SMM APM AA AB AAH RAJ AM AN RAS. Analyzed data in consultation with statistician: KSP TA TS GHG. Contributed to meta-analysis in consultation with statistician who performed meta-analysis: TA TS GHG. Analyzed non-pooled data: KSP GHG. Interpreted data: KSP TA DM TS AM JNL JYY SJD GHG. Wrote first draft: KSP TA DM. Reviewed and contributed to revisions of draft manuscript: KSP TA DM TS SMM APM AA AB AAH RAJ AM AN RAS NB IAD JNL JJY SJD GHG. Major contributors to final manuscript: KSP TA DM GHG. Approved final version of manuscript: KSP TA DM TS SMM APM AA AB AAH RAJ AM AN RAS NB IAD JNL JJY SJD GHG. Attended all or some of weekly teleconferences and face-to-face meetings over two years: KSP TA DM TS SMM APM AA AB AAH RAJ AM AN RAS NB IAD JNL JJY SJD GHG. Led end-of-grant knowledge translation: DM. Consultation on end-of-grant knowledge translation: KSP. Guarantors affirming that this manuscript is an honest, accurate, and transparent account of the study being reported; that no important aspects of the study have been omitted; and that any discrepancies from the study as planned have been explained: KSP GHG.

References

1. Canadian Institute for Health Information (2009) Health Care in Canada 2009: A decade in review. Ottawa, Ont. Available: https://secure.cihi.ca/free_products/HCIC_2009_Web_e.pdf Accessed 2013 July 11.
2. O'Reilly J, Busse R, Hakkinen U, Or Z, Street A, et al. (2012) Paying for hospital care: the experience with implementing activity-based funding in five European countries. Health Econ Policy Law 7: 73–101.
3. Canadian Institute for Health Information, Activity-Based Funding Unit. (2010) A primer on activity-based funding. Ottawa (ON): The Institute Available: http://www.cihi.ca/CIHI-ext-portal/pdf/internet/primer_activity_based_fund_en Accessed 2013 July 22.
4. Busse R, Geissler A, QuentinW, Wiley M, eds. (2011) Diagnosis-Related Groups in Europe: Moving towards Transparency, Efficiency and Quality in Hospitals. Maidenhead, England: World Health Organization on behalf of European Observatory on Health Systems and Policies Series, McGraw Hill, Open University Press. Available: http://www.euro.who.int/__data/assets/pdf_file/0004/162265/e96538.pdf Accessed 2014 March 21.
5. Palmer KS, Martin D, Guyatt GH (2013) Prelude to a systematic review of activity-based funding of hospitals: potential effects on cost, quality, access, efficiency, and equity. Open Medicine 7: e94–e97.
6. Tan SS, Serden L, Geissler A, van Ineveld, M., Redekop K, et al. (2011) DRGs and cost accounting: Which is driving which? In: Busse R, Geissler A, QuentinW, Wiley M, eds. Diagnosis-Related Groups in Europe: Moving towards Transparency, Efficiency and Quality in Hospitals. Maidenhead, England: World Health Organization on behalf of European Observatory on Health Systems and Policies Series, McGraw Hill, Open University Press. Available: http://www.euro.who.int/__data/assets/pdf_file/0004/162265/e96538.pdf Accessed: 2014 March 21.
7. Mayes R (2007) The origins, development, and passage of Medicare's revolutionary prospective payment system. J Hist Med Allied Sci 62: 21–55.
8. (1983) Medicare program; prospective payments for Medicare inpatient hospital services–HCFA. Interim final rule with comment period. Fed Regist 48: 39752–39890.
9. Canadian Institute for Health Information (2013) The Why, the What and the How of Activity-Based Funding in Canada: A Resource for Health System Funders and Hospital Managers. Ottawa, ON: The Institute. Available: https://secure.cihi.ca/free_products/ActivityBasedFundingManualEN-web_Nov2013.pdf Accessed 2013 July 21.
10. Tan SS, van Ineveld M, Redekop K, Hakkaart-van Roijen L (2010) Structural reforms and hospital payment in the Netherlands. Euro Observer 12(3): 7–9. Available: http://eurodrg.projects.tu-berlin.de/publications/Structural reforms and hospital payment in the Netherland1.pdf Accessed 2014 March 21.
11. Kobel C, Thuilliez J, Bellanger M, Pfeiffer K-P (2011) DRG systems and similar patient classification systems in Europe. In: Busse R, Geissler A, QuentinW, Wiley M, eds. Diagnosis-Related Groups in Europe: Moving towards Transparency, Efficiency and Quality in Hospitals [Internet]. Maidenhead, England: World Health Organization on behalf of European Observatory on Health Systems and Policies Series, McGraw Hill, Open University Press. pp. 37–58. Available: http://www.euro.who.int/__data/assets/pdf_file/0004/162265/e96538.pdf Accessed 2014 March 20.
12. Chulis GS (1991) Assessing Medicare's prospective payment system for hospitals. Med Care Rev 48: 167–206.
13. US Congress, Office of Technology Assessment (1995) Hospital Financing in Seven Countries. OTA-BP-H-148, Washington, DC: U.S. Government Printing Office, p. 139. Available: http://ota.fas.org/reports/9562.pdf Accessed 2014 September 24.
14. Biorn E, Hagen TP, Iversen T, Magnussen J (2010) How different are hospitals' responses to a financial reform? The impact on efficiency of activity-based financing. Health Care Manag Sci 13: 1–16.
15. Yin J, Luras H, Hagen TP, Dahl FA (2013) The effect of activity-based financing on hospital length of stay for elderly patients suffering from heart diseases in Norway. BMC Health Serv Res 13: 172.
16. Schuetz P, Albrich WC, Suter I, Hug BL, Christ-Crain M, et al. (2011) Quality of care delivered by fee-for-service and DRG hospitals in Switzerland in patients with community-acquired pneumonia. Swiss Med Wkly 141: w13228.
17. Carroll NV, Erwin WG (1990) Effect of the prospective-pricing system on drug use in Pennsylvania long-term-care facilities. Am J Hosp Pharm 47: 2251–2254.
18. Qian X, Russell LB, Valiyeva E, Miller JE (2011) "Quicker and sicker" under Medicare's prospective payment system for hospitals: new evidence on an old issue from a national longitudinal survey. Bull Econ Res 63: 1–27.
19. Dafny LS (2005) How do hospitals respond to price changes? American Economic Review 95: 1525–1547.
20. Berta P, Callea G, Martini G, Vittadini G (2009) The Effects of Upcoding, Cream Skimming and Readmission on the Italian Hospitals Efficiency: a Population-based Investigation. Munich Personal RePEc Archive; 17671: 1–42. Available: http://mpra.ub.uni-muenchen.de/17671/1/MPRA_paper_17671.pdf Accessed 2014 March 20.
21. Newhouse JP (1989) Do unprofitable patients face access problems? Health Care Financ Rev 11: 33–42.
22. Ellis RP (1998) Creaming, skimping and dumping: provider competition on the intensive and extensive margins. J Health Econ 17: 537–555.
23. Sutherland JM, Repin N, Crump TR (2012) Reviewing the potential roles of financial incentives for funding healthcare in Canada. Ottawa (ON): Canadian Foundation for Healthcare Improvement. Available: http://www.cfhi-fcass.ca/publicationsandresources/researchreports/ArticleView/12-12-21/bec64e56-ce47-43c9-b05c-98186051731d.aspx Accessed 2014 March 20.
24. Moreno-Serra R, Wagstaff A (2010) System-wide impacts of hospital payment reforms: evidence from Central and Eastern Europe and Central Asia. J Health Econ 29: 585–602.
25. Eijkenaar F, Emmert M, Scheppach M, Schoffski O (2013) Effects of pay for performance in health care: a systematic review of systematic reviews. Health Policy 110: 115–130.
26. Fleiss JL (1993) The statistical basis of meta-analysis. Stat Methods Med Res 2: 121–145.
27. Higgins JP, Thompson SG, Deeks JJ, Altman DG (2003) Measuring inconsistency in meta-analyses. BMJ 327: 557–560.
28. Researchers of the Italian Group of Pharmaco-epidemiology in the Aged (GIFA) (1996) [Characteristics of hospitalization of aged patients before and after introduction of the prospective payment (DRG-ROD system)]. Ann Ital Med Int 11: 220–227.
29. Brizioli E, Fraticelli A, Marcobelli A, Paciaroni E (1996) Hospital payment system based on diagnosis related groups in Italy: early effects on elderly patients with heart failure. Arch Gerontol Geriatr 23: 347–355.
30. Busato A, von Below G (2010) The implementation of DRG-based hospital reimbursement in Switzerland: A population-based perspective. Health Res Policy Syst 8: 31.
31. Carroll NV, Erwin WG (1987) Patient shifting as a response to Medicare Prospective Payment. Med Care 25: 1161–1167.
32. Cutler DM (1995) The Incidence of Adverse Medical Outcomes under Prospective Payment. Econometrica 63: 29–50.
33. DesHarnais S, Chesney J, Fleming S (1988) Trends and regional variations in hospital utilization and quality during the first two years of the prospective payment system. Inquiry 25: 374–382.
34. DesHarnais S, Hogan AJ, McMahon LF, Jr., Fleming S (1991) Changes in rates of unscheduled hospital readmissions and changes in efficiency following the introduction of the Medicare prospective payment system. An analysis using risk-adjusted data. Eval Health Prof 14: 228–252.
35. DesHarnais S, Kobrinski E, Chesney J, Long M, Ament R, et al. (1987) The early effects of the prospective payment system on inpatient utilization and the quality of care. Inquiry 24: 7–16.
36. DesHarnais SI, Schumacher D (1991) The effects of the Medicare PPS on vulnerable subgroups of psychiatric patients treated in short-term general hospitals. QRB Qual Rev Bull 17: 261–268.
37. DesHarnais SI, Wroblewski R, Schumacher D (1990) How the medicare prospective payment system affects psychiatric patients treated in short-term general hospitals. Inquiry 27: 382–388.
38. Draper D, Kahn KL, Reinisch EJ, Sherwood MJ, Carney MF, et al. (1990) Studying the effects of the DRG-based prospective payment system on quality of care. Design, sampling, and fieldwork. JAMA 264: 1956–1961.
39. Easton LS, Cogen R, Fulcomer M (1991) Effect of Medicare prospective payment system on a home health agency: changes in patient population and services provided. Appl Nurs Res 4: 107–112.
40. Eggers PW (1987) Prospective payment system and quality: early results and research strategy. Health Care Financ Rev Spec No: 29–37.
41. Epstein AM, Bogen J, Dreyer P, Thorpe KE (1991) Trends in length of stay and rates of readmission in Massachusetts: implications for monitoring quality of care. Inquiry 28: 19–28.
42. Farrar S, Yi D, Sutton M, Chalkley M, Sussex J, et al. (2009) Has payment by results affected the way that English hospitals provide care? Difference-in-differences analysis. BMJ 339: b3047.
43. Fitzgerald JF, Fagan LF, Tierney WM, Dittus RS (1987) Changing patterns of hip fracture care before and after implementation of the prospective payment system. JAMA 258: 218–221.
44. Fitzgerald JF, Moore PS, Dittus RS (1988) The care of elderly patients with hip fracture. Changes since implementation of the prospective payment system. N Engl J Med 319: 1392–1397.
45. Frick U, Barta W, Binder H (2001) [Hospital financing in in-patient psychiatry via DRG-based prospective payment–The Salzburg experience]. Psychiatr Prax 28 Suppl 1: S55–62.
46. Friedman B, Farley D (1995) Strategic responses by hospitals to increased financial risk in the 1980s. Health Serv Res 30: 467–488.
47. Fuchs PC, Gustafson ME (1986) Significance of nosocomial infection rates in the era of DRGs. Infect Control 7: 506–507.
48. Gaumer GL, Stavins J (1992) Medicare use in the last ninety days of life. Health Serv Res 26: 725–742.
49. Gay EG, Kronenfeld JJ (1990) Regulation, retrenchment–the DRG experience: problems from changing reimbursement practice. Soc Sci Med 31: 1103–1118.
50. Gay EG, Kronenfeld JJ, Baker SL (1994) Increasing home health service referrals, boon or bane? Home Health Care Serv Q 14: 49–67.
51. Gerety MB, Soderholm-Difatte V, Winograd CH (1989) Impact of prospective payment and discharge location on the outcome of hip fracture. J Gen Intern Med 4: 388–391.

52. Gianfrancesco FD (1990) Prospective payment system and other effects on post-hospital services. Health Care Financ Rev 12: 37–54.
53. Guterman S, Eggers PW, Riley G, Greene TF, Terrell SA (1988) The first 3 years of Medicare prospective payment: an overview. Health Care Financ Rev 9: 67–77.
54. Helms CM (1987) A pseudo-epidemic of septicemia among Medicare patients in Iowa. Am J Public Health 77: 1331–1332.
55. Hing E (1989) Effects of the prospective payment system on nursing homes. Vital Health Stat 13: 1–38.
56. Jauss M, Hamann GF, Claus D, Misselwitz B, Kugler C, et al. (2010) [Billing based on a case-based lump sum for stroke. Did this lead to discharge of patients in a worse clinical condition?]. Nervenarzt 81: 218–225.
57. Kahn KL, Keeler EB, Sherwood MJ, Rogers WH, Draper D, et al. (1990) Comparing outcomes of care before and after implementation of the DRG-based prospective payment system. JAMA 264: 1984–1988.
58. Kanda K, Mezey M (1991) Registered nurse staffing in Pennsylvania nursing homes: comparison before and after implementation of Medicare's Prospective Payment System. Gerontologist 31: 318–324.
59. Kane JT, Gallaher AJ, Davis DM, Cummings V (1987) Diagnostic-related groups: their impact on an inpatient rehabilitation program. Arch Phys Med Rehabil 68: 833–836.
60. Keeler EB, Rubenstein LV, Kahn KL, Draper D, Harrison ER, et al. (1992) Hospital characteristics and quality of care. JAMA 268: 1709–1714.
61. Kerr GD, Dunt D, Gordon IR (1998) Effect of casemix funding on outcomes in patients admitted to hospital with suspected unstable angina. Med J Aust 168: 57–60.
62. Leibson C, Naessens JM, Krishan I, Campion ME, Ballard D (1990) Disposition at discharge and 60-day mortality among elderly people following shorter hospital stays: a population-based comparison. Gerontologist 30: 316–322.
63. Leibson CL, Naessens JM, Campion ME, Krishan I, Ballard DJ (1991) Trends in elderly hospitalization and readmission rates for a geographically defined population: pre- and post-prospective payment. J Am Geriatr Soc 39: 895–904.
64. Lewis MA, Leake B, Leal-Sotelo M, Clark V (1987) The initial effects of the prospective payment system on nursing home patients. Am J Public Health 77: 819–821.
65. Long MJ, Chesney JD, Ament RP, DesHarnais SI, Fleming ST, et al. (1987) The effect of PPS on hospital product and productivity. Med Care 25: 528–538.
66. Long MJ, Chesney JD, Fleming ST (1989) Were hospitals selective in their product and productivity changes? The top 50 DRGs after PPS. Health Serv Res 24: 615–641.
67. Long MJ, Chesney JD, Fleming ST (1990) A reassessment of hospital product and productivity changes over time. Health Care Financ Rev 11: 69–77.
68. Louis DZ, Yuen EJ, Braga M, Cicchetti A, Rabinowitz C, et al. (1999) Impact of a DRG-based hospital financing system on quality and outcomes of care in Italy. Health Serv Res 34: 405–415.
69. Manton KG, Liu K (1990) Recent changes in service use patterns of disabled Medicare beneficiaries. Health Care Financ Rev 11: 51–66.
70. Manton KG, Vertrees JC, Wrigley JM (1990) Changes in health service use and mortality among U.S. elderly in 1980–1986. J Aging Health 2: 131–156.
71. Manton KG, Woodbury MA, Vertrees JC, Stallard E (1993) Use of Medicare services before and after introduction of the prospective payment system. Health Serv Res 28: 269–292.
72. Mayer-Oakes SA, Oye RK, Leake B, Brook RH (1988) The early effect of Medicare's prospective payment system on the use of medical intensive care services in three community hospitals. JAMA 260: 3146–3149.
73. Morrisey MA, Sloan FA, Valvona J (1988) Medicare prospective payment and posthospital transfers to subacute care. Med Care 26: 685–698.
74. Onder G, Bernabei R, Cesari M, Gambassi G (2001) Prospective payment system and hospitalization for pneumonia in Italy. Arch Intern Med 161: 1918–1919.
75. Palmer RM, Saywell RM, Jr., Zollinger TW, Erner BK, LaBov AD, et al. (1989) The impact of the prospective payment system on the treatment of hip fractures in the elderly. Arch Intern Med 149: 2237–2241.
76. Pfeiffer D, Christian P (1987) Impact of the federal prospective payment system upon long-term care related Medicare patients. J Health Hum Resour Adm 10: 115–146.
77. Ray WA, Griffin MR, Baugh DK (1990) Mortality following hip fracture before and after implementation of the prospective payment system. Arch Intern Med 150: 2109–2114.
78. Rich MW, Freedland KE (1988) Effect of DRGs on three-month readmission rate of geriatric patients with congestive heart failure. Am J Public Health 78: 680–682.
79. Rogers WH, Draper D, Kahn KL, Keeler EB, Rubenstein LV, et al. (1990) Quality of care before and after implementation of the DRG-based prospective payment system. A summary of effects. JAMA 264: 1989–1994.
80. Schmidt SM, Guo L, Scheer SJ (2002) Changes in the status of hospitalized stroke patients since inception of the prospective payment system in 1983. Arch Phys Med Rehabil 83: 894–898.
81. Shmueli A, Intrator O, Israeli A (2002) The effects of introducing prospective payments to general hospitals on length of stay, quality of care, and hospitals' income: the early experience of Israel. Soc Sci Med 55: 981–989.
82. Sloan FA, Morrisey MA, Valvona J (1988) Case shifting and the Medicare Prospective Payment System. Am J Public Health 78: 553–556.
83. South M (1997) Reduction in length of hospital stay for acute childhood asthma associated with the introduction of casemix funding. Med J Aust 167: 11–13.
84. Stromberg L, Ohlen G, Svensson O (1997) Prospective payment systems and hip fracture treatment costs. Acta Orthop Scand 68: 6–12.
85. Van Gelder S, Bernstein J (1986) Home health care in the era of hospital prospective payment: some early evidence and thoughts about the future. Pride Inst J Long Term Home Health Care 5: 3–11.
86. von Eiff W, Schuring S, Greitemann B, Karoff M (2011) [REDIA–impacts of DRG introduction in the acute sector on medical rehabilitation]. Rehabilitation (Stuttg) 50: 214–221.
87. Weinberger M, Ault KA, Vinicor F (1988) Prospective reimbursement and diabetes mellitus. Impact upon glycemic control and utilization of health services. Med Care 26: 77–83.
88. Wells KB, Rogers WH, Davis LM, Kahn K, Norquist G, et al. (1993) Quality of care for hospitalized depressed elderly patients before and after implementation of the Medicare Prospective Payment System. Am J Psychiatry 150: 1799–1805.
89. Xiao J, Lee A, Vemuri SR, Beaver C (2000) An assessment of the effects of casemix funding on hospital utilisation: a Northern Territory perspective. Aust Health Rev 23: 122–136.
90. Brereton L, Vasoodaven V (2010) The Impact of the NHS Market: an overview of the literature. London: Civitas Available: http://www.civitas.org.uk/nhs/download/Civitas_LiteratureReview_NHS_market_Feb10.pdf Accessed 2014 March 24.
91. Roland M, Rosen R (2011) English NHS embarks on controversial and risky market-style reforms in health care. N Engl J Med 364: 1360–1366.
92. Enthoven AC (1991) Internal market reform of the British National Health Service. Health Aff (Millwood) 10: 60–70.
93. LoGerfo JP (1990) The prospective payment system and quality. No skeletons in the closet. JAMA 264: 1995–1996.
94. Street A, Vitikainen K, Bjorvatn A, Hvenegaard A (2007) Introducing activity-based financing: a review of experience in Australia, Denmark, Norway and Sweden [Internet]. CHE research paper 30. Centre for Health Economics, University of York Available: http://www.york.ac.uk/media/che/documents/papers/researchpapers/rp30_introducing_activity-based_financing.pdf Accessed 2013 September 15.
95. Cohen M, McGregor M, Ivanova I, Kinkaid C (2013) Beyond the hospital walls: Activity-based funding versus integrated health care reform [Internet]. Vancouver, BC: Canadian Centre for Policy Alternatives, Available: http://www.policyalternatives.ca/sites/default/files/uploads/publications/BC Office/2012/01/CCPA-BC_ABF_2012.pdf Accessed 2013 July 2.
96. Canadian Institute for Health Information (2013) Evaluating the Impact of Activity-Based Funding on Health System Performance. Ottawa, Ont.; The Institute, Available: http://www.cihi.ca/CIHI-ext-portal/pdf/internet/EVALUATING_IMPACT_ABF_EN Accessed 2013 July 11.
97. Sutherland JM (2011) Hospital payment mechanisms an overview and options for Canada. CHSRF Series on Cost Drivers and Health System Efficiency: Paper 4. Ottawa, ON: Canadian Health Services Research Foundation. Available: http://www.cfhi-fcass.ca/Libraries/Hospital_Funding_docs/CHSRF-Sutherland-HospitalFundingENG.sflb.ashx Accessed 2014 March 21.
98. Ettelt S, Thomson S, Nolte E, Mays N (2006) Reimbursing highly specialised hospital services: the experience of activity-based funding in eight countries. A report commissioned the Department of Health and prepared by the London School of Hygiene and Tropical Medicine, London. Available: http://researchonline.lshtm.ac.uk/5510/ Accessed 2014 September 21.
99. Coulam RF, Gaumer GL (1991) Medicare's prospective payment system: a critical appraisal. Health Care Financ Rev Annu Suppl: 45–77.
100. Laderman M, Loehrer S, McCarthy D (2013) The Effect of Medicare Readmissions Penalties on Hospitals' Efforts to Reduce Readmissions: Perspectives from the Field. In: The Commonwealth Fund. New York, NY: The Commonwealth Fund. Available: http://www.commonwealthfund.org/Blog/2013/Feb/The-Effect-of-Medicare-Readmissions-Penalties-on-Hospitals.aspx Accessed 2014 March 21.
101. Averill RF, McCullough EC, Hughes JS, Goldfield NI, Vertrees JC, et al. (2009) Redesigning the Medicare Inpatient PPS to Reduce Payments to Hospitals with High Readmission Rates. Health Care Financing Review 30: 1–15.
102. Centers for Medicare & Medicaid Services Readmissions Reduction Program (2013) In: CMS.gov Centers for Medicare & Medicaid Services. Baltimore, MD Centers for Medicare & Medicaid Services. Available: http://www.cms.gov/Medicare/Medicare-Fee-for-Service-Payment/AcuteInpatientPPS/Readmissions-Reduction-Program.html Accessed 2014 March 21.
103. U.S. Department of Health & Human Services (2013 May 14) Medicare Fraud strike force charges 89 individuals for approximately $223 million in false billing. In: HHS.gov U.S. Department of Health & Human Services, Available: http://www.hhs.gov/news/press/2013pres/05/20130514a.html Accessed 2014 March 21.
104. Bresnick J (2013 Aug 15) Knee and hip replacement readmissions may cost $265,000. In: EHRIntelligence.com. Danvers, MA. Xtelligent Media, LLC. Available from: http://ehrintelligence.com/2013/08/15/knee-and-hip-replacement-readmissions-may-cost-265000/ Accessed 20114 March 21.

105. Office of Inspector General. (ND) Management Challenge 5: Fighting Fraud and Waste in Medicare Parts A & B. In: Top management & performance challenges. U.S Department of Health & Human Services. Available from: http://oig.hhs.gov/reports-and-publications/top-challenges/2013/challenge05.asp Accessed 2014 March 21.
106. Carlson J (2013) Faulty gauge? Mod Healthc 43: 6–7, 1.
107. Dishonest Hospitals Sidestep Medicare Readmission Penalties by Submitting Claims for Inappropriate Observation Stays (2013) In: Nolan Auerbach and White: Medicare Fraud BLOG. [place unknown]. Available: http://medicare-fraud.net/dishonest-hospitals-sidestep-medicare-readmission-penalties-by-submitting-claims-for-inappropriate-observation-stays/ Accessed 2014 March 21.
108. Center for Public Integrity (2013) Cracking the codes. Washington, DC: Center for Public Integrity, Available: https://s3.amazonaws.com/iw-files/documents/pdfs/CPI+Cracking+the+Codes.pdf Accessed 2014 March 24.
109. U.S. Department of Health and Human Services (HHS), Office of Inspector General. (2014 February) Adverse events in skilled nursing facilities: national incidence among Medicare beneficiaries. Report No.: OEI-06-11-00370. Available: https://oig.hhs.gov/oei/reports/oei-06-11-00370.pdf Accessed 2014 March 24.
110. DeJong G (2010) Bundling acute and postacute payment: from a culture of compliance to a culture of innovation and best practice. Phys Ther 90: 658–662.
111. Buntin MB, Colla CH, Escarce JJ (2009) Effects of payment changes on trends in post-acute care. Health Serv Res 44: 1188–1210.
112. Murkofsky RL, Phillips RS, McCarthy EP, Davis RB, Hamel MB (2003) Length of stay in home care before and after the 1997 Balanced Budget Act. JAMA 289: 2841–2848.
113. Hussey PS, Ridgely MS, Rosenthal MB (2011) The PROMETHEUS bundled payment experiment: slow start shows problems in implementing new payment models. Health Aff (Millwood) 30: 2116–2124.
114. Ackerly DC, Grabowski DC (2014) Post-acute care reform–beyond the ACA. N Engl J Med 370: 689–691.
115. Welch WP (1998) Bundled Medicare payment for acute and postacute care. Health Aff (Millwood) 17: 69–81.
116. Long MJ, Chesney JD, Fleming ST (1993) Profitable and unprofitable DRGs: the implications for access. Health Serv Manage Res 6: 61–69.
117. Day B (2007) Letter from the National Health Service Consultants Association. In: CUPE 50 [Internet]. Ottawa, ON: CUPE. Available from: http://cupe.ca/health-care/NHSCAletter Accessed 2014 March 21.
118. Abler S, Verde P, Stannigel H, Mayatepek E, Hoehn T (2011) Effect of the introduction of diagnosis related group systems on the distribution of admission weights in very low birthweight infants. Archives of Disease in Childhood-Fetal and Neonatal Edition 96: F186–F189.

Increasing Incidence of Hospital-Acquired and Healthcare-Associated Bacteremia in Northeast Thailand: A Multicenter Surveillance Study

Maliwan Hongsuwan[1], Pramot Srisamang[2], Manas Kanoksil[3], Nantasit Luangasanatip[1], Anchalee Jatapai[1], Nicholas P. Day[1,4], Sharon J. Peacock[1,5,6], Ben S. Cooper[1,4], Direk Limmathurotsakul[1,7]*

1 Mahidol-Oxford Tropical Medicine Research Unit, Faculty of Tropical Medicine, Mahidol University, Bangkok, Thailand, **2** Department of pediatrics, Sappasithiprasong Hospital, Ubon Ratchathani, Thailand, **3** Department of pediatrics, Udon Thani Hospital, Udon Thani, Thailand, **4** Center for Tropical Medicine, Nuffield Department of Clinical Medicine, University of Oxford, Oxford, United Kingdom, **5** Department of Microbiology and Immunology, Faculty of Tropical Medicine, Mahidol University, Bangkok, Thailand, **6** Department of Medicine, Cambridge University, Addenbrooke's Hospital, Cambridge, United Kingdom, **7** Department of Tropical Hygiene, Faculty of Tropical Medicine, Mahidol University, Bangkok, Thailand

Abstract

Background: Little is known about the epidemiology of nosocomial bloodstream infections in public hospitals in developing countries. We evaluated trends in incidence of hospital-acquired bacteremia (HAB) and healthcare-associated bacteremia (HCAB) and associated mortality in a developing country using routinely available databases.

Methods: Information from the microbiology and hospital databases of 10 provincial hospitals in northeast Thailand was linked with the national death registry for 2004–2010. Bacteremia was considered hospital-acquired if detected after the first two days of hospital admission, and healthcare-associated if detected within two days of hospital admission with a prior inpatient episode in the preceding 30 days.

Results: A total of 3,424 patients out of 1,069,443 at risk developed HAB and 2,184 out of 119,286 at risk had HCAB. Of these 1,559 (45.5%) and 913 (41.8%) died within 30 days, respectively. Between 2004 and 2010, the incidence rate of HAB increased from 0.6 to 0.8 per 1,000 patient-days at risk ($p<0.001$), and the cumulative incidence of HCAB increased from 1.2 to 2.0 per 100 readmissions ($p<0.001$). The most common causes of HAB were *Acinetobacter* spp. (16.2%), *Klebsiella pneumoniae* (13.9%), and *Staphylococcus aureus* (13.9%), while those of HCAB were *Escherichia coli* (26.3%), *S. aureus* (14.0%), and *K. pneumoniae* (9.7%). There was an overall increase over time in the proportions of ESBL-producing *E. coli* causing HAB and HCAB.

Conclusions: This study demonstrates a high and increasing incidence of HAB and HCAB in provincial hospitals in northeast Thailand, increasing proportions of ESBL-producing isolates, and very high associated mortality.

Editor: Linda Anne Selvey, Curtin University, Australia

Funding: The work was supported by the Wellcome Trust of Great Britain (grant number 089275/Z/09/Z). BSC was supported by The Medical Research Council and Department for International Development (grant number MR/K006924/1). SJP receives support from the NIHR Cambridge Biomedical Research Centre. DL is supported by an Intermediate Wellcome Trust Fellowship (grant number 101103/Z/13/Z). The funder has no role in the study design, data collection and analysis, decision to publish, or preparation of the manuscript.

Competing Interests: The authors have declared that no competing interests exist.

* Email: direk@tropmedres.ac

Introduction

Nosocomial infections are the most frequent adverse event in healthcare delivery worldwide, but there is a paucity of information about their epidemiology from developing countries [1]. This is particularly true for nosocomial bacteremia which are frequently used as indicators of trends in overall nosocomial infection in developed countries because of the availability of clear definitions and clinical relevance [2,3]. A recent comprehensive systematic review found only 13 studies of bloodstream infection from developing countries between 1995 and 2008, with only six studies in the Southeast Asia region and none from the Western Pacific region [1]. For example, the reported incidence rates of hospital-acquired bacteremia (HAB) through active surveillance were 1.0 per 1,000 patient-days in a district hospital in Kenya between 2002–2009 [4], and 1.2 per 1,000 patient-days in a university hospital in Iran in 2006 [5]. This lack of information is a consequence, at least in part, of the paucity of reliable surveillance systems for such outcomes in resource-limited settings. Moreover, published literature from developing countries is often from better resourced or university hospitals [4,5], and may not provide a reliable basis for generalization to public hospitals in those countries.

In this study, we combined multiple sources of routine surveillance data including microbiology databases, hospital admission databases and the national death registry from a sample of provincial hospitals in northeast Thailand [6]. Our objectives were to demonstrate trends in incidence, antibiotic-resistance and mortality associated with HAB and healthcare-associated bacteremia (HCAB) over a seven year period.

Materials and Methods

Study population

Northeast Thailand consists of 20 provinces, covers 170,226 km^2 and had an estimated population in 2010 of 21.4 million. Each province has a provincial hospital that provides care to people living within its catchment area and acts as a referral hospital for smaller district hospitals. The number of beds per provincial hospital ranges from 200 to 1000, and all provincial hospitals are equipped with intensive care units (ICUs). Severely ill patients presenting to district hospitals are often referred to provincial hospitals. Provincial hospitals are equipped with a microbiology laboratory that provides a bacterial culture service, while district hospitals normally do not have such facilities. All microbiology laboratories in provincial hospitals use standard methodologies for bacterial identification and susceptibility testing provided by the Bureau of Laboratory Quality and Standards, Ministry of Public Health, Thailand [7].

Study design

We conducted a retrospective, multicenter surveillance study of all provincial hospitals in northeast Thailand. The data were collected as previously described [2]. In brief, the director of each hospital was contacted and given information on the study. For those hospitals that agreed to participate, data were collected from the microbiology and hospital databases between Jan 2004 to Dec 2010. Admission number (AN) was used as the record linkage between the two databases, and hospital number (HN) was used to identify individuals who had repeated admissions. The death registry for northeast Thailand between Jan 2004 to Jan 2011 was obtained from the Ministry of Interior, Thailand, and used to identify patients who were discharged from hospital and died within 30 days after discharge from the hospital. Ethical permission for this study was obtained from the Ethical and Scientific Review Committees of Faculty of Tropical Medicine, Mahidol University, and of the Ministry of Public Health, Thailand. Written consent was given by the director of the hospitals to use the routine hospital database for research. Consent was not sought from the patients as this was a retrospective study, and the Ethical and Scientific Review Committees approved the process.

Data collection

The microbiology laboratory data collected were HN, AN, specimen type, specimen date, culture result, and antibiotic susceptibility profile (antibiogram). Hospital data were collected from the routine in-patient discharge report (Report 501), which is regularly completed by attending physicians and reported to the Ministry of Public Health, Thailand, as part of national morbidity and mortality reporting system. The data collected were HN, AN, national identification 13-digit number, gender, age, admission date, discharge date, and outcome. A single outcome variable is required by this reporting system, which is completed by the attending physicians and categorized as cured, improved, not improved, transfer to another hospital, refusal of treatment, or died. Date of death was also extracted from this record. Data collected from the death registry obtained from the Ministry of Interior were national identification 13-digit number and date of death. Data are not suitable for public deposition due to ethical restrictions. Raw database requests may be made to the director of each participating hospital (Table S1).

Definitions

Bacteremia was classified as community-acquired bacteremia (CAB), HAB or HCAB. CAB was defined as the isolation of a pathogenic organism from blood taken in the first 2 days of admission and without a hospital stay in the 30 days prior to admission [2]. HAB was defined as the isolation of a pathogenic organism from blood taken after the first 2 days of admission [8,9]. HCAB was defined as the isolation of a pathogenic organism from blood taken in the first 2 days of admission and with a hospital stay within 30 days prior to the admission [8,9]. Patients at risk of HCAB were those with a hospital stay within 30 days prior to the admission. Patients were considered at risk of HAB after they stayed in the hospital for more than 2 days. Because of the difficulty in establishing their clinical significance, organisms frequently associated with contamination including coagulase-negative *staphylococci*, viridans group *streptococci*, *Corynebacterium* spp., *Bacillus* spp., *Diptheroid* spp., *Micrococcus* spp., and *Propionibacterium* spp. were excluded from the analysis [10]. Organisms that produced an extended-spectrum β lactamase (ESBL) were defined using standard methodologies for bacterial identification and susceptibility testing provided by the Bureau of Laboratory Quality and Standards, Ministry of Public Health, Thailand [7]. All patients with bacteremia caused by *B. pseudomallei* were categorized as CAB because this organism is not a cause of HAB or HCAB [11]. Polymicrobial infection was defined in patients who had more than one species of pathogenic organisms isolated from the blood during the same episode. Information on patients with a first CAB episode has been published previously [2]. In this study, patients with a first episode of HAB or HCAB were evaluated in relation to epidemiology and mortality.

The 30-day mortality of HAB was determined on the basis of a record of death within 30 days of the positive blood culture taken as recorded in the routine hospital database or by a record of death in the national death registry. The 30-day mortality of HCAB was defined as death within 30 days of the admission date. The incidence rate of HAB was calculated as the number of HAB per 1,000 patient-days at risk. The cumulative incidence of HCAB was calculated as the number of HCAB per 100 readmissions. To avoid the assessment of multiple outcomes for a single patient, in the event that a patient had more than one episode of bacteremia (either HAB and/or HCAB) only the first episode was included in the study.

Statistical analysis

All analyses were performed using STATA version 12.0 (StataCorp LP, College station, Texas). Poisson regression models were used to calculated incidence rate ratios, and logistic regression models were used to calculated odds ratios. Fisher's exact test was used to compare categorical variables. The Mann-Whitney test was used to compare continuous variables. A non-parametric test for trend was used to assess change in proportion over time and stratified by hospital (using the npt_s command in STATA).

Results

All 20 provincial hospitals in northeast Thailand were contacted to participate in this study. Agreement was obtained from 15 (75%) hospitals, of which 10 had microbiological laboratory and hospital databases as electronic files in a readily accessible format (Figure S1). Of the 10 hospitals included in the analysis, 3 (30%) had data available for the period 2004–2010, 1 (10%) between 2006–2010, 2 (20%) between 2007–2010, 3 (30%) between 2008–2010, and 1 (10%) between 2009–2010 (Tables 1 and 2). The median bed number was 450 beds (range 300 to 1,000 beds). A total of 1,969,474 admission records from 1,372,446 patients were evaluated, of which 21,438 (1.1%) admission records had at least one blood culture positive for pathogenic organisms during admission. A total of 3,451 (16.1%) episodes were defined as hospital-acquired bacteremia (HAB), 2,302 (10.7%) episodes were healthcare-associated bacteremia (HCAB) and 15,685 (73.2%) episodes were community-acquired bacteremia (CAB). Multiple episodes of HAB and HCAB were noted in 26 and 102 patients, respectively. Only the first episodes of HAB and HCAB in 3,424 and 2,184 patients, respectively, were included in further analysis.

Incidence of HAB and HCAB

The average incidence rate for HAB during the 7-year study period was 0.7 per 1,000 patient-days, with an overall increase in rate over time. The incidence rate of HAB increased from 0.6 in 2004 to 0.8 per 1,000 patient-days in 2010 ($p<0.001$) (Table 1).

Of 1,969,474 admission records, 119,286 (10.1%) had a hospital stay within 30 days prior to admission and were at risk of HCAB. The cumulative incidence for HCAB during the 7-year study period was 1.8 per 100 readmissions, with an overall increase in the cumulative incidence over time. The cumulative incidence of HCAB increased from 1.2 in 2004 to 2.0 per 100 readmissions in 2010 ($p<0.001$) (Table 2). The incidence rate of HAB and HCAB varied by hospitals (Figure S2 and S3), but the overall increasing trends were observed in most hospitals.

Demographic risk factors for HAB and HCAB

Of 3,424 patients with a primary episode of HAB, 2,000 (58.4%) were male and 1,424 (41.6%) were female. The median age was 51 years (interquartile range [IQR] 16–67 years, range 0–88 years). The median time from hospital admission to bacteremia was 8 days (IQR 4–15 days, range 3–105 days). The median length of stay for patients with HAB was longer than patients who were at risk of, but did not develop HAB (18 vs. 4 days, $p<0.001$). The overall incidence rate of HAB was higher in males than in females (0.8 vs. 0.6 per 1,000 patient-days, incidence rate ratio [IRR] 1.21; 95% confidence interval [CI] 1.13 to 1.30, $p<0.001$) (Figure 1). The incidence rates of HAB were highest in infants (1.1 per 1,000 patient-days), and in those older than 80 years of age (0.9 per 1,000 patient-days).

Of 2,184 patients with a primary episode of HCAB, 1,166 (53.4%) were male and 1,018 (46.6%) were female. Median age was 57 years (IQR 41–70 years, range 0–89 years). The median time between prior and study admission was 11 days (IQR 6–19 days, range 1–30 days). The median length of stay for patients with HCAB was longer than patients who were at risk of, but did not present with HCAB (6 vs. 3 days, $p<0.001$). Male gender was associated with a higher risk of HCAB (odds ratio [OR] 1.29; 95%CI 1.18 to 1.40, $p<0.001$) (Figure 2). The incidence rates of

Table 1. Incidence rates of hospital-acquired bacteremia (HAB) and associated death rate between 2004 and 2010 in northeast Thailand.

Year	Total number of hospitals with available data	Total number of hospital admissions	Total number of hospital admissions at risk of HAB*	Total number of patients with HAB	Deaths associated with HAB	30-day mortality associated with HAB	Incidence rate for HAB (per 1,000 patient-days)
2004	3	129,376	74,272	212	90	42.5%	0.6
2005	3	138,816	79,254	292	120	41.1%	0.8
2006	4	187,812	102,948	259	100	38.6%	0.5
2007	6	241,208	129,574	366	185	50.5%	0.6
2008	9	372,564	199,154	640	281	43.9%	0.7
2009	10	453,791	239,814	840	388	46.2%	0.8
2010	10	445,907	244,427	815	395	48.5%	0.8
Overall	10	1,969,474	1,069,443	3,424	1,559	45.5%	0.7

*Patients at risk of HAB were patients who stayed in the hospital longer than 2 days.

Table 2. Cumulative incidence of healthcare-associated bacteremia (HCAB) and associated death rate between 2004 and 2010 in northeast Thailand.

Year	Total number of hospitals with available data	Total number of hospital admissions	Total number of hospital admission at risk of HCAB*	Total number of patients with HCAB	Deaths associated with HCAB	30-day mortality associated with HCAB	Cumulative incidence for HCAB (per 100 readmissions)
2004	3	129,376	7,259	86	44	51.2%	1.2
2005	3	138,816	8,266	125	41	32.8%	1.5
2006	4	187,812	10,960	157	68	43.3%	1.4
2007	6	241,209	14,234	272	117	43.0%	1.9
2008	9	372,564	22,601	435	198	45.5%	1.9
2009	10	453,790	26,969	527	206	39.1%	2.0
2010	10	445,907	28,997	582	239	41.1%	2.0
Overall	10	1,969,474	119,286	2,184	913	41.8%	1.8

*Patients at risk of HCAB were patients who had a hospital stay within 30 days prior to the admission.

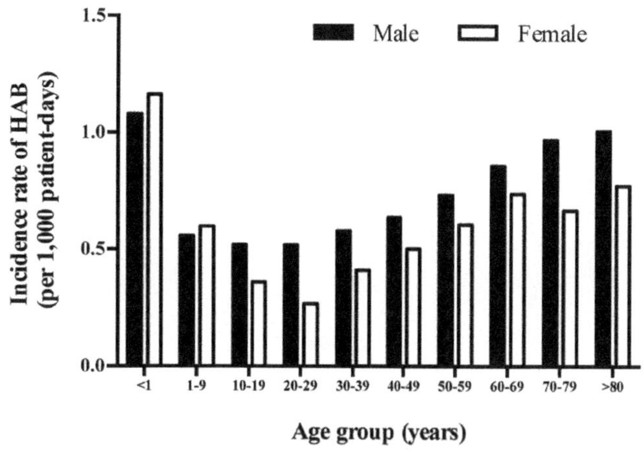

Figure 1. Age- and gender- specific incidence rates of hospital-acquired bacteremia (HAB) between 2004 and 2010 in north-east Thailand.

HCAB were high in infants (1.1 per 100 readmission), and very high in those older than 30 years of age (Figure 2).

Pathogenic organisms associated with HAB and HCAB

Of all pathogenic organisms causing HAB, 2,313 (67.6%) were Gram-negative bacteria, 885 (25.8%) were Gram-positive bacteria, 81 (2.4%) were fungi, 3 (0.1%) were *Mycobacterium* spp., and 141 (4.1%) were polymicrobial (Table 3). The most common pathogens identified were *Acinetobacter* spp. (16.2%), *Klebsiella pneumoniae* (13.9%), *Staphylococcus aureus* (13.9%), *Escherichia coli* (12.6%), and *Pseudomonas* spp. (10.5%). Amongst *S. aureus* HABs, the proportion of methicillin-resistant *S. aureus* (MRSA) was 37.0% (176/476). Corresponding proportions of extended-spectrum β lactamase (ESBL)-producing *E. coli* and *K. pneumoniae* were 38.9% (169/434) and 59.3% (283/477), respectively.

Of all pathogenic organisms causing HCAB, 1,470 (67.3%) were Gram-negative bacteria, 592 (27.1%) were Gram-positive bacteria, 24 (1.1%) were fungi, 4 (0.2%) were *Mycobacterium* spp., and 94 (4.3%) were polymicrobial (Table 3). The most common pathogens identified were *E. coli* (26.3%), *S. aureus* (14.0%), *K. pneumoniae* (9.7%), *Pseudomonas* spp. (9.4%) and *Acinetobacter* spp. (5.7%). The proportion of ESBL-producing *E. coli*, ESBL-

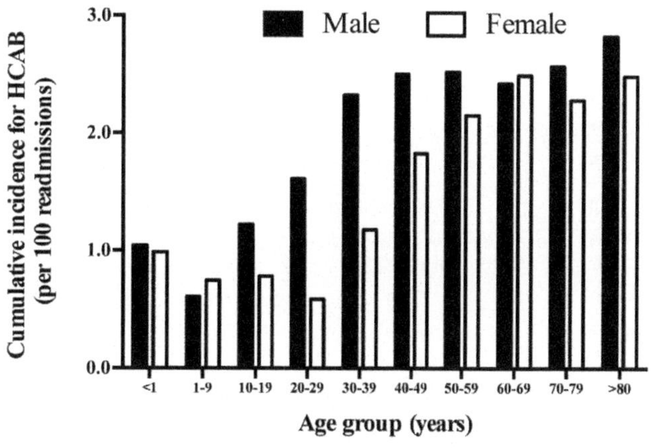

Figure 2. Age- and gender- specific cumulative incidence rates of healthcare-associated bacteremia (HCAB) between 2004 and 2010 in northeast Thailand.

Table 3. Pathogenic organisms associated with hospital-acquired bacteremia (HAB) or healthcare-acquired bacteremia (HCAB).

Organisms	HAB	HCAB
Gram negative bacteria	2,313 (67.6%)	1,470 (67.3%)
Acinetobacter spp.	554 (16.2%)	124 (5.7%)
Escherichia coli		
ESBL -ve	265 (7.7%)	400 (18.3%)
ESBL +ve	169 (4.9%)	175 (8.0%)
Klebsiella pneumoniae		
ESBL -ve	194 (5.7%)	141 (6.5%)
ESBL +ve	283 (8.3%)	70 (3.2%)
Klebsiella spp.	122 (3.6%)	55 (2.5%)
Enterobacter spp.	155 (4.5%)	44 (2.0%)
Pseudomonas spp.	358 (10.5%)	205 (9.4%)
Other Gram-negative bacteria	213 (6.2%)	256 (11.7%)
Gram positive bacteria	885 (25.8%)	592 (27.1%)
Staphylococcus aureus		
Methicillin-susceptible	300 (8.8%)	231 (10.6%)
Methicillin-resistant	176 (5.1%)	74 (3.4%)
Enterococcus spp.	173 (5.1%)	74 (3.4%)
Other Gram positive bacteria	236 (6.9%)	213 (9.8%)
Fungi	81 (2.4%)	24 (1.1%)
Cryptococcus spp.	16 (0.5%)	20 (0.9%)
Candida spp.	59 (1.7%)	4 (0.2%)
Penicillium spp.	6 (0.2%)	-
Histoplasma spp.	1 (0.0%)	-
Mycobacterium spp.	3 (0.1%)	4 (0.2%)
Polymicrobial infection	141 (4.1%)	94 (4.3%)
Overall	3,424 (100.0%)	2,184 (100.0%)

producing *K. pneumoniae* and MRSA were 30.4% (175/575), 33.2% (70/211), and 24.3% (74/305), respectively.

There were no differences in the patterns of common pathogens identified among different provinces or over the study period. However, there was an overall increase in the proportions of ESBL-producing *E. coli* over time. From 2004 to 2010, the proportion of ESBL-producing *E. coli* causing HAB rose from 33.3% (10/30) to 51.5% (51/99) ($p = 0.005$), and that causing HCAB rose from 20.8% (5/24) to 32.9% (48/146) ($p < 0.001$). The rising trend of ESBL-producing *E. coli* was observed in most hospitals. We did not observe a clear overall trend in the proportions of ESBL-producing *K. pneumoniae* or MRSA.

Mortality associated with HAB and HCAB

Death within 30-days of the positive blood culture taken was identified in 1,559 patients with HAB, giving an overall 30-day mortality of 45.5% (Table 1). Considering all patients who were admitted for more than 2 days, the 30-day mortality of those with HAB was higher than those without HAB (45.5% [1,559/3,424] vs. 5.5% [45,807/833,818], $p < 0.001$). Death in HAB patients occurred rapidly, with 749 of 1,559 deaths (48.0%) occurring within two days of the bacteremia, 89 (5.7%) on day 3, and 74 (4.8%) on day 4. Death in HAB patients occurred in hospital in 58.4% (911/1,559) of cases, the reminder occurring after hospital discharge. There was no change in the 30-day mortality associated with HAB over time ($p = 0.58$).

Death within 30 days of admission with an episode of HCAB was identified in 913 patients, giving an overall 30-day mortality of 41.8% (Table 2). Considering all patients who had a hospital stay within 30 days prior to the admission, the mortality of those with HCAB was significantly higher than those without HCAB (41.8% [913/2,184] vs. 13.0% [15,168/117,102], $p < 0.001$). Death in HCAB patients also occurred rapidly, with 410 of 913 deaths (45.7%) occurring within the first two days of admission, 54 (6.0%) on day 3, and 46 (5.1%) on day 4. Death in HCAB patients occurred in hospital in 43.2% (394/913) of cases, the reminder occurring after hospital discharge. There was no change in the 30-day mortality associated with HCAB over time ($p = 0.36$).

Discussion

Our study showed that nosocomial infection is an increasing and important problem in northeast Thailand. The total number of deaths associated with HAB and HCAB in 2010 in our study ($n = 634$) were much higher than the total number of reported deaths due to important notifiable diseases such as dengue hemorrhagic fever ($n = 139$), influenza ($n = 126$), and leptospirosis ($n = 43$) during the same period countrywide [12]. There was a 32.3% increase in the incidence rate of HAB and 66.8% in the cumulative incidence of HCAB between 2004 and 2010 in northeast Thailand. These estimates reinforce the need for improved surveillance and prevention of nosocomial infection in developing countries.

An incidence rate of HAB in the participating hospitals in 2010 of 0.8 per 1,000 patient-days is higher than recent estimates in high-income countries, including 0.7 per 1,000 patient-days in Canada between 2007–2010 [13], 0.6 per 1,000 patient-days in the USA in 2005 [14], and 0.6 per 1,000 patient-days in Estonia between 2004–2005 [15]. The Thai data are consistent with a recent review showing that other parameters used to estimate the burden of nosocomial infection in developing countries, such as prevalence of healthcare associated infections and ICU-acquired infections, are substantially higher than in developed countries [1]. The recent surveillance study conducted by the International Nosocomial Infection Control Consortium (INICC) also found that rates of central line associated bloodstream infection (CLAB) were significantly higher in ICUs in developing countries (6.8 per 1,000 central line-days) versus those reported in US ICUs (2.0 per 1,000 central line-days) [16]. Our HAB incidence rate is, however, lower than HAB rates reported through active surveillance in some developing countries, including 1.0 per 1,000 patient-days in Kenya between 2002–2009 [4], and 1.2 per 1,000 patient-days in Iran in 2006 [5]. It is possible that active surveillance may improve the detection of HAB and nosocomial infection in our geographical region.

During the study period, *Acinetobacter* spp. was the most common pathogen associated with HAB, followed by *K. pneumoniae* and *S. aureus*. *Acinetobacter* spp. is increasingly recognized as an important cause of nosocomial infection [17], and our study confirms the importance this species as a leading cause of nosocomial infection in developing tropical countries [1,4,18]. The proportion of MRSA causing HAB in our setting (37%) was higher than that reported from developed countries [13,15,19], and is consistent with a previous review of developing countries [1]. An increase in the proportion of ESBL-producing *E. coli* causing HAB in our study is alarming, and is consistent with our previous report of an increase in the proportion of ESBL-producing organisms causing CAB in the same setting [6].

This study highlights an increasing incidence of HCAB in developing countries. We used the total number of patients with readmission as a denominator to estimate the cumulative incidence of HCAB rather than the total number of patients with bacteremia [8,9,20]. Our estimates showed that healthcare-associated infection was an increasing cause of readmission. The high proportion of MRSA, ESBL-producing *E. coli* and ESBL-producing *K. pneumoniae* amongst organisms causing HCAB was relatively similar to that causing HAB. Much lower resistance levels were seen in organisms causing CAB [6]. This is consistent with previous reports of HCAB in developed countries [8,9,20].

The observed increase in incidence of both HAB and HCAB could be due to a combination of an increase in the incidence of nosocomial infection associated with a rise in the number of at-risk patients (for example aging patients and those with invasive interventions), and an increase in detection of HAB and HCAB due to improved healthcare practice over time. There is evidence that the incidence rate of CLAB in developing countries can be substantially reduced using a multi-dimensional infection control approach including a bundle of interventions, education, outcome surveillance, process surveillance, feedback on CLAB rate and performance feedback [21–27].

The overall 30-day mortality with HAB of 45.5% in our setting is much higher than that typically reported in high-income countries [13,15,28], but lower than the reported in-hospital mortality of 53% from a rural district hospital in Kenya [4]. The overall 30-day mortality with HCAB of 41.8% in our setting is also much higher than typically seen in high-income countries [8,9,20]. In addition to patient-related factors, the higher mortality typically seen in developing countries may be related to the proportion of antimicrobial-resistant pathogens, empirical antibiotic regimens used, and sub-optimal severe sepsis management in resource-limited settings [4,29]. It is also possible that practice in high-income countries can detect milder bacteremia cases such as cases due to intravenous device that is then rapidly removed, while the practice in low-income countries may be less likely to achieve this. The high mortality observed in our study also reflects post-dischage ascertainment of patient outcomes using the national death registry. We found that in 47.2% of fatal cases of HAB or HCAB death occurred after hospital discharge. This reflects a preference amongst people in the study area to die at home. Further studies need to explore how to reduce the mortality of patients with HAB and HCAB in resource-limited areas.

A limitation of this study is that more complete clinical data were not available. As data on central line days were not available, the incidence rate of CLAB per 1,000 central line days could not be estimated and benchmarked against other prospective studies [30–47]. As data on process surveillance were not available, the reasons for the increased incidence of HAB could not be systematically assessed [32,41,48,49]. Another potential limitation is that blood cultures may not have been performed for all patients with a likelihood of nosocomial infection, and this might lead to an underestimation in the incidence of HAB and HCAB among participating hospitals. In addition, data on hospitalization in other hospitals not participating in the study (for example, a district hospital or a private hospital in the province) were not available, which could have resulted in an underestimation of the incidence of HAB and HCAB in our study. It is also possible that some patients with HAB and HCAB in our study may have had contaminated cultures and were incorrectly counted. However, the high mortality in patients with HAB and HCAB suggested that true infection was more likely than culture contamination. Although our data showed that, in general, patients with HAB and HCAB stayed in the hospital longer than those without, the analysis did not take account of the high mortality associated with HAB and HCAB. The length of stay would be further extended if death of patients with HAB and HCAB could be reduced. Additional costs and extra length of stay attributable to HAB and HCAB will be further evaluated using health economic models [50,51].

Although monitoring of nosocomial infection in developing countries is hampered by incomplete routine notification, our study has shown that careful evaluation of readily available routinely collected databases can provide valuable information on the incidence and trend of HAB and HCAB. The methodology used in our study could be applied to other geographical areas where microbiological facilities are available to provide a more comprehensive global picture of the importance of nosocomial infection as a cause of death.

Supporting Information

Figure S1 Location of participating hospitals. These were situated in: (1) Loei, (2) Udon Thani, (3) Nong Khai, (4) Nakhon Phanom, (5) Chaiyaphum, (6) Mahasarakarm, (7) Yasothorn, (8) Buriram, (9) Sisaket, and (10) Ubon Ratchathani.

Figure S2 Trend in hospital-acquired bacteremia (HAB) in ten provincial hospitals in Thailand.

Figure S3 Trend in healthcare-associated bacteremia (HCAB) in ten provincial hospitals in Thailand.

Table S1 List of participating hospitals.

Acknowledgments

We gratefully acknowledge the Bacterial Infection in North East Thailand (BINET) network for providing microbiological and hospital admission data. BINET are comprised of Chalavit Limpavithayakula, Chatchawan Namsorn, Chadaporn Paungmala (Amnatchareon hospital), Chan Tantiwaraporn, Somsak Kitisriworapun, Kanyapak Panjaiya, Kridsada Sirichaisit (Buengkarn hospital), Chalit Thongprayoon, Somchai Jittai, Rattana Jirajaruporn (Buriram hospital), Sompong Charoenwat, Some Prasarn, Wiset Phosawang, Peeraphorn Lamworaphong (Chaiyaphum hospital), Pramoth Boonjian, Pattarawadee Wongmeema, Sunthorn Thongbai (Loei hospital), Sunthorn Yontrakul, Piyalak Siritaratiwat, Supanne Pisuttimarn (Mahasarakham hospital), Udom Pedphuwadee (Mukdaharn hospital), Somkid Suriyalert, Pichai Thongtaradol, Somsri Viriyaphun (Nakhon Phanom hospital), Kittisak Danwiboon, Kanjana Kehatan, Wannakorn Dechnorasing (Nongkhai hospital), Narong Uentrakul (Roi Ed hospital), Somsak Chaosirikul, Anek Jaddee, Soontorn Romaneeyapech (Sisaket hospital), Thongchai Triwiboonwanich, Saowarat Deekae, Vorathep Wuttisil (Surin hospital), Pramot Srisamang, Nittaya Teerawattanasook (Ubon Ratchathani hospital), Pichart Dolchalermyuttana, Yaowalau Loottrakul, Sayrung Sripavatakul (Udon Thani hospital), Charan Thongthap, Pongsathorn Siripoulsak, Chainakhon Kaewluang (Yasothorn hospital). We thank Mayura Malasit and Jintana Suwannapruk for their administrative support. We gratefully acknowledge the support provided by staff at the Mahidol-Oxford Tropical Medicine Research Unit and all participating hospitals. We thank Chutawat Luangsa-ard, Kraiwuth Sriporamanont, Mongkol Fungprasertkul and Dean Sherwood for computational support.

Author Contributions

Conceived and designed the experiments: MH PS MK AJ NPD SJP DL. Performed the experiments: MH MK AJ DL. Analyzed the data: MH AJ DL. Contributed to the writing of the manuscript: MH PS MK NL AJ NPD SJP BSC DL.

References

1. Allegranzi B, Bagheri Nejad S, Combescure C, Graafmans W, Attar H, et al. (2011) Burden of endemic health-care-associated infection in developing countries: systematic review and meta-analysis. Lancet 377(9761): p.228–41.
2. Vrijens F, Hulstaert F, Van de Sande S, Devriese S, Morales I, et al. (2010) Hospital-acquired, laboratory-confirmed bloodstream infections: linking national surveillance data to clinical and financial hospital data to estimate increased length of stay and healthcare costs. J Hosp Infect 75(3): p.158–62.
3. Wenzel RP, Edmond MB (2001) The impact of hospital-acquired bloodstream infections. Emerg Infect Dis 7(2): p.174–7.
4. Aiken AM, Mturi N, Njuguna P, Mohammed S, Berkley JA, et al. (2011) Risk and causes of paediatric hospital-acquired bacteraemia in Kilifi District Hospital, Kenya: a prospective cohort study. Lancet 378(9808): p.2021–7.
5. Askarian M, Mahmoudi H, Assadian O (2013) Incidence of Nosocomial Infections in a Big University Affiliated Hospital in Shiraz, Iran: A Six-month Experience. Int J Prev Med 4(3): p.366–72.
6. Kanoksil M, Jatapai A, Peacock SJ, Limmathurotsakul D (2013) Epidemiology, microbiology and mortality associated with community-acquired bacteremia in northeast Thailand: a multicenter surveillance study. PLoS One 8(1): p. e54714.
7. Opartkiattikul N, Bejrachandra S (2002) The external quality assessment schemes in Thailand. Rinsho Byori 50(2): p.121–5.
8. Shorr AF, Tabak YP, Killian AD, Gupta V, Liu LZ, et al. (2006) Healthcare-associated bloodstream infection: A distinct entity? Insights from a large U.S. database. Crit Care Med 34(10): p.2588–95.
9. Rodriguez-Bano J, Lopez-Prieto MD, Portillo MM, Retamar P, Natera C, et al. (2010) Epidemiology and clinical features of community-acquired, healthcare-associated and nosocomial bloodstream infections in tertiary-care and community hospitals. Clin Microbiol Infect 16(9): p.1408–13.
10. Hall KK, Lyman JA (2006) Updated review of blood culture contamination. Clin Microbiol Rev 19(4): p.788–802.
11. Wiersinga WJ, Currie BJ, Peacock SJ (2012) Melioidosis. N Engl J Med 367(11): p.1035–44.
12. Epidemiology BO (2011) Annual Epidemiology Surveillance Report 2010.
13. Fortin E, Rocher I, Frenette C, Tremblay C, Quach C (2012) Healthcare-associated bloodstream infections secondary to a urinary focus: the Quebec provincial surveillance results. Infect Control Hosp Epidemiol 33(5): p.456–62.
14. Lee MC, Saxinger L, Forgie SE, Taylor G (2010) Trends in nosocomial bloodstream infections following health care restructuring in Alberta between 1999 and 2005. Can J Infect Dis Med Microbiol 21(1): p. e1–5.
15. Mitt P, Adamson V, Loivukene K, Lang K, Telling K, et al. (2009) Epidemiology of nosocomial bloodstream infections in Estonia. J Hosp Infect 71(4): p.365–70.
16. Rosenthal VD, Bijie H, Maki DG, Mehta Y, Apisarnthanarak A, et al. (2012) International Nosocomial Infection Control Consortium (INICC) report, data summary of 36 countries, for 2004–2009. Am J Infect Control 40(5): p.396–407.
17. Peleg AY, Hooper DC (2010) Hospital-acquired infections due to gram-negative bacteria. N Engl J Med 362(19): p.1804–13.
18. Pereira CA, Marra AR, Camargo LF, Pignatari AC, Sukiennik T, et al. (2013) Nosocomial bloodstream infections in Brazilian pediatric patients: microbiology, epidemiology, and clinical features. PLoS One 8(7): p. e68144.
19. Johnson AP (2011) Methicillin-resistant Staphylococcus aureus: the European landscape. J Antimicrob Chemother 66 Suppl 4: p. iv43–iv48.
20. Son JS, Song JH, Ko KS, Yeom JS, Ki HK, et al. (2010) Bloodstream infections and clinical significance of healthcare-associated bacteremia: a multicenter surveillance study in Korean hospitals. J Korean Med Sci 25(7): p.992–8.
21. Rosenthal VD, Maki DG, Rodrigues C, Alvarez-Moreno C, Leblebicioglu H, et al. (2010) Impact of International Nosocomial Infection Control Consortium (INICC) strategy on central line-associated bloodstream infection rates in the intensive care units of 15 developing countries. Infect Control Hosp Epidemiol 31(12): p.1264–72.
22. Rosenthal VD, Ramachandran B, Villamil-Gomez W, Armas-Ruiz A, Navoa-Ng JA, et al. (2012) Impact of a multidimensional infection control strategy on central line-associated bloodstream infection rates in pediatric intensive care units of five developing countries: findings of the International Nosocomial Infection Control Consortium (INICC). Infection 40(4): p.415–23.
23. Rosenthal VD, Duenas L, Sobreyra-Oropeza M, Ammar K, Navoa-Ng JA, et al. (2013) Findings of the International Nosocomial Infection Control Consortium (INICC), part III: effectiveness of a multidimensional infection control approach to reduce central line-associated bloodstream infections in the neonatal intensive care units of 4 developing countries. Infect Control Hosp Epidemiol 34(3): p.229–37.
24. Jaggi N, Rodrigues C, Rosenthal VD, Todi SK, Shah S, et al. (2013) Impact of an international nosocomial infection control consortium multidimensional approach on central line-associated bloodstream infection rates in adult intensive care units in eight cities in India. Int J Infect Dis 17(12): p. e1218–24.
25. Leblebicioglu H, Ozturk R, Rosenthal VD, Akan OA, Sirmatel F, et al. (2013) Impact of a multidimensional infection control approach on central line-associated bloodstream infections rates in adult intensive care units of 8 cities of Turkey: findings of the International Nosocomial Infection Control Consortium (INICC). Ann Clin Microbiol Antimicrob 12: p.10.
26. Higuera F, Rosenthal VD, Duarte P, Ruiz J, Franco G, et al. (2005) The effect of process control on the incidence of central venous catheter-associated bloodstream infections and mortality in intensive care units in Mexico. Crit Care Med 33(9): p.2022–7.
27. Rosenthal VD, Guzman S, Pezzotto SM, Crnich CJ (2003) Effect of an infection control program using education and performance feedback on rates of intravascular device-associated bloodstream infections in intensive care units in Argentina. Am J Infect Control 31(7): p.405–9.
28. Klevens RM, Edwards JR, Richards CL Jr, Horan TC, Gaynes RP, et al. (2007) Estimating health care-associated infections and deaths in U.S. hospitals, 2002. Public Health Rep 122(2): p.160–6.
29. Cheng AC, West TE, Limmathurotsakul D, Peacock SJ (2008) Strategies to reduce mortality from bacterial sepsis in adults in developing countries. PLoS Med 5(8): p. e175.
30. Duenas L, Bran de Casares A, Rosenthal VD, Jesus Machuca L (2011) Device-associated infections rates in pediatrics and neonatal intensive care units in El Salvador: findings of the INICC. J Infect Dev Ctries 5(6): p.445–51.
31. Guanche-Garcell H, Requejo-Pino O, Rosenthal VD, Morales-Perez C, Delgado-Gonzalez O, et al. (2011) Device-associated infection rates in adult intensive care units of Cuban university hospitals: International Nosocomial Infection Control Consortium (INICC) findings. Int J Infect Dis 15(5): p. e357–62.
32. Hu B, Tao L, Rosenthal VD, Liu K, Yun Y, et al. (2013) Device-associated infection rates, device use, length of stay, and mortality in intensive care units of 4 Chinese hospitals: International Nosocomial Control Consortium findings. Am J Infect Control 41(4): p.301–6.
33. Kubler A, Duszynska W, Rosenthal VD, Fleischer M, Kaiser T, et al. (2012) Device-associated infection rates and extra length of stay in an intensive care unit of a university hospital in Wroclaw, Poland: International Nosocomial Infection Control Consortium's (INICC) findings. J Crit Care 27(1): p.105 e5–10.
34. Navoa-Ng JA, Berba R, Galapia YA, Rosenthal VD, Villanueva VD, et al. (2011) Device-associated infections rates in adult, pediatric, and neonatal

intensive care units of hospitals in the Philippines: International Nosocomial Infection Control Consortium (INICC) findings. Am J Infect Control 39(7): p.548–54.
35. Rasslan O, Seliem ZS, Ghazi IA, El Sabour MA, El Kholy AA, et al. (2012) Device-associated infection rates in adult and pediatric intensive care units of hospitals in Egypt. International Nosocomial Infection Control Consortium (INICC) findings. J Infect Public Health 5(6): p.394–402.
36. Tao L, Hu B, Rosenthal VD, Gao X, He L (2011) Device-associated infection rates in 398 intensive care units in Shanghai, China: International Nosocomial Infection Control Consortium (INICC) findings. Int J Infect Dis 15(11): p. e774–80.
37. Rosenthal VD, Guzman S, Orellano PW (2003) Nosocomial infections in medical-surgical intensive care units in Argentina: attributable mortality and length of stay. Am J Infect Control 31(5): p.291–5.
38. Rosenthal VD, Guzman S, Crnich C (2004) Device-associated nosocomial infection rates in intensive care units of Argentina. Infect Control Hosp Epidemiol 25(3): p.251–5.
39. Moreno CA, Rosenthal VD, Olarte N, Gomez WV, Sussmann O, et al. (2006) Device-associated infection rate and mortality in intensive care units of 9 Colombian hospitals: findings of the International Nosocomial Infection Control Consortium. Infect Control Hosp Epidemiol 27(4): p.349–56.
40. Ramirez Barba EJ, Rosenthal VD, Higuera F, Oropeza MS, Hernandez HT, et al. (2006) Device-associated nosocomial infection rates in intensive care units in four Mexican public hospitals. Am J Infect Control 34(4): p.244–7.
41. Rosenthal VD, Maki DG, Salomao R, Moreno CA, Mehta Y, et al. (2006) Device-associated nosocomial infections in 55 intensive care units of 8 developing countries. Ann Intern Med, 2006. 145(8): p.582–91.
42. Leblebicioglu H, Rosenthal VD, Arikan OA, Ozgultekin A, Yalcin AN, et al. (2007) Device-associated hospital-acquired infection rates in Turkish intensive care units. Findings of the International Nosocomial Infection Control Consortium (INICC). J Hosp Infect 65(3): p.251–7.
43. Mehta A, Rosenthal VD, Mehta Y, Chakravarthy M, Todi SK, et al. (2007) Device-associated nosocomial infection rates in intensive care units of seven Indian cities. Findings of the International Nosocomial Infection Control Consortium (INICC). J Hosp Infect 67(2): p.168–74.
44. Cuellar LE, Fernandez-Maldonado E, Rosenthal VD, Castaneda-Sabogal A, Rosales R, et al. (2008) Device-associated infection rates and mortality in intensive care units of Peruvian hospitals: findings of the International Nosocomial Infection Control Consortium. Rev Panam Salud Publica 24(1): p.16–24.
45. Rosenthal VD (2008) Device-associated nosocomial infections in limited-resources countries: findings of the International Nosocomial Infection Control Consortium (INICC). Am J Infect Control 36(10): p. S171 e7–12.
46. Salomao R, Rosenthal VD, Grimberg G, Nouer S, Blecher S, et al. (2008) Device-associated infection rates in intensive care units of Brazilian hospitals: findings of the International Nosocomial Infection Control Consortium. Rev Panam Salud Publica 24(3): p.195–202.
47. Madani N, Rosenthal VD, Dendane T, Abidi K, Zeggwagh AA, et al. (2009) Health-care associated infections rates, length of stay, and bacterial resistance in an intensive care unit of Morocco: findings of the International Nosocomial Infection Control Consortium (INICC). Int Arch Med 2(1): p.29.
48. Friedman C, Richter D, Skylis T, Brown D (1984) Process surveillance: auditing infection control policies and procedures. Am J Infect Control 12(4): p.228–32.
49. Baker OG (1997) Process surveillance: an epidemiologic challenge for all health care organizations. Am J Infect Control 25(2): p.96–101.
50. Higuera F, Rangel-Frausto MS, Rosenthal VD, Soto JM, Castanon J, et al. (2007) Attributable cost and length of stay for patients with central venous catheter-associated bloodstream infection in Mexico City intensive care units: a prospective, matched analysis. Infect Control Hosp Epidemiol 28(1): p.31–5.
51. Rosenthal VD, Guzman S, Migone O, Crnich CJ (2003) The attributable cost, length of hospital stay, and mortality of central line-associated bloodstream infection in intensive care departments in Argentina: A prospective, matched analysis. Am J Infect Control 31(8): p.475–80.

9

Screening for Older Emergency Department Inpatients at Risk of Prolonged Hospital Stay: The Brief Geriatric Assessment Tool

Cyrille P. Launay[1], Laure de Decker[2], Anastasiia Kabeshova[1], Cédric Annweiler[1,3], Olivier Beauchet[1,4]*

1 Department of Neuroscience, Division of Geriatric Medicine, UPRES EA 4638, UNAM, Angers University Hospital, Angers, France, **2** Department of Geriatrics, EA 1156–12, Nantes University Hospital, Nantes, France, **3** Robarts Research Institute, Schulich School of Medicine and Dentistry, the University of Western Ontario, London, Ontario, Canada, **4** Biomathics, Paris, France

Abstract

Background: The aims of this study were 1) to confirm that combinations of brief geriatric assessment (BGA) items were significant risk factors for prolonged LHS among geriatric patients hospitalized in acute care medical units after their admission to the emergency department (ED); and 2) to determine whether these combinations of BGA items could be used as a prognostic tool of prolonged LHS.

Methods: Based on a prospective observational cohort design, 1254 inpatients (mean age ± standard deviation, 84.9±5.9 years; 59.3% female) recruited upon their admission to ED and discharged in acute care medical units of Angers University Hospital, France, were selected in this study. At baseline assessment, a BGA was performed and included the following 6 items: age ≥85years, male gender, polypharmacy (i.e., ≥5 drugs per day), use of home-help services, history of falls in previous 6 months and temporal disorientation (i.e., inability to give the month and/or year). The LHS in acute care medical units was prospectively calculated in number of days using the hospital registry.

Results: Area under receiver operating characteristic (ROC) curves of prolonged LHS of different combinations of BGA items ranged from 0.50 to 0.57. Cox regression models revealed that combinations defining a high risk of prolonged LHS, identified from ROC curves, were significant risk factors for prolonged LHS (hazard ratio >1.16 with P>0.010). Kaplan-Meier distributions of discharge showed that inpatients classified in high-risk group of prolonged LHS were discharged later than those in low-risk group (P<0.003). Prognostic value for prolonged LHS of all combinations was poor with sensitivity under 77%, a high variation of specificity (from 26.6 to 97.4) and a low likelihood ratio of positive test under 5.6.

Conclusion: Combinations of 6-item BGA tool were significant risk factors for prolonged LHS but their prognostic value was poor in the studied sample of older inpatients.

Editor: Leocadio Rodríguez-Mañas, Hospital Universitario de Getafe, Spain

Funding: The authors report no current funding sources for this study.

Competing Interests: O. Beauchet is affiliated with Biomathics, Paris. There are no patents, products in development or marketed products to declare.

* Email: olbeauchet@chu-angers.fr

Introduction

Older adults are the fastest increasing group of patients admitted to hospital, often through emergency departments (ED) [1,2]. Compared to younger inpatients, multimorbidity and related-disabilities leading to a high disease burden characterize the older inpatients group [3–5]. Because hospital is largely configured for single acute disease rather than multimorbidity and related disability, age-related high burden disease is one of the main challenges faced by hospitals [6]. Thus, assessing and addressing the needs of the growing number of older inpatients with a greater range of acute and chronic diseases causing disability but not mortality is mandatory [6–8].

Adapted care plan of older inpatients are based on multidimensional, interdisciplinary diagnostic process to determine the medical, psychological, and functional capabilities called comprehensive geriatric assessment (CGA) [3]. CGA allows a coordinated and integrated plan for treatment, and thus may prevent complicated medical pathway characterized, for instance, by prolonged length of hospital stay (LHS) [4,3,9]. Early screening of older inpatients at risk of prolonged LHS based on CGA approach is the first step of an adapted care plan of older inpatients because it improves the medical decision-making process, and thus the care pathway [4,10].

Benefits of CGA have been confirmed through a meta-analysis reporting a reduction of admissions and readmissions to hospital [11]. Recently, it has been reported that an early intervention made by geriatricians of a mobile geriatric team (MGT) using a 6-item brief CGA (BGA) reduced LHS in older inpatients [12]. The 6-item BGA has been developed in response to the difficulty of systematic implementation of CGA in daily practice for every older inpatient admitted to ED [4,13,14]. It has been shown that CGA cannot be applied to every older inpatient, and that the best compromise could be the use of two-step approach [15]. The first step is the screening of older inpatients at high risk of adverse outcomes such as prolonged LHS by non-geriatricians using a brief and accurate screening tool applicable during clinical practice, and the second step is a CGA by geriatricians with a diagnostic and therapeutic purpose [15,16].

We recently showed that different combinations of the 6-item BGA tool (i.e., age ≥85 years, gender male, polypharmacy, non-use of home services, history of falls and cognitive decline) were risk factors for prolonged LHS in a cohort of 424 older patients admitted to acute care medical units following ED discharge [16,17]. Among these different combinations, history of falls and cognitive decline were major predictors for prolonged LHS. We also reported that the maximum number of items to predict prolonged LHS was 4. Indeed, the combination of a history of falls, male gender, cognitive impairment and age under 85 years, identified older patients at highest risk of prolonged LHS. These results allowed the identification of 3 levels of risk of prolonged LHS (i.e., high, intermediate and low) according to different combinations of the BGA 6 items. The aims of this study were 1) to confirm that combinations of BGA items were significant risk factors for prolonged LHS among geriatric patients hospitalized in acute care medical units after their admission to the ED; and 2) to determine whether these combinations of BGA items could be used as a prognostic tool of prolonged LHS.

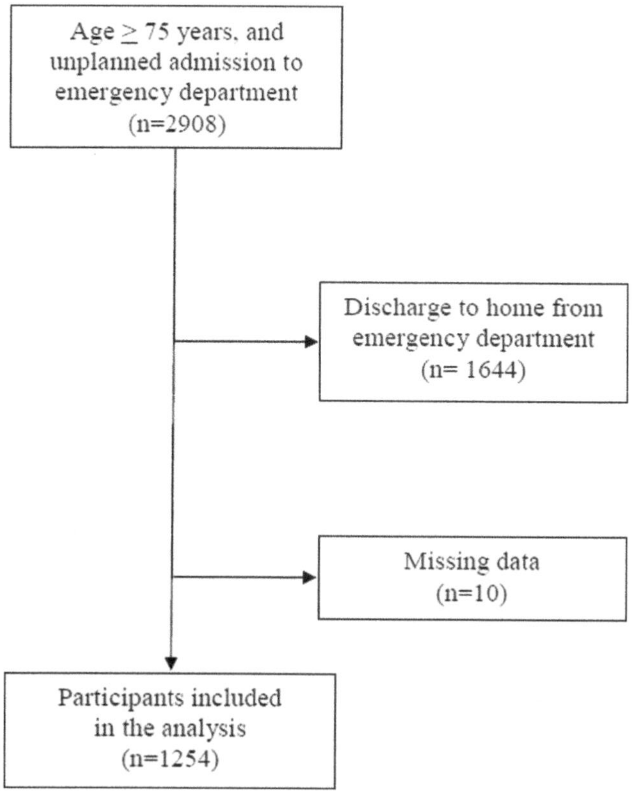

Figure 1. Flow chart showing the selection of participants included in the analysis.

Methods

Recruitment of participants

Between January and December 2012, 2908 older adults aged 75 years and over were admitted to the ED of Angers University Hospital, France. Among them, 1264 (43.5%) were discharged in acute care medical units. None of them declined to be part of the study. Inclusion criteria were: unplanned admissions in ED followed by discharge in acute care medical units, age of 75 years and over, not identified as treatment-limiting decision and willingness to participate. A total of 10 participants have missing data and were excluded form the analysis. In final, 1254 participants (mean age ± standard deviation, 84.9±5.9 years; 59.3% female) were included in the study (Figure 1).

Assessment of participants

The 6-item BGA was performed upon the admission to ED. It was composed of the following items: age coded as a binary variable (i.e.,≥ or <85 years), gender, polypharmacy defined as ≥ 5 drugs per day, use of formal and/or informal home-help services coded as a binary variable (i.e., yes or no), history of falls in previous 6 months coded as a binary variable (i.e., yes or no), and temporal disorientation defined as the inability to give the month and/or year coded as a binary variable (i.e., yes or no). We chose these items because each of them has been separately associated with a prolonged LHS and because we previously reported that their combinations predicted prolonged LHS [16–20]. The place of life (i.e., home versus institution) and the reasons for admission to ED were also recorded because these parameters have both been associated with prolonged LHS [18–20]. Reasons for admission were categorized using two complementary approaches. First, we distinguished acute organ failure versus non-acute organ failure. Second, we specified the nature of the acute organ failure in four subgroups based on the prevalence of related diseases in our sample of participants: 19.5% (n = 156) cardio-vascular diseases, 18.4% (n = 147) respiratory diseases, 16.2% (n = 129) digestive diseases, 12.0% (n = 96) neuropsychiatric diseases and 33.9% (n = 271) other acute diseases. In addition, the use of psychoactive drugs including benzodiazepines, antidepressants or neuroleptics was noted.

Definition of endpoints

The risk of prolonged LHS was estimated using two consecutive strategies. First, *a priori* combinations of BGA items as previously reported to determine 3 levels of risk of prolonged LHS [16,17]. High risk of prolonged LHS was defined by the combination of cognitive decline + history of falls. Intermediate risk was defined by the finding of cognitive decline, or history of falls, or the combination of age ≥85years + male gender + polypharmacy + no use of home services. Low risk of prolonged LHS was defined by the combination of 3 items or less among age ≥85years, male gender male, polypharmacy, and no use of home services. No information was provided to the physicians in charge of the patients. Second, we explored all other possible combinations of BGA items using the receiver operating characteristic (ROC) curve. A new classification into three levels of risk of prolonged LHS was therefore built using areas under ROC separated into three parts (i.e., highest, intermediate and lowest values). The three best combinations for each part were used to define the risk of prolonged LHS. The LHS was prospectively calculated using the administrative registry of the University Hospital and corresponded to the delay in days between the first day of

Table 1. Baseline characteristics of participants (n = 1254).

Characteristics	Value	[95% confidence interval]
Age (years)		
Mean ±SD	84.9±5.9	[84.6–85.3]
≥85 years	671 (53.5)	[50.7–56.3]
Male gender, n (%)	511 (40.7)	[38.0–43.5]
Number of drugs daily taken		
Mean ±SD	6.7±3.2	[6.6–6.9]
≥5, n (%)	929 (74.1)	[71.7–76.5]
Use of psychoactive drugs*, n (%)	646 (51.1)	[48.8–54.3]
History of falls during the past 6 months, n (%)	468 (37.3)	[34.6–40.0]
Temporal disorientation†, n (%)	415 (33.1)	[30.5–35.7]
Non-use of formal and/or informal home services‡	310 (24.7)	[22.3–27.1]
Living at home	875 (69.7)	[67.2–72.3]
Acute organ failure as reason for admission to Emergency Department, n (%)	799 (63.3)	[61.0–66.4]
Cardio-vascular diseases, n (%)	156 (19.5)	[16.8–22.3]
Respiratory diseases, n (%)	147 (18.4)	[15.7–21.1]
Digestive diseases, n (%)	129 (16.2)	[13.6–18.7]
Neuropsychiatric diseases, n (%)	96 (12.0)	[9.8–14.3]
Other diseases, n (%)	271 (33.9)	[30.6–37.2]
Length of hospital stay (days), mean ±SD	8.8±8.4	[8.3–9.2]

SD: standard deviation.
*: Use of benzodiazepines or antidepressants or neuroleptics.
†: Inability to give the month and/or year.
‡: Formal (i.e., health and/or social professional) or informal (i.e., family and/or friends).

admission to ED and the last day of hospitalization in the acute care medical units. Prolonged LHS was defined as being in the highest tertile of LHS (i.e.,>13 days).

Statistical analysis

First, the participants' baseline characteristics were summarized using means and standard deviations or frequencies and percentages, as appropriate. Second, areas under ROC curve of prolonged LHS was calculated for each item and all possible combinations. Third, univariate and multiple Cox regression models were performed to examine the association between prolonged LHS (dependent variable) and the different combinations of BGA items (independent variables) stratified in three risk-levels (low, intermediate, high). For multiple Cox regression models, two types of models were distinguished: those using low-risk level of prolonged LHS as reference and the others. In both cases, there was an adjustment on the place of life and the reasons for admission to ED. Two kind of adjustment were done for reasons of admission using either acute organ failure as independent variable or the nature of acute organ failures (i.e., cardio-vascular diseases, respiratory diseases, digestive diseases, neuropsychiatric diseases and other diseases). Exponential of negative coefficients were calculated for each model. The model produced a survival function that provided the probability of discharge of hospital at a given time for the features supplied for independent variables. Fourth, we studied the elapsed time to discharge from acute care medical units by survival Kaplan-Meier curves and log-rank test. Because only discharge to acute care medical unit was examined, the analysis was censored to 21 days. Fifth, sensitivity, specificity, positive (PPV) and negative (NPV) predictive values, likelihood ratios of positive (LR+) and negative (LR-) tests of each BGA item and all possible combinations of prolonged LHS were calculated. P-values <0.05 were considered statistically significant. All statistics were performed using SPSS (version 19.0; SPSS, Inc., Chicago, IL) and RStudio.

Standard Protocol Approvals, Registrations, and Participant Consents

The study was conducted in accordance with the ethical standards set forth in the Helsinki Declaration (1983). All participants recruited in this study provided a verbal informed consent because the study did not change the usual clinical practice. The verbal informed consent was obtained from the patients themselves in the presence of their trusted person, usually a family member, who helped them to make decision. The participant consent was recorded in the digital file of patients. The entire study protocol and the consent procedure were approved by the Ethical Committee of Angers, France.

Results

The baseline characteristics of participants are presented in Table 1. More than half of patients were aged 85 years and over. A total of 74.1% took 5 and over different drugs per day. Nearly one third had a history of falls in the past 6 months or had temporal disorientation. One quarter of participants were isolated, and more than two thirds lived at home. A total of 63.3% patients were admitted to ED for an acute organ failure. The main causes of acute organ failure were cardiovascular diseases (19.5%), respiratory diseases (18.4%), digestive diseases (16.2%) and neuropsychiatric diseases (12.0%). The mean LHS was around 9 days. A total of 157 patients (12.5%) died during hospitalization.

Table 2. Area under Receiver operating characteristic curve and prognostic values of brief geriatric assessment items and their combinations* for prolonged length of hospital stay† (n = 1254).

	Area under ROC	Sensitivity(%)	Specify(%)	PPV (%)	NPV (%)	LR+	LR-	Number of individuals classified			
								TP	FP	FN	TN
6 items of the brief geriatric assessment, considered separately											
Age≥85 years	0.50	53.02	46.34	23.55	75.99	0.99	1.01	158	513	140	443
Male gender	0.50	40.94	59.31	23.87	76.31	1.00	1.00	122	389	176	576
Polypharmacy‡	0.51	76.17	26.57	24.43	78.15	1.04	0.90	227	702	71	254
Non-use of home help services§	0.52	27.85	76.26	26.77	77.22	1.17	0.95	83	227	215	729
History of falls¶	0.52	39.93	63.49	25.43	77.23	1.09	0.95	119	349	179	607
Temporal disorientation#	0.55	40.94	69.35	29.40	79.02	1.34	0.58	122	293	176	663
Combinations of the 6 items of the brief geriatric assessment **											
A priori combinations††											
Low risk											
Male + polypharmacy‡ + non-use of home services§	0.54	9.40	91.95	26.67	76.50	1.17	0.99	28	77	270	879
Age≥85 years + polypharmacy‡ + non-use of home services§	0.53	9.06	94.46	33.75	76.92	1.63	0.96	27	53	271	903
Age≥85 years + male + non-use of home services§	0.52	3.69	96.13	22.92	76.20	0.95	1.00	11	37	287	919
Intermediate risk											
History of falls	0.52	39.93	63.49	25.43	77.23	1.09	0.95	119	349	179	607
Temporal disorientation#	0.55	40.94	69.35	29.40	79.02	1.34	0.58	122	293	176	663
Age ≥85years + male + polypharmacy‡ + non-use of home services§	0.54	2.35	97.38	21.88	76.19	0.90	1.00	7	25	291	931
High risk											
History of falls + temporal disorientation#	0.56	18.46	86.30	29.57	77.25	1.35	0.95	55	131	243	825
Newly identified combinations											
Low risk											
Polypharmacy‡ + non-use of home help services§	0.53	17.79	84.21	25.98	76.67	1.13	0.98	53	151	245	805
Polypharmacy‡ + history of falls	0.53	31.88	75.00	28.44	77.93	1.28	0.91	95	239	203	717
Age≥85 years + polypharmacy‡ + history of falls	0.53	17.79	83.89	25.60	76.60	1.10	0.98	53	154	245	802
Intermediate risk											
Age≥85 years + polypharmacy‡ + temporal disorientation#	0.56	15.44	86.72	26.59	76.69	1.16	0.98	46	127	252	829
Male + polypharmacy‡ + temporal disorientation#	0.56	12.08	92.26	32.73	77.10	1.56	0.95	36	74	262	882
Age≥85 years + male + polypharmacy‡ + temporal disorientation#	0.56	5.37	95.26	28.57	76.46	1.28	0.99	16	40	232	915
High risk											
History of falls + temporal disorientation# + Polypharmacy‡	0.57	12.75	91.32	31.40	77.05	1.47	0.96	38	83	260	873

Table 2. Cont.

	Area under ROC	Sensitivity(%)	Specify(%)	PPV (%)	NPV (%)	LR+	LR-	Number of individuals classified			
								TP	FP	FN	TN
History of falls + temporal disorientation# + Polypharmacy‡ + male	0.57	5.03	96.55	31.25	76.53	1.46	0.98	15	33	283	923
Age≥85 years + polypharmacy‡ + non-use of home help services§	0.57	4.03	99.27	63.16	76.84	5.50	0.97	12	7	286	949

ROC: Receiver operating characteristic curve; PPV: Positive predictive value; NPV: Negative predictive value; LR+: Likelihood ration of positive test; LR-: Likelihood ration of negative test; TP: True positive; FP: False positive; TN: True negative; FN: False negative;
*: Only three best models (i.e., highest value of ROC) by level (i.e., Low, intermediate and high risk) are shown;
†: Defined being in the highest tertile of length of hospital saty (i.e.,>13 days);
‡: Defined by a number of drugs taken per day above 4;
§: Living alone without using any formal or informal home services and social help;
¶: during the past 6 months;
#: Inability to give the month and/or year;
**: Only combination involving at least 10 participants were considered;
††: Combinations described in previous published study (Beauchet et al. J Emerg Med. 2013; 45: 739–45).

They were older than those who did not die (mean age ± standard deviation, 86.2±5.4 years versus 84.7±5.9 with P = 0.004) and there were fewer women in this group (49.0% versus 60.4%, P = 0.007). In addition, they had a longer LHS compared to those who did not die (11.3±10.5 days versus 8.4±8.1 days with P< 0.001).

Among BGA items, the best predictor of prolonged LHS was temporal disorientation, this item having the highest value of ROC curve (0.55) (Table 2). The combination 'history of falls' plus 'temporal disorientation', defining the *a priori* high risk of prolonged LHS identified in our previous publication [16], had the highest value of ROC curve (0.56). Its sensitivity and PPV were low (18.46% and 29.57) but the specificity and NPV were high (86.30% and 77.25). The LR+ and LR- were calculated at 1.35 and 0.95. Compared to this *a priori* classification, new combinations defining high risk of prolonged LHS had highest values of ROC curve. The sensitivity of all combinations of this level of risk was low under 13.0% but the specificity was high above 90.0%. In addition, the highest LR+ of 5.50 was shown for a combination involving 'age ≥85 years' plus 'polypharmacy' plus 'non-use of home-help services'.

Univariate and Cox regression models adjusted on acute organ failure and place of life showed that patients classified *a priori* with low risk of prolonged LHS had indeed a significantly shorter LHS (unadjusted Hazard Ratio [HR] = 0.82 with P = 0.001, and adjusted HR = 0.80 with P<0.001), whereas those with high risk of prolonged LHS had a longer LHS (unadjusted HR = 1.27 with P = 0.003, adjusted HR = 1.29 with P = 0.002 and fully adjusted HR = 1.44 with P<0.001) (Table 3). In addition, fully adjusted Cox model (i.e., using the group at low risk of prolonged LHS as reference) shown that patients in intermediate risk group (HR = 1.20 with P = 0.006) had also prolonged LHS. Classification of risk of prolonged LHS based on newly identified combinations underscored that only high risk level predicted a prolonged LHS (unadjusted HR = 1.40 with P<0.001, adjusted HR = 1.43 with P<0.001 and fully adjusted HR = 1.47 with P<0.001). As shown in Table 4, adjustment for the nature of acute organ failures did not alter our results. Indeed, intermediate risk and high risk of prolonged LSH predicted effectively a prolonged LSH with *a priori* combinations (HR>1.15 and P<0.015), whereas only high risk level predicted prolonged LSH with new combinations (HR> 1.46 and P<0.001).

Generated Kaplan-Meier plot of the probability of discharge from acute care medical units is reported Figures 2 et 3. While using *a priori* combinations of BGA items (Figure 2), comparison of survival curves showed that inpatients considered at low risk of prolonged LHS were faster discharged from acute care medical units than those in intermediate (P = 0.013) and high-risk groups (P<0.001). Furthermore, patients in intermediate risk of prolonged LHS were also faster discharged from acute care medical units than those in high-risk group (P = 0.026). The new classification showed similar results (Figure 3), except for the comparison of discharge between patients in low-risk group and those in intermediate-risk group which was not significant (P = 0.931). Comparison of survival curves showed that inpatients considered at low risk of prolonged LHS were faster discharged from acute care medical units than those in high-risk group (P< 0.001). Furthermore, patients with intermediate risk of prolonged LHS were also faster discharged from acute care medical units than those in high-risk group (P<0.001).

Table 3. Cox regression models showing the association between the length of hospital stay (dependent variable) and combinations of brief geriatric assessment items (independent variables) separated into three risk-levels (i.e., low risk, intermediate risk, and high risk of prolonged length of hospital stay) (n = 1254).

Combinations of the 6-item brief geriatric assessment, stratified in three levels of risk (low, intermediate, high)	**HR [95% CI] (P-Value)**		
	Model 1	**Model 2**	**Model 3**
A priori combinations*			
Low-risk level: Three items among age ≥85years, male gender, polypharmacy† and non-use of home services‡	**0.82** [0.74; 0.92]	**0.80** [0.71; 0.91]	1.00(Ref)
	(**0.001**)	(**0.001**)	
Intermediate-risk level: History of falls§, or temporal disorientation, or (age ≥85years + male gender + polypharmacy† + non-use of home services‡)	1.06 [0.95; 1.18]	1.06 [0.95; 1.19]	**1.20** [1.05; 1.36]
	(0.325)	(0.323)	(**0.006**)
High-risk level: history of falls§ + temporal disorientation	**1.27** [1.09; 1.49]	**1.29** [1.09; 1.51]	**1.44** [1.20; 1.73]
	(**0.003**)	(**0.002**)	(**<0.001**)
Newly identified combinations			
Low-risk level: polypharmacy† + (non-use of home-help services‡ or age ≥85years or history of falls§) + (absence of temporal disorientation)	0.93 [0.82; 1.06]	0.90 [0.79; 1.02]	1.00(Ref)
	(0.291)	(0.104)	
Intermediate-risk level: combinations other than low- or high-level combinations	0.91 [0.81; 1.02]	0.93 [0.82; 1.04]	1.05 [0.91; 1.19]
	(0.096)	(0.208)	(0.519)
High-risk level: temporal disorientation + polypharmacy† + (history of falls§ or (age ≥85years or non use of home help services‡))	**1.40** [1.17; 1.68]	**1.43** [1.19; 1.72]	**1.47** [1.20; 1.81]
	(**<0.001**)	(**<0.001**)	(**<0.001**)

Model 1: Unadjusted model.
Model 2: Model adjusted on organ failure and place of life.
Model 3: Low risk of prolonged length of hospital stay used as reference, with adjustment on organ failure and place of life.
*: Combinations described previously (Beauchet et al. J Emerg Med. 2013; 45: 739–45).
†: Defined by a number of drugs taken per day above 4.
‡: Living alone without using any formal or informal home services and social help.
§: In past 6 months.
¶: Inability to give the month and/or year.
Hazard ratio and p-value significant (i.e., <0.05) indicated in bold.

Discussion

Our results show that combinations of BGA items were significant risk factors for prolonged LHS in geriatric patients admitted to ED and discharged to acute care medical units. However, the prognostic value for prolonged LHS of these combinations of BGA items was poor, whatever the BGA items or their combinations used.

The main findings of our study is the discrepancy between the fact that combinations of BGA items were risk factors for prolonged LHS and their poor prognostic value for this endpoint. Limitations of risk factors as a prognostic tool have been previously reported [21–23]. The conclusions of these publications was that risk factors should exhibit a much stronger association with the studied endpoint (e.g., prolonged LHS in our case) than they ordinarily show in epidemiological studies if it is to provide a basis for prediction in individual patients. Our results are, therefore, in total concordance with this assumption. Indeed, even if HR of certain combinations of BGA items were significant risk factors for prolonged LHS, the magnitude of their values was low below 2, which is consistent with a poor prognostic value for prolonged LHS. This apparent paradoxical result (i.e., a significant risk factor having a poor prognostic value) is in relation with the fact that a risk factor is assessed by comparing the risk of studied outcome at each end of the distribution of the risk factor. While using this statistical approach the effect of being highly exposed to the factor is compared with the effect of being slightly exposed. Thus, comparison is done on jointly exclusive groups of individuals. The main consequence of this approach is that the group of individuals in the middle of distribution, which represents the majority of individuals, is ignored. Because the aim in screening tool is to identify a group of individuals with a high risk relative to everyone, there is necessary a discrepancy between to be a significant risk factor associated with the studied outcome and to be a poor prognostic risk factor for this outcome.

Combinations of BGA items were significant risk factors for prolonged LHS among studied geriatric inpatients. The strength of this association was greater when specific items were combined underscoring a stronger association while using newly identified combinations compared to *a priori* combinations [16]. This result may be explained by the fact that the BGA items, and specifically the combinations defining the high-risk level, are markers of frailty, which is a status previously identified as a risk factor for prolonged LHS [16,17,5]. Frailty in older adults usually refers to a physiological vulnerability medical that expose to adverse health, functional and social outcomes [24]. Despite the lack of consensus on the definition of frailty, there is a broad agreement that frailty is characterized by an accumulation of deficits related to a combined action of aging and morbidities [25–27]. Under the action of the morbidities and/or ageing that generate disabilities, this dynamic process, occurring from reduced physiological resources, results in

Table 4. Cox regression models showing the association between the length of hospital stay (dependent variable) and combinations of brief geriatric assessment items (independent variables) separated into three risk-levels (i.e., low risk, intermediate risk, and high risk of prolonged length of hospital stay) with separated models for reasons for admission to emergency department (n = 1254).

Combinations of the 6-item brief geriatric Assessment stratified in three levels of risk (low, intermediate, high)	**HR [95% CI] (P-Value)***				
	Cardio vascular disease	**Respiratory disease**	**Digestive disease**	**Neuropsychological disease**	**Other diseases**
A priori combinations†					
Low-risk level: three items among age ≥85years, male gender, polypharmacy‡ and non-use of home-help services§	1.00(Ref)	1.00(Ref)	1.00(Ref)	1.00(Ref)	1.00(Ref)
Intermediate-risk level: history of falls, or temporal disorientation#, or (age ≥85years + male gender + polypharmacy‡ + non-use of home-help services§)	**1.17** [1.04; 1.32]	**1.19** [1.06; 1.35]	**1.18** [1.04; 1.33]	**1.17** [1.04; 1.32]	**1.21** [1.07; 1.37]
	(0.012)	**(0.004)**	**(0.008)**	**(0.010)**	**(0.003)**
High-risk level: history of falls + temporal disorientation#	**1.39**[1.17; 1.65]	**1.44** [1.21; 1.70]	**1.41** [1.19; 1.67]	**1.40** [1.18; 1.65]	**1.46** [1.22; 1.74]
	(<0.001)	**(<0.001)**	**(<0.001)**	**(<0.001)**	**(<0.001)**
Newly identified combinations					
Low-risk level: polypharmacy‡ + (non use of home help services§ or age ≥85years or history of falls) + (absence of temporal disorientation)	1.00(Ref)	1.00(Ref)	1.00(Ref)	1.00(Ref)	1.00(Ref)
Intermediate-risk level: combinations other than low- or high-level combinations	1.05 [0.92; 1.19]	1.03 [0.91; 1.18]	1.04 [0.92; 1.19]	1.05 [0.92; 1.19]	1.04 [0.91; 1.18]
	(0.509)	(0.614)	(0.520)	(0.484)	(0.609)
High-risk level: temporal disorientation# + polypharmacy‡ + (history of falls or (age ≥85years + non-use of home-help services§))	**1.47** [1.19; 1.80]	**1.48** [1.20; 1.81]	**1.48** [1.20; 1.82]	**1.47** [1.20; 1.81]	**1.48** [1.21; 1.82]
	(<0.001)	**(<0.001)**	**(<0.001)**	**(<0.001)**	**(<0.001)**

All models used low-risk level as reference value.
*: adjustment on place of life.
†: Combinations described previously (Beauchet et al. J Emerg Med. 2013; 45: 739–45).
‡: Defined by a number of drugs taken per day above 4.
§: Living alone without using any formal or informal home services and social help.
¶: In past 6 months.
#: Inability to give the month and/or year.
Hazard ratio and p-value significant (i.e., <0.05) indicated in bold.

impaired adaptation to stress such as a hospitalization. As a consequence frail older adults are more prone to prolonged LHS than non-frail older ones [16,25–29].

Our results also show that the risk of prolonged LHS did not increase in a simple cumulative way according to the combination of items. Considered separately, older age, male gender, polypharmacy and the absence of home-help services have been previously associated with prolonged LHS [10,16,28–30]. The highest risk was not reported with the combination of all 6 items. Moreover, high risk of prolonged LHS was found with several combinations rather than one. This results is probably the consequence of a complex interplay of BGA items which are direct or indirect markers of geriatric syndromes, morbidities or functional decline, and where the interaction between medical and change of the environment of an individuals (i.e., hospital and more precisely acute care unit in our study) exposes patients to a major risk of prolonged LHS [16,28,29]. Indeed, the latter parameter underscores the inability of changes of frail individuals due to poor physiological resources. In addition, the heterogeneity of health conditions among geriatric population may also account for the various combinations related to a high risk of prolonged LHS [2,8,16].

Among the BGA items, we confirmed in the studied sample of inpatients that the history of falls and temporal disorientation were strongly related to prolonged LHS, and thus were part of most combinations defining the high risk of prolonged LHS [16–18]. In addition, the risk of prolonged LHS increased when both these items were associated. Falls usually cause and/or result from gait and/or balance disorders, which are themselves identified risk factors for prolonged LHS [31–33]. This specific association has been underscored using Timed Up & Go (TUG), which is a basic assessment of functional mobility and measures the time needed to rise from a chair, walk 3 meters, turn around and return to a seated position [33]. It has been reported that longer TUG was a marker of prolonged LHS in older patients [10,18]. Furthermore, the association between temporal disorientation and prolonged LHS may be explained by the fact that temporal disorientation is a surrogate measure of severe cognitive disorders, either acute (i.e., delirium) and/or chronic (i.e., dementia) [17]. Because these both cognitive disorders have been identified as risk factors for prolonged LHS, they could explain the prolonged LHS reported in our study [10,18]. Our results also highlighted that the risk of prolonged LHS increased when history of falls was combined with temporal disorientation. This is in concordance with previous results showing that individuals combining cognitive decline and

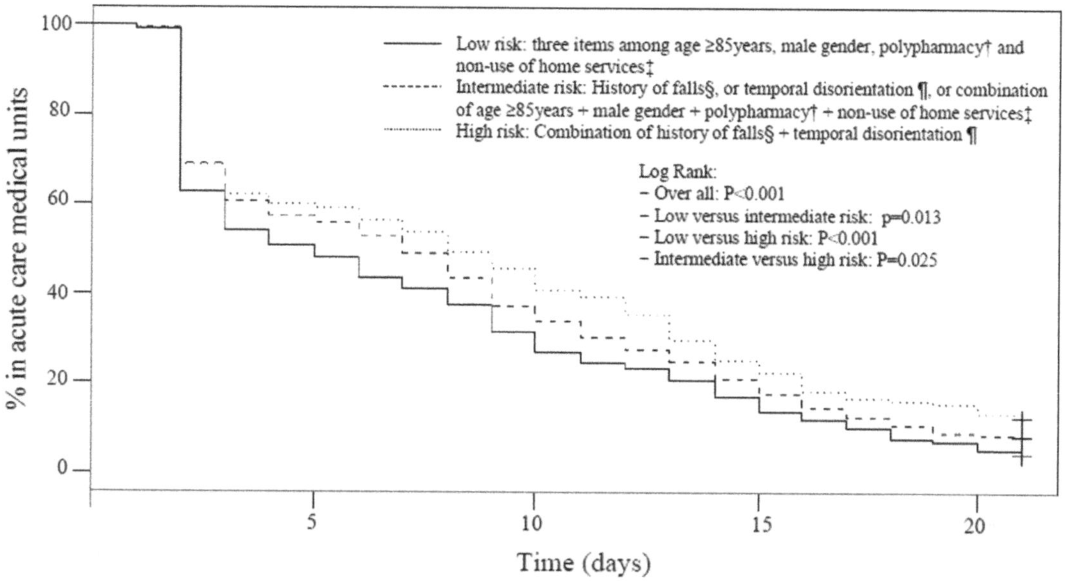

Figure 2. Kaplan-Meier estimates of the probability of discharge from acute care medical units among older inpatients (n = 12,054) using *a priori combinations of the 6 items of the brief geriatric assessment.** *: Combinations described previously (Beauchet et al. J Emerg Med. 2013; 45: 739–45). †: Defined by a number of drugs taken per day above 4. ‡: Living alone without using any formal or informal home services and social help. §: In past 6 months. ¶: Inability to give the month and/or year.

mobility disorders were more at risk of adverse outcomes than those having only one disorder, and that LHS increases with the accumulation of risk factors [18–20]. Finally, this strong association of history of falls and temporal disorientation with prolonged LHS may be explained by the fact that both these disorders are common ways of expression of diseases, whatever their nature. Older adults' health and functional status is heterogeneous because of the various cumulative effects of chronic diseases and physiologic decline, contributing to a vicious cycle of increased frailty, the frailty being defined as a clinically recognizable state of increased vulnerability [24–27]. The expression of this vulnerability is often a decrease in gait and cognitive performance, the clinical symptoms of this decline being falls and temporal disorientation [24,25].

The poor prognostic value of the 6-item BGA is in concordance with results of previous studies exploring the predictive value of clinical parameters for the occurrence of adverse health events in older adults. Prognostic value of prior tools, such as the

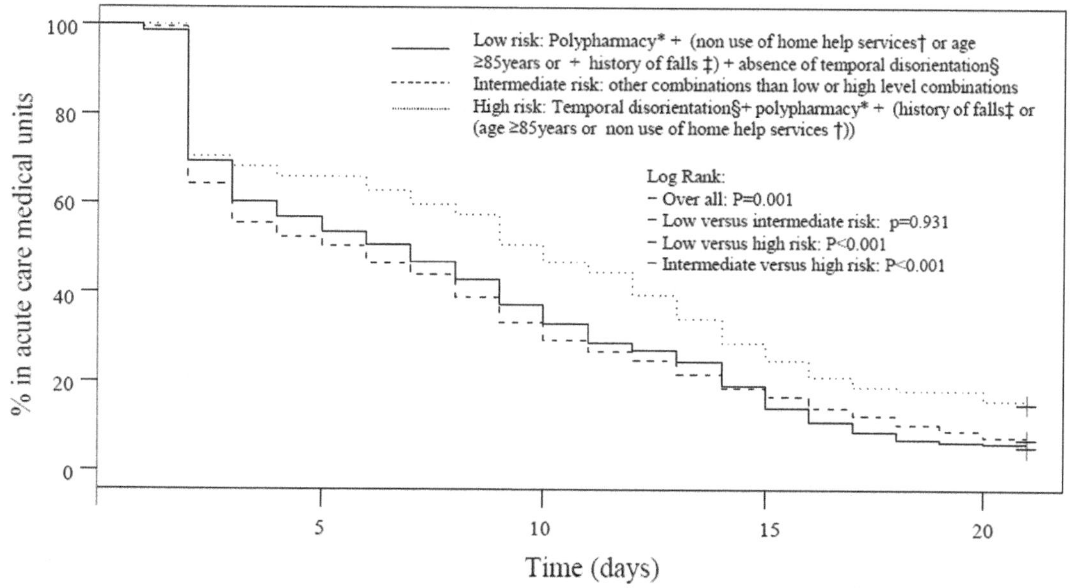

Figure 3. Kaplan-Meier estimates of the probability of discharge from acute care medical units among older inpatients (n = 12,054) using newly identified combinations of the 6 items of the brief geriatric assessment. *: Defined by a number of drugs taken per day above 4. †: Living alone without using any formal or informal home services and social help. ‡: In past 6 months. §: Inability to give the month and/or year.

Identification of Seniors At Risk (ISAR) score and the triage risk stratification tool (TRST), which are the main tools validated in ED users aged 65 years and older, have been examined [34,35]. Like our results, it has been reported that these tools have a poor prognostic value for adverse health outcomes in ED (i.e., death, institutionalisation, readmission) [34,35]. Developing one single tool to predict LHS remains a complex challenge but an objective to reach. A perspective for the prediction of frailty-related adverse outcomes such as prolonged LHS could come from non-linear statistical methods [36–38]. For instance, artificial neural networks (ANNs) are data analysis tools that have been developed to overcome limitations of linear models [36]. Because they apply non-linear statistic to pattern recognition, ANNs are particularly adapted to "chaotic" behavior like frailty-related adverse outcomes. Nowadays, the advance of ANNs combined with improvement of computers technology open new perspectives in diagnostic support aids for helping physicians to take the best decision for their patients [37,38].

Some limitations of this study need to be considered. First, participants were included from a single centre and, thus, they were probably not representative of all older adults admitted to ED. Secondly, although we were able to control for many characteristics likely to modify the LHS, residual potential confounders might still be present. We limited this confounding bias by adjusting our results on organ failure and place of life because these covariables are strong determinants of prolonged LHS [17–18]. Third, there was a potential recall bias about the history of falls, which is well known in the elderly. Falls are usually underreported because of a cognitive decline of fallers who forget to report the falls, and depends on the occurrence of fall-related adverse health outcomes [39].

In conclusion, combinations of 6 BGA items were significant risk factors for prolonged LHS with a risk that did not increase linearly with the accumulation of items, underscoring that some specific combinations of BGA items were greater risk factors than others. Unfortunately, their prognostic value was poor. Further research is required to improve the prognostic value of clinical tools for the identification of adverse events among older adults hospitalized in medical and surgical care units. A perspective may rely on the use of ANNs.

Acknowledgments

The authors would like to thank the patients for their participation in the study.

Author Contributions

Conceived and designed the experiments: CPL OB. Performed the experiments: CPL LDD AK. Analyzed the data: CPL LDD CA AK OB. Contributed reagents/materials/analysis tools: CPL CA AK OB. Wrote the paper: CPL LDD CA AK OB.

References

1. Aminzadeh F, Dalziel WB (2002) Older adults in the emergency department: a systematic review of patterns of use, adverse outcomes, and effectiveness of interventions. Ann Emerg Med 393: 238–247.
2. Xu KT, Nelson BK, Berk S (2009) The changing profile of patients who used emergency department services in the United States: 1996 to 2005. Ann Emerg Med 546: 805–810.
3. Stuck AE, Iliffe S (2011) Comprehensive geriatric assessment for older adults. BMJ 343: 6799.
4. Conroy SP, Ansari K, Williams M, Laithwaite E, Teasdale B, et al (2013) A controlled evaluation of comprehensive geriatric assessment in the emergency department: the 'Emergency Frailty Unit'. Age Ageing 431: 109–114.
5. Drame M, Jovenin N, Novella JL, Lang PO, Somme D, et al. (2008) Predicting early mortality among elderly patients hospitalised in medical wards via emergency department: the SAFES cohort study. J Nutr Health Aging 12: 599–604.
6. Barnett K, Mercer SW, Norbury M, Watt G, Wyke S, et al. (2012) Epidemiology of multimorbidity and implications for health care, research, and medical education: a cross-sectional study. Lancet 380: 37–43
7. Gill TM, Gahbauer EA, Han L, Allore HG (2010) Trajectories of disability in the last year of life. N Engl J Med 362: 1173–1180.
8. Wolff JL, Starfield B, Anderson G (2002) Prevalence, expenditures, and complications of multiple chronic conditions in the elderly. Arch Intern Med 162: 2269–2276.
9. Yoo JW, Seol H, Kim SJ, Yang JM, Ryu WS, et al. (2013) Effects of hospitalist-directed interdisciplinary medicine floor service on hospital outcomes for seniors with acute medical illness. Geriatr Gerontol Int 14: 71–77.
10. Lang PO, Heitz D, Hedelin G, Dramé M, Jovenin N, et al. (2006) Early markers of prolonged hospital stays in older people: a prospective, multicenter study of 908 inpatients in French acute hospitals. J Am Geriatr Soc 547: 1031–1039.
11. Ellis G, Whitehead MA, Robinson D, O'Neill D, Langhorne P (2011) Comprehensive geriatric assessment for older adults admitted to hospital: meta-analysis of randomised controlled trials. BMJ 343: 1034–1036.
12. Launay C, Annweiler C, de Decker L, Kabeshova A, Fantino B at al. (2013) Early hospital discharge of older adults admitted to the emergency department: effect of different types of recommendations made by a mobile geriatric team. J Am Geriatr Soc 616: 1031–1033.
13. Graf CE, Zekry D, Giannelli S, Michel JP, Chevalley T (2010) Efficiency and applicability of comprehensive geriatric assessment in the emergency department: a systematic review. Aging Clin Exp Res 234: 244–254
14. Somme D, Rousseau C (2013) Standardized geriatric assessment or comprehensive gerontological assessment: where do we stand? Rev Med Interne 342: 114–122.
15. McCusker J, Dendukuri N, Tousignant P, Verdon J, Poulin de Courval L, et al. (2003) Rapid two-stage emergency department intervention for seniors: impact on continuity of care. Acad Emerg Med 103: 233–243
16. Beauchet O, Launay CP, Fantino B, Lerolle N, Maunoury F, et al. (2013) Screening for Elderly Patients Admitted to the Emergency Department Requiring Specialized Geriatric Care. J Emerg Med 455: 739–745.
17. Launay C, Haubois G, Hureaux-Huynh R, Gautier J, Annweiler C, et al. (2014) Older adults and emergency department: who is at risk of hospitalization? Geriatr Psychol Neuropsychiatr Vieil 12: 43–49.
18. Lim SC, Doshi V, Castasus B, Lim JK, Mamun K (2006) Factors causing delay in discharge of elderly patients in an acute care hospital. Ann Acad Med Singapore 351: 27–32
19. Byrne DG, Chung SL, Bennett K (2010) Age and outcome in acute emergency medical admissions. Age Ageing 396: 694–698
20. Hastings SN, Whitson E, Purser JL, Sloane RJ, Johnson KS (2009) Emergency department discharge diagnosis and adverse health outcomes in older adults. J Am Geriatr Soc 5710: 1856–1861
21. Wald NJ, Hackshaw AK, Frost CD (1999) When can a risk factor be used as a worthwhile screening test? BMJ 319: 1562–1565.
22. Ware JH (2006) The limitations of risk factors as prognostic tools. N Engl J Med 355: 2615–2617.
23. Pepe MS, Janes H, Longton G, Leisenring W, Newcomb P (2004) Limitations of the odds ratio in gauging the performance of a diagnostic, prognostic, or screening marker. Am J Epidemiol 159: 882–890.
24. Sternberg SA, Wershof Schwartz A, Karunananthan S, Bergman H, Mark Clarfield A (2011) The identification of frailty: a systematic literature review. J Am Geriatr Soc 59: 2129–2138.
25. Berrut G, Andrieu S, Araujo de Carvalho I, Baeyens JP, Bergman H, et al. (2013) Promoting access to innovation for frail old persons. IAGG (International Association of Gerontology and Geriatrics), WHO (World Health Organization) and SFGG (Société Française de Gériatrie et de Gérontologie) Workshop–Athens January 20–21, 2012 Tool (GFST). J Nutr Health Aging 17: 688–693
26. Rockwood K, Bergman H (2012) FRAILTY: A Report from the 3(rd) Joint Workshop of IAGG/WHO/SFGG, Athens, January 2012. Can Geriatr J 15: 31–36.
27. Ravindrarajah R, Lee DM, Pye SR, Gielen E, Boonen S, et al European Male Aging Study Group (2013) The ability of three different models of frailty to predict all-cause mortality: results from the European Male Aging Study (EMAS). Arch Gerontol Geriatr 57: 360–368.
28. Rozzini R, Sleiman I, Maggi S, Noale M, Trabucchi M (2009) Gender differences and health status in old and very old patients. J Am Med Dir Assoc 108: 554–558.
29. Beauchet O, Launay C, de Decker L, Fantino B, Kabeshova A, et al. (2013) Who is at risk of long hospital stay among patients admitted to geriatric acute care unit? Results from a prospective cohort study. J Nutr Health Aging 178: 695–699.
30. de Decker L, Launay C, Annweiler C, Kabeshova A, Beauchet O (2013) Number of drug classes taken per day may be used to assess morbidity burden in older inpatients: a pilot cross-sectional study. J Am Geriatr Soc 617: 1224–1255.

31. Beauchet O, Dubost V, Revel Delhom C, Berrut G, Belmin J (2011) How to manage recurrent falls in clinical practice: guidelines of the French Society of Geriatrics and Gerontology. J Nutr Health Aging 151: 79–84.
32. Rossat A, Fantino B, Nitenberg C, Annweiler C, Poujol L, et al. (2010) Risk factors for falling in community-dwelling older adults: which of them are associated with the recurrence of falls? J Nutr Health Aging 149: 787–791.
33. Podsiadlo D, Richardson S (1991) The timed "Up & Go": a test of basic functional mobility for frail elderly persons. J Am Geriatr Soc 39: 142–148.
34. McCusker J, Bellavance F, Cardin S, Trépanier S, Verdon J, et al. (1999) Detection of older people at increased risk of adverse health outcomes after an emergency visit: the ISAR screening tool. J Am Geriatr Soc 47: 1229–1237.
35. Meldon SW, Mion LC, Palmer RM, Drew BL, Connor JT, et al. (2003) A brief risk-stratification tool to predict repeat emergency department visits and hospitalizations in older patients discharged from the emergency department. Acad Emerg Med 10: 224–232.
36. Akl A, Ghoneim M (2011) Forcasting the Clinical Outcome: Artificial Neural Networks or Multivariate Statistical Models?, Artificial Neural Networks - Methodological Advances and Biomedical Applications, Prof. Kenji Suzuki (Ed.); InTech, ISBN: 978-953-307-243-2.
37. Baxt WG (1995) Application of artificial neural networks to clinical medicine. Lancet 346: 1135–1138.
38. Baxt WG, Skora J (1996) Prospective validation of artificial neural network trained to identify acute myocardial infarction. Lancet 347: 12–15.
39. Cummings SR, Nevitt MC, Kidd S (1988) Forgetting falls. The limited accuracy of recall of falls in the elderly. J Am Geriatr Soc 367: 613–616.

Implementation of Patient Safety and Patient-Centeredness Strategies in Iranian Hospitals

Asgar Aghaei Hashjin[1,2]*, Dionne S. Kringos[1], Jila Manoochehri[3], Hamid Ravaghi[2], Niek S. Klazinga[1]

1 Department of Public Health, Academic Medical Center (AMC)/University of Amsterdam, Amsterdam, the Netherlands, 2 Department of Health Services Management, School of Health Services Management and Information Sciences, Iran University of Medical Sciences, Tehran, Iran, 3 Department of Quality Improvement, Tehran Heart Center Hospital, Tehran University of Medical Sciences, Tehran, Iran

Abstract

Objective: To examine the extent of implementation for patient safety (PS) and patient-centeredness (PC) strategies and their association with hospital characteristics (type, ownership, teaching status, annual evaluation grade) in Iran.

Methods: A cross-sectional study through an adapted version of the MARQuIS questionnaire, eliciting information from hospital and nursing managers in 84 Iranian hospitals on the implementation of PS and PC strategies in 2009–2010.

Results: The majority of hospitals reported to have implemented 84% of the PS and 72% of the PC strategies. In general, implementation of PS strategies was unrelated to the type of hospital, with the exception of health promotion reports, which were more common in the Social Security Organization (SSO), and MRSA testing, which was reported more often in nonprofit hospitals. MRSA testing was also more common among teaching hospitals compared to non-teaching hospitals. The higher grade hospitals reported PS strategies significantly more frequently than lower grade hospitals. Overall, there was no significant difference in the reported implementation of PC strategies across general and specialized hospitals; except for the provision of information in different languages and recording of patient's diet which were reported significantly more often by general than specialized hospitals. Moreover, patient hotel services were more common in private compared to public hospitals.

Conclusions: Despite substantial reporting of PS and PC strategies, there is still room for strengthening standard setting on safety, patient services and patient-centered information strategies in Iranian hospitals. To assure effective implementation of PS and PC strategies, enforcing standards, creating a PS and PC culture, increasing organizational responsiveness, and partnering with patients and their families need more attention.

Editor: Hassan Ashktorab, Howard University, United States of America

Funding: The authors received no specific funding for this work.

Competing Interests: The authors have declared that no competing interests exist.

* Email: a.aghaeihashjin@amc.uva.nl

Introduction

Despite the considerable developments in health care, patient safety (PS) and patient-centeredness (PC) still remain a topic of concern in health care systems world-wide [1]. Patient complaints, unsafe patient care, medical errors and adverse events are still prevalent in most health care systems, and the risk of patient harm and complications remain unacceptably high and costly in both developed and developing countries [2–4]. The risk of hospital related infections in some developing countries is reported to be 20 times higher than in developed countries and unsafe injections have been reported as high as 70% [5]. Up to 18% of hospitals' inpatient admissions are associated with patient harm and 3% of them have been reported to result to death or permanent disability in some Eastern Mediterranean Region's countries. In the United States, serious adverse events occurred in 3.7% of the hospitalizations [6]. Some countries report that patient related complications annually cost the health care budget billions [7].

Less information is available concerning PS and patient-related complaints in Iran. Over the years reports of patient harm, adverse events, medical error, unsafe injections, hazardous treatments threaten the safety of patients and result in iatrogenic complications. The Institute of Medicine estimated that up to 98,000 Americans die from medical errors annually, and hospital-associated infections cause or contribute to 99,000 deaths each year in the United States [6], [8]. An estimated 24,500 people die annually due to medical errors in Iran [9], [10]. The prevalence of hospital acquired infections is reported as high as 8–10% in Iranian hospitals [11]. A lack of attention to patients, patient involvement and the limited implementation of patient rights principles was also reported [12].

In response to the existing PS and PC problems, the Iranian Ministry of Health and Medical Education (MOHME) developed and implemented various strategies in recent years in several stages. The political agenda is currently paying more attention to the reduction of patient harm, ensuring quality, safety and the

Table 1. The characteristics of study population.

Hospitals	Ownership					Teaching status				Annual evaluation grade				
	Gov.	PFP	SSO	PNP	Total	Non-tea.	Non-tea. +Tea.	Non-tea.+ Tea.+Res.	Total	Ex.	1	2	3	Total
General	35	11	21	5	**72**	35	33	4	**72**	4	59	5	1	**69**
Specialized	11	1	0	0	**12**	1	8	3	**12**	0	12	0	0	**12**
Total	46	12	21	5	**84**	36	41	7	**84**	4	71	5	1	**81**

Gov. = Governmental, PFP = Private for-profit, PNP = Private nonprofit, SSO = Social Security Organization, Non-tea. = Non-teaching, Tea. = Teaching, Res. = Research, Ex. = Excellent.

improvement of PC. To reach this mission, the MOHME statutorily implemented hospital licensing, annual hospital performance evaluations and routine inspections for all hospitals since 1997 [13]. Moreover, the MOHME compiled the Patients' Bill of Rights in 2002 to improve patient-centered care and assed it by the Policy Council in 2009. It obliged all hospitals to implement

Table 2. The extent of overall reported implementation of patient safety strategies by the type of hospitals.

Strategy		The reported implementation level of patient safety strategies by the type of hospitals n (%)			P-value
		Total	General hospitals	Specialized hospitals	
Assigning responsibility	Responsible personnel for hospital infection control	79 (100)	67 (100)	12 (100)	–
	Responsible personnel for patient safety	51 (68.9)	42 (67.7)	9 (75)	0.559
	Responsible personnel for blood transfusion	64 (84.2)	56 (86.2)	8 (72.7)	0.528
	Responsible personnel for antibiotic use policy	56 (71.8)	47 (70.1)	9 (81.8)	0.723
	Responsible personnel for prevention of decubitus	50 (66.7)	40 (63.5)	10 (83.3)	0.406
	Responsible personnel for clinical waste management	68 (86.1)	58 (86.6)	10 (83.3)	0.295
	Responsible personnel for health promotion	68 (86.1)	56 (83.6)	12 (100)	0.318
Specific strategies for standard setting	Policies in place to prevent falls	33 (43.4)	26 (40.6)	7 (58.3)	0.523
	Hand washing policy	49 (62.8)	42 (63.6)	7 (58.3)	0.328
	MRSA testing	20 (26)	17 (26.2)	3 (25)	0.688
	Identifying patients in the emergency room	13 (15.9)	11 (15.7)	2 (16.7)	0.984
	Identifying admitted patients	21 (25)	18 (25)	3 (25)	0.701
	Availability of clinical guidelines/protocols	75 (89.3)	63 (87.5)	12 (100)	0.432
	Ratified clinical guidelines	54 (71.1)	46 (71.9)	8 (66.7)	0.096
	Updating of clinical guidelines	39 (56.5)	33 (55.9)	6 (60)	0.058
	Drug storage locked	67 (81.7)	55 (78.6)	12 (100)	0.207
	High risk drugs storage separately	71 (86.6)	62 (87.3)	9 (81.8)	0.624
	Checking drug expiration date routinely	82 (98.8)	70 (98.6)	12 (100)	0.679
Reporting strategies on outcomes	Reports on control of hospital infections	79 (100)	67 (100)	12 (100)	–
	Reports on patient safety	46 (61.3)	38 (60.3)	8 (66.7)	0.650
	Reports on blood transfusion policies	58 (75.3)	50 (75.8)	8 (72.7)	0.605
	Reports on antibiotic use policy	47 (62.7)	41 (64.1)	6 (54.5)	0.439
	Reports on prevention of decubitus	49 (64.5)	39 (60.9)	10 (83.3)	0.212
	Reports on clinical waste management	65 (85.5)	56 (86.2)	9 (81.8)	0.827
	Reports on health promotion	59 (75.6)	53 (79.1)	6 (54.5)	0.208

Table 3. The extent of overall implementation level of patient-centeredness strategies by the type of hospitals.

Strategy		The reported implementation level of patient-centeredness strategies by the type of hospitals n (%)			P-value
		Total	General hospitals	Specialized hospitals	
Patient services	Possibility to contact with family or friends by patient	50 (62.5)	43 (63.2)	7 (58.3)	0.660
	Possibility to contact with family doctor or GP by patient	48 (60.8)	41 (61.2)	7 (58.3)	0.618
	Providing meals for family and relatives of patients	67 (81.7)	57 (81.4)	10 (83.3)	0.875
	Providing room/bed for family and relatives of patients	56 (67.5)	50 (70.4)	6 (50)	0.245
	Offering single room upon request	40 (48.8)	36 (51.4)	4 (33.3)	0.269
	Access to internet in or outside the room	15 (18.1)	13 (18.3)	2 (16.2)	0.907
	Access to tel. in the room with instructions in other languages	54 (65.1)	45 (63.4)	9 (75)	0.672
	Access to TV and satellite in the room	68 (82.9)	56 (80)	12 (100)	0.235
	Providing daily newspaper for patients	12 (14.5)	9 (12.7)	3 (25)	0.434
	Access to smoking room	11 (13.4)	9 (12.9)	2 (16.7)	0.865
	Having coordinator for patients affairs	46 (55.4)	40 (56.3)	6 (50)	0.650
	Having coordinator for discharge of patients	44 (53)	39 (54.9)	5 (41.7)	0.389
	Having transport services for patients	17 (20.5)	14 (19.7)	3 (25)	0.894
	Providing medicines if needed after discharge	73 (88)	62 (87.3)	11 (91.7)	0.355
	Recording of patient's diet preferences	82 (97.6)	71 (98.6)	11 (91.7)	0.045
	Offering a choice of the meals to patients	19 (22.6)	16 (22.2)	3 (25)	0.764
	Offering a choice in the timing of the meals	13 (15.5)	12 (16.7)	1 (8.3)	0.502
	Visit of patients by family or relatives	80 (96.4)	69 (95.8)	11 (100)	0.788
Patient information, involvement and empowerment	Providing information in different languages	67 (79.8)	60 (83.3)	7 (58.3)	0.016
	Written policy for patient involvement in decision making	58 (69.9)	51 (71.8)	7 (58.3)	0.625
	Possibility to give information to patients in their language	67 (79.7)	57 (79.1)	10 (83.3)	0.470
	Having a procedure for the requirements before admission	40 (48.8)	35 (49.3)	5 (41.7)	0.408
	Possibility to contact with the patient's doctor before admission	12 (14.3)	9 (12.5)	3 (25)	0.227
	Patients and their family involvement in care decision making	51 (60.7)	43 (59.7)	8 (66.7)	0.856
	Providing written information regarding to patient's treatment	43 (51.2)	35 (48.6)	8 (66.7)	0.264
	Written policy for informed consent to interventions/treatments	74 (89.2)	63 (88.7)	11 (91.7)	0.763
Patient rights	Have patient rights department	61 (73.5)	51 (71.8)	10 (83.3)	0.631
	Written policy regarding confidentiality of patient information	78 (92.9)	66 (91.7)	12 (100)	0.584
	Written policy for patients' privacy	79 (95.2)	67 (94.4)	12 (100)	0.701
	Written policy for patients' access to their health record	80 (96.4)	68 (95.8)	12 (100)	0.468
	Written policy for appropriate religious support	75 (90.4)	64 (90.1)	11 (91.7)	0.425
	Patient rights posted in a place visible to all patients and visitors	83 (98.8)	71 (98.6)	12 (100)	0.681

and post the Bill in a place where it is visible to the public [12]. In addition, in 2009, the MOHME implemented "Clinical Governance" principles as a framework to improve quality of care, PS and PC in all hospitals. The MOHME also started to pilot the "Patient Safety Friendly Hospital Initiative (PSFHI)" plan for the first time in a limited number of hospitals in 2010, which was in line with WHO plans. The ambition was that these hospitals should try to obtain the first level of PSFHI standards by meeting "critical standards" [14]. Most recently, in 2011, the MOHME revised the "national hospital evaluation program" based on PS and PC principles and compiled the "Hospital Accreditation Standards in Iran" to ensure safety and improve patient-centeredness in hospitals [15]. In this manual, an extensive emphasis has been bestowed on patient safety, patient's rights and patient-centered care in hospitals.

Although there have been some efforts to improve PS and PC in Iranian hospitals, there is very few information available on the actual implementation of specific strategies. This study therefore aims to explore:

Table 4. The associations between implementation of patient safety and patient-centeredness strategies and the type of hospitals.

Strategy		Extent of reported implementation level of patient safety and patient-centeredness strategies by the type of hospitals n (%)			P-value (Cramer's V coefficient)
		Total	General hospitals	Specialized hospitals	
Patient safety	–	–	–	–	–
Patient-centeredness	Providing information in different languages	67 (79.8)	60 (83.3)	7 (58.3)	0.016 (0.31)
	Recording of patient's diet preferences	82 (97.6)	71 (98.6)	11 (91.7)	0.045 (0.27)

1- The reported level of implementation of PS and PC strategies in Iranian hospitals in 2009–2010.
2- The association of the reported level of implementation of PS and PC strategies with the key characteristics of hospitals including type, ownership, teaching status and annual evaluation grade.

Methods

This is a descriptive cross-sectional study based on a self-reported questionnaire survey. A questionnaire was distributed to hospital and nursing managers in a purposive sample of Iranian hospitals eliciting information on the implementation of PS and PC strategies in 2009 and 2010.

The study questionnaire

Data was collected by using an existing validated (from the MARQuIS - Methods of Assessing Response to Quality Improvement Strategies – project) questionnaire [16]. We translated the questionnaire from English into Persian (Farsi). We then adapted the questions to the Iranian health care situation and added some questions on the characteristics of hospitals. We did not re-validate the questionnaire due to time and financial constraints. The questionnaire included in total 57 questions regarding the implementation of 25 PS and 32 PC strategies. The PS and PC strategies were categorized both in three groups. Each group included relevant detailed questions. Four questions on the characteristics of hospitals which are known to be influential in the implementation of PS and PC strategies were included in the questionnaire. They related to the type of hospital (multi-specialty/general, or single specialty/specialized); ownership status of hospitals (university (governmental), Social Security Organization (SSO), private for-profit and private nonprofit (including military and charity organizations); teaching status (non-teaching, non-teaching and teaching, or non-teaching, teaching and research); and the obtained annual evaluation grade (ranging from excellent, 1, 2 to 3).

Pilot and sampling

After verifying the content of the translated and adapted questionnaire, it was piloted in 5 hospitals (including 3 public governmental, 1 private for-profit and 1 SSO hospital). Necessary changes and further improvements were made based on the responses received from the pilot hospitals. Subsequently, the questionnaires were distributed among 145 general and specialized hospitals across the country. These hospitals were selected by using a purposive sampling method and based on hospitals' willingness to be involved in this research project.

Statistics

We examined the extent of implementation of the selected PS and PC strategies based on the positive responses received from the respondents for specific strategies. To examine the relationship between the extent of implementation and characteristics of hospitals we conducted cross tabulations in SPSS. We applied Cramer's V coefficient based on Pearson chi-squared test to measure association between the variables. Our criterion for the statistical differences was $p<0.05$.

The study was approved by the Deputy of Research and Technology of the Iran University of Medical Sciences (Code: 958/1635996).

Results

Study population

Of the 145 hospitals that initially participated in this study, we received questionnaires from 102 hospitals (70.3% response rate). We excluded 18 questionnaires from the final analysis due to incomplete or unreliable answers. This resulted in a total of 84 questionnaires from 72 general and 12 specialty hospitals on which we based our analysis. The characteristics of the included hospitals are shown in table 1.

The majority of hospitals were owned either by university (government) (55%) or by the SSO (25%). Forty three percent of hospitals (n = 36) were non-teaching, forty nine percent (n = 41) of them non-teaching and teaching hospitals and only seven hospitals were involved in research areas besides their non-teaching and teaching activities. Eighty five percent of hospitals were given the second highest rating in the annual evaluation program and 5% the highest rating. There is only one participating hospital that received the lowest rating (grade 3). The hospitals have on average 206 beds (range: 32–620 beds; SD = 137).

The implementation of patient safety and patient-centeredness strategies in general

Patient safety strategies. From the total number of 25 PS strategies, 21 items were reported to have been highly implemented in the majority of the participating hospitals (see table 2). All hospitals acknowledged having assigned infection control personnel and to reporting hospital infections regularly. Ninety nine

Table 5. The associations between implementation of patient safety and patient-centeredness strategies and the ownership of hospitals.

Strategy		Extent of reported implementation level of patient safety and patient-centeredness strategies by the ownership of hospitals n (%)					P-value (Cramer's V coefficient)
		Total	University	SSO	PFP	PNP	
Patient safety	Reports on health promotion	59 (75.6)	26 (65)	20 (95.2)	11 (91.7)	(40)	0.019 (0.31)
	MRSA testing	20 (26)	10 (22.2)	2 (11.1)	4 (44.4)	4 (80)	0.033 (0.30)
Patient-centeredness	Providing room/bed for family and relatives of patients	56 (67.5)	23 (50)	16 (80)	12 (100)	5 (100)	0.012 (0.31)
	Access to internet	15 (18.1)	8 (17.4)	1 (5)	3 (25)	3 (60)	0.021 (0.30)
	Having coordinator for patients affairs	46 (55.4)	22 (47.8)	13 (65)	9 (75)	2 (40)	0.020 (0.30)
	Possibility to contact with the patient's doctor before admission	12 (14.3)	5 (10.9)	0 (0)	5 (41.7)	2 (40)	0.025 (0.29)
	Offering a choice of the meals to patients	19 (22.6)	6 (13)	0 (0)	10 (83.3)	3 (60)	0.000 (0.50)
	Offering a choice in the timing of the meals	13 (15.5)	6 (13)	1 (4.8)	5 (41.7)	1 (20)	0.006 (0.33)

PFP = private for-profit; PNP = private nonprofit.

percent (82) of hospitals reported having a system to routinely check drug expiration dates. In contrast, a number of specific strategies for standard setting have been reported to be less implemented in hospitals. For example few hospitals reported to have specific policies to prevent patients' falling (43%), and MRSA testing was compulsory in only 26% of hospitals. Sixteen percent of hospitals reported to have procedures in place for patient identification in the emergency department and 25% for identifying patients admitted.

Patient-centeredness strategies. There was large variation in the reported level of implementation of various PC strategies (ranging from 13–99%). Twenty-three PC strategies (out of 32) were reported to be implemented in the majority of hospitals (see table 3).

The strategies related to patient rights had the highest reported implementation rate (>89%). The least implemented strategy in this group was having a separate patient rights department, which was present in74% of the hospitals. The provision of some patient and family hotel services (including access to internet, daily newspaper, smoking room, transport services, and choice and timing of the meals) were rarely implemented in hospitals (<23% reported implementation rate). In contrast, some other hotel services such as access to telephone and TV in the room were more common among (65% and 83% respectively) the hospitals.

The association between implementation of patient safety or patient-centeredness strategies and characteristics of hospitals

Patient safety strategies and characteristics of hospitals. The implementation of PS strategies appears unrelated to the type of hospital (table 4). However, the SSO hospitals reported implementation of reports on health promotion significantly more often than the total average reported rates. The hospitals owned by nonprofit organizations reported MRSA testing significantly more often than the total average rate of all hospitals (table 5). The hospitals that are not involved in teaching and research activities, reported the presence of the antibiotic use policy significantly more often than the hospitals involved in teaching and research activities. In contrast, table 6 shows MRSA testing is reported significantly more often by hospitals involved in research, besides their teaching and therapeutic activities. The differences in the implementation rates of the majority of PS strategies were not associated with differences in hospital grades. However, the hospitals with a higher grade reported significantly more often to having responsible personnel available for clinical waste management and health promotion. Higher grade hospitals reported more often to have clinical waste management procedures in place and to perform health promotion activities than lower grade hospitals (see table 7).

Patient-centeredness strategies and characteristics of hospitals. There is no significant difference between general and specialized hospitals in the reported implementation rates of PC strategies with the exception of providing information in different languages and recording of the patient's diet preference. The general hospitals reported significantly more often to have implemented these strategies than specialized hospitals (see table 4). The patient services strategies including provision of a room/bed for the relatives of patients, possibility to contact the patient's family doctor/specialist before admission, offering a choice of meals and timing of meals to patients, were reported to be implemented significantly more often in private (both for-profit and nonprofit) hospitals compared to the total average rate of all

Table 6. The associations between implementation of patient safety and patient-centeredness strategies and the teaching and research status of hospitals.

Strategy		Extent of reported implementation level of patient safety and patient-centeredness strategies by the teaching status of hospitals n (%)				P-value (Cramer's V coefficient)
		Total	Non-teaching	Non-teaching & teaching	Non-teaching & teaching & research	
Patient safety	Reports on antibiotic use policy	47 (62.7)	23 (76.7)	21 (53.8)	3 (50)	0.020 (0.28)
	MRSA testing	20 (26)	6 (19.4)	10 (25.6)	4 (57.1)	0.001 (0.35)
Patient-centeredness	Providing daily newspaper for patients	12 (14.5)	4 (11.4)	4 (9.8)	4 (57.1)	0.021 (0.26)
	Having coordinator for patients affairs	46 (55.4)	26 (74.3)	18 (43.9)	2 (28.6)	0.002 (0.32)
	Having transport services for patients	17 (20.5)	7 (20)	6 (14.6)	4 (57.1)	0.007 (0.29)

hospitals (as shown in the table 5). The association was strongest (Cramer's V = 0.50) in case of offering a choice of the meals to patients in the private hospitals (83% compared to average rate of 23%). It seems that the rate of implementation of PC strategies is unrelated to the annual evaluation grade of hospitals.

Discussion

This is the first study to our knowledge that provides comprehensive insight in the (reported) implementation of PS and PC strategies in Iranian hospitals. However, the study has some limitations. First, the authors tried to include a representative sample of hospitals in the study as much as possible. Although the sample size of the study was relatively small especially with regard to the limited number of hospitals with lower annual evaluation grades (grade 2 and 3) and the hospitals owned by nonprofit organizations, the total number of these groups of hospitals is limited in the country. Another limitation concerns the validity of the questionnaire. Due to time and funding constraints, the questionnaire was not re-validated, which seems acceptable given the minor changes that were made compared to the original validated version. Another limitation of the study was the 30% non-response and those who had to be excluded from the final analysis due to incomplete or unreliable data. Finally, the study was based on a purposive sampling method and a self-reported questionnaire; potentially producing biased results.

Our study identified that the strategies related to assigning responsibilities, outcomes reporting, patient rights and the majority of patient services were reported to be most often implemented by all hospitals. However, the specific strategies which were related to standard setting and some patient hotel services were reported less commonly in Iranian hospitals. These findings are mostly in line with the MARQuIS study [17], [18] which reported similar results concerning the implementation of PS and PC strategies in hospitals in European countries (Belgium, the Czech Republic, France, Ireland, the Netherlands, Poland, Spain, UK). Surprisingly, this study also reported that MRSA testing and choice of timing of the meals were less common strategies in European countries. Our findings related to patient identification strategies are different from the MARQuIS study. We found patient identification strategies were less commonly applied in Iranian hospitals, while in the MARQuIS study a relatively higher implementation rate was reported. Our study has also found a meaningful association between ownership status and annual evaluation grade of hospitals and the implementation of PS and PC strategies. The strategies which are (statutorily) part of the Iranian annual evaluation program were more often reported to be implemented compared to the other non-obligatory strategies. In addition, the rate of implementation for (some of) the patient hotel services was significantly more often reported in the private (both for-profit and nonprofit) hospitals compared to other hospitals.

Attention to the specific strategies for standard setting and patient hotel services

Although the majority of PS and PC strategies assessed in our study were reported to be widely implemented, there were less frequent implementation rates reported for strategies related to standard setting and (some) patient services. Identifying patients in hospital, MRSA testing, policies for preventing patient falls were less common PS strategies reported to be implemented by hospitals. Moreover, the implementation of a number of patient hotel services was reported to be significantly lower in hospitals compared to other strategies. Although our findings are in line with the lower implementation rates, some PS and PC strategies reported in a few countries [17–19]. There is a concern about suboptimal implementation rates. More attention needs to be given to the implementation of these strategies to complete the cycle of PS and PC care in hospitals. These strategies have been reported in other studies to be important factors in improving safety and PC in hospitals. They have also been identified as the main PS and PC issues in hospitals around the world [20–24].

Emphasize the effectiveness of strategies in practice

Although the overall reported implementation rate of the majority of the PS and PC strategies was relatively high, a continuous debate concerning the actual impact of these strategies for improving safety and PC in hospitals. A gap remains between the reported implementation rate and the effectiveness of strategies in practice. The evidence from the relevant literature shows that the strategies in some cases have not been effectively implemented. For instance, although 100% of hospitals in our study reported

Table 7. The associations between implementation of patient safety and patient-centeredness strategies and the annual evaluation grade of hospitals.

Strategy		Extent of reported implementation level of patient safety and patient-centeredness strategies by the annual evaluation grade of hospitals n (%)					P-value (Cramer's V coefficient)
		Total	Excellent1	Grade 1	Grade 2	Grade 3	
Patient safety	Responsible personnel for clinical waste management	65 (85.5)	4 (100)	58 (86.6)	3 (75)	0 (0)	0.022 (0.31)
	Responsible personnel for health promotion	65 (85.5)	4 (100)	58 (86.6)	3 (75)	0 (0)	0.003 (0.36)
	Reports on clinical waste management	62 (84.9)	4 (100)	55 (85.9)	3 (75)	0 (0)	0.001 (0.39)
	Reports on health promotion	56 (74.7)	4 (100)	49 (74.2)	3 (75)	0 (0)	0.04 (0.30)
	Availability of clinical guidelines/protocols	73 (90.1)	2 (50)	66 (93)	4 (80)	1 (100)	0.042 (0.28)
Patient-centeredness	–	–	–	–	–	–	–

having responsible personnel and routinely reports for infection control in place, several studies identified that the hospital infection rate in Iran is still remarkably higher than the infection rate in European countries (8–10% compared to 5%) [25], [26]. In addition, almost all hospitals reported to having posted the Patients' Bill of Rights and to implementing the patient rights principles. Some report that patient rights principles are not fully implemented by all health care providers [27]. Our study thus suggests that reporting a higher rate of strategies implementation does not guarantee safety and better patient care. Such efforts should be supported by legal embedding and enforcement of strategies, creating an organizational responsiveness and culture of safety and PC [28–30]. Truly partnering with patients and their families can also be effective [2], [30], [31], [32].

How is the implementation of patient safety and patient-centeredness strategies associated with characteristics of hospitals?

Our study showed that there are meaningful associations between the implementation of PS and PC strategies and the characteristics of hospitals, which is in line with related research in this field. A study has revealed that the hospital characteristics may predict the implementation of PS and PC strategies [33]. In our study the implementation rates of patient hotel services were reported significantly more often in the private (for-profit and nonprofit) hospitals. This may suggest that private hospitals in Iran are more service-oriented and thus more interested in implementation of hotel services. The financial incentives for hospitals clearly play a role in the implementation of PC strategies especially with regard to hotel services. The results showed that the hospitals were involved in teaching and research activities besides non-teaching activities, reported higher implementation of some specific PS strategies (i.e. MRSA testing). Although it is difficult to speak of a pattern because of the limited number of the hospitals involved in both non-teaching, teaching and research activities, these hospitals appear to be more safety-oriented.

Finally, our results revealed that the hospitals with higher evaluation grades, reported a significantly higher implementation rate of the strategies compared to the lower grade hospitals. Hospitals in our study reported a higher implementation rate with regard to obligatory PS strategies which were subjected to the Iranian hospital evaluation program. The commitment to PS strategies by the higher graded hospitals is required in order to achieve a higher evaluation grade. The obligation of hospitals to implement specific strategies can be a potential incentive for planning and implementing PS or PC strategies.

Conclusion

Although the implementation of a number of PS and PC strategies were widely reported by Iranian hospitals, there is room for improvement and strengthening of the implementation of specific strategies related to standard setting and patient services. The association of PS and PC strategies with characteristics of hospitals (type, ownership, teaching status and annual evaluation grade) provides a mixed picture. The implementation of PS and PC strategies are influenced by the characteristics of these hospitals. The safety strategies which are statutorily obligated by the government were more frequently implemented in the higher grade hospitals. The PC strategies were more common in the private (for-profit and nonprofit) hospitals, which appear to be more service-oriented. Despite the reporting of relatively high implementation rates for the majority of strategies, the effectiveness of PS and PC strategies in hospitals still needs improvement.

An effective implementation of PS and PC initiatives may depend on the legal embedding and enforcement of standards, creating an organizational responsiveness to demands of patients, creating a PS and PC culture in hospitals and partnering with patients and their families.

Acknowledgments

The authors are grateful to Dr. Mehdi Jafari, Dr. Seysed Hesam Seyedin, Mr. Saeidreza Azamy and Mrs. Seyran Naghdi for facilitating the data collection for this study. The authors would also like to thank Professor Dr. Karien Stronks for supporting this research project at the Department of Public Health, Academic Medical Center (AMC) - University of Amsterdam.

Author Contributions

Conceived and designed the experiments: AAH NSK DSK. Performed the experiments: AAH HR NSK DSK JM. Analyzed the data: AAH NSK DSK. Contributed reagents/materials/analysis tools: AAH NSK HR JM. Contributed to the writing of the manuscript: AAH NSK DSK.

References

1. World Health Organization (WHO) (2013) Patient safety assessment manual. Available: http://applications.emro.who.int/dsaf/emropub_2011_1243.pdf. Accessed 9 August 2013.
2. Australian Commission on Safety and Quality in Health Care (ACSQHC) (2010) Patient-centred care: improving quality and safety by focusing care on patients and consumers, Discussion paper draft for public consultation, September. Available: http://www.podiatrywa.com.au/news/146-Patient-CentredCarePaperweb.pdf. Accessed 13 February 2013.
3. Institute for Patient- and Family-Centered Care website (2013) Available: http://www.ipfcc.org. Accessed 7 July 2013.
4. Wong J, Beglaryan H (2004) Strategies for Hospitals to Improve Patient Safety. A Review of the Research February, The Change Foundation. Available: http://www.providence.on.ca/wp-content/uploads/2012/05/Change-Foundation-Improve-Patient-Safety.pdf. Accessed 14 February 2013.
5. World Health Organization (WHO) (2013) 10 facts on Patient Safety. Available: http://www.who.int/features/factfi les/patient_safety/en/index.html. Accessed 8 June 2013.
6. James JT (2013) A New, Evidence-based Estimate of Patient Harms Associated with Hospital Care, Journal of Patient Safety: September; Volume 9 - Issue 3 - p 122–128 doi: 10.1097/PTS.0b013e3182948a69.
7. World Health Organization (WHO): Patient safety (2013) Available: http://www.emro.who.int/entity/patient-safety/. Accessed 7 June 2013.
8. Pollack A (2010) Rising Threat of Infections Unfazed by Antibiotics. New York Times, Feb. 27.
9. Zargarzadeh AH (2013) Medication Safety in Iran. J Pharm Care; 1(4): 125–126.
10. Sheikhtaheri A, Sadoughi F, Ahmadi M, Moghaddasi H (2013) Developing Iranian patient safety indicators: an essential approach for improving safety of health care. Asian Biomedicine June; Vol. 7 No. 3, 365–373, doi: 10.5372/1905-7415.0703.188.
11. Zahraei SM, Eshrati B, Masoumi Asl H, Pezeshki Z (2012) Epidemiology of Four Main Nosocomial Infections in Iran during March 2007– March 2008 based on the Findings of a Routine Surveillance System. Arch Iran Med; 15(12): 764–766.
12. Joolaee S, Hajibabaee F (2012) Patient rights in Iran: A review article. Nurs Ethics 19: 45 originally published online 2 December 2011, doi:10.1177/0969733011412100.
13. Aghaei Hashjin A, Delgoshaei B, Kringos DS, Tabibi SJ, Manoochehri J, et al. (2014) Implementation of hospital quality assurance policies in Iran. Submitted for publication in 2014.
14. World Health Organization (WHO): Patient safety friendly hospitals (2013) Available: http://www.emro.who.int/patient-safety/countries/country-activities-islamic-republic-of-iran.html. Accessed at 10 June 2013.
15. Iranian Ministry of Health and Medical Education (MOHME) (2011) Hospital Accreditation Standards in Iran. Tehran.
16. Assessing of the effectiveness of quality improvement strategies in Europe: the MARQuIS project (2006) Available: http://www.marquisquestionnaire.nl/marquis/print/printallgeneral.asp. Accessed 25 July 2006.
17. Lombarts MJ, Rupp I, Vallejo P, Suñol R, Klazinga NS (2009) Application of quality improvement strategies in 389 European hospitals: results of the MARQuIS project. BMJ journal of Quality & Safety in Health Care, vol. 18, supplement 1.
18. Groene O, Lombarts MJ, Klazinga N, Alonso J, Thompson A, Suñol R (2009) Is patient-centredness in European hospitals related to existing quality improvement strategies? Analysis of a cross-sectional survey (MARQuIS study). BMJ journal of Quality & Safety in Health Care, vol. 18, supplement 1: i44–i50 doi:10.1136.
19. Lombarts MJ, Rupp I, Vallejo P, Klazinga NS, Sunol R (2009) Differentiating between hospitals according to the "maturity" of quality improvement systems: a new classification scheme in a sample of European hospitals. BMJ journal of Quality & Safety in Health Care, vol. 18, supplement 1.
20. Griese BR, Frazier CR (2011) Patient Identification: Simple Measures, Big Benefits: Ensuring patient identification means avoiding financial loss and accreditation - and keeping patients safe. Advance health care network, February 17. Available: http://healthcare-executive-insight.advanceweb.com/Columns/Case-Files-Legal-Issues-for-Healthcare-Executives/Patient-Identification-Simple-Measures-Big-Benefits.aspx. Accessed 23 September 2013.
21. World Health Organization (WHO) (2007) Patient identification. Patient Safety Solutions, vol. 1, solution 2, May.
22. Deleo FR, Otto M, Kreiswirth BN, Chambers HF (2010) Community-associated meticillin-resistant Staphylococcus aureus. Lancet; 375: 1557–1568.
23. Askari E, Soleymani F, Arianpoor A, Tabatabai SM, Amini AR, et al. (2012) Epidemiology of mecA-Methicillin Resistant Staphylococcus aureus (MRSA) in Iran: A Systematic Review and Meta-analysis. Iranian Journal of Basic Medical Sciences Sep-Oct; 15(5): 1010–1019.
24. Grundmann H, Aires-de-Sousa M, Boyce J, Tiemersma E (2006) Emergence and resurgence of methicillinresistant Staphylococcus aureus as a public-health threat. Lancet, 368: 874–85.
25. Zahraei SM, Eshrati B, Masoumi Asl H, Pezeshki Z (2012)Epidemiology of Four Main Nosocomial Infections in Iran during March 2007– March 2008 based on the Findings of a Routine Surveillance System. Arch Iran Med; 15(12): 764–766.
26. Askarian M, Gooran NR (2003) National nosocomial infection surveillance system-based study in Iran: additional hospital stay attributable to nosocomial infections. American Journal of Infection Control, Dec; 31(8): 465–8.
27. Joolaee S, Hajibabaee F (2011) Patient rights in Iran: A review article. Nurs Ethics 2012, 19: 45 DOI: 10.1177/0969733011412100.
28. Wagner C, Smits M, Sorra J, Huang CC (2013)Assessing patient safety culture in hospitals across countries. International Journal of Quality in Health Care Jul; 25(3): 213–21. doi: 10.1093.
29. Aghaei Hashjin A, Ravaghi H, Kringos DS, Ogbu UC, Fischer C, et al. (2014) Using Quality Measures for Quality Improvement: The Perspective of Hospital Staff. PLOS ONE, January 23, DOI: 10.1371/journal.pone.0086014.
30. Verbeek-Van Noord I, Wagner C, Twisk JWR, De Bruijne MC (2013) Is culture associated with patient safety in the emergency department? A study of staff perspectives, Int J Qual Health Care (2014) 26 (1): 64–70 first published online December 10, doi:10.1093/intqhc/mzt087.
31. Groene O, Sunol R, Klazinga NS, Wang A, Dersarkissian M, et al. (2014) Involvement of patients or their representatives in quality management functions in EU hospitals: implementation and impact on patient-centred care strategies, Int J Qual Health Care first published online March 9, doi:10.1093/intqhc/mzu022.
32. Hrisos S, Thomson R (2013) Seeing It from Both Sides: Do Approaches to Involving Patients in Improving Their Safety Risk Damaging the Trust between Patients and Healthcare Professionals? An Interview Study. PLOS ONE, November 06, DOI: 10.1371/journal.pone.0080759.
33. Longo DR, Hewett JE, Ge B, Schubert S (2007) Hospital patient safety: characteristics of best-performing hospitals. Journal of Healthcare Management May-Jun; 52(3): 188–204; discussion 204–5.

11

Impact of Appropriate Antimicrobial Therapy for Patients with Severe Sepsis and Septic Shock – A Quality Improvement Study

Paula K. O. Yokota[1], Alexandre R. Marra[1]*, Marines D. V. Martino[2], Elivane S. Victor[3], Marcelino S. Durão[1], Michael B. Edmond[4], Oscar F. P. dos Santos[1]

1 Division of Medical Practice, Hospital Israelita Albert Einstein, São Paulo, Brazil, **2** Laboratory of Microbiology, Hospital Israelita Albert Einstein, São Paulo, Brazil, **3** Statistics Department, Instituto Israelita de Ensino e Pesquisa (IIEP), Hospital Israelita Albert Einstein, São Paulo, Brazil, **4** Department of Internal Medicine, Virginia Commonwealth University School of Medicine, Richmond, Virginia, United States of America

Abstract

Background: There is ample literature available on the association between both time to antibiotics and appropriateness of antibiotics and clinical outcomes from sepsis. In fact, the current state of debate surrounds the balance to be struck between prompt empirical therapy and care in the choice of appropriate antibiotics (both in terms of the susceptibility of infecting organism and minimizing resistance arising from use of broad-spectrum agents). The objective of this study is to determine sepsis bundle compliance and the appropriateness of antimicrobial therapy in patients with severe sepsis and septic shock and its impact on outcomes.

Material: This study was conducted in the ICU of a tertiary care, private hospital in São Paulo, Brazil. A retrospective cohort study was conducted from July 2005 to December 2012 in patients with severe sepsis and septic shock.

Results: A total of 1,279 patients were identified with severe sepsis and septic shock, of which 358 (32.1%) had bloodstream infection (BSI). The inpatient mortality rate was 29%. In evaluation of the sepsis bundle, over time there was a progressive increase in serum arterial lactate collection, obtaining blood cultures prior to antibiotic administration, administration of broad-spectrum antibiotics within 1 hour, and administration of appropriate antimicrobials, with statistically significant differences in the later years of the study. We also observed a significant decrease in mortality. In patients with bloodstream infection, after adjustment for other covariates the administration of appropriate antimicrobial therapy was associated with a decrease in mortality in patients with severe sepsis and septic shock ($p = 0.023$).

Conclusions: The administration of appropriate antimicrobial therapy was independently associated with a decline in mortality in patients with severe sepsis and septic shock due to bloodstream infection. As protocol adherence increased over time, the crude mortality rate decreased, which reinforces the need to implement institutional guidelines and monitor appropriate antimicrobial therapy compliance.

Editor: Heiman Frank Louis Wertheim, Oxford University, Viet Nam

Funding: The authors have no support or funding to report.

Competing Interests: The authors have declared that no competing interests exist.

* Email: alexandre.marra@einstein.br

Background

Severe sepsis and septic shock are worrisome manifestations of systemic infection and the leading causes of hospitalization in intensive care units (ICUs), where an estimated 19 million cases occur worldwide each year, resulting in the death of one in four of these patients [1,2]. According to the Ministry of Health of Brazil, severe sepsis and septic shock are responsible for an average of 41% of the total yearly in-hospital mortality for adults from 2008 through August 2013. Case mortality is 46% in the southeast region [3], which reinforced our desire to participate in the Surviving Sepsis Campaign beginning in 2004, as well as the "Stop Sepsis, Save Lives" project [4,5].

According to the international guidelines, for the immediate treatment of severe sepsis or septic shock, antibiotic administration should occur within the first hour of recognition as it directly impacts in mortality [2]. Since 2006, we have utilized the sepsis bundle in our ICU [6], the treatment recommendations were organized in two bundles: a resuscitation bundle (6 tasks to begin immediately and to be accomplished within 6 hours) and a management bundle (4 tasks to be completed within 24 hours) [4]; however, there is no evaluation of the appropriateness of antimicrobial therapy after collecting blood cultures in sepsis bundle studies, which is one of the main measures to reduce mortality in critically ill patients suffering from infectious processes. When longer time frames to appropriate antibiotic therapy are observed there is an increased risk of death [7–9].

Thus, the objectives of the study were to determine i) the sepsis bundle compliance, ii) as well as the appropriateness of antimicrobial therapy for patients with severe sepsis and septic shock, as well as impact on outcomes.

Methods

This study was conducted in the ICU of a tertiary care, private hospital in São Paulo, Brazil. This open model ICU is a 41-bed medical-surgical unit with approximately 10,500 patient-days yearly.

A retrospective cohort study was conducted from July 2005 to December 2012 in patients with severe sepsis and septic shock to analyze the impact of appropriate antimicrobial therapy. This study was a quality improvement project that was approved by the Institutional Review Board (IRB) of Hospital Israelita Albert Einstein. The requirements for informed consent were waived by our IRB in accordance of the Code of Federal Regulation and of the Privacy Rule. This project includes data from our previous sepsis bundle study from July 2005 to December 2009 [6] with the addition of observations for the period from January 2010 to December 2012 in order to evaluate whether sustained implementation of the sepsis bundle in our ICU could effectively reduce mortality in severe sepsis and septic shock patients.

Sepsis was defined as infection plus two or more of the following SIRS criteria: T>38°C or <36°C; heart rate >90/min; respiratory rate >20 breaths/min (or Paco2<32 mm Hg); or WBC count, >12,000 cells/μL or <4,000 cells/μL (or >10% band forms) [10]. Severe sepsis was defined as sepsis plus organ dysfunction, hypotension, or hypoperfusion abnormalities, including lactic acidosis, oliguria, or encephalopathy. Septic shock was defined as sepsis-induced hypotension (ie, systolic BP, <90 mm Hg or a drop of >40 mm Hg in the absence of other cause of hypotension) plus hypoperfusion abnormalities despite adequate fluid resuscitation [10] (Appendix S1) Infection was defined according to the definitions of the International Sepsis Forum [11] and adjudicated by the patient's physician.

The data collected included age, gender, admission date, the time when severe sepsis or septic shock was diagnosed, location before ICU admission, hospital and ICU length of stay, organ dysfunction at the time of diagnosis, APACHE II score on admission, and outcome status (death was defined as in-hospital mortality). As per the Surviving Sepsis Campaign, "time zero" was defined as the time of diagnosis of severe sepsis or septic shock.

Once a patient meets the bundle initiation criteria, the 6-hour bundle was initiated by collecting serum arterial lactate and obtaining blood cultures before antibiotic administration (Appendix S1). From the time of severe sepsis (time zero), broad-spectrum antibiotics are to be administered within 1 hour (since every hour of delay increases the risk of poorer outcomes). Hypotension and/or elevated lactate are treated with IV fluids; in the event of persistent hypotension despite fluid resuscitation (septic shock) and/or lactate >4 mmol/L (>36 mg/dL), maintaining adequate central venous pressure and central venous oxygen saturation are indicated. Patients who do not have septic shock and elevated lactate >4 mmol/L (>36 mg/dL) do not require measurement of central venous pressure and central venous oxygen saturation.

The first 24-hour management bundle includes optimization of glycemic control, respiratory inspiratory plateau pressure, and determination of the need for corticosteroids and drotrecogin alfa (activated) [4]. However, we did not perform analysis for the 24-hour sepsis bundle for patients with severe sepsis or septic shock because there have been changes in the recommendations (e.g., glycemic control, and use of activated protein C) [2,6].

Our hospital has an electronic system for activating a team dedicated to diagnosing and treating severe sepsis and septic shock patients immediately. The ICU doctor and the nurse manager are simultaneously notified. The development of this sepsis team was part of implementing the sepsis bundle. Our hospital also has had a rapid response team since 2007 [6]. The rapid response team is alerted based on the following criteria: respiratory problems such as acute decrease in oxygen saturation <90% and change in respiratory rate to <8/minute or >28/minute; circulatory problems: decrease in systolic arterial pressure to <90 mmHg associated with symptoms; and change in heart rate to <40 bpm or >130 bpm; neurologic problems: decreasing consciousness levels or seizures; or a serious concern with the patient's overall condition (patient claims to be feeling unwell or has the sensation "something is not right"), and change in color, diaphoresis, or coolness of the extremities. Some of these described signs are the same as those noted in sepsis patients [6,12].

Antimicrobial therapy

Antimicrobial therapy was considered appropriate if the bacteria identified in blood culture was susceptible to at least one of the antibiotics administered within 24 hours after the collection of culture. If the isolated microorganism was not susceptible by in vitro testing to the antibiotic used, the therapy was considered inadequate [7].

The microbiology laboratory has an alert system to notify physicians of patients with positive blood cultures and their gram stain results.

Microbiological methods

All samples were identified by manual or automated method and confirmed using the Vitek 2 (bio-Merieux Vitek, Inc., Hazelwood, MO) system. To determine the prevalence of antimicrobial resistance, the same organism with identical antimicrobial profiles from the same or different anatomic sites in the same patient were considered a single isolate. Antimicrobial susceptibility testing was performed by an automated method or by disk diffusion as described by the Clinical and Laboratory Standards Institute (CLSI) [13].

Statistical analysis

Differences over time were evaluated by autoregressive time series models. The order of the models was determined according to the analysis of the partial autocorrelation function of residuals. The summary of the year was presented as means ± standard deviations or as absolute frequencies and percentages. Significance of changes was evaluated by trend effects. All tests of significance are two-tailed and alpha was set at 0.05.

To analyze the impact of inadequate antimicrobial therapy on mortality in the 358 patients with bloodstream infection, models were constructed by binary logistic regression in single and multiple approaches, only with data collected between 2010 and 2012. The variables with $p \leq 0.10$ in the simple analysis models were evaluated via multivariate analysis. The association of independent variables was expressed as odds ratios with 95% confidence intervals.

Analyses were performed with the Statistical Package for the Social Sciences 17.0 (Chicago, IL, USA).

Results

The total cohort, shown in Figure S1, consisted of 1,279 consecutive patients, where 57.7% (N = 738) were male, mean age ± standard deviation (SD) 67±18 years, mean APACHE II score

Table 1. Demographic and clinical characteristics of severe sepsis and septic shock patients from July 2005 to December 2012.

Variables	Before protocol		After protocol													
	07/05 a 04/06		05/06 a 12/06		2007		2008		2009		2010		2011		2012	
	(n = 100)		(n = 73)		(n = 140)		(n = 134)		(n = 117)		(n = 197)		(n = 240)		(n = 279)	
	n	%	n	%	n	%	n	%	n	%	n	%	n	%	n	%
Septic shock	88	88.0	62	84.9	108	77.1	100	75.2	68	58.1	116	58.9	152	63.3	182	65.2
APACHE	25	±8	25	±9	24	±7	23	±6	21	±6	19	±7	21	±7	23	±7
Age	63	±20	66	±20	67	±19	67	±17	67	±18	69	±18	67	±18	66	±18
Serum arterial lactate	72	72.0	68	93.2	121	86.4	123	92.5	96	82.1	183	92.9	231	96.3	274	98.2
Blood culture prior to antibiotic administration	44	44.0	42	57.5	67	47.9	99	74.4	85	72.6	171	86.8	232	96.7	270	96.8
Positive blood culture	23	43.4%	27	34.6%	37	39.4%	41	37.3%	31	28.7%	52	30.4%	75	32.3%	72	26.7%
Broad-spectrum antibiotic within 1 h	58	58.0	46	63.0	105	75.0	103	77.4	73	62.4	105	53.3	137	57.1	228	81.7
Central venous oxygen saturation ($ScvO_2 \geq 70\%$)	50	50.0	34	46.6	60	42.9	64	48.1	66	56.4	59	95.2	100	76.9	103	64.8
Appropriate antibiotic therapy	13	56.5%	19	70.4%	19	51.4%	32	78.0%	26	83.9%	40	76.9	52	69.3	59	81.9
Mortality Rate	54	54.0	30	41.1	55	39.3	55	41.4	19	16.2	61	31.0	46	19.2	49	17.6

-Analyses of antimicrobial appropriateness and value of central venous oxygen saturation were performed with the total of 199 and 358 patients, respectively.

Table 2. Comparison between patients with and without positive blood cultures.

Variables	**Blood culture**		**p**
	Negative (N = 758)	**Positive (N = 358)**	
Male - n (%)	432 (57.%)	221 (61.7%)	0.134
Organ dysfunction – n (%)			
Liver	39 (5.1%)	27 (7.5%)	0.113
Cardiologic	492 (64.9%)	273 (76.3%)	$<$0.001
Renal	286 (37.7%)	138 (38.5%)	0.793
Hematologic	277 (36.5%)	134 (37.4%)	0.774
Respiratory	529 (69.8%)	210 (58.7%)	$<$0.001
Neurologic	260 (34.3%)	119 (33.2%)	0.727
Metabolic acidosis on admission	252 (33.2%)	133 (37.2%)	0.200
Mortality rate – n (%)	185 (24.4%)	101 (28.2%)	0.174
Apache II - mean (±SD)	16.8 (±10.1)	18.1 (±10.2)	0.005
Age - mean (±SD)	67.5 (±18.3)	64.2 (±17.9)	0.050

163 patients without blood culture collected during the study period.

of 18±10, mean length of stay 33±71 days, mean time to administration of antibiotic was 2.5±3.6 hours, mean serum arterial lactate 27±24 mg/dL, and mean ± central venous oxygen saturation 76.2±11.4%. The total number of deaths was 371 (29.0%).

In analysis of sepsis bundle performance by year (table 1), there was a significant progressive increase in serum arterial lactate collection, administration of broad-spectrum antibiotic within 1 hour, and treatment with appropriate antimicrobial therapy. We also observed a significant decrease in crude mortality (figure S2).

In our cohort, 163 patients (12.7%) did not have blood culture collected. Of the 1,116 patients with blood cultures collected, 358 (32.1%) were positive. Comparing patients with and without positive blood cultures, cardiac dysfunction and a high APACHE II score were more prevalent in patients with positive blood cultures (p-value <0.001 and 0.005, respectively, table 2). Older patients and those with respiratory dysfunction were more likely to have negative blood cultures (p-value <0.001 and 0.05, respectively).

For all patients with severe sepsis and septic shock, higher APACHE II scores were an independent predictor of mortality (Table 3). Patients with circulatory dysfunction, renal dysfunction, hematologic dysfunction, and respiratory dysfunction also had increased odds of death. Mortality was significantly lower in patients who had blood cultures obtained, and in those for whom serum arterial lactate was measured.

In the subset of patients with bloodstream infection, the APACHE II score were also remained an independent predictor of death (Table 4). Patients with renal and neurological dysfunction also had increased odds of death. After adjustment for other covariates, the administration of appropriate antimicrobial therapy was associated with a decreased risk of mortality (OR 0.54, p = 0.023) (Table 4). Higher APACHE II scores and the presence of polymicrobial infection were associated with inadequate antimicrobial therapy (p<0.001 and p = 0.016, respectively) (Table 5).

Among the 358 patients with positive blood cultures, 333 (93.0%) had monobacterial infections (table 6). The most common pathogens were *Escherichia coli* (n = 101, 28.2%), *Streptococcus pneumoniae* (n = 31, 8.7%). Bacteria belonging to the ESKAPE group were represented as follows: *Staphylococcus aureus* (n = 24, 6.7%), *Klebsiella pneumoniae* (n = 20, 5.6%), *Pseudomonas aeruginosa* (n = 18, 5.0%), *Enterobacter* spp (n = 10, 2.8%), *Enterococcus faecium* (n = 2, 0.6%), *Acinetobacter baumannii* (n = 4, 1.1%). Considering fungal infections, 5 patients (1.5%) had *Candida* bloodstream infection; of these, 2 patients had *Candida albicans*, 2 patients had *Candida parapsilosis*, and one patient *Candida krusei*. Among the monomicrobial infection cases 74.2% (n = 247) received adequate antimicrobial therapy. One reason for inadequate therapy was fungal bloodstream infection (83.3%, n = 5). There were few cases of polymicrobial bloodstream infections (N = 25, 7.0%). More than a half of these cases received adequate antimicrobial therapy (n = 13, 52.0%). Highly resistant organisms not covered by usual empiric therapy as represented by the ESKAPE pathogen group could be expected to be associated with inadequate therapy; however, we were not able to demonstrate this by the multivariate analysis (table 5).

Discussion

With improvement of compliance to the sepsis bundle over time, we demonstrate an association with reduced mortality. Not surprisingly, risk factors for death include the APACHE II score, as well as the presence of other disorders that contribute to severe worsening of the patient's general condition [1].

In addition to implementing the sepsis protocol at our institution (May 2006), practical bedside contact with evidence-based medicine and attendance at several scientific meetings by the multidisciplinary team also contributed in improving the care of these patients. Over the period of analysis, changes in treatment, such as the utilization of Activated protein C followed by its suspension reflect the need for continuous learning and improving based on the state of the science [6].

Another important fact, demonstrated by logistic regression, is that despite the implementation of the measures incorporated in the sepsis bundle, such as collecting serum arterial lactate and timely administration of antibiotics, it was antimicrobial appropriateness that contributed to decreased mortality in severe sepsis and septic shock patients. Over the past two years, our mortality rate in severe sepsis and septic shock patients was below 20% as

Table 3. Risk factors associated with death in all patients with severe sepsis or septic shock.

Variables	Survival (N=908)	Death (N=371)	Univariate analysis				Multivariate analysis			
			OR	CI 95%		P	OR	CI 95%		p
	N (%)	N (%)		Min	Max			Min	Max	
Age (years), mean ± SD	65.9±18	69.2±18	1.010	1.003	1.017	**0.004**	1.004	0.997	1.012	0.263
APACHE II, mean ± SD	16.2±9	21.8±10	1.060	1.046	1.074	**<0.001**	1.052	1.037	1.067	**<0.001**
Liver dysfunction	48 (5.2)	20 (5.3)	1.021	0.597	1.745	0.940				
Cardiac dysfunction	595 (97.8)	287 (77.3)	1.797	1.360	2.376	**<0.001**	1.439	1.048	1.976	**0.025**
Renal dysfunction	307 (33.8)	204 (54.9)	2.391	1.869	3.060	**<0.001**	1.792	1.371	2.341	**<0.001**
Hematologic dysfunction	307 (33.8)	155 (41.7)	1.405	1.096	1.800	**0.007**	1.684	1.270	2.234	**<0.001**
Respiratory dysfunction	576 (63.4)	255 (68.7)	1.267	0.979	1.640	**0.072**	1.693	1.265	2.266	**<0.001**
Neurologic dysfunction	283 (31.2)	142 (38.2)	1.369	1.064	1.762	**0.015**	1.286	0.976	1.694	0.073
Blood cultures prior to antibiotic administration	830 (91.4)	286 (77.0)	0.316	0.226	0.442	**<0.001**	0.380	0.264	0.546	**<0.001**
Broad-spectrum antibiotic within 1 hour	585 (64.4)	206 (55.5)	0.689	0.539	0.881	**0.003**	0.771	0.589	1.010	0.060
Serum arterial lactate	884 (97.4)	350 (94.3)	0.452	0.249	0.823	**0.009**	1.383	1.037	1.845	**0.027**
Central venous oxygen saturation	493 (54.3)	255 (68.7)	1.850	1.433	2.389	**<0.001**	0.392	0.203	0.757	**0.005**

OR = Odds Ratio; CI = Confidence Interval; APACHE: Acute Physiology and Chronic Health Evaluation II.

Table 4. Risk factors associated with death for patients with severe sepsis or septic shock and documented bloodstream infection.

Variables	Survival (N=257)	Death (N=101)	Univariate analysis				Multivariate analysis			
			OR	CI 95%		P	OR	CI 95%		p
	N (%)	N (%)		Min	Max			Min	Max	
Age (years), mean ± SD	64.5±17	63.2±19	0.996	0.983	1.009	0.521				
APACHE II, mean ± SD	16.9±10	21.0±11	1.041	1.017	1.066	**0.001**	1.029	1.004	1.055	**0.022**
Liver dysfunction	19 (7.4)	08 (7.9)	1.078	0.456	2.547	0.865				
Cardiac dysfunction	189 (73.5)	84 (83.2)	1.778	0.985	3.208	**0.056**	1.392	0.746	2.595	0.299
Renal dysfunction	81 (31.5)	57 (56.4)	2.815	1.754	4.518	**<0.001**	2.432	1.472	4.018	**0.001**
Hematologic dysfunction	89 (34.6)	45 (44.6)	1.517	0.949	2.425	**0.082**	1.583	0.953	2.628	0.076
Respiratory dysfunction	144 (56.0)	66 (65.3)	1.480	0.917	2.387	0.108				
Neurologic dysfunction	74 (28.8)	45 (44.6)	1.987	1.234	3.200	**0.005**	1.908	1.153	3.158	**0.012**
Broad-spectrum antibiotic within 1 hour	160 (62.3)	60 (59.4)	0.887	0.554	1.420	0.618				
Adequate antimicrobial therapy	197 (76.7)	63 (62.4)	0.505	0.308	0.829	**0.007**	0.536	0.314	0.916	**0.023**
Serum arterial lactate	252 (98.1)	97 (96.0)	0.481	0.127	1.829	0.283				
Central venous oxygen saturation	161 (62.6)	71 (70.3)	1.411	0.859	2.317	0.174				

OR = Odds Ratio; CI = Confidence Interval; APACHE = Acute Physiology and Chronic Health Evaluation II.

Table 5. Risk factors associated with inadequate antimicrobial therapy in patients with severe sepsis or septic shock patients who had documented bloodstream infection.

Variables	Adequate antimicrobial therapy		Univariate analysis				Multivariate analysis			
	No (N=98)	Yes (N=260)	OR	CI 95%		p	OR	CI 95%		p
	N (%)	N (%)		Min	Max			Min	Max	
Male	63 (28.5)	158 (71.5)	1.162	0.717	1.882	0.542				
Age (years), mean ± SD	65±20	64±17	1.005	0.991	1.018	0.495				
APACHE II, mean ± SD	21±11	17±10	1.044	1.02	1.069	**<0.001**	1.048	1.023	1.074	**<0.001**
Liver dysfunction	05 (18.5)	22 (81.5)	0.582	0.214	1.581	0.288				
Cardiac dysfunction	78 (28.6)	195 (71.4)	1.3	0.738	2.289	0.363				
Renal dysfunction	37 (26.8)	101 (73.2)	0.955	0.592	1.541	0.85				
Hematologic dysfunction	39 (29.1)	95 (70.9)	1.148	0.713	1.849	0.57				
Respiratory dysfunction	55 (26.2)	155 (73.8)	0.866	0.542	1.386	0.55				
Neurologic dysfunction	32 (26.9)	87 (73.1)	0.964	0.588	1.581	0.885				
Polymicrobial infection	12 (48.0)	13 (52.0)	2.651	1.165	6.032	**0.02**	2.954	1.227	7.115	**0.016**
ESKAPE pathogen causing bloodstream infection	44 (33.3)	88 (66.7)	1.593	0.992	2.558	**0.054**	1.436	0.872	2.366	0.155

OR = Odds Ratio; CI = Confidance Interval; APACHE = Acute Physiology and Chronic Health Evaluation II.
ESKAPE = ***Enterococcus, Staphylococcus aureus, Klebsiella pneumoniae, Pseudomonas aeruginosa, Enterobacter spp.***

Table 6. The most prevalent microorganisms from monomicrobial bloodstream infections and clinical outcome stratified by adequacy of antimicrobial therapy during the study period.

Microorganisms		All organisms					Resistant organisms				
		N (%)	Death		Survival		N (%)	Death		Survival	
			Adequate ATB	Inadequate ATB	Adequate ATB	Inadequate ATB		Adequate ATB	Inadequate ATB	Adequate ATB	Inadequate ATB
			N (%)	N (%)	N (%)	N (%)		N (%)	N (%)	N (%)	N (%)
Fungi (N=5, 1.5%)	*Candida albicans*	02	-	01	01	-	no	-	-	-	-
		(40.0)		(50.0)	(50.0)						
	Candida krusei	01	-	-	-	01	01*	-	-	-	01
		(20.0)				(100.0)	(100.0)				(100.0)
	Candida parapsilosis	02	-	02	-	-	no	-	-	-	-
		(40.0)		(100.0)							
Gram negative (N=190; 57.1%)	*Escherichia coli*	101	13	05	77	06	07**	01	04	02	-
		(53.1)	(12.8)	(4.9)	(76.2)	(6.1)	(6.9)	(14.2)	(57.3)	(28.5)	
	Pseudomonas aeruginosa	18	07	04	06	01	08#	02	04	02	-
		(10.0)	(38.9)	(22.2)	(33.3)	(5.6)	(44.4)	(25.0)	(50.0)	(25.0)	
	Acinetobacter spp	8	02	01	04	01	01#	-	01	-	-
		(4.2)	(25.0)	(12.5)	(50.0)	(12.5)	(12.5)		(100.0)		
	Klebsiella spp	24	03	04	13	04	10**	01	03	03	03
		(12.6)	(12.5)	(16.6)	(54.3)	(16.6)	(41.2)	(10.0)	(30.0)	(30.0)	(30.0)
Gram positive (N=138; 41.4%)	*Staphylococcus aureus*	24	07	04	02	11	11##	06	04	01	-
		(17.3)	(29.2)	(16.6)	(8.4)	(45.8)	(45.8)	(54.5)	(36.3)	(9.2)	
	Enterococcus spp	11	04	00	04	03	01###	-	-	01	-
		(7.9)	(36.3)	(0.0)	(36.3)	(27.4)	(9.2)			(100.0)	
	Coagulase-negative staphylococci	44	13	08	16	07	35##	11	08	11	05
		(26.1)	(29.5)	(18.2)	(36.4)	(15.9)	(79.5)	31.4)	(22.9)	(31.4)	(14.3)

*resistant to fluconazole.
**resistant to 3rd and 4th generation cephalosporins.
#resistant to carbapenems.
##resistant to methicillin.
###resistant to vancomycin.

compared to 55% prior to the implementation of the sepsis bundle [6].

Over time, after implementation of the bundle, we observed improved compliance with the protocol (Figure S2); in 2012 we had 54% compliance with the sepsis bundle, and a 17% mortality rate. The correct antibiotics, administered at the right time, contribute to an effective recovery of the patient. It also acts as a measurable and actionable safety metric, which reduces mortality by decreasing the time of exposure to the organism and its toxins. This has been the target of study of several groups around the world [14–17]. However, the indiscriminate use of antibiotics may lead, for example, to the development of antimicrobial resistance and an increase in *Clostridium difficile* infections. In addition, some antimicrobials have side effects that require caution and rational prescribing [7–9].

While empiric antibiotic therapy is important [17], targeted therapy based on culture results should also be a goal. However, sepsis bundle evaluation studies have not examined the appropriateness of the antimicrobial therapy administered [18].

Because identification of pathogens in cultures is time intensive, one of the ways that our institution found to speed up the process of communicating blood cultures results was for laboratory staff to call the physicians responsible for the patient.

Of the ESKAPE pathogens [19,20], which have paramount importance due to the their pathogenesis, transmission mode and antimicrobial resistance, the most common was *E.coli*. However, the incidence of *S. aureus* (MRSA) and *E. faecium* (VRE) cases was low (Table 6).

Regarding the appropriateness of antibiotic selection for the cases with positive blood culture, our data show a fair rate of treatment adequacy, but in relation to fungal infections of the five cases identified 60.0% (3/5) died and none were receiving adequate therapy (Table 6). In the APACHE II study [21], calculations were done only on the day of admission. One explanation to justify why patients with higher APACHE II were associated with inadequate antimicrobial therapy was in the first 24 hours there was an underestimation of the severity of these patients and the appropriate antimicrobial therapy. If we had calculated the prognostic score on our patients at the time of severe sepsis and septic shock diagnosis, the APACHE score would likely be very different. Recently, in a similar study evaluating etiology, antimicrobial therapy and outcome of patients with severe sepsis, quick identification of the source of infection, proper sampling for microbiological analyses, and the rapid administration of adequate antimicrobial therapy were shown to be crucial management points [22].

Study Limitations

A limitation of our study is that it was performed at a single private medical facility so it may not be generalizable to other hospitals (e.g., public facilities). In addition, data was retrospectively collected from medical records; however because of the sepsis bundle protocol these septic patients were followed prospectively. Lastly, we did not include microbiologic data from sites other than blood cultures with regards to assessing appropriateness of antimicrobial therapy. However, cultures from nonsterile sites (e.g., respiratory tract) are more difficult to interpret since in many cases the organisms are colonizing rather than causing true infection.

Implications for policy and practice

Other improvements that were taking place may have impacted our study findings. Since 2007 our hospital has been engaged in zero tolerance for healthcare associated infections. We have observed a significant reduction in ventilator-associated pneumonia and in central venous associated bloodstream infections [23,24]. We also implemented other ICU best practices during the study period, including a glycemic control protocol [25]. We adopted intermediate glucose control, because we believe that tight glucose control is difficult to accomplish in routine intensive care unit settings and is associated with a significant increase in the incidence of hypoglycaemia [25,26]. However, it is interesting to note that the best practices for the care of patients with severe sepsis and septic shock were improving over time in our ICU. This affirms our belief that the sepsis bundle needs to be considered as the intervention decreasing mortality in septic shock and severe sepsis because of the better care and the prompt recognition of these patients in hospital [6].

Conclusions

Appropriate antimicrobial therapy and implementation of the sepsis bundle in patients with severe sepsis and septic shock due to bloodstream infection was associated with a 46% reduction in mortality. Assessment of appropriate antimicrobials should be incorporated into the Surviving Sepsis Campaign as a quality metric [18].

Supporting Information

Figure S1 Flow-diagram - Cohort selection of total patients, septic shock patients and bloodstream infection.

Figure S2 Proportion of patients with severe sepsis and septic shock who died and sepsis bundle compliance.

Appendix 1 Sepsis definitions.

Author Contributions

Conceived and designed the experiments: PKOY ARM MSD OFPS. Performed the experiments: PKOY MDVM ESV. Analyzed the data: PKOY ARM ESV. Contributed reagents/materials/analysis tools: PKOY ARM ESV. Wrote the paper: PKOY ARM MDVM ESV MSD MBE. Provided support to implement the sepsis bundle: OFPS.

References

1. Angus DC, van der Poll T (2013) Severe sepsis and septic shock. N Engl J Med 369: 840–851.
2. Dellinger RP, Levy MM, Rhodes A, Annane D, Gerlach H, et al. (2013) Surviving sepsis campaign: international guidelines for management of severe sepsis and septic shock: 2012. Crit Care Med 41: 580–637.
3. Ministério da Saúde. Informações de Saúde. DATASUS. Taxa de mortalidade hospitalar por local de internação – Brasil 2008 a agosto 2013. Brasília: Ministério da Saúde, DATASUS. Available: http://tabnet.datasus.gov.br/cgi/tabcgi.exe?sih/cnv/niuf.def. Accessed: 2013 Oct 21.
4. Dellinger RP, Carlet JM, Masur H, Gerlach H, Calandra T, et al. (2004) Surviving Sepsis Campaign guidelines for management of severe sepsis and septic shock. Crit Care Med 32: 858–873.
5. Global Sepsis Alliance. World sepsis day. Jena: Center for Sepsis Control and Care. Available: http://www.world-sepsis-day.org. Accessed 2013 Oct 25.
6. Shiramizo SC, Marra AR, Durão Jr MS, Paes ÂT, Edmond MB, et al. (2011) Decreasing mortality in severe sepsis and septic shock patients by implementing a sepsis bundle in a hospital setting. PLoS One 6 (11): e26790.
7. Ibrahim EH, Sherman G, Ward S, Fraser VJ, Kollef M (2000) The influence of inadequate antimicrobial treatment of bloodstream infections on patient outcomes in the ICU setting. Chest 118: 146–155.

8. Zaragoza R, Artero A, Camarena JJ, Sancho S, Gonzales R, et al. (2003) The influence of inadequate empirical antimicrobial treatment on patients with bloodstream infections in an intensive care unit. Clin Microbiol Infect 9: 412–418.
9. Kang CI, Kim SH, Kim HB, Park SW, Choe YJ, et al. (2003) *Pseudomonas aeruginosa* bacteremia: risk factors for mortality and influence of delayed receipt of effective antimicrobial therapy on clinical outcome. Clin Infect Dis 37: 745–751.
10. Bone RC, Balk RA, Cerra FB, Dellinger RP, Fein AM, et al. (1992) Definitions for sepsis and organ failure and guidelines for the use of innovative therapies in sepsis. The ACCP/SCCM Consensus Conference Committee. American College of Chest Physicians/Society of Critical Care Medicine. Chest 101: 1644–1655.
11. Calandra T, Cohen J (2005) International Sepsis Forum Definition of Infection in the ICU Consensus Conference. The International sepsis forum consensus conference on definitions of infection in the intensive care unit. Crit Care Med 33: 1538–48.
12. Gonçales PDS, Polessi JA, Bass LM, Santos GPD, Yokota PKO, et al. (2012) Reduced frequency of cardiopulmonar arrest by rapid response teams. Einstein (São Paulo) 10: 442–448.
13. Clinical and Laboratory Standards Institute (2006) Performance Standards for antimicrobial susceptibility testing: sixteenth informational supplement. CLSI document M100-S16.Wayne, PA: CLSI.
14. Proudfoot AG, McAuley DF, Hind M, Griffiths MJD (2011) Translational research: what does it mean, what has it delivered and what might it deliver? Curr Opin Crit Care 17: 495–503.
15. Cardoso T, Ribeiro O, Aragão I, Costa-Pereira A, Sarmento A (2013) The impact of healthcare-associated infection on mortality: failure in clinical recognition is related with inadequate antibiotic therapy. PloS ONE 8(3): e58418.
16. Zubert S, Funk DJ, Kumar A (2010) Antibiotics in sepsis and septic shock: like everything else in life, timing is everything. Crit Care Med 38: 1211–1212.
17. Gaieski DF, Mikkelsen ME, Band RA, Pines JM, Massone R, et al. (2010) Impact of time to antibiotics on survival in patients with severe sepsis or septic shock in whom early goal-directed therapy was initiated in the emergency department. Crit Care Med 38: 1045–1053.
18. Barochia AV, Cui X, Eichacker PQ (2013) The surviving sepsis campaign's revised sepsis bundles. Curr Infect Dis Rep 15: 385–393.
19. Rice LB (2008) Federal funding for the study of antimicrobial resistance in nosocomial pathogens: no ESKAPE. J Infect Dis 197: 1079–1081.
20. Boucher HW, Talbot GH, Bradley JS, Edward JE Jr, Gilbert D, et al. (2009) Bad bugs, no drugs: no ESKAPE! An update from the infectious diseases society of America. Clin Infect Dis 48: 1–12.
21. Knaus WA, Draper EA, Wagner DP, Zimmerman JE (1985) APACHE II: a severity of disease classification system. Crit Care Med 13: 818–829.
22. Nygård ST, Langeland N, Flaatten HK, Fanebust R, Haugen O, et al. (2014) Aetiology, antimicrobial therapy and outcome of patients with community acquired severe sepsis: a prospective study in a Norwegian university hospital. BMC Infect Dis 14: 121.
23. Marra AR, Cal RG, Silva CV, Caserta RA, Paes AT, et al. (2009) Successful prevention of ventilator-associated pneumonia in an intensive care setting. Am J Infect Control 37: 619–625.
24. Marra AR, Cal RG, Durão MS, Correa L, Guastelli LR, et al. (2010) Impact of a program to prevent central line-associated bloodstream infection in the zero tolerance era. Am J Infect Control 38: 434–439.
25. Durao MS, Marra AR, Moura DF, Almeida SM, Fernandes CJ, et al. (2010) Tight glucose control versus intermediate glucose control: a quasi-experimental study. Anaesth Intensive Care 38: 1–7.
26. Finfer S, Chittock DR, Su SY, Blair D, Foster D, et al. (2009) Intensive versus conventional glucose control in critically ill patients. N Engl J Med; 360: 1283–1297.

Writing In and Reading ICU Diaries: Qualitative Study of Families' Experience in the ICU

Maité Garrouste-Orgeas[1,2]*, Antoine Périer[3,4], Philippe Mouricou[5], Charles Grégoire[1], Cédric Bruel[1], Sandie Brochon[1], François Philippart[1], Adeline Max[1], Benoit Misset[1,6]

1 Medical-Surgical ICU, Saint Joseph Hospital Network, Paris, France, **2** IAME, UMR 1137, Paris Diderot University, Sorbonne Paris Cité, Paris, France, **3** Maison des Adolescents, University Hospital Cochin, Paris, France, **4** INSERM U-669, University Paris Sud and University Paris Descartes, UMR-S0669, Paris, France, **5** Management department, ESSCA School of Management PRES UNAM, Boulogne- Billancourt, France, **6** University Paris Descartes, Paris, France

Abstract

Purpose: Keeping an ICU patient diary has been reported to benefit the patient's recovery. Here, we investigated the families' experience with reading and writing in patient ICU diaries kept by both the family and the staff.

Methods: We conducted a qualitative study involving 32 semi-structured in-depth interviews of relatives of 26 patients (34% of all family members who visited patients) who met our ICU-diary criterion, i.e., ventilation for longer than 48 hours. Grounded theory was used to conceptualise the interview data via a three-step coding process (open coding, axial coding, and selective coding).

Results: Communicative, emotional, and humanising experiences emerged from our data. First, family members used the diaries to access, understand, and assimilate the medical information written in the diaries by staff members, and then to share this information with other family members. Second, the diaries enabled family members to maintain a connection with the patient by documenting their presence and expressing their love and affection. Additionally, families confided in the diaries to maintain hope. Finally, family members felt the diaries humanized the medical staff and patient.

Conclusions: Our findings indicate positive effects of diaries on family members. The diaries served as a powerful tool to deliver holistic patient- and family-centered care despite the potentially dehumanising ICU environment. The diaries made the family members aware of their valuable role in caring for the patient and enhanced their access to and comprehension of medical information. Diaries may play a major role in improving the well-being of ICU-patient families.

Editor: Fiona Harris, University of Stirling, United Kingdom

Funding: The authors received no specific funding for this work.

Competing Interests: The authors have declared that no competing interests exist.

* Email: mgarrouste@hpsj.fr

Introduction

For family members, having a patient in the intensive care unit (ICU) is a highly stressful experience. The French FAMIREA group reported symptoms of anxiety and depression in 69% and 35% of family members, respectively; as well as post-traumatic stress symptoms in 33% [1]. Restricted visitation policies [2,3], poor communication with the staff [4], poor comprehension of the medical information about the patient [4], participation in decision-making about patient care [5], lack of support from the staff, and fear for the patient contribute to cause distress in family members [6]. High levels of distress in family members have been reported not only during the ICU stay, but also during the next several months [7].

Strategies designed to help family members actively provide support to themselves and to the patient include broad visitation policies [8,9,10], involvement in nursing care [11], and participation in keeping a patient diary during the ICU stay [12,13]. ICU diaries were introduced in the 1980s in Denmark by nurses, as a patient debriefing tool for use after ICU discharge. ICU staff participation seemed important to the effect of diaries in decreasing anxiety among family members [14]. ICU diaries are usually kept by both staff members and family members. Studies have assessed the impact of ICU diaries on long-term outcomes of patients [15,16,17,18,19,20] and families [13]. The use of ICU diaries was associated with decreased symptoms of anxiety, depression [18], and posttraumatic stress in both patients [17] and families [12,21] at various time points after ICU discharge. The diaries enabled survivors to make sense of their ICU experience [22]. Qualitative studies established that ICU diaries were useful in describing the patient's environment in the ICU; building a time line of health-related events; inserting the time line of the patient's experience within that of the family, community, and world events; demonstrating the continuity of the patient's life; expressing feelings and emotions; and documenting the presence, commitment, and supportive role of the staff and family [12,23,24]. Despite this growing empirical evidence, family members' experience with ICU diaries has rarely been investigated. To learn from family members how writing in and reading ICU diaries affected their experience in the ICU, we conducted a qualitative study based on an inductive grounded theory approach. Our findings provide new insights into the benefits of ICU diaries for families.

Methods

Design

We conducted a qualitative study to obtain new insights into a topic about which little published information was available. More specifically, to shed light on the families' account of their situation, we chose the grounded theory approach. The methods and procedures of grounded theory involve cycles of data collection and analysis to identify interrelations among concepts, which eventually aggregate into an integrative theory [25,26]. The study was approved by the appropriate ethics committee (*Pitié-Salpêtrière Comité de Protection des Personnes*).

Context

The substantive area in which we have performed our study was the 10-bed medical-surgical unit of the Saint Joseph Hospital Network in Paris, France. This ICU has placed strong emphasis on family-centred care, with around-the-clock visitation [7] and participation of family members in patient care [9]. All the patients were admitted to the same ICU and received care from the same staff.

Content and use of the diaries

Since 2009, ICU diaries are kept by the ICU staff (physicians, nurses, and nursing assistants) and families [10]. The diaries were not part of the official clinical records of the patients. The ICU diary is in a folder placed in plain view in the patient's room. ICU staff attended lectures and discussions on writing in the diaries. There was a single diary per patient, which was used by both the staff and the family. Patients ventilated for more than 48 hours had a diary created as soon as possible by their ICU physician. All physicians in the unit could create diaries. The physician started the diary with an account of the initial medical event. Then, all staff members could write about events experienced by the patient in the ICU; they wrote in the diaries during their normal working hours, including those spent in ICU meetings about patient care. The ICU staff addressed personally to the patient. Both positive and negative changes could be recorded in the diary, although physicians were not obligated to provide complete medical information. Nosocomial and iatrogenic events were entered as part of the medical information about the patient. Relatives were invited directly to write freely in the diaries, without guidance from the ICU staff. The only instruction given to families and staff members about diary entries was to refrain from writing about confidential matters that should not be shared among the patient, all relatives, and the staff. Staff members were free to express compassion and their hope, or the absence thereof, that the patient would recover. Our previous study about the experience of the staff with ICU diaries showed that most of the staff members read the entries by the families [27]. No patients wrote in the diaries. At ICU discharge, the diary was given to the patient if he or she had recovered and to the family otherwise.

Data collection and analysis procedures

In keeping with our focus on the family members' experience with the ICU diaries, we conducted semi-structured interviews of families' members. We used the grounded theory approach [25,26], which involves moving back and forth between data collection and analysis until the emergence of a theory that fits the data.

The participants were selected via theoretical sampling: that is, we included individuals likely to provide the information we needed. The data obtained from the first study participants determined which new categories of participants we needed to include [28]. Thus the sample size is governed by the spectrum of data needed to develop a theory, which cannot be determined before data collection starts. The goal is not to obtain a statistically representative sample. Family members were defined as all relatives and friends who visited the patient. We interviewed families if French was their native language and their patient stayed longer than 48 hours in the ICU, and had an ICU diary. Several family members could be included for the same patient, as experience might differ according to the relationship with the patient. For each family member, we recorded age, gender, relationship with the patient, and educational level. The data recorded for each patient were age, gender, reason for ICU admission, severity of illness assessed using the Simplified Acute Physiological Score (SAPS II) based on the worst physical and laboratory data during the first 24 hours in the ICU [29] and type of admission (medical, scheduled surgical, or emergent surgical).

The main investigator (MGO) invited the family members to participate in the study. Each family member was interviewed at patient ICU discharge to ensure that the full ICU experience was captured, while avoiding the inconvenience and possible distress associated with having to return to the ICU after discharge. Prior to the interview, each participant gave written informed consent to the audio-recorded interview. An in-depth semi-directive interview was conducted by either a psychologist (MT) or a physician (MGO), both of whom were trained in qualitative data collection. The psychologist was hired specifically for the study and did not belong to the ICU staff. The physician (MGO) is on the ICU staff and dedicates most of her time to research; she does not participate in bedside patient care. In accordance with Charmaz guidelines [25], the interview guide was composed of informational questions followed by reflective and feeling-oriented questions (Table 1). Each interview lasted about 1 hour and was conducted in a quiet room in the hospital. The interviews were recorded and transcribed. To simplify the data analysis process, the data rendered anonymous only after data analysis was complete.

First round of data collection

We first interviewed 22 family members between November 2012 and June 2013. We analysed their data and developed a provisional theory. As the study was exploratory, we used a three-step analysis process to move from a descriptive coding scheme to a more analytical one, through progressively increasing abstraction. For data analysis, we used the insider-outsider approach: researchers with experience in research in the ICU worked jointly with researchers who were new to this field. This approach strengthens the trustworthiness of research results by interconnecting interpretations made by people having different levels of understanding of both empirical research and the ICU context of care. Consequently, the analysis was done by MGO and two other individuals (AP and PM), who were not on the ICU staff and who had previously been trained in grounded theory procedures.

Open coding was the first step. We developed a fine-grained coding scheme by collaboratively analysing the interview transcripts during a workshop. Each workshop participant (MGO, AP, PM) then coded the interviews independently. The results were compared and discrepancies resolved by consensus. The first version of the coding scheme had 46 categories and sub-categories.

Table 1. Interview guide.

1. Can you tell me how you used the diary during your family member's stay in the ICU?
2. Can you tell me what you wrote? And perhaps also why?
3. How did it make you feel to write in the diary?
4. Do you see a connection between how the diary was used and the course of your family member's health condition?
5 Have you thought about the possibility that others will read what you wrote? How does that affect you?
6. Have you read what the staff members wrote during the ICU stay? How did that make you feel?
7. Have you talked about the diary to family members or friends?
8*. What do you think about the design of the diary (format, materials used, appearance)?

* This question was included in the first interview guide then removed after the preliminary analysis.

In accordance with Creswell [30], at this stage of the analysis, we began to identify the most illustrative excerpts for later access and possible inclusion in the study report.

Results of the preliminary analysis

Our preliminary analysis established that most interviewees both read and wrote in the diaries. Therefore, the analysis could not use one or the other of these two activities (reading and writing) as the central focus. Furthermore, the lead researcher initially felt that family perceptions about the design of the diary (format, material, and appearance) would be of interest. However, the interviewees consistently felt satisfied with the design of the diaries. Consequently, the question in the interview guide about diary design was removed. No other questions in the guide were removed, added, or changed.

Second round of data collection

We interviewed 10 additional family members between July 2013 and October 2013. The data collection procedure was the same as for the first round, except for the removal of the interview-guide question on diary design.

We performed axial coding to view the data from a higher degree of abstraction and to uncover deeper patterns. Several subcategories were subsequently relabeled and reorganized as first-order properties of the emerging data structure. Comparison of the data from each new second-round interviewee to the existing data identified three categories, as detailed in the results section. During this phase, we also used in vivo coding (i.e., we used interviewees' words to label categories) to conceptualize the ICU experience based on the family members' perceptions. Saturation was defined as failure of data from new interviewees to generate new properties or induce changes in the data structure.

Finally, the third step consisted in selective coding to integrate and synthesise the categories derived from the analysis. In line with our research question, we paid special attention to the outcomes of the previously defined categories. These findings are reported in the results section ("Family Experience in Context" subheading). The analysis was performed in French. All quotes were translated for publication by an American physician and medical writer.

Results

We interviewed 32 family members. Our sample was composed of 34% of the family members who visited patients ventilated for more than 48 hours. Their main characteristics and those of the corresponding patients are shown in Tables 2 and 3, respectively. The final data structure contained 13 first-order concepts, six second-order themes, and three aggregate dimensions: communication, emotional experience and humanization experience of the staff and patient (Table 4).

A communicative experience

The diaries, historically conceived as a patient debriefing tool, had major effects on family members by enhancing access to and assimilation of medical information about the patient (13/32 families members, 41%) and by helping to share various types of information among family members (5/32, 16%).

Access to and assimilation of medical information about the patient

Although the families attached considerable importance to information delivered orally by the staff, they felt that information written in the diaries was more reliable and more powerful, particularly in the area of medical information. Family members who read entries signed by the physicians no longer felt the need to check by asking questions of other staff members. *'There is no need to ask the same thing over and over again ...we don't ask about the information in the diary, because it's written down'* (31-year-old daughter). Family members sometimes felt the information was insufficient or irregularly provided. *'I'd like the doctor to write in the diary more often; an entry every day would work for me: I'd know what he thinks from day to day about the changes in my father's condition'* (48-year-old daughter). The family members did not focus only on the information written by the physicians: entries by other staff members were also read with interest, as they bore witness to what happened at times when no family members were in the room. *'The diary let me know what happened at night, when I wasn't there'* (45-year-old mother). Some family members, however, seemed reluctant to read entries intended for the patient and to intrude into the intimate patient-staff member relationship (4/32, 12%) *'When I read the entries by the staff members, I feel they're not intended for us and that I'm reading something that's none of my business'* (74-year-old spouse).

In addition to facilitating access to medical information, the families felt that the diary improved comprehension of the information, because the staff, particularly the physicians, made greater use of everyday terms for the written entries than for the oral information. Furthermore, a very powerful characteristic of the diaries was the possibility for the family members to read the entries as often as they wished, which helped them to assimilate the information. In addition, they could read the entries again at the time of their choosing and at their own pace, when the conditions were optimal for them, and they could rebuild the patient's story and assess the changes over time whenever they felt the need and

Table 2. Characteristics of the 32 family members interviewed for the study.

Variables	Data
Age in years, mean±SD	54.6±13.0
Female gender, n (%)	27 (84)
Relationship with the patient, n (%)	
Spouse	11 (34.3)
Grown child	10 (31.2)
Sibling	4 (12.5)
Other	7 (21.8)
Occupation, n (%) *	
Tertiary-sector employees**	15 (65.2)
Retired	7 (30.4)
Educational level, n (%)	
No formal education	7 (21.8)
Completed secondary education	5 (15.6)
2 years of higher education	1 (3.1)
3 years of higher education	16 (50)
5–8 years of higher education	3 (9.3)

*10 family members had never had paid jobs.
**Tertiary-sector: production of services (trade, administration, transportation, finance, services to corporations and individuals, healthcare, education, and social work).

regardless of the course of the patient's clinical condition. *'Since it's written down, we can read it as often as we want to – and to be honest, I've read the diary at least 15 times, and when I read your first entry I understood it but I read it again and again because each time I needed to read everything from the beginning'* (21-year-old daughter).

Sharing information among families members

The diary served as a channel of communication among the family members. It allowed all family members to have access to the medical information and to obtain news about the patient on a daily basis. *'I just write that in the diary, so that the people who come to visit after me know, even if they don't necessarily have all the information'* (45-year-old sister-in-law). The main function of the

Table 3. Characteristics of the 26 patients whose family members were interviewed for the study.

Variables	
Age in years, mean±SD, Median (25th–75th)	71±11, 73 [64–78]
Male gender, n%	19 (73.1)
Type of patient, n (%)	
Medical	16 (61.5)
Unscheduled surgical	8 (30.8)
cheduled surgical	2 (7.7)
SAPS II, mean±SD	49±19
Predicted hospital mortality (%)	11 (43%)
ICU stay in days, Median (25th–75th)	29 [15–44]
ICU mortality, n (%)	8 (30.8)
Reasons for admission, n (%)	
Shock	10 (38.5)
Acute respiratory disease	6 (23.1)
OPD	1 (3.9)
oma	5 (19.2)
cute renal disease	3 (11.5)
onitoring	1 (3.9)

SAPS II, Simplified Acute Physiology Score, version II; ICU, intensive care unit; COPD, chronic obstructive pulmonary disease.

Table 4. Data structure.

1st Order Concepts	2nd Order Themes	Aggregate Dimensions
Written information is more reliable than information delivered orally by the physicians.	To access and assimilate the information	Communicative experience
The use of everyday terms in the diary entries and the ability to read the entries as many times as desired improves assimilation of the information		
Cooperation between the family and staff to write the patient's story	Sharing of information	
Concern about being intrusive may be a barrier to writing in the diary		
The diary serves as a communication tool among family members		
Keeping the patient alive by expressing active feelings for him/her in writing	To bear witness to one's presence	Emotional experience
The diary allows the family members to record their presence at the patient's side.		
The diary is used as a journal in which fears and anxieties can be released	To confide and keep hope alive	
Supportive statements by the staff allow the family to project into the future, after the ICU stay.		
The diary serves as a medium for developing a warm relationship with the staff.	New way of perceiving the staff	Humanisation experience
The diary bears witness to the commitment of the staff, which goes beyond medical care		
The diary shows how the staffs take the patient into consideration.	New way of perceiving the patient	
The patient recovers the status of a living individual.		

diary was to provide opportunities for cooperation between the staff and family in the service of the patient and to record the medical and non-medical events that would allow the patient to rebuild the gap in his or her life and the connection with the family members. *'…so the diary lets him know what happened day by day in our family, who came to visit him, what happened to him, what progress he made'* (62-year-old spouse). Additional diary entries are provided in the online-only supplement (Table 5).

An emotional experience

The ICU stay is usually a severely traumatic experience for families. The diary helped the families understand and cope with potentially overwhelming emotional experiences. The diary produced strong emotions in the family members as they documented their presence at the patient's side, expressed their affection or love for the patient (19/32, 59%), confided their intimate feelings, and struggled to maintain hope (13/32, 41%).

Documenting presence, expressing love or affection

The dated and signed diary entries bore witness to the presence of the family members at the patient's side. *'That way he'll realise that he's not fighting this alone… as I explain to him in the diary, I can't be physically present – instead, I'm physically present in the diary'* (35-year-old daughter). The vulnerability of the patient encouraged the family members to say things they had never said before. *'I felt the need to tell him that I love him, that I have always loved him, although we've been living separately for several years'* (53-year-old wife). The written diary entries served as complements to what was said to the patient. The diary created greater continuity of communication over time, by leading the family member to engage in an intimate inner dialogue with the patient. *'Writing in the diary was life-giving for me – it's as if, since he couldn't answer me or hear me, he came to life through the writing'* (62-year-old sister-in-law). Communication usually took the form of a dialogue with the patient, although occasionally the diary served as a personal journal in which the family members confided their fears, anxieties, enthusiasm, or optimism. *'Using the diary allowed me to resume the dialogue with him. I continued to talk to him as if he were there. And the day I started writing in the diary, I began to be able to talk to him'* (62-year-old wife). Once the dialogue was established, the personal history with the family member could continue to unfold. A connection was formed with the outside world, and the family circle concept regained its meaning. *'When I sit down (by his side) and write in the diary, time seems to stop and I feel I can finally settle down and take a brief look at the short day I spent with him'* (35-year-old daughter).

Confiding in the diary and maintaining hope

The diary offered a means of organising the inner dialogue with oneself or others, of putting names on emotions that were often powerful and overwhelming, and of expressing those emotions by incorporating them into a narrative. In this way, the writer began to find some distance from the strong emotions. *'I also felt I was confiding in the diary. I was able to say things, my feelings for him that he couldn't hear me describe, all my pain, all the joy I felt at seeing that he was a tiny bit better…. I could open my heart to it – the diary became my confidante'* (45-year-old mother). The diary was the only document shared by the family and staff in the service of the patient. The continuous communication via the diary influenced the family's relationship with the staff, and the wishes for recovery expressed by the staff generated hope in the family members that an improvement was possible, thus changing the family's experience. *'I believe that a doctor who writes 'today, you were able to do this, well, I think that's far more powerful than just saying it. I believe the doctor chose his words and thought carefully about what to write, so the words really mean something So that helped me a lot'* (62-year-old wife). As shown by the verbatim passage below, another factor that maintained hope was the better emotional regulation that resulted from writing in the diary. *'…It's thanks to being able to write in this diary… Writing gave me hope - it felt as if I was talking to him (in the diary), so nothing was lost.'* And the wife of this patient continued: *'And little by little, that made me more confident, and I'd say to myself "We're going to make it, we're going to make it"'* (62-year-old wife). However, changes in the condition of the patient affected the way the families used the diary, as illustrated by the two excerpts below. In the first case, as the condition of the patient improved, his wife wrote less often in

Table 5. Diary entries related to the communication experience.

Themes	Entries
Having access to information about the patient's health condition	Sister, 73: In general, we already knew, because they informed us, but we were glad they wrote it down and didn't hide anything, and it was in everyday language.
	Daughter, 21: Actually, in the conclusions, we had an overview of the situation, and in the entries we could discover things we hadn't heard, because it wasn't from a medical viewpoint ... So it was the little details that added a bit to what I'd heard in the full meetings.
	Wife, 68: I think the diary is just perfect, because every day we can see what's new, what the doctors and nurses came to do or told him, what they think, what they wrote each time.
	Sister-in-law, 45: For me, regularly, I would read it, and that way I could get information about what was happening.
	Daughter, 21: We read everything and at least we could follow what was happening – even though we get information during the meetings and over the phone, we can see what happened, so the information is more detailed.
Assimilating the medical information	Wife, 52: We can also see the changes between the first few days when the situation was really critical, the time when we could finally really have a conversation with him when he woke up, when he recovered complete consciousness...we can see the changes, we see what's happening, we see what happened.
	Daughter, 35: So actually, I need some time to adjust. It's true that being able to settle down to write what the doctors tell us and taking the time to analyse the situation – that helps me understand the course of my father's condition ... Reading makes it much easier for me to realise what's going on and makes things much more concrete, so I can understand the reality of the care that he's getting and that I don't fully grasp but that I sort of feel.
	Daughter, 51: Entries were made in it (the diary) at admission, so we knew exactly what happened when he arrived...there is no ambiguity, we don't need to ask the same questions over and over, we know what was done, what happened... so the relationship with the doctors and nurses is easier.
	Daughter, 70: I was able to grasp the medical information more serenely, because I had enough time - because I was alone, so when they talked I had to pay careful attention ....
	Sister-in-law, 62: We either softened the information given by the doctors a bit or on the contrary we catastrophized. So reading the diary corrects that and put things in their proper place.
Sharing of information	Wife, 47: People who write do so because they want to leave a message, and people who read want to receive it ... I think it's really a communication tool! I'd say even a tool for communion, it brings us together...
	Sister, 51: My niece and I, the two of us come regularly, and when there's a serious difficulty, when we need to communicate – well, sometimes it serves as a connection to my niece – yes, I've left documents for her.
	Wife, 74: Writing in the diary allowed me to connect with the other members of the family.
	Husband, 68: It's interesting for the person who is in the hospital and who wants to read it to know what the experience was like.
	Sister-in-law, 62: It's really interesting to see entries by both the staff and the family members, whoever they are – I agree that it's important to have a daily record of what happened to the patient, to fill the gaps during the times he was unconscious.

the diary. *'It's the fact of being conscious or not – as long as he was unconscious, in an artificial coma, I used the diary to write his story ... when he regained consciousness, I continued the story a bit, but with fewer details – the need wasn't as great'* (52-year-old wife). In the second case, the patient's condition deteriorated and her daughter became aware that she would be unable to read the messages. *'It's not that I gave up, but I thought, she won't read it - she wouldn't read it, so... it's not that it was useless, not at all, but I was troubled when I took the diary this time, for the first time'* (21-year-old daughter). Additional diary entries are provided in the online-only supplement (Table 6).

A humanising experience

The last dimension of the diary-related experience as perceived by the family was humanisation of the staff, together with an awareness that the staff viewed the patient as a living human being (8/32, 25%). The diary changed the way the family members viewed the staff and, through the support expressed by the staff, changed the way they viewed the patient (8/32, 25%).

Change in perceptions of the staff

The diary changed the families' perceptions of the staff. The contribution of the staff to keeping the diary and the time devoted by staff members to the diary outside the regular working hours were seen by the families as signs of consideration, emotional involvement, and empathy. *'You're a doctor, you took care of her too, but you also took the time to write about your concerns and your joys and to give your encouragements, and we will never forget all that'* (21-year-old daughter). The family members no longer perceived the staff as only healthcare professionals but also saw them as people like them, since they expressed emotions. In this way, reading the diary humanised the staff members, particularly the physicians. *'I think it's important that the doctors communicate at our level...but at least they take the time, they create a level field. It's not the doctor speaking, it's the human being, who gives information – and obviously it's medical – but it's a human being speaking to another human being'* (35-year-old daughter).

Change in perceptions of the patients

The consideration and support given by the staff to the patient resulted in humanisation of the patient. The entries by the staff portrayed the patient as a living human being at a time when the family had difficulty recognising their loved one in the very ill and usually unconscious person connected to multiple catheters, tubes, and machines. The staff members wrote directly to the patient, describing the changes in his or her clinical condition, thus

Table 6. Diary entries related to the emotional experience.

Themes	Entries
Documenting one's presence	Wife, 62: So I'd let him know what our grandchildren were up to, that they were back in school – but I felt the most important thing was to let him know I was there.
	Wife, 54: Apart from that, the diary was a way to let him know about what happened while he was away! and to send him all the text messages he got from his friends and co-workers, to write exactly what they sent.
	Wife, 53: Words spoken are forgotten but writings remain – so I wanted him to know everything I had to say to him – that what we lived through together was very very special – I wanted him to know that, well, he was the love of my life… I wanted to confirm that I really meant what I said to him, so that he'd know, so that he could read it, so that this little diary that he will keep reminds him every day that I was there, despite all the things that happened between us, that whatever happens I'll be at his side – I'll always be at his side. So it had to be written down, so that it would stay there forever. If at any point in time I became unable to visit him here, he'd know that in spite of everything I was at his side and that I was always at his side as soon as I found out he was seriously ill – that's it.
	Daughter, 21: It was really good for me and I said to myself that if she could read it, then she'd be happy to know that we supported her and that her family held her in our thoughts.
	Daughter, 45: I write in the diary every day that I come to the ICU – I write and it's a bit like sending a message to my father at the same time.
	Wife, 72: It's as if I can be part of his life – it's life that's surrounding him, I'm here, I show him that I'm here – he senses that and maybe he'll sense it even more strongly a bit later on.
	Wife, 52: The thing is that at that time, if the person dies while in the artificial coma, we don't know what will happen – actually, we don't know any longer what kind of connection we have to the person or what will happen. And so the diary – it's really like an everyday connection, a connection through what's possible day to day – and it's the diary that allowed that connection.
	Wife, 62: Well I think it connected me to the staff – it made me feel, sort of, that I was still talking with my husband.
	Wife, 70: It's sort of also to make a connection among ourselves, the family, our children, his grandchildren. And life going on all around, life at home, cultural happenings that he's sort of putting on the back burner for now but that I try to maintain a bit.
	Wife, 52: It helped my son, my youngest who is 19 and hadn't seen his father for 15 years – and the first time he visited he didn't know what to say to him – so I said, write, then afterward you'll read it to him – so he wrote in the diary and later on he read it to his father – and I believe we say some things but when we write other things can come to mind, things we think about and that take shape as we write – but for me, I always read everything I wrote to him, I read it to him afterwards, always – he knows every word I ever wrote in the diary.
Confiding in the diary and maintaining hope	Wife, 70: A bit like a journal. To express my feelings, what I want to say to him, what I've been doing – while he's in the hospital, but me, what I do in the meantime, how I manage to get on with the difference in my life.
	Wife, 53: I need to talk, I need to speak up, and it meant a lot to me to have this diary so that I could talk about my feelings at the very moment they were there.
	Wife, 62: Actually, for me, it was more like a haven – I don't know how to explain it. To me it was almost like a private journal I could confide in - and like a hand stretched out to me – something like that, sort of like a dialogue.… Because I'd read the little notes that were in the diary and when I read that today he was better than yesterday, well, that was fantastic.
	Daughter, 35: The diary meant that there was hope for later on – that's just it! (yes!) – it was exactly that connection, I'd write in it every day, because I wanted him to know what happened day by day and what he went through, him and also us, what we went through because of his treatment, and to show him what road, what journey he had travelled – to say, well, it was touch-and-go, but we can see the future, we were thinking about the future … I need to write every day, every time I visit I write to him, sometimes not much, other times I'll write two pages, sometimes ten lines or so because sometimes he's not doing very well and then it's not easy to write that he's not doing well because then we're not feeling well either – so we just write 'you're not doing well today, and we hope tomorrow you'll be better' – but that helps, because we hope that tomorrow will be better and that opens up the possibility of hope – it helps us move forward.
	Wife, 80: And more than anything else, it keeps our spirits up, because everyone writes a really kind note, and that feels good. It lifts our spirits, because with all the little notes by the doctors, they say 'we took good care of you, today you're better, but this or that happened, you had a little bit of heart trouble, but it's going to sort itself out'… Every time, it boosts our spirits. They don't say 'unfortunately, you're not doing as well as yesterday but we'll take care of you…' It's sort of hopeful and I find that's lovely.

humanising the patient in the minds of the family members. *'When I read what the staff members wrote, I really feel they're taking care of a person who is alive'* (62-year-old sister-in-law). The ICU environment and the severity of the illness cast a veil over the patient's dignity and humanity, and this veil was lifted by the writings of the staff. This change in the way the patient was perceived helped the family get through the ICU stay. *'The diary breathes strength into us, strength and a kind of serenity, of confidence, since what was written also was a source of confidence'* (42-year-old daughter). Additional diary entries are provided in the online-only supplement (Table 7).

The families' experience in context

In sum, grounded theory analysis of the interview data suggested the following model (Figure 1). The families perceived the diaries as promoting the acquisition and assimilation of medical information and, in collaboration with the staff, as providing an account of the patient's stay in the ICU. By documenting their presence, the diary connects the family members to the patient and ensures continuity of the family story during the ICU stay. Participating in the diary arouses strong emotions in the family members and allows them to express those emotions, thereby gaining distance and improving their emotional regulation capabilities. Finally, the diary changes the family

Table 7. Diary entries related to the humanisation experience.

Themes	Entries
Change in the way staff are viewed	Wife, 70: Me, I think it helps, it really establishes a connection, a connection between you and us… it's personal and individual. It's individualised, like the care that's given here…
	Daughter, 21: I thanked one of the nurses this morning – she didn't have to write in the diary, no one had an obligation to write in the diary, but for us, for us, me personally, I was touched to see what you wrote, to see the entries… that's what we talked about with my father, that we found that really human, that for once the patient was being taken care of and the family was being taken care of too.
	Son, 41: I found the idea original and nice and that it really gave a human quality to the ICU, for the families and even more so for the patient, in our case, since my mother asked, asked insistently to see the diary … it really gives a human character to this unit, which is awfully rough.
	Daughter, 35: To see that when we aren't here, because we can't be here all the time, and fortunately they take care of my father, and I feel this emotional aspect is very important – information isn't everything – that's what I realised when a nursing aide wrote 'I took care of you, I gave you comfort care – I did this, I gave you a massage …', things like that! It feels good, and also they write in the diary, they take the time, the time to write, because we know that in an ICU, in intensive care, time is valuable, there's a lot to do, and I find it extraordinary that they give us some of their time.
	Daughter, 42: I don't know why, but it made me stronger – it made me stronger because I realised they were people - the people who wrote were reliable, they did something, they did what was best – and they were going to try to solve this problem.
	Wife, 75: It's a good thing that it's the doctor. The first time, I said 'wow' and I thought there are patients and they still take the time to write, that's it – they still take the time to write.
	Daughter, 45 (The diary is) moving, because each person leaves a bit of their heart in it and a bit of the connection they may have with him. So it's moving and it's interesting too, because the different people who write discover little things about one another. Some reveal more than others, but it's clear that for everyone some of their emotions seep into the diary.
Change in the way the patient is viewed	Daughter, 35: It helped me a lot to read what the staff members wrote, for several reasons. One was a feeling of being acknowledged, because I felt they were giving special attention to my father.
	Daughter, 42: It's that we get the feeling that we have some control over the events, it's like a log, he was given a log book so now we have a task to accomplish, finally something to do – to recapitulate what is happening – so that way we don't feel completely helpless, it helps to no longer feel so helpless when we come to see someone who – we don't know whether he can hear us, whether he can't hear us …
	Daughter, 45: Because I think we give the staff information that's rather private on the person's life … the diary also replaces those exchanges, when we can't meet. There are nurses, nursing aides, other healthcare personnel that we don't see because we don't come at the same times … but with the diary, everyone gets the information, and to take into account a person who can't communicate, who can't explain things, it recreates a connection. Let everyone take a piece of it, because everyone takes a piece, but in some way it humanises the person who is lying down in bed with all those tubes – and in a way, it reassures us, because it's also sort of for us, the fear we can have is that the kind of care that's given is a bit too… dehumanised. It's the machines that scare us – they make us realise that so much depends on the machines and on the staff, so we're not sure whether there's still a place for humanity in all that.

members' perceptions of the staff and contributes to humanize their ICU experience.

Discussion

We investigated the experience of ICU-patient family members related to ICU diaries kept by both the family and the ICU staff. We identified three main domains of the diary experience: communication, in which the diary served as an ever-present source of reliable information about the medical condition of patient; expression of emotions, which strengthened the connection to the patient during the ICU stay and helped with emotional regulation; and humanisation of both the staff and the patient.

Routinely creating ICU diaries as a clinical intervention remains controversial [19,31]. Our study adds new insights about the benefits to families during the ICU stay and, to our knowledge, is the first investigation of this point, as most of the earlier studies focused on the patients. Analyses of the diary contents have shown how families use the diaries to communicate their emotions and feelings to the patients [12] and ICU staff [24]. Our results are consistent with this earlier work, as they indicate that reading and writing in the diaries arouse strong emotions in the family members and allow them to express those emotions. The feeling of loss due to absence of the patient from the daily family routine of communication and activities [32] was alleviated by the ability to communicate with the patient via entries in the diary. Thus, the family remained connected to the patient, who continued to be viewed as a living human being. In addition, the diary served as evidence that the family was actively present. The diary ensured that the patient remained included within the family story, so that the structure of the family remained intact. The ability to confide in the diary may have improved the regulation of emotions and contributed to the well-being of the families. This effect may explain the previously reported beneficial impact of diaries during the post-ICU period [12,21].

Diaries improved both family-staff and within-family communication. Communication is central to family satisfaction [4]. Receiving clear medical information about the patient's status is among the most important family needs [33]. However, the high prevalence of symptoms of post-traumatic stress, anxiety, and depression, most notably within the first few days after ICU admission [7], affects the family members' perceptions of communication. Quantitative and qualitative studies established that family satisfaction was related to the organisational culture [34], quality of information [4], and perceived ICU climate. Comprehension was improved by delivery of the information in a variety of formats (oral and written) [35] and by availability of the staff for communicating with families [4]. ICU diaries provide written information in everyday language, which can be read as often as desired. Our study showed that families felt the diaries helped them to understand the patient's condition and to assimilate the medical information. ICU diary content varies across countries with or without staff participation [14,21,36]. In our ICU, the physicians contribute to the narration of the patient's illness in the diary. The families felt that the information written by physicians in the diaries was more powerful and more trustworthy

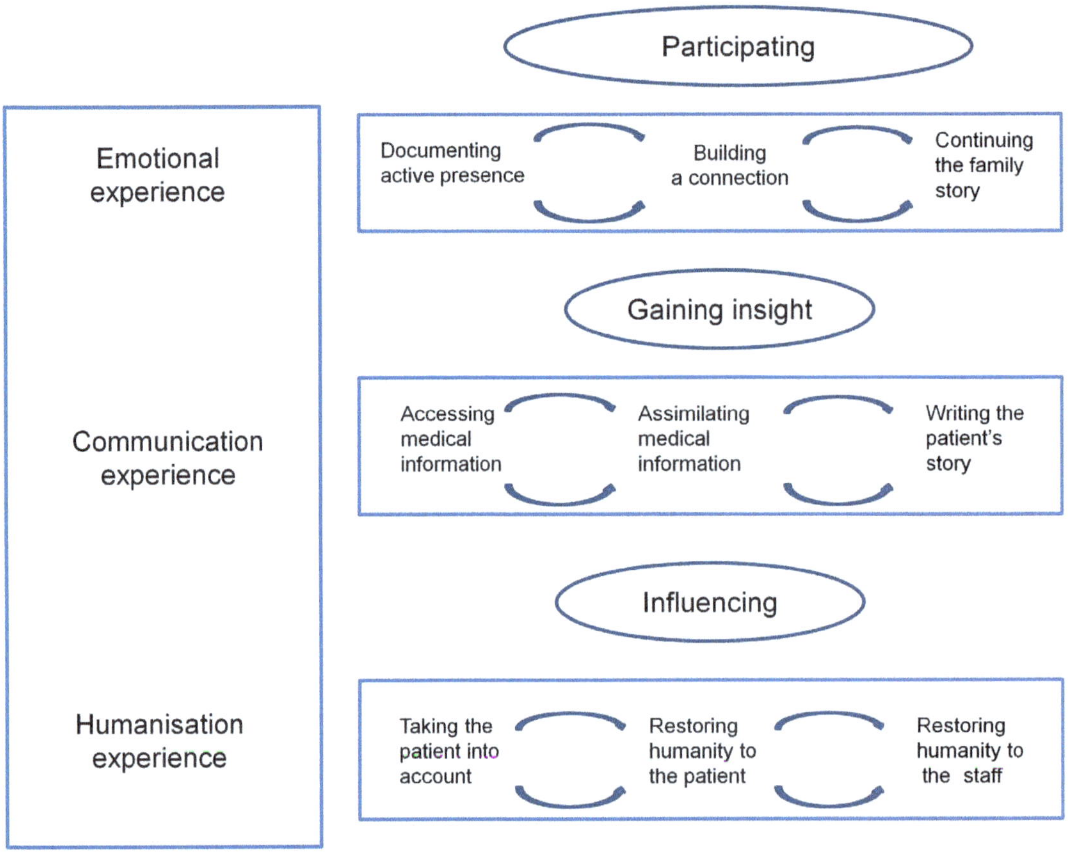

Figure 1. Components of the ICU-diary experience that helped to humanize the ICU experience for the families. For family members, participating in an ICU diary generated an emotional experience that built a connection with the patient and ensured continuation of the family story in the ICU. The diary enhanced the communication experience by providing medical information and describing the patient's story. The diary humanized the ICU.

than oral information. Thus, having the physicians contribute to the ICU diaries may help to improve the family's comprehension of the patient's situation. The diaries also improved communication within the family by ensuring that all family members had access to personal and medical information.

The families indicated that the diary was a tool of humanization of the ICU. The use of the diary by the staff to communicate with the patient indicated to the families that the staff members were compassionate and empathetic, thereby providing reassurance that the patient was safe and in good hands. Furthermore, the respect and compassion expressed by the staff generated hope in the family members. In an earlier study by our group [27] staff members reported that writing in the diaries helped them 'to humanize their roles by emphasising the dimension of sensitivity and empathy in their interactions with the patient and the family'. In addition, awareness that the staff viewed the patient as a living human being humanised the patient in the eyes of the families. A critical illness not only causes fear that the patient might die, but also induces distress due to a perception that the patient has lost some of his or her humanity. Seen in the unfamiliar and somewhat frightening ICU environment, connected to machines, and often unable to communicate, the patient is not easily recognised by the family as their loved one, they know so well. The ability of the diary to restore the patient's humanity in the eyes of the family illustrates the differences between, and complementarity of, care and treatment. For family members who are made vulnerable by the critical illness of their relative, the diary serves as a powerful tool for improving holistic family-centred care.

Some methodological aspects are important to discuss. To take into account the possible role for subjectivity inherent in qualitative analyses, we used an insider-outsider approach, with three people, of whom two did not belong to the ICU staff and usually worked outside the ICU setting. The use of theoretical sampling with the inclusion of new interviewees in an approach that goes back and forth between the data and the analysis allows the uncovering of a theory [28]. The participation of both family members and all ICU staff members in the diaries, the specific instructions given to diary writers, and the inclusion of medical information in the diaries may limit the general applicability of our findings. The high educational level of our sample may limit the general applicability of our results. Finally, we did not take family dynamics into account.

Conclusions

This study produced important insights about the usefulness of ICU diaries to families. The diary served as a vector that connected the patient, family, and staff into a single coherent story. It contributed to support the family members in the ICU and to restore the functional and social role of the family. The medical information given by physicians in the diary was greatly appreciated by the families, who felt it improved their comprehension. Physician participation in ICU diaries probably deserves to be encouraged.

Acknowledgments

We thank all the families who participated in the study and the staff members of our ICU for their participation. We thank A. Wolfe, MD, for helping to prepare this manuscript; and Malika Talbi, who contributed to perform the interviews. We also thank Claire Launay, Yasminka Pichon and Adrien Pichon, who transcribed the interviews.

Author Contributions

No other contribution. Conceived and designed the experiments: MGO AP BM. Performed the experiments: MGO. Analyzed the data: MGO AP PM. Contributed reagents/materials/analysis tools: MGO CB FP AM BM CG SB. Wrote the paper: MGO AP PM.

References

1. Azoulay E, Pochard F, Kentish-Barnes N, Chevret S, Aboab J, et al. (2005) Risk of post-traumatic stress symptoms in family members of intensive care unit patients. Am J Respir Crit Care Med 171: 987–994.
2. Berwick DM, Kotagal M (2004) Restricted visiting hours in ICUs: time to change. JAMA 292: 736–737.
3. Giannini A, Miccinesi G, Leoncino S (2008) Visiting policies in Italian intensive care units: a nationwide survey. Intensive Care Medicine 34: 1256–1262.
4. Azoulay E, Chevret S, Leleu G, Pochard F, Barboteu M, et al. (2000) Half the families of intensive care unit patients experience inadequate communication with physicians. Crit Care Med 28: 3044–3049.
5. Azoulay E, Pochard F, Chevret S, Adrie C, Annane D, et al. (2004) Half the family members of intensive care unit patients do not want to share in the decision-making process: a study in 78 French intensive care units. Crit Care Med 32: 1832–1838.
6. Davidson JE, Powers K, Hedayat KM, Tieszen M, Kon AA, et al. (2007) Clinical practice guidelines for support of the family in the patient-centered intensive care unit: American College of Critical Care Medicine Task Force 2004–2005. Critical Care Medicine 35: 605–622.
7. McAdam JL, Fontaine DK, White DB, Dracup KA, Puntillo KA (2012) Psychological symptoms of family members of high-risk intensive care unit patients. American Journal of Critical Care: an official publication, American Association of Critical-Care Nurses 21: 386–393; quiz 394.
8. Garrouste-Orgeas M, Philippart F, Timsit JF, Diaw F, Willems V, et al. (2008) Perceptions of a 24-hour visiting policy in the intensive care unit. Critical Care Medicine 36: 30–35.
9. Giannini A, Marchesi T, Miccinesi G (2011) Andante moderato: signs of change in visiting policies for Italian ICUs. Intensive Care Medicine 37: 1890.
10. Giannini A, Garrouste-Orgeas M, Latour JM (2014) What's new in ICU visiting policies: can we continue to keep the doors closed? Intensive Care Medicine 40: 730–733.
11. Garrouste-Orgeas M, Willems V, Timsit JF, Diaw F, Brochon S, et al. (2010) Opinions of families, staff, and patients about family participation in care in intensive care units. J Crit Care 25: 634–640.
12. Garrouste-Orgeas M, Coquet I, Perier A, Timsit JF, Pochard F, et al. (2012) Impact of an intensive care unit diary on psychological distress in patients and relatives. Critical Care Medicine 40: 2033–2040.
13. Egerod I, Christensen D, Schwartz-Nielsen KH, Agard AS (2011) Constructing the illness narrative: a grounded theory exploring patients' and relatives' use of intensive care diaries. Critical Care Medicine 39: 1922–1928.
14. Kloos JA, Daly BJ (2008) Effect of a Family-Maintained Progress Journal on anxiety of families of critically ill patients. Crit Care Nurs Q 31: 96–107; quiz 108–109.
15. Egerod I, Bagger C (2010) Patients' experiences of intensive care diaries–a focus group study. Intensive Critical Care Nursing: the Official Journal of the British Association of Critical Care Nurses 26: 278–287.
16. Hale M, Parfitt L, Rich T (2010) How diaries can improve the experience of intensive care patients. Nursing Management 17: 14–18.
17. Jones C, Backman C, Capuzzo M, Egerod I, Flaatten H, et al. (2010) Intensive care diaries reduce new onset post traumatic stress disorder following critical illness: a randomised, controlled trial. Critical Care 14: R168.
18. Knowles RE, Tarrier N (2009) Evaluation of the effect of prospective patient diaries on emotional well-being in intensive care unit survivors: a randomized controlled trial. Crit Care Med 37: 184–191.
19. Aitken LM, Rattray J, Hull A, Kenardy JA, Le Brocque R, et al. (2013) The use of diaries in psychological recovery from intensive care. Critical Care 17: 253.
20. Hodge B (2013) The use of symptom diaries in outpatient care. Fam Pract Manag 20: 24–28.
21. Jones C, Backman C, Griffiths RD (2012) Intensive care diaries and relatives' symptoms of posttraumatic stress disorder after critical illness: a pilot study. American Journal of Critical Care: an Official Publication, American Association of Critical-Care Nurses 21: 172–176.
22. Ewens B, Chapman R, Tulloch A, Hendricks JM (2014) ICU survivors' utilisation of diaries post discharge: a qualitative descriptive study. Aust Crit Care 27: 28–35.
23. Roulin MJ, Hurst S, Spirig R (2007) Diaries written for ICU patients. Qual Health Res 17: 893–901.
24. Di Gangi S, Naretto G, Cravero N, Livigni S (2013) A narrative-based study on communication by family members in intensive care unit. J Crit Care 28: 483–489.
25. Charmaz K (1990) 'Discovering' chronic illness: using grounded theory. Soc Sci Med 30: 1161–1172.
26. Strauss AL, Corbin JM (1998) Basics of Qualitative Research. Grounded Theory Procedures and Techniques. 2nd ed. London: Sage Publications.
27. Perier A, Revah-Levy A, Bruel C, Cousin N, Angeli S, et al. (2013) Phenomenologic analysis of healthcare worker perceptions of intensive care unit diaries. Critical Care 17: R13.
28. Coyne I (1996) Sampling in qualitative research. Purposeful and theoritical sampling: merging or clear boundaries? Journal of Advanced Nursing 26: 623–630.
29. Le Gall JR, Lemeshow S, Saulnier F (1993) A new Simplified Acute Physiology Score (SAPS II) based on a European/North American multicenter study. JAMA 270: 2957–2963.
30. Creswell J (2009) Research design: qualitative, quantitative, and mixed methods approaches. Thousand Oaks, California: Sage Publications.
31. Mehlhorn J, Freytag A, Schmidt K, Brunkhorst FM, Graf J, et al. (2014) Rehabilitation interventions for postintensive care syndrome: a systematic review. Crit Care Med 42: 1263–1271.
32. Urizzi F, Correa A (2007) Relatives' experience of intensive care: the other side of hospitalization. Rev Latino Am Enfermagem 15: 598–604.
33. Molter NC (1979) Needs of relatives of critically ill patients: a descriptive study. Heart Lung 8: 332–339.
34. Dodek P, Heyland D, Cook D, Rocket G, Kutsogiannis D, et al. (2012) The relationship between organizational culture and family satisfaction in critical care. Crit Care Med. 40: 1506–1512.
35. Stephenson PL (2006) Before the teaching begins: Managing patient anxiety prior to providing education. Clin J Oncol Nurs 10: 241–245.
36. Egerod I, Schwartz-Nielsen KH, Hansen GM, Laerkner E (2007) The extent and application of patient diaries in Danish ICUs in 2006. Nursing in Critical Care 12: 159–167.

13

Prevalence of Comorbidities and Their Impact on Hospital Management and Short-Term Outcomes in Vietnamese Patients Hospitalized with a First Acute Myocardial Infarction

Hoa L. Nguyen[1,2*], Quang Ngoc Nguyen[3], Duc Anh Ha[4], Dat Tuan Phan[3], Nguyen Hanh Nguyen[1], Robert J. Goldberg[5]

1 Institute of Population, Health and Development, Ha Noi, Viet Nam, **2** Oxford University Clinical Research Unit, Ho Chi Minh City, Viet Nam, **3** Viet Nam National Heart Institute, Ha Noi, Viet Nam, **4** Ministry of Health, Ha Noi, Viet Nam, **5** Department of Quantitative Health Sciences, University of Massachusetts Medical School, Worcester, Massachusetts, United States of America

Abstract

Background: Cardiovascular disease is one of the leading causes of morbidity and mortality in Vietnam. We conducted a pilot study of Hanoi residents hospitalized with a first acute myocardial infarction (AMI) at the Vietnam National Heart Institute in Hanoi for purposes of describing the prevalence of cardiovascular (CVD) and non-CVD comorbidities and their impact on hospital management, in-hospital clinical complications, and short-term mortality in these patients.

Methods: The study population consisted of 302 Hanoi residents hospitalized with a first AMI at the largest tertiary care medical center in Hanoi in 2010.

Results: The average age of study patients was 66 years and one third were women. The proportions of patients with none, any 1, and $\geq$ 2 CVD comorbidities were 34%, 42%, and 24%, respectively. Among the CVD comorbidities, hypertension was the most commonly reported (59%). There were decreasing trends in the proportion of patients who were treated with effective cardiac medications and coronary interventions as the number of CVD comorbidities increased. Patients with multiple CVD comorbidities tended to develop acute clinical complications and die at higher rates during hospitalization compared with patients with no CVD comorbidities (Odds Ratio: 1.40; 95% Confidence Interval: 0.40–4.84).

Conclusions: Our data suggest that patients with multiple cardiac comorbidities tended to experience high in-hospital death rates in the setting of AMI. Full-scale surveillance of Hanoi residents hospitalized with AMI at all Hanoi hospitals is needed to confirm these findings. Effective strategies to manage Vietnamese patients hospitalized with AMI who have multiple comorbidities are warranted to improve their short-term prognosis.

Editor: Chiara Lazzeri, Azienda Ospedaliero-Universitaria Careggi, Italy

Funding: This study was partially funded by the Global Health Office, University of Massachusetts Medical School, Worcester, MA, USA. Additional support was provided by internal funding. The funders had no role in study design, data collection and analysis, decision to publish, or preparation of the manuscript.

Competing Interests: The authors have declared that no competing interests exist.

* Email: hoanguyen@phad.org

Introduction

The prevalence of persons with multiple comorbidities in the general population is increasing, even in low-middle income countries (LMICs) [1,2,3]. Data from the International Network for Demographic Evaluation of Populations and Their Health including 8 Asian sites in Vietnam, Bangladesh, Thailand, Indonesia, and India in 2005 showed that 23% of men and 32% of women aged 25–64 years reported having at least 1 chronic health condition, and 5% of men and 9% of women reported having 2 or more chronic conditions [2]. Patients hospitalized with acute myocardial infarction (AMI) also have a variety of cardiovascular (CVD) and non-CVD comorbidities present [4,5,6,7,8]. Previous studies have suggested that CVD and non-CVD comorbidities exert a negative impact on in-hospital complications and mortality in patients hospitalized with AMI, though these studies have been primarily conducted in high-income countries [4,5,6,7,8,9].

Vietnam is an LMIC, which has been undergoing an important epidemiological transition. The overall morbidity and mortality from Non-Communicable Diseases (NCDs) has been rising rapidly over the last two decades and the NCDs have become a major societal problem. CVD is now the leading cause of death in

Vietnam, accounting for approximately one quarter of all deaths annually. Moreover, the major risk factors for CVD are either on the rise or at disturbing levels in the Vietnamese population [10]. Data from the International Network for Demographic Evaluation of Populations and Their Health in 2005 showed that the prevalence of persons with 2 or more chronic conditions was approximately 6% for Vietnamese men and 7% for women [2].

Despite the important impact of multiple comorbidities on the prognosis of patients hospitalized with AMI, to the best of our knowledge no studies have reported the prevalence of CVD and non-CVD comorbidities and their impact on hospital management practices and short-term outcomes among adults hospitalized with AMI in Vietnam. The objectives of this observational study were to describe the prevalence of several CVD and non-CVD comorbidities and their impact on hospital management, in-hospital clinical complications, and mortality in patients hospitalized with a first AMI during 2010 at the Vietnam National Heart Institute in Hanoi.

Methods

Ethics Statement

The Institutional Review Board at the Institute of Population, Health and Development approved this study. The study was conducted with a waiver of patient consent approved by the institute's Institutional Review Board. Patient records/information was anonymized and de-identified prior to analysis.

Study Setting

This study was carried out at the Vietnam National Heart Institute [11]. This facility is a 250 bed- tertiary care medical center in Hanoi (2009 census = 6.5 million), which treats the majority of Hanoi residents hospitalized with acute coronary disease and other NCDs.

Case Ascertainment Approaches

Computerized printouts of patients discharged from the Vietnam National Heart Institute in 2010 with possible AMI were obtained and International Classification of Disease codes for possible AMI (I20-I25) were reviewed. Cases of possible AMI were independently validated according to predefined criteria for AMI by two cardiologists. The diagnosis of AMI was made on the basis of criteria developed by the World Health Organization which includes a suggestive clinical history, serum enzyme elevations above the hospital's normal range (normal ranges: Troponin I< 0.5 ng/ml, Troponin T<0.01 ng/ml, CK-MB <7–25 U/L, CK: Male: 38–174 U/L, Female: 26–140 U/L), and serial electrocardiographic (ECG) findings during hospitalization consistent with the presence of AMI; at least 2 of these 3 criteria needed to be present for an AMI to have occurred [12]. A total of 315 residents of the city of Hanoi who satisfied criteria for the diagnosis of AMI were identified. Since the majority (302 patients) of this population was hospitalized for a first AMI (96%), we restricted our patient population to those with an initial AMI based on the review of information obtained from hospital medical records. Our patient population was also further classified into those with ST segment elevation AMI (STEMI) and non-ST segment elevation AMI (NSTEMI), using standard classification techniques [13]. Each of the ECG's of patients with possible AMI was reviewed by a physician under the guidance of a senior cardiologist. A small number of patients with AMI (n = 21) were not able to be classified as STEMI or NSTEMI due to the poor quality of reviewed ECGs.

Data Collection

We reviewed the paper medical records of all patients who were admitted with discharge diagnoses suggestive of AMI and reviewed each of their hospital charts. For each independently validated case of AMI who satisfied our geographic eligibility criteria, a variety of socio-demographic, clinical, and medical care related information was collected from the review of the medical record and abstracted onto a standardized case-report form by trained study physicians. Information was collected about patient's age, sex, previously diagnosed comorbidities, admission heart rate, blood pressure, serum glucose and serum lipid levels, AMI type (STEMI vs. NSTEMI), receipt of effective cardiac medications during the index hospitalization (e.g., Angiotensin converting enzyme inhibitors-ACEIs; Angiotensin II receptor blockers-ARBs, beta blockers) and coronary interventional procedures (e.g., percutaneous coronary intervention -PCI, coronary artery bypass surgery -CABG), clinically significant in-hospital complications (e.g., heart failure, stroke, atrial fibrillation), hospital discharge status, and length of hospital stay.

Comorbidities in the present study were defined as those chronic conditions that were previously diagnosed, and had been documented, in the medical history section of reviewed hospital charts, and did not include any conditions that may have been newly diagnosed during the patient's hospital admission. Thus, there were no clinical or laboratory criteria that were used to make the final diagnoses for these conditions. Comorbidities in this patient population were categorized into 2 groups: CVD and non-CVD comorbidities. Seven CVD comorbidities were considered including atrial fibrillation, coronary heart disease -CHD (prior angina, CHD, MI, CABG, and PCI), diabetes, heart failure, hypertension, hyperlipidermia, and stroke. Six non-CVD comorbidities including anemia, asthma, cancer, chronic obstructive pulmonary disease (COPD), gastro-intestinal (GI) bleeding/peptic ulcer, and chronic renal disease were examined. The selection of these conditions was made based on findings from previous studies that have examined the associations of these comorbdiities with the prognosis of patients hospitalized with AMI [4,5,6,7,8] and based on their prevalence in this patient sample.

The primary outcome of the present study was the in-hospital case- fatality rate (CFR). Secondary outcomes included hospital management practices (e.g., use of aspirin, ACEIs/ARBs, beta blockers, statins, PCI, and CABG), hospital clinical complications (e.g., atrial fibrillation, heart failure, cardiogenic shock), and hospital length of stay. In terms of hospital clinical complications, atrial fibrillation included the documentation of new atrial fibrillation in the hospital medical record or occurrence of typical electrocardiographic changes consistent with this diagnosis. Heart failure was indicated by clinical or radiographic evidence of pulmonary edema or bilateral basilar rales with an S3 gallop. Cardiogenic shock was defined as a systolic blood pressure of less than 90 mmHg in the absence of hypovolemia and associated with cyanosis, cold extremities, changes in mental status, persistent oliguria, or congestive heart failure.

Data Analysis

The overall prevalence of single and multiple comorbidities in this population was calculated in a standard manner. The number of CVD comorbidities was categorized into 3 categories (0, 1, and ≥2) and the number of non-CVD comorbidites was categorized into 2 categories (0 and ≥1). Data were presented as percentages for categorical variables and compared using the chi-square or Fisher exact tests if expected values were less than 5; medians (inter quartile range- IQR) for continuous variables were calculated and compared using the Kruskal-Wallis tests.

Logistic regression models were used to examine the impact of number of comorbidities on in-hospital CFRs. A multivariable logistic regression model was adjusted for several patient associated characteristics that significantly differed according to number of comorbidities in unadjusted analyses (age, MI characteristic: STEMI vs. NSTEMI). The most common clusters of co-existing comorbidities were identified and in-hospital CFRs associated with these clusters were reported. Two-sided analytic tests were used and a p value less than 0.05 was considered to be statistically significant. All analyses were performed using STATA 11.0 (StataCorp. TX).

Results

The study population consisted of 302 Hanoi residents hospitalized with a first AMI at the VNHI in 2010. The average age of study patients was 66 years and one third were women. Seventy three percent of patients developed an STEMI. The overall in-hospital mortality was 7.0%.

Prevalence of CVD and Non-CVD Comorbidities

The mean and median number of CVD comorbidities in this population were 0.9 and 1 respectively (range: 0-3; only 2 patients had 3 conditions). Two thirds of patients had at least 1 CVD comorbidity previously diagnosed. The proportions of patients with none, any 1, and any 2 or more CVD comorbidities were 34%, 42%, and 24%, respectively. Among the cardiac comorbid conditions examined, hypertension was the most commonly reported (59%) followed by diabetes (17%) (Figure 1).

The majority (90%) of patients had none of the non-CVD comorbidities examined and only 10% had any 1 or more non-CVD comorbidities previously diagnosed. Among the non-CVD comorbidities, GI bleeding/ulcer was the most commonly reported (7%) (Figure 1). Since the prevalence of non-CVD comorbidities was very low in this population, we did not perform further analyses according to the number of non-CVD comorbidities present.

Study Population Characteristics

Patients with any CVD comorbidity were significantly older and more likely to have developed a NSTEMI than patients without any previously diagnosed CVD comorbidity (Table 1). On admission, patients with any CVD comorbidity had significantly higher blood pressure results, higher plasma glucose levels, but lower estimated glomerular filtration rate (eGFR) findings compared to patients without any CVD comorbidity.

Hospital Management Practices

Overall, during the first 24 hours after hospital admission, the use of aspirin and lipid lowering agents was high (>90%) as was the use of ACE inhibitors (~70%); however, the use of beta-blockers was comparatively low (~30%) (Table 2).

During the first 24 hours after hospital admission, although there were no statistically significant differences in medication utilization both singly and in combination in relation to the number of CVD comorbidities previously diagnosed, there was a decreasing trend in the proportion of patients who received effective cardiac medications as the number of cardiac comorbidities increased (Table 2). Similarly, the proportion of patients undergoing PCI tended to decrease with increasing number of CVD comorbidities present (63% to 53%). Similar findings were

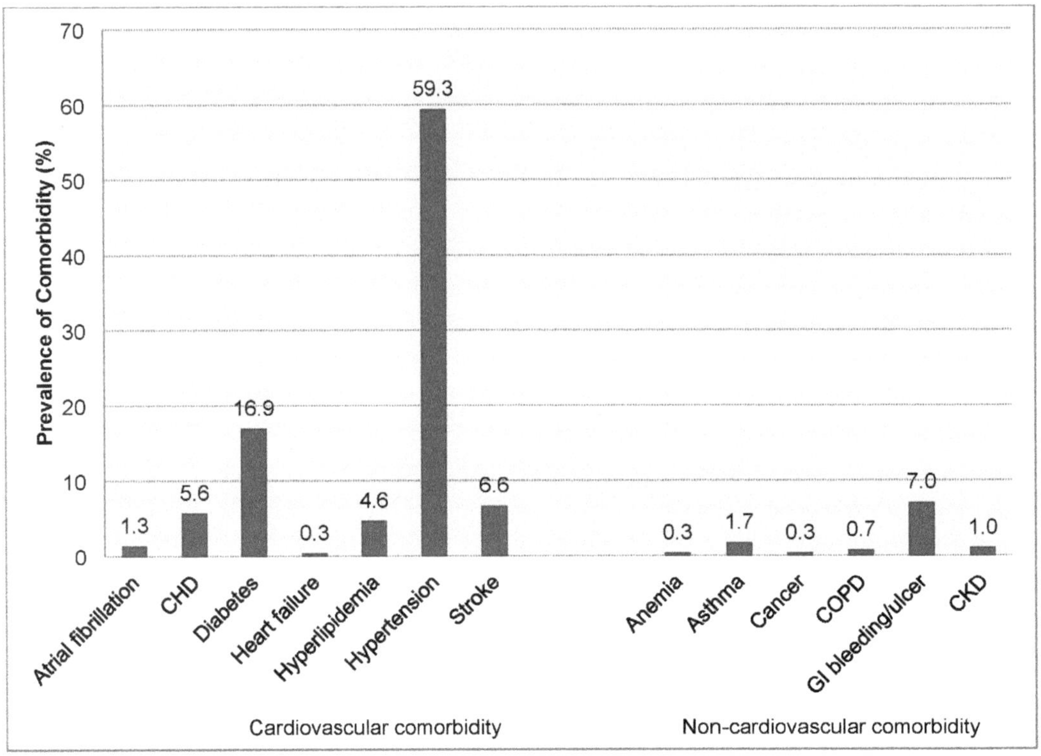

Figure 1. Prevalence of Selected Cardiovascular and Non-Cardiovascular Comorbidities among Patients Hospitalized with Acute Myocardial Infarction. CHD, coronary heart disease; COPD, chronic obstructive pulmonary disease; GI, gastro-intestinal; CKD, chronic kidney disease.

Table 1. Study Population Characteristics According to Number of Cardiovascular Comorbidities.

	0 (n = 103)	1 (n = 127)	≥2 (n = 72)	p value*
Age (mean, SD), years	63(13)	68(11)	67(10)	0.003
Male	76(73.8)	83(65.4)	42(58.3)	0.10
Ethnicity (n,%)				
Kinh**	100(97.1)	127(100)	69(95.8)	0.09
Minority	3(2.9)	0(0)	3(4.2)	
MI characteristic (n,%)				
STEMI¶	80(83.3)	84(72.4)	43(62.3)	0.010
Non-STEMI	16(16.7)	32(27.6)	26(37.7)	
Clinical parameters on admission (median, IQR)				
Heart rate (beats/min)	82(72–97)	87(72–102)	90(79–102)	0.16
Systolic blood pressure (mmHg)	120(100–130)	120(110–145)	130(120–140)	0.002
Diastolic blood pressure (mmHg)	70(60–80)	80(70–90)	80(70–90)	0.008
Laboratory findings on admission (median, IQR)				
Cholesterol (mmol/L)	4.5(3.9–5.0)	4.6(4.0–5.1)	4.4(4.0–5.3)	0.84
LDL (mmol/L)	2.7(2.1–3.1)	2.8(2.3–3.1)	2.6(2.2–3.4)	0.71
Glucose (mmol/L)	6.8(5.4–9.0)	7.5(5.7–9.0)	8.5(6.1–12.2)	0.008
eGFR (ml/min/1.73 m^2)°	75(62–92)	67(52–80)	68(54–89)	0.002
Cardiovascular comorbidity (n,%)				
Atrial fibrillation	NA	2(1.6)	2(2.8)	
Coronary heart disease	NA	4(3.1)	13(18.1)	
Diabetes	NA	10(7.9)	41(56.9)	
Heart failure	NA	0(0)	1(1.4)	
Hypertension	NA	108(85)	71(98.6)	
Hyperlipidemia	NA	1(0.8)	13(18.1)	
Stroke	NA	2(1.6)	18(25)	

SD: Standard deviation; IQR: Inter quartile range; STEMI: ST segment elevation AMI; LDL: Low Density Lipoprotein
**The Kinh people are the majority ethnic group in Vietnam, comprising 87% of the population (census 2009)
¶data missing in 21 patients
°eGFR: glomerular filtration rate was calculated based on CKD-EPI Equation
*p values from chi-square or Fisher exact tests for categorical variables and Kruskal-Wallis tests for continuous variables.

observed when we examined the use of medications and cardiac procedures during the entire hospitalization.

In-Hospital Clinical Complications

During hospitalization, although there were no statistically significant differences with regards to the risk of developing important clinical complications in relation to the number of CVD comorbidities, there was an increasing trend in the development of heart failure (from 11% to 18%), and recurrent angina (4% to 7%) as the number of CVD comorbidities increased (Table 2). However, there was a decreased likelihood of developing cardiogenic shock (5% to 3%) and ventricular fibrillation/cardiac arrest (7% to 4%) as the number of CVD comorbidities increased.

During hospitalization, although there were no statistically significant differences in terms of the risk of dying according to the number of CVD comorbidities, the crude in-hospital CFRs tended to be lower in patients with any 1 CVD comorbidity compared to those without any CVD comorbidity (5.5% vs. 6.8%, Table 2). After adjusting for age and AMI associated characteristic (STEMI vs. NSTEMI), there was a 29% lower risk of dying for patients with any 1 cardiac condition compared with patients without any CVD condition (adjusted OR: 0.71; 95%CI: 0.22–2.31).

On the other hand, the crude in-hospital CFR tended to be higher in patients with 2 or more CVD conditions compared to those without any CVD condition (9.7% vs. 6.8%, Table 2). After adjusting for age and AMI related characteristic, patients with multiple CVD comorbidities were 40% more likely to have died during hospitalization compared to patients without any cardiac condition (adjusted OR: 1.40; 95%CI: 0.40–4.84). Hospital length of stay did not differ according to the number of CVD comorbidities previously diagnosed.

Common Clusters of CVD Comorbidities

The most common clusters of CVD comorbidities included "hypertension + diabetes" (n = 40,13.3%), "hypertension + stroke" (n = 18, 6.0%), "hypertension + CHD" (n = 12, 4.0%), and "hypertension + hyperlipidemia" (n = 13, 4.3%); the in-hospital CFRs for these clusters were 5.0%, 9.5%, 25.0% and 7.7%, respectively. Hypertension was included in all common clusters, and the in-hospital CFR for patients with both hypertension and CHD conditions was the highest, being approximately 3 times as high as that of the whole study population (overall CFR of 7.0%).

Table 2. Study Outcomes According to Number of Cardiovascular Comorbidities.

	0 (n = 103)	1 (n = 127)	≥2 (n = 72)	p value*
Management in the first 24 hours after admission (n,%)				
Aspirin	100(97.1)	123(96.9)	65(90.3)	0.06
ACE Is	73(70.9)	91(71.7)	51(70.8)	0.99
Beta blockers	26(25.2)	25(19.7)	11(15.3)	0.26
Lipid lower agents	96(94.1)	118(92.9)	62(86.1)	0.14
All 4 medications	23(22.3)	22(17.3)	10(13.9)	0.34
Percutaneous coronary intervention	64(62.7)	74(58.3)	38(52.8)	0.42
Management during hospitalization (n,%)				
Aspirin	102(99.0)	127(100)	71(98.6)	0.46
ACE Is/ARB	86(83.5)	111(87.4)	58(80.6)	0.42
Beta blockers	34(33.0)	41(32.3)	16(22.2)	0.24
Lipid lower agents	97(94.2)	118(92.9)	63(87.5)	0.25
All 4 medications	30(29.1)	36(28.3)	16(22.2)	0.56
Hospital cardiac procedures (n,%)				
Cardiac catheterization	84(81.6)	95(74.8)	54(75.0)	0.42
Percutaneous coronary intervention	73(70.9)	87(68.5)	47(65.3)	0.74
Coronary artery bypass surgery	3(3.0)	1(0.8)	0(0)	0.36
Hospital complications (n,%)				
Atrial fibrillation	2(1.9)	2(1.6)	0(0)	0.68
Cardiogenic shock	5(4.9)	5(3.9)	2(2.8)	0.87
Heart failure	11(10.7)	15(11.8)	13(18.1)	0.32
Recurrent angina	4(3.9)	6(4.7)	5(6.9)	0.65
Stroke	0(0)	1(0.8)	0(0)	0.99
Ventricular fibrillation or cardiac arrest	7(6.8)	6(4.7)	3(4.2)	0.76
In-hospital case-fatality rates (n,%)	7(6.8)	7(5.5)	7(9.7)	0.53
Length of hospital stay (median, IQR), days	4(3–7)	4(2–5)	4(2–6)	0.17

ACE-Is: Angiotensin converting enzyme inhibitors; ARBs: Angiotensin II receptor blockers
*p values from chi-square or Fisher exact tests for categorical variables and Kruskal-Wallis tests for continuous variables.

Discussion

The results of our pilot study in Hanoi, Vietnam showed that approximately two thirds of patients hospitalized with a first AMI at the largest tertiary care center in Hanoi had at least 1 CVD comorbidity present. In terms of non-CVD comorbidity, the majority of our study sample had none, and only a tenth had any 1 or more of these conditions. Patients with multiple CVD comorbidities were more likely to be older, to have developed a NSTEMI, and tended to be at higher risk for dying during hospitalization compared with patients without any CVD comorbidity.

Prevalence of CVD and Non-CVD Comorbidities

Our study showed that nearly one half of patients hospitalized with a first AMI had any 1, and a quarter had any 2 or more, CVD comorbidities; only one tenth of the study population had at least 1 non-CVD comorbidity previously diagnosed. Both the average number of comorbidities, and prevalence of multiple comorbidities, in our study population were lower than those reported in studies from high-income countries [4,5,6,7,8,9] including Spain, Denmark, the United States and Switzerland. These differences may be explained partially by the fact that our study population was relatively younger and included only patients hospitalized with their first AMI. However, given the aging Vietnamese population, and the increasing adoption of a western style diet and various lifestyle practices, it is expected that the prevalence of patients with multiple chronic conditions will continue to increase in Vietnam. Inasmuch, monitoring trends in the frequency of individual and multiple comorbidities among patients hospitalized with AMI will be of continued importance to inform health systems and practitioners to design and provide more optimal patient care for these complex patients.

In our study, hypertension was found to be the most prevalent cardiac condition followed by diabetes. These findings are consistent with the results of other studies in LMICs [14,15,16,17] and in high-income countries [4,5,6,7,8] where the prevalence of hypertension has ranged from approximately 50%–75%, and the prevalence of diabetes has ranged from 17%–46% in patients hospitalized with AMI. However, the prevalence of hyperlipidemia in our study was relatively low (5%) compared to that of other LMICs where the prevalence has ranged from 15–30% [14,15,16,17]. GI bleeding/ulcer was found to be the most common non-CVD comorbidity in our patient population and other conditions were found at extremely low rates. These findings are in contrast to those observed in high-income countries [4,7,8] where chronic kidney disease, COPD, and depression have been noted in a significant proportion of these diverse study populations. For example, data from more than 30,000 patients with an acute coronary syndrome in the nationwide AMIS Plus registry in Switzerland between 2002–2012 showed that 7%, 6%, and 2% of patients reported having kidney disease, chronic lung disease, and a GI ulcer, respectively [9]. Similarly, in a study of more than 5,000 patients hospitalized with AMI in Spain between 2003–2009, the prevalence rates of kidney disease, chronic lung disease, depression, and GI ulcer were 11%, 16%, 4%, and 0.5%, respectively, in 2009 [4]. Previous studies from LMICs [14,15,16,17] have failed to report the frequency of non-CVD comorbidities, so we were unable to compare our findings with the data from other LMICs.

Factors Associated with Multiple Comorbidities

In our study population, patients with multiple cardiac comorbidities were more likely to be older, to have developed a NSTEMI, and to have higher serum glucose, but lower eGFR findings, compared with patients without any cardiac comorbidity. This finding is consistent with previous studies in the setting of AMI [4,5,6,7,8,9], as well as studies in general population samples from LMICs [1,2,3,18]. For example, in the Worcester Heart Attack Study of nearly 3,000 patients hospitalized with AMI in central Massachusetts (United States) between 2003–2007, patients with multiple chronic conditions were more likely to be older, female, to have developed an NSTEMI, and to have higher serum glucose, but lower eGFR and serum cholesterol levels, at the time of hospital admission compared to those without any cardiac comorbidity [8]. Identifying patient characteristics associated with multiple cardiac comorbidities is important to inform interventions designed to decrease the prevalence of multiple comorbidities in these individuals.

Hospital Management Practices

Although there were no statistically significant differences in hospital management practices in relation to the number of chronic conditions previously diagnosed in the present study, our results suggest that there was a decreasing trend in the receipt of effective cardiac medications and PCI as the number of cardiac comorbidities increased, consistent with the findings from several developed countries [7,8,9]. For example, a study of nearly 3,000 patients with AMI in 53 hospitals in Ontario, Canada between 1999–2003 demonstrated that the number of pre-existing conditions was inversely associated with the receipt of coronary reperfusion therapy [7]. Similarly, data from the AMIS Plus registry found that patients with multiple (CVD and non-CVD) comorbidities were less likely to have received effective cardiac medications and coronary reperfusion therapy compared to patients with no comorbidity [9].

Patients with multiple comorbidities are challenging to treat due to issues related to possible medication contraindications and their high rates of adverse events. Current management guidelines in Vietnam focus only on patients with a single condition and not on those with multiple conditions. Thus, developing comprehensive management strategies for these patients is urgently needed. One such approach to consider would be a patient-and family centered approach to care throughout the health system [19].

In-hospital Complications and Death Rates

Our data showed that as the number of CVD comorbidities increased, the risk of developing heart failure and cardiogenic shock increased, as did the number of patients who died during hospitalization. These findings are consistent with previous studies [4,5,8,9]. For example, a nationwide study in Denmark including more than 200,000 patients hospitalized with a first AMI between 1984–2008 found that patients with multiple comorbidities experienced higher short- and long-term mortality compared to patients without multiple comorbidities [5].

In the present study, we also found that the risk of ventricular fibrillation or cardiac arrest tended to decrease as the number of CVD comorbidities increased. Similar findings have been reported in patients with other conditions, such as heart failure, in which the risk of non-sudden death and total mortality increased as the number of comorbidities increased, whereas the risk of sudden death/ventricular fibrillation decreased [20].

There are several potential explanations for these findings. First, patients with multiple comorbidities tend to be older and female, and older age and female sex have been found to be independent risk factors for mortality in patients with AMI [21,22,23,24]. Second, patients with multiple comorbidities may misinterpret the symptoms of AMI and delay seeking timely medical care. Furthermore, patients with multiple comorbidities were less likely to be treated with effective medications and coronary interventions that may increase their risk of dying in hospital [7,8,9]. Finally, patients with multiple comorbidities tend to develop clinical complications that can contribute to higher mortality. More educational approaches and interventional efforts targeted at patients with multiple comorbidities are needed to improve their hospital outcomes.

Common Clusters of Multiple CVD Comorbidities

Our study found that the most common clusters of chronic CVD comorbidities were "hypertension and diabetes", "hypertension and stroke", "hypertension and CHD", and "hypertension and hyperlipidemia". These findings are in line with the results of other studies in patients with AMI from high-income countries [8], as well as data from general population samples [25]. Identifying the common patterns of chronic comorbidities in patients hospitalized with AMI will help in the design of effective management strategies in these difficult to treat patients.

Study Strengths and Limitations

This study is the first to have examined the prevalence of CVD and non-CVD comorbidities and their impact on short-term outcomes in patients hospitalized with AMI in Vietnam. The study has several limitations that must be kept in mind in interpreting our study results, however. First, since the population included only patients hospitalized at one hospital, the Vietnam National Heart Institute in Hanoi, the generalizability of our findings to patients admitted to other hospitals in Hanoi is limited and unknown. Since the sample size in the present study was small, we were underpowered to detect meaningful differences in other patient characteristics, hospital management practices, and short-term outcomes. Third, due to the nature of the study's retrospective design, we likely underestimated the prevalence of comorbidities in our study population. We also did not have information on several patient-associated characteristics (e.g., socioeconomic status, psychological factors, body mass index) which may have confounded some of the observed associations [1,3]. We had very limited information on medication contraindications; therefore, we were unable to carry out an analysis restricted to patients without contraindications to the medications examined, and likely underestimated the use of appropriate medications. Finally, because patients who died before hospitalization for AMI were not included, our findings are only generalizable to patients hospitalized with AMI.

Conclusions

In summary, our findings highlight the importance of identifying patients hospitalized with AMI who have multiple CVD comorbidities to provide better care to these high risk and complex patients, and therefore, improve their short-term prognosis. Continued monitoring of trends in multiple comorbidities in patients hospitalized with AMI and other conditions of major public health importance, such as stroke, cancer, and chronic lung disease, in Vietnam remains of considerable clinical and public health importance.

Acknowledgments

We thank the doctors and nurses at the Vietnam National Heart Institute for their support and help.

Author Contributions

Conceived and designed the experiments: HLN RJG. Performed the experiments: HLN QNN DAH DTP NHN. Analyzed the data: HLN RJG. Wrote the paper: HLN RJG.

References

1. Hosseinpoor AR, Bergen N, Mendis S, Harper S, Verdes E, et al. (2012) Socioeconomic inequality in the prevalence of noncommunicable diseases in low- and middle-income countries: results from the World Health Survey. BMC public health 12: 474.
2. Van Minh H, Ng N, Juvekar S, Razzaque A, Ashraf A, et al. (2008) Self-reported prevalence of chronic diseases and their relation to selected sociodemographic variables: a study in INDEPTH Asian sites, 2005. Preventing chronic disease 5: A86.
3. Boutayeb A, Boutayeb S, Boutayeb W (2013) Multi-morbidity of non communicable diseases and equity in WHO Eastern Mediterranean countries. International journal for equity in health 12: 60.
4. Gili M, Sala J, Lopez J, Carrion A, Bejar L, et al. (2011) [Impact of comorbidities on in-hospital mortality from acute myocardial infarction, 2003-2009]. Revista espanola de cardiologia 64: 1130–1137.
5. Schmidt M, Jacobsen JB, Lash TL, Botker HE, Sorensen HT (2012) 25 year trends in first time hospitalisation for acute myocardial infarction, subsequent short and long term mortality, and the prognostic impact of sex and comorbidity: a Danish nationwide cohort study. BMJ 344: e356.
6. McManus DD, Nguyen HL, Saczynski JS, Tisminetzky M, Bourell P, et al. (2012) Multiple cardiovascular comorbidities and acute myocardial infarction: temporal trends (1990–2007) and impact on death rates at 30 days and 1 year. Clinical epidemiology 4: 115–123.
7. Parker AB, Naylor CD, Chong A, Alter DA (2006) Clinical prognosis, pre-existing conditions and the use of reperfusion therapy for patients with ST segment elevation acute myocardial infarction. The Canadian journal of cardiology 22: 131–139.
8. Chen HY, Saczynski JS, McManus DD, Lessard D, Yarzebski J, et al. (2013) The impact of cardiac and noncardiac comorbidities on the short-term outcomes of patients hospitalized with acute myocardial infarction: a population-based perspective. Clinical epidemiology 5: 439–448.
9. Radovanovic D, Seifert B, Urban P, Eberli FR, Rickli H, et al. (2014) Validity of Charlson Comorbidity Index in patients hospitalised with acute coronary syndrome. Insights from the nationwide AMIS Plus registry 2002–2012. Heart 100: 288–294.
10. Ministry of Health (2010) Health Statistic Year Book 2009. Hanoi, Vietnam: Ministry of Health
11. Nguyen HL, Ha DA, Phan DT, Nguyen QN, Nguyen VL, et al. (2014) Sex differences in clinical characteristics, hospital management practices, and in-hospital outcomes in patients hospitalized in a vietnamese hospital with a first acute myocardial infarction. PloS one 9: e95631.
12. Tunstall-Pedoe H, Kuulasmaa K, Mahonen M, Tolonen H, Ruokokoski E, et al. (1999) Contribution of trends in survival and coronary-event rates to changes in coronary heart disease mortality: 10-year results from 37 WHO MONICA project populations. Monitoring trends and determinants in cardiovascular disease. Lancet 353: 1547–1557.
13. McManus DD, Gore J, Yarzebski J, Spencer F, Lessard D, et al. (2011) Recent trends in the incidence, treatment, and outcomes of patients with STEMI and NSTEMI. Am J Med 124: 40–47.
14. Butala NM, Desai MM, Linnander EL, Wong YR, Mikhail DG, et al. (2011) Gender differences in presentation, management, and in-hospital outcomes for patients with AMI in a lower-middle income country: evidence from Egypt. PloS one 6: e25904.
15. Song XT, Chen YD, Pan WQ, Lu SZ (2007) Gender based differences in patients with acute coronary syndrome: findings from Chinese Registry of Acute Coronary Events (CRACE). Chinese medical journal 120: 1063–1067.
16. Srichaiveth B, Ruengsakulrach P, Visudharom K, Sanguanwong S, Tangsubutr W, et al. (2007) Impact of gender on treatment and clinical outcomes in acute ST elevation myocardial infarction patients in Thailand. Journal of the Medical Association of Thailand = Chotmaihet thangphaet 90 Suppl 1: 65–73.
17. Pagidipati NJ, Huffman MD, Jeemon P, Gupta R, Negi P, et al. (2013) Association between gender, process of care measures, and outcomes in ACS in India: results from the detection and management of coronary heart disease (DEMAT) registry. PloS one 8: e62061.
18. Miszkurka M, Haddad S, Langlois EV, Freeman EE, Kouanda S, et al. (2012) Heavy burden of non-communicable diseases at early age and gender disparities in an adult population of Burkina Faso: World Health Survey. BMC public health 12: 24.
19. Boyd CF, Fortin M (2010) Future of Multimorbidiity Research: How should Understanding of Multimorbidity Inform Health System Design? Public Health Reviews 32: 451–474.
20. Clarke B, Howlett J, Sapp J, Andreou P, Parkash R (2011) The effect of comorbidity on the competing risk of sudden and nonsudden death in an ambulatory heart failure population. The Canadian journal of cardiology 27: 254–261.
21. Nguyen HL, Saczynski JS, Gore JM, Waring ME, Lessard D, et al. (2011) Long-term trends in short-term outcomes in acute myocardial infarction. The American journal of medicine 124: 939–946.
22. Vaccarino V, Parsons L, Every NR, Barron HV, Krumholz HM (1999) Sex-based differences in early mortality after myocardial infarction. National Registry of Myocardial Infarction 2 Participants. N Engl J Med 341: 217–225.
23. Wenger NK, Shaw LJ, Vaccarino V (2008) Coronary heart disease in women: update 2008. Clin Pharmacol Ther 83: 37–51.
24. Heer T, Schiele R, Schneider S, Gitt AK, Wienbergen H, et al. (2002) Gender differences in acute myocardial infarction in the era of reperfusion (the MITRA registry). Am J Cardiol 89: 511–517.
25. Sinnige J, Braspenning J, Schellevis F, Stirbu-Wagner I, Westert G, et al. (2013) The prevalence of disease clusters in older adults with multiple chronic diseases—a systematic literature review. PloS one 8: e79641.

14

Netrin-1 and Semaphorin 3A Predict the Development of Acute Kidney Injury in Liver Transplant Patients

Lidia Lewandowska[2], Joanna Matuszkiewicz-Rowińska[2], Calpurnia Jayakumar[1], Urszula Oldakowska-Jedynak[3], Stephen Looney[4], Michalina Galas[3], Małgorzata Dutkiewicz[5], Marek Krawczyk[3], Ganesan Ramesh[1]*

1 Vascular Biology Center, Georgia Regents University, Augusta, GA, United States of America, **2** Department of Nephrology, Dialysis & Internal Diseases, Medical University of Warsaw, Warsaw, Poland, **3** Department of General, Transplant and Liver Surgery, Medical University of Warsaw, Warsaw, Poland, **4** Department of Biostatistics and Epidemiology, Georgia Regents University, Augusta, GA, United States of America, **5** Department of General and Nutritional Biochemistry, Medical University of Warsaw, Warsaw, Poland

Abstract

Acute kidney injury (AKI) is a serious complication after liver transplantation. Currently there are no validated biomarkers available for early diagnosis of AKI. The current study was carried out to determine the usefulness of the recently identified biomarkers netrin-1 and semaphorin 3A in predicting AKI in liver transplant patients. A total of 63 patients' samples were collected and analyzed. AKI was detected at 48 hours after liver transplantation using serum creatinine as a marker. In contrast, urine netrin-1 (897.8±112.4 pg/mg creatinine), semaphorin 3A (847.9±93.3 pg/mg creatinine) and NGAL (2172.2±378.1 ng/mg creatinine) levels were increased significantly and peaked at 2 hours after liver transplantation but were no longer significantly elevated at 6 hours after transplantation. The predictive power of netrin-1, as demonstrated by the area under the receiver-operating characteristic curve for diagnosis of AKI at 2, 6, and 24 hours after liver transplantation was 0.66, 0.57 and 0.59, respectively. The area under the curve for diagnosis of AKI was 0.63 and 0.65 for semaphorin 3A and NGAL at 2 hr respectively. Combined analysis of two or more biomarkers for simultaneous occurrence in urine did not improve the AUC for the prediction of AKI whereas the AUC was improved significantly (0.732) only when at least 1 of the 3 biomarkers in urine was positive for predicting AKI. Adjusting for BMI, all three biomarkers at 2 hours remained independent predictors of AKI with an odds ratio of 1.003 (95% confidence interval: 1.000 to 1.006; $P = 0.0364$). These studies demonstrate that semaphorin 3A and netrin-1 can be useful early diagnostic biomarkers of AKI after liver transplantation.

Editor: Giovanni Camussi, University of Torino, Italy

Funding: This work was supported by an R01 grant (1R01DK083379 - 01A3) to Ganesan Ramesh from NIH-NIDDK. The funders had no role in study design, data collection and analysis, decision to publish, or preparation of the manuscript.

Competing Interests: Dr. Ramesh has filed a provisional patent through Georgia Regents University for discovering semaphorin3A and a patent was awarded to Dr. Ramesh and Pennsylvania State University for discovering netrin-1 as an early diagnostic biomarker of injury and disease. The details are as follows: Ganesan Ramesh: "Netrin-1 as a Biomarker of Injury and Disease", Provisional Patent Filed on 1/20/2009. Application No: 61/145,764. Ganesan Ramesh: "Netrin-1 as a Biomarker of Injury and Disease", Provisional Patent Filed on 7/31/2009. Application No: 61/230,346. Ganesan Ramesh: "Semaphorin 3A as a Biomarker of injury and Disease" Provision Patent Filed. Application #61/711,007.

* Email: gramesh@gru.edu

Introduction

Acute kidney injury (AKI) is a serious complication after liver transplantation. Several studies have demonstrated that development of AKI has been associated with increased length of hospital stay, morbidity, and mortality [1–3]. The incidence of post liver transplantation AKI has been reported in the range of 50–94% [2–5]. The mechanisms of renal dysfunction in liver transplant recipients are not clearly understood. Calcineurin inhibitors are generally perceived as the most prominent cause; however, the liver transplant procedure itself represents a significant surgical/ hemodynamic/inflammatory trauma that, on its own can cause renal dysfunction [1]. Development of therapies has been hindered by lack of early diagnostic biomarkers. Creatinine and creatinine clearance are late markers of AKI, and changes in these parameters occur only after substantial injury has already occurred. Even a stable creatinine level does not exclude structural kidney damage. Moreover, in the settings of end stage liver disease, creatinine was found to be an unreliable marker of renal function [6]. Several studies have examined urinary neutrophil gelatinase-associated lipocalin (NGAL), IL-8, IL-18 and liver fatty acid binding protein (L-FABP) as biomarkers of AKI in orthotopic liver transplantation (OLT) patients [7,8]. However, their usefulness has not been translated to theclinic. The recent identification of new biomarkers e.g., netrin-1 and semaphorin 3A (sema3A) for the diagnosis of AKI have shown significant promise in a variety of clinical settings [9–12]. However, the use of these biomarkers for the detection of AKI in patients undergoing OLT has not been explored. Netrin-1 and sema3A are neuronal guidance cues known to regulate axons to find their target during development [13–16]. However, these molecules are also expressed in adult tissues, including kidney. Recent studies show that netrin-1 plays a protective role in kidney injury, whereas sema3A may have a pathogenic role [17–19]. Therefore, in this study, we examined these newly identified biomarkers, netrin-1 and sema3A, in OLT patient urine to determine whether they can predict the early development of AKI, much before serum creatinine levels are increased.

Materials and Methods

Patients

All patients over 18 years old who underwent an OLT at the University of Warsaw Medical Center, Poland were eligible for the study. The age of the patient populationranged from 19 to 64 years. The inclusion criteria included liver insufficiency, acute or chronic, such that liver transplantation was required. Patients were excluded from the study if they were unable to provide consent and if they had had a previous transplant procedure. A total of 68 patients were recruited, out of which 4 patients were excluded due to a second transplant procedure and 1 patient was excluded due to incomplete collection of urine samples. I All donors over age 60 years and donors aged 50–59 years with at least two of the three following criteria (1) cause of death was cerebrovascular accident; 2) preexisting history of systemic hypertension; and 3) terminal serum creatinine >1.5 mg/d were identified as extended donor criteria (EDC)). Whether or not the organ donor was an EDC did not appear to affect whether the receipient did or did not develop AKI. Ten patients had preexisting renal dysfunction (mean basal serum creatinine concentration 2.14±1.19 mg/dl; range 1.26–5.31 mg/dl). All transplanted patients received either tacrolimus, cyclosporine, or mycophenolate mofetil as immunosuppressive therapy. All eligible patients were consented according to proper procedures over an 18-month period (2010–2011) were enrolled at the hospital. All study enrollment procedures and subsequent data collection and acquisition were approved by the Institutional Review Board at the Medical University of Warsaw. Written informed consent was obtained from the patients or their legal guardian if they were not capable of consenting before enrollment. The sample processing and data analysis were carried out at Georgia Regents University and were approved by Institutional Review Board.

Sample collection and processing

Pre-operative blood and urine samples (ten milliliters) were collected from each patient within 24 hours of OLT. Additional urine samples (10 milliliter) were collected at 2, 6 and 24 hr after OLT (measured from the time the operation ended). Blood samples were collected at 2, 6 and 24 hr, then every 24 hr thereafter until day 7 after surgery. Collected urine samples were centrifuged at 10000 G for 10 minutes, and the supernatant liquid was aliquoted and stored at −80°C. Blood samples were centrifuged at 10000 RPM for ten minutes, and serum was stored at −80°C.

Biomarker Measurement

Biomarkers were measured on individual, not pooled, samples. Urine netrin-1 levels were measured with a specific enzyme-linked immunosorbent assay (ELISA) kit (Cat #MBS725887, MyBiosource, Inc., San Diego, CA) that specifically detects human netrin-1. Urine sema3A levels were measured with a specific ELISA kit (Cat #MBS732622, MyBiosource, Inc., San Diego, CA). All measurements were made in a blinded fashion. The inter- and intra-assay coefficient variations were 5–10%, corresponding to that reported by the kit manufacturer. Urine NGAL levels were measured using a commercially available ELISA kit (Human Lipocalin-2/NGAL, R&D Systems, Minneapolis, MN, cat no. DLCN20).

Serum creatinine levels were measured daily by the hospital's central laboratory as part of routine peri-operative care, but we performed additional measurements corresponding to same time-points used here for the biomarker measurements, and then additionally for 7 days of follow-up observation. A combination of retrospective and prospective chart reviews was performed to collect demographic and pertinent clinical data. AKI was defined as an increase in serum creatinine level by 50% or greater compared to pre-operative values that occurred within 72 hours of the OLT. Results were also analysed according to the definition of AKI, which was based on the Risk, Injury, Failure, Loss, End-Stage Renal Disease (RIFLE) classification [20,21].

Statistical Analyses

SAS version 9.3 was used for all analyses (SAS Institute, Cary, NC, 2010), and a significance level of 0.05 was used throughout, controlling for multiple comparisons whereever necessary. Demographics and clinical outcomes were compared between patients who developed AKI and patients who did not. Continuous variables were compared using the two-sample *t* test, and categorical variables were compared using Fisher's exact test. Estimates of mean values of serum creatinine and urinary netrin levels by a group at various time points were calculated using repeated-measures ANOVA, which accounts for correlations of measurements from the same individuals across time. Least square (LS) means and their standard errors (SEMs) are reported. Spearman correlation coefficients were used to examine the correlation between urinary netrin concentrations at various time points (baseline and at 2, 6, and 24 hours after surgery) and the following clinical outcomes: percent change in serum creatinine level, liver transplantation surgery time, length of hospital stay after surgery and days of AKI.

To measure the sensitivity and specificity for urinary netrin-1, a conventional receiver-operating characteristic (ROC) curve was generated for urinary netrin at 2, 6, and 24 hours after liver transplantation. We calculated the area under the curve (AUC) to ascertain the utility of netrin-1 as a biomarker. An area of 0.5 is expected by chance, whereas a value of 1.0 signifies a perfect biomarker. The optimal urinary netrin time point was selected to maximize prediction at the earliest time possible, thus weighing the AUC, timing of measurement, and *P* value from the predictive logistic model. We then identified the values of urinary netrin level that provided 95% sensitivity, 95% specificity, and optimal sensitivity and specificity using the ROC curve at the best time point.

Univariable and multivariable logistic regression analyses were then performed to assess predictors of AKI. Potential independent predictor variables included urinary netrin concentration at the best time point, age, sex, BMI, surgery time, hospital length of stay and urine output on day 1. Variables were retained in the final model if $P \leq 0.05$.

Results

Patient Characteristics and Renal Function Changes

During the enrollment period, 83 subjects underwent a liver transplant at our institution. Of these, 63 subjects met the inclusion criteria for this study. AKI occurred in 35 patients (56%) within a 3-day period. No significant differences were noted between the two groups with respect to gender, BMI, surgery time, or hospital stay (Table 1). Patients who developed AKI were significantly older at baseline compared with those who did not

($P = 0.0475$) and had significantly greater percent change in serum creatinine post surgery ($P<0.0001$), lower urine output on Day 1 ($P = 0.0286$), and greater need for dialysis ($P = 0.0419$). Figure 1 shows the changes of serum creatinine concentrations after liver transplantation for patients who developed AKI and those who did not. During the first 6 hours after transplantation, serum creatinine did not differ significantly between the two groups. Significant differences between groups were seen by 24 hours after surgery and were maintained until 7 days after surgery.

Associations of Biomarkers with Patient Characteristics

Netrin-1 level, but not sema 3A and NGAL levels, was positively associated with patient age at 2 and 6 hours post-surgery (Table 2). Netrin, sema3A and NGAL levels were not significantly associated with any post-surgery outcome at baseline or at 2, 6, or 24 h following liver transplant (Table 2).

Urinary Netrin-1 and Sema3A Levels Predict AKI after Liver Transplantation

The currently used, but late, diagnostic biomarker for AKI, serum creatinine, begins to rise significantly at 24 hr after liver transplant surgery and remains elevated for the remaining study period in patients categorized as AKI (Figure 1). In contrast, urinary netrin-1 and sema3A levels increased significantly ($P = 0.0106$ and $P = 0.0012$, respectively) and peaked at 2 hours following liver transplant surgery in patients who developed AKI and were no longer significantly elevated at 6 hours after surgery (Figure 2 A and B). Patients who did not develop AKI experienced a much smaller increase in concentration of these biomarker after surgery, which did not differ significantly from baseline. However, the netrin-1 level was relatively higher in the AKI group as compared to the non-AKI group at baseline but this did not reach statistical significance.

Conventional ROC curves for AKI *versus* no AKI were generated for urinary netrin-1, sema3A and NGAL at 2, 6, and 24 hours after surgery. The AUCs of the three ROC curves for netrin-1 were 0.658 ($P = 0.0123$), 0.570 ($P = 0.3342$), and 0.594 ($P = 0.1919$), respectively. The AUCs of the three ROC curves for sema3A were 0.631 ($P = 0.0680$), 0.560 ($P = 0.4057$), and 0.523 ($P = 0.7528$) respectively. The AUCs of the three ROC curves were 0.651 ($P = 0.0306$), 0.605 ($P = 0.1369$), and 0.603 ($P = 0.1563$), respectively. Thus, the time point for optimal urinary concentration for all three biomarkers was at 2 hours after surgery. Figure 3 displays the unadjusted ROC curve for the three biomarkers at 2 hours after liver transplantation. The sensitivities and specificities for the three biomarkers at optimal concentrations obtained at the 2-hour time point with different combination analyses are listed in Table 3, corresponding to 95% sensitivity, optimal sensitivity and specificity and 95% specificity. All three biomarkers performed equally well when analysed individually. The simultaneous occurrence of levels of 2 urine biomarkers above a designated threshold did not improve the AUC for the prediction of AKI (e.g., when biomarkers were taken in pairs, i.e., 2 by 2), while the AUC improved significantly only when at least 1 of the 3 biomarker urine levels was above threshold.

Among the 35 subjects who developed AKI, 17 (27%) were classified as being in the risk (R) category, 9 (14%) in the injury (I) category, and 9 (14%) in the failure (F) category, on the basis of RIFLE criteria. Analysis of netrin-1 concentrations by RIFLE classification revealed that the injury group differed from no AKI at 2 hours and 6 hours after OLT (all $P<0.0070$; Figure 3). No other significant differences were found among the RIFLE groups. However, analysis of sema3A concentrations by RIFLE classification revealed that the risk group differed significantly from no AKI at 2 hours ($P = 0.0026$; Figure 4).

Univariable logistic regression identified that age ($P = 0.0471$), urine output on Day 1 ($P = 0.0265$), and higher netrin-1 concentrations at 2 hours ($P = 0.0369$) are significantly associated with higher odds of AKI. A stepwise logistic regression analysis was used to determine the most parsimonious model, given a set of potential variables for predicting AKI. Potential variables for this model included age, sex, BMI, urine output on Day 1, surgery time, hospital length of stay and netrin-1 level at the selected optimal time point (i.e., 2 hours after liver transplant surgery). The final model revealed that BMI and biomarker concentrations at 2 hours after surgery were the only significant independent predictors of AKI in our cohort. The estimated odds ratio for every 1- pg/mg of urinary creatinine increase of netrin-1 at 2 hours after surgery was 1.003 (95% confidence interval: 1.000 to 1.006; $P = 0.0364$). The estimated odds ratio for every 1 unit increase in BMI was 1.198 (95% CI: 1.030 to 1.394; $P = 0.0194$). The estimated odds ratio for every 1- pg/mg of urinary creatinine

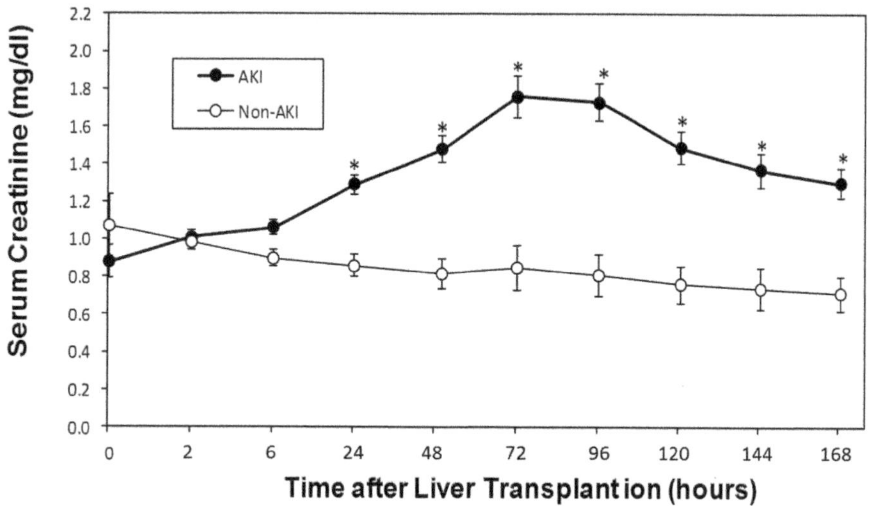

Figure 1. Changes in serum creatinine (LS mean ± SE) at various time points after liver transplantation in the non-AKI and AKI group. *$p \leq 0.0001$ for differences between groups by repeated measures ANOVA.

Table 1. Descriptive statistics of patient characteristics.

Parameter	AKI	No AKI	*P*
N	35	28	–
Age, yr	49.0±11.2	42.4±13.5	0.0475[a]
Male, %	66	70	0.6870[b]
BMI	26.8±6.3	24.0±4.2	0.0735[a]
Surgery time, h	7.1±1.4	6.9±1.3	0.6339[a]
Creatinine change, %	245.7±98.7	13.9±13.6	<0.0001[a]
Urine output (day 1), ml/24 h	1699.8±1178.2	2687.6±1735.6	0.0286[a]
Duration of AKI, d	3.3±2.0	–	–
Hospital stay, d	19.3±18.5	14.0±5.6	0.1359[a]
Dialysis, %	20	4	0.0419[b]

Means ± standard deviation (SD) are reported for continuous measures, percentages are reported for categorical variables.
[a]Welch modified two-sample *t* test.
[b]Fisher exact test.

increase of sema3A at 2 hours after surgery was 1.004 (95% confidence interval: 1.001 to 1.007; $P = 0.0166$). The estimated odds ratio for every 1 unit increase in BMI was 1.238 (95% CI: 1.049 to 1.460; $P = 0.0113$). The estimated odds ratio for every 1 ng/mg of urinary creatinine increase of NGAL at 2 hours after surgery was 1.001 (95% confidence interval: 1.000 to 1.002; $P = 0.0069$). The estimated odds ratio for every 1 unit increase in BMI was 1.225 (95% CI: 1.043 to 1.439; $P = 0.0135$).

Discussion

In this study, we validated two new biomarkers that have never been studied in liver transplant patients for the diagnosis of AKI. Based on our earlier studies, we chose to examine biomarkers at very early time points i.e., 2, 6 and 24 hr, after transplantation. Our results show that both netrin-1 and sema3A were able to predict the development of AKI similar to known established biomarkers such as NGAL. Our analysis, based on RIFLE classification, shows that the netrin-1 level is much higher in the injury group whereas the sema3A levels is elevated in the risk, injury and failure groups. Interestingly, different combinations of biomarkers did not improve the sensitivity and specificity, as compared to the individual biomarkers, except when at least one marker was considered positive for the prediction of AKI.

Post-operative serum creatinine level begins to rise by 24 hr and remain significantly elevated until day 7 in the AKI group as compared to the non-AKI group. Interestingly, however, we found that the pre-operative serum creatinine level tends to be lower in the AKI group than in the non-AKI group although the difference did not reach statistical significance. The baseline creatinine difference before surgery suggests that AKI patients did not harbor any renal dysfunction prior to transplantation, which was further supported by the similar low basal levels of NGAL and sema3A in both groups. It is interesting to note that pre-operative urine netrin-1 levels tended to be higher in the AKI group as compared to the non-AKI group. However, the reason behind this elevation is unknown. Using serum creatinine elevation to define AKI, we found statistically significant elevation in post-operative urine netrin-1, sema3A and NGAL levels at 2 hr, which then decreases in the subsequent time points. These results are remarkably similar to earlier studies in cardiac bypass surgery patients for netrin-1 and sema3A [9,12] and in liver transplant patients for NGAL [22]. ROC curve analysis showed that urine netrin-1 levels had a slightly better diagnostic performance as compared to sema3A and NGAL levels, however, it did not reach statistical significance. A number of studies recently evaluated NGAL, but not netrin-1 and sema3A, as a biomarker of AKI in the OLT population. In 2009, Niemann et al. evaluated plasma NGAL levels in 59 patients undergoing OLT and found that elevation in NGAL levels measured at two hours after reperfusion was predictive of AKI [22]. Among those patients with pre-operative serum creatinine levels of <1.5 mg/dL, the plasma NGAL level at two hours post-perfusion was associated with the subsequent development of AKI. The following year, Portal et al. evaluated both urinary and serum NGAL levels in 95 patients undergoing OLT and found that post-operative serum NGAL (but not urinary NGAL) was a predictor of severe AKI using multiple logistic regression analysis [23]. In 2011, Wagener et al. examined urinary NGAL/creatinine ratios in

Table 2. Spearman correlation coefficients of netrin with clinical characteristics.

	Age	Percent Change in Serum Creatinine	Surgery Time	Hospital Length of Stay	Days AKI
Baseline	0.20	0.10	0.01	−0.08	0.19
2 h	0.30[a]	0.15	−0.04	0.04	0.21
6 h	0.32[a]	0.08	0.11	0.02	0.09
24 h	0.08	0.03	0.03	−0.15	0.12

[a]$P \leq 0.05$.

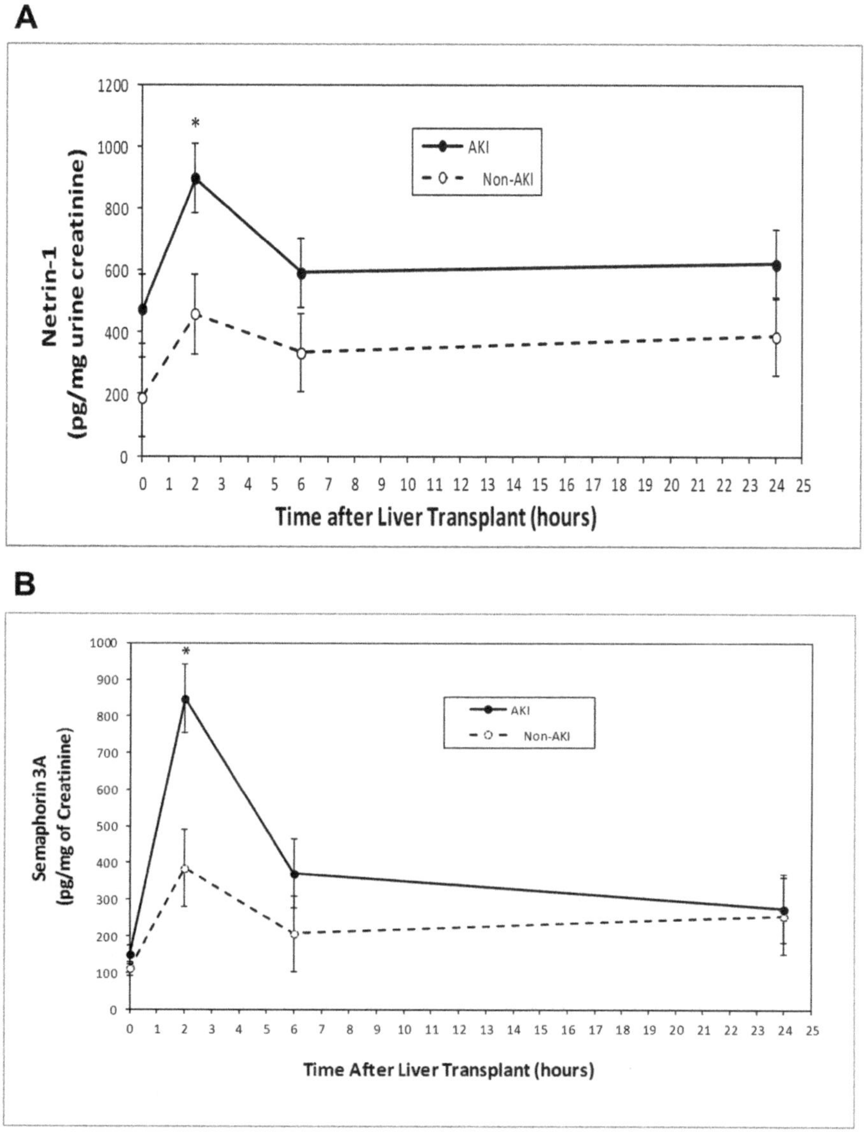

Figure 2. Changes in urinary netrin-1 (A) and sema3A (B) concentrations at various time points after liver transplant surgery in non-AKI and AKI patients. Error bars are LS mean ± SEM. *$P = <0.001$ for differences between groups (non-AKI and AKI) by repeated-measures ANOVA.

Table 3. Test characteristics for various combinations of biomarkers at 2 hr post-surgery.

Biomarker or Combination	AUC	Sensitivity	Specificity	Positive Predictive Value	Negative Predictive Value
SEMA at 464.5	0.631	0.57	0.79	0.77	0.59
NETRIN at 621.9	0.658	0.47	0.82	0.76	0.56
NGAL at 1225.3	0.651	0.51	0.89	0.86	0.60
SEMA + NETRIN	0.582	0.34	0.82	0.71	0.50
SEMA + NGAL	0.707	0.49	0.93	0.89	0.59
NETRIN + NGAL	0.625	0.29	0.96	0.91	0.52
At Least 1 Positive	**0.732**	**0.71**	**0.75**	**0.78**	**0.68**
At Least 2 Positive	0.664	0.54	0.79	0.76	0.58
All 3 Positive	0.625	0.29	0.96	0.91	0.52

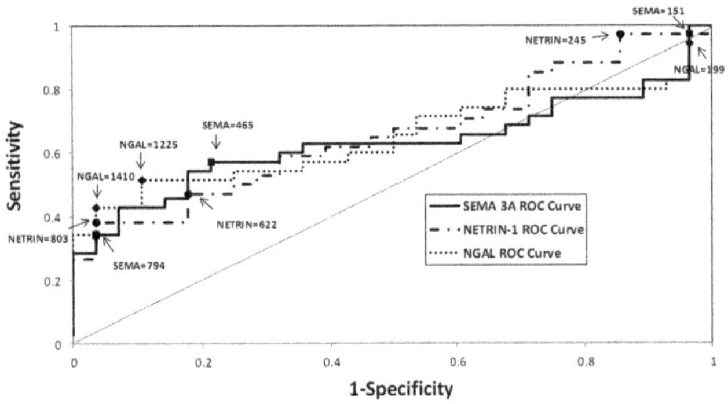

Figure 3. ROC curve analysis for urinary semaphorin 3A, Netrin-1, and NGAL at 2 hours after liver transplantation. The values are urinary concentrations at 2 hours after liver transplant, which correspond to 95% sensitivity, optimal sensitivity and specificity, and 95% specificity, respectively, for each biomarker.

92 patients undergoing OLT [24]. Elevations in urinary NGAL/creatinine ratios were detected three hours after reperfusion and were more pronounced in patients who developed AKI. Urinary NGAL/creatinine ratios were evaluated again in a recent study by Jeong et al. [25]. Elevated urinary NGAL/creatinine ratios were seen two hours after reperfusion in 11 patients who developed AKI after liver transplantation from a living, related donors and peak elevation was preceded by a rise in serum creatinine in these patients by 19 hours. However, NGAL itself has a varying degree of performance in different settings. Therefore, there is a need to study other biomarkers to determine their relative performance and to see whether a combination of biomarkers can be used for the diagnosis of AKI.

It is interesting to note that the baseline level of netrin-1 in the AKI group was relatively higher than the non-AKI group. The reason for this difference is not clear. However it could be due to the presence of higher levels of renal stressors including circulating factors, hemodymic changes or other unknown factors that may have influence netrin-1 expression in this group. Further studies are required to determine the significance of this observation.

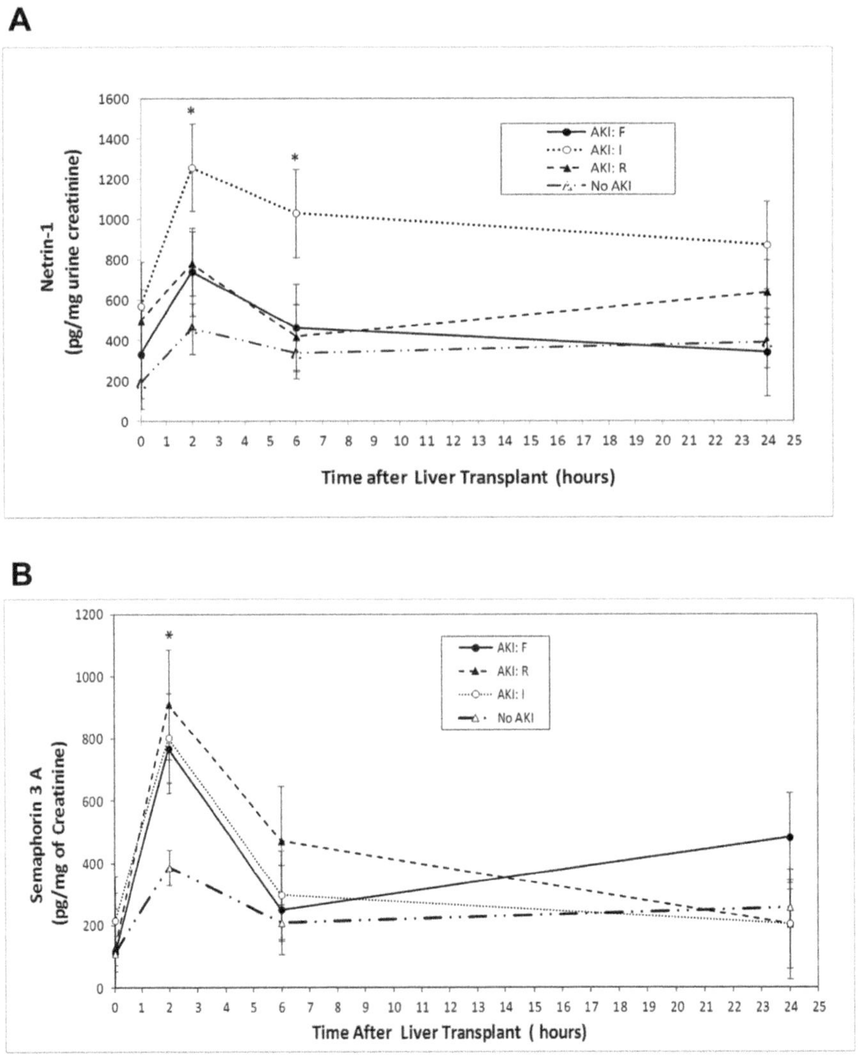

Figure 4. Changes in urinary netrin-1 (A) and sema3A (B) concentrations at various time points after liver transplant surgery in non-AKI and AKI patients, stratified by RIFLE categories. *$p \leq 0.0070$ for differences between groups (non-AKI and each of the RIFLE categories) by repeated-measures ANOVA.

Previous studies suggest that netrin-1 is also induced and excreted after kidney transplantation [10] as well other forms of AKI. The induction of netrin-1 was localized in the proximal tubular epithelial cells in response to injury [26], whereas sema3A expression is localized in distal and collecting tubules [12], which is similar to NGAL expression. Based on previous studies, urine netrin-1 most likely comes from proximal tubular epithelium of the kidney. The contribution of serum netrin-1 to urine netrin-1 is unlikely due to its large size (72 KDa). Similarly, the mature form of sema3A has a molecular weight of 95 KDa, which may not be filtered under normal conditions. However, it is also possible that due to a change in hemodynamics, netrin-1 and sema3A may be filtered from the blood and may contribute to urine netrin-1 and sema3A levels in the disease state. This needs to be clarified by future studies. Animal studies show that netrin-1 plays a protective role in epithelial cells [18,19] whereas sema3A may have a pathogenic role [17] in kidney disease. The molecular mechanism of sema3A induction is less clear. However, netrin-1 expression was shown to be regulated at the translational level [27]. Recently, two biomarkers, insulin like growth factor binding protein-1 (IGFBP-1) and tissue inhibitor of metalloprotease-2 (TIMP-2), were shown to have high specificity and sensitivity for detecting AKI in two different studies, as compared to other previously described biomarkers such as NGAL, KIM-1, IL-18, NAG and liver fatty acid binding protein-1 [28,29]. However, the performance of IGFBP-1 and TIMP-2 was not validated in OLT patients. Moreover, no studies have compared these biomarkers with netrin-1 and sema3A. Further studies are needed to determine whether netrin-1 and sema3A, either alone or in combination with IGFBP-1 and TIMP-2, can perform better for early diagnosis of AKI in different settings.

Our study has several noteworthy strengths. First, the incidence of AKI in our OLT patient population is 56%, which is similar to what was reported in the literature [5,22,25,30]. Second, netrin-1 and sema3A were examined in an OLT patient population for the first time. Third, netrin-1 performed better than NGAL and sema3A performed similarly to NGAL. Fourth, by examining earlier time points, we found peaks levels of biomarkers that would have been overlooked in previous studies [8]. Our study also has limitations. It is a single-center study. Second, the AUC achieved with all three biomarkers is moderate. Third, the absence of an evaluation of renal function (e.g., serum creatinine, eGFR) months after OLT makes it difficult to know the real clinical impact of the early netrin-1 and sema3a urine levels on the long-term outcome of renal function in OLT recipients.

Conclusion

The present study establishes the utility of measuring the newly discovered biomarkers netrin-1 and sema3A as biomarkers of AKI in liver transplantation patients. This work should prompt further research into the use of these biomarkers along with urine NGAL to detect AKI prior to the randomization of therapeutic strategies in clinical studies. Given the prevalence of AKI associated with OLT and its associated morbidity and mortality, therapeutic studies based on the diagnosis of AKI using a panel of biomarkers including netrin-1, sema3A, IGFBP-1 and TIMP-2 [28] may be possible in the future.

Author Contributions

Conceived and designed the experiments: LL JM GR. Performed the experiments: LL CJ UO MG. Analyzed the data: LL SL JM GR. Contributed reagents/materials/analysis tools: UO MG MD MK GR. Wrote the paper: LL JM CJ GR.

References

1. Lima EQ, Zanetta DM, Castro I, Massarollo PC, Mies S, et al. (2003) Risk factors for development of acute renal failure after liver transplantation. Ren Fail 25: 553–560.
2. Bilbao I, Charco R, Balsells J, Lazaro JL, Hidalgo E, et al. (1998) Risk factors for acute renal failure requiring dialysis after liver transplantation. Clin Transplant 12: 123–129.
3. Cabezuelo JB, Ramirez P, Rios A, Acosta F, Torres D, et al. (2006) Risk factors of acute renal failure after liver transplantation. Kidney Int 69: 1073–1080.
4. Utsumi M, Umeda Y, Sadamori H, Nagasaka T, Takaki A, et al. (2013) Risk factors for acute renal injury in living donor liver transplantation: evaluation of the RIFLE criteria. Transpl Int 26: 842–852.
5. Barri YM, Sanchez EQ, Jennings LW, Melton LB, Hays S, et al. (2009) Acute kidney injury following liver transplantation: definition and outcome. Liver Transpl 15: 475–483.
6. Caregaro L, Menon F, Angeli P, Amodio P, Merkel C (1994) Limitations of serum creatinine level and creatinine clearance as filtration markers in cirrhosis. Arch Intern Med 154: 201–205.
7. Li Y, Zhu M, Xia Q, Wang S, Qian J, et al. (2012) Urinary neutrophil gelatinase-associated lipocalin and L-type fatty acid binding protein as diagnostic markers of early acute kidney injury after liver transplantation. Biomarkers 17: 336–342.
8. Sirota J, Walcher A, Faubel S, Jani A, McFann K, et al. (2013) Urine IL-18, NGAL, IL-8 and serum IL-8 are biomarkers of acute kidney injury following liver transplantation. BMC Nephrology 14: 17.
9. Ramesh G, Krawczeski CD, Woo JG, Wang Y, Devarajan P (2010) Urinary netrin-1 is an early predictive biomarker of acute kidney injury after cardiac surgery. Clin J Am Soc Nephrol 5: 395–401.
10. Ramesh G, Kwon O, Ahn K (2010) Netrin-1: a novel universal biomarker of human kidney injury. Transplant Proc 42: 1519–1522.
11. Mishra J, Dent C, Tarabishi R, Mitsnefes MM, Ma Q, et al. (2005) Neutrophil gelatinase-associated lipocalin (NGAL) as a biomarker for acute renal injury after cardiac surgery. Lancet 365: 1231–1238.
12. Jayakumar C, Ranganathan P, Devarajan P, Krawczeski CD, Looney S, et al. (2013) Semaphorin 3A Is a New Early Diagnostic Biomarker of Experimental and Pediatric Acute Kidney Injury. PLoS ONE 8: e58446.
13. Huber AB, Kolodkin AL, Ginty DD, Cloutier JF (2003) Signaling at the growth cone: ligand-receptor complexes and the control of axon growth and guidance. Annu Rev Neurosci 26: 509–563.
14. Barallobre MJ, Pascual M, Del Rio JA, Soriano E (2005) The Netrin family of guidance factors: emphasis on Netrin-1 signalling. Brain Res Brain Res Rev 49: 22–47.
15. Furne C, Rama N, Corset V, Chedotal A, Mehlen P (2008) Netrin-1 is a survival factor during commissural neuron navigation. Proc Natl Acad Sci U S A 105: 14465–14470.
16. de Wit J, Verhaagen J (2003) Role of semaphorins in the adult nervous system. Prog Neurobiol 71: 249–267.
17. Tapia R, Guan F, Gershin I, Teichman J, Villegas G, et al. (2007) Semaphorin3a disrupts podocyte foot processes causing acute proteinuria. Kidney Int 73: 733–740.
18. Wang W, Reeves WB, Ramesh G (2008) Netrin-1 and kidney injury. I. Netrin-1 protects against ischemia-reperfusion injury of the kidney. Am J Physiol Renal Physiol 294: F739–F747.
19. Wang W, Reeves WB, Pays L, Mehlen P, Ramesh G (2009) Netrin-1 overexpression protects kidney from ischemia reperfusion injury by suppressing apoptosis. Am J Pathol 175: 1010–1018.
20. Ricci Z, Cruz DN, Ronco C (2011) Classification and staging of acute kidney injury: beyond the RIFLE and AKIN criteria. Nat Rev Nephrol 7: 201–208.
21. Bellomo R, Ronco C, Kellum JA, Mehta RL, Palevsky P (2004) Acute renal failure - definition, outcome measures, animal models, fluid therapy and information technology needs: the Second International Consensus Conference of the Acute Dialysis Quality Initiative (ADQI) Group. Crit Care 8: R204–R212.
22. Niemann CU, Walia A, Waldman J, Davio M, Roberts JP, et al. (2009) Acute kidney injury during liver transplantation as determined by neutrophil gelatinase-associated lipocalin. Liver Transpl 15: 1852–1860.
23. Portal AJ, McPhail MJ, Bruce M, Coltart I, Slack A, et al (2010) Neutrophil gelatinase-associated lipocalin predicts acute kidney injury in patients undergoing liver transplantation. Liver Transpl 16: 1257–1266.
24. Wagener G, Minhaz M, Mattis FA, Kim M, Emond JC, et al. (2011) Urinary neutrophil gelatinase-associated lipocalin as a marker of acute kidney injury after orthotopic liver transplantation. Nephrol Dial Transplant 26: 1717–1723.

25. Jeong TD, Kim S, Lee W, Song GW, Kim YK, et al. (2012) Neutrophil gelatinase-associated lipocalin as an early biomarker of acute kidney injury in liver transplantation. Clin Transplant 26: 775–781.
26. Reeves WB, Kwon O, Ramesh G (2008) Netrin-1 and kidney injury. II. Netrin-1 is an early biomarker of acute kidney injury. Am J Physiol Renal Physiol 294: F731–F738.
27. Jayakumar C, Mohamed R, Ranganathan PV, Ramesh G (2011) Intracellular Kinases Mediate Increased Translation and Secretion of Netrin-1 from Renal Tubular Epithelial Cells. PLoS ONE 6: e26776.
28. Kashani K, Al Khafaji A, Ardiles T, Artigas A, Bagshaw S, et al. (2013) Discovery and validation of cell cycle arrest biomarkers in human acute kidney injury. Critical Care 17: R25.
29. Bihorac A, Chawla LS, Shaw AD, Al Khafaji A, Davison DL, et al. (2014) Validation of Cell-Cycle Arrest Biomarkers for Acute Kidney Injury Using Clinical Adjudication. Am J Respir Crit Care Med 189: 932–939.
30. Rimola A, Gavaler JS, Schade RR, el Lankany S, Starzl TE, et al. (1987) Effects of renal impairment on liver transplantation. Gastroenterology 93: 148–156.

Comparison of Regression Methods for Modeling Intensive Care Length of Stay

Ilona W. M. Verburg[1]*, Nicolette F. de Keizer[1], Evert de Jonge[2], Niels Peek[1,3]

1 Department of Medical Informatics, Academic Medical Center, University of Amsterdam, Amsterdam, the Netherlands, **2** Department of Intensive Care, Leiden University Medical Center, Leiden, the Netherlands, **3** Health eResearch Centre, Centre for Health Informatics, University of Manchester, Manchester, United Kingdom

Abstract

Intensive care units (ICUs) are increasingly interested in assessing and improving their performance. ICU Length of Stay (LoS) could be seen as an indicator for efficiency of care. However, little consensus exists on which prognostic method should be used to adjust ICU LoS for case-mix factors. This study compared the performance of different regression models when predicting ICU LoS. We included data from 32,667 unplanned ICU admissions to ICUs participating in the Dutch National Intensive Care Evaluation (NICE) in the year 2011. We predicted ICU LoS using eight regression models: ordinary least squares regression on untransformed ICU LoS,LoS truncated at 30 days and log-transformed LoS; a generalized linear model with a Gaussian distribution and a logarithmic link function; Poisson regression; negative binomial regression; Gamma regression with a logarithmic link function; and the original and recalibrated APACHE IV model, for all patients together and for survivors and non-survivors separately. We assessed the predictive performance of the models using bootstrapping and the squared Pearson correlation coefficient (R^2), root mean squared prediction error (RMSPE), mean absolute prediction error (MAPE) and bias. The distribution of ICU LoS was skewed to the right with a median of 1.7 days (interquartile range 0.8 to 4.0) and a mean of 4.2 days (standard deviation 7.9). The predictive performance of the models was between 0.09 and 0.20 for R^2, between 7.28 and 8.74 days for RMSPE, between 3.00 and 4.42 days for MAPE and between −2.99 and 1.64 days for bias. The predictive performance was slightly better for survivors than for non-survivors. We were disappointed in the predictive performance of the regression models and conclude that it is difficult to predict LoS of unplanned ICU admissions using patient characteristics at admission time only.

Editor: Jorge I.F. Salluh, D'or Institute of Research and Education, Brazil

Funding: The NICE foundation (http://www.stichting-nice.nl) pays the department of Medical Informatics, Academic Medical Center for the processing and analyses of the data in the NICE registry. The NICE board assesses each study application on the registry, including this study, on scientific quality, feasibility, and privacy aspects.

Competing Interests: Two coauthors (E. de Jonge and N. de Keizer) are members of the board of NICE.

* Email: i.w.verburg@amc.uva.nl

Introduction

Hospitals face continuous pressure to improve quality and reduce costs. The care provided by intensive care units (ICUs) is complex and the associated costs are high, so ICUs are particularly interested in assessing, comparing and improving their performance. To do this they often use case-mix adjusted outcome measures, such as in-hospital mortality and length of stay (LoS) on the ICU. ICU LoS can serve as an indicator for efficiency of care as it is strongly related to ICU costs. Prognostic models, such as APACHE II [1,2], SAPS II [3] and APACHE IV [2,4] have been proposed and widely implemented to adjust hospital mortality for ICU case-mix. However, the predictive performance for LoS of existing models is poor [5–8] and little consensus exists on the best method for predicting this outcome.

Existing models for predicting ICU LoS, such as the commonly used APACHE IV [6] model, make use of ordinary least squares (OLS) regression on untransformed ICU LoS [9,10] or log-transformed ICU LoS [11–13]. These models make no distinction between ICU survivors and non-survivors, although the association between patient characteristics and ICU LoS is often strikingly different for these two groups. For instance, comorbidities tend to prolong the LoS of survivors, while accelerating death in non-survivors. The fact that ICU LoS is often positively skewed also causes problems for OLS regression, which assume symmetrical error distributions. Although, regression methods for modeling positively skewed data have been proposed [14], these models have not been used to predict ICU LoS. Previously, researchers have examined the performance of a range of regression models to analyze hospital LoS in a cohort of patients undergoing coronary artery bypass graft (CABG) surgery [15]. Patient who experienced an unplanned admission to the ICU, are more heterogeneous in terms of case-mix than those admitted following CABG surgery. Patients undergoing elective surgery (planned admissions) require a different ICU indication, often monitoring for a fixed ICU LoS, than patients, who experience an unplanned ICU admission. Furthermore, ICU mortality is higher for patients with an unplanned ICU admission than for CABG patients.

In this study, we investigated the feasibility of predicting individual patient LoS following an unplanned admission to the ICU for medical reasons or following emergency surgery. These patients form an heterogeneous population with a substantial mortality rate. We developed the prognostic models for all patients together and for survivors and non-survivors separately. Patients, who leave the ICU alive are often discharged at set times of day, leading to a multimodal distribution of observed ICU LoS. Hence, we investigated whether cyclical terms (cosine and sine functions of discharge time) [16] increased the predictive power of our models. We compared OLS regression, generalized linear models (GLMs), and Cox proportional hazards (CPH) regression on data from the NICE ICU registry [17]. We included patient characteristics, but no structural or organizational characteristics of the ICUs, so that our models could potentially be used to correct for case-mix when comparing institutions.

Materials and Methods

Data

Since 1996, the Dutch National Intensive Care Evaluation (NICE) registry has collected data on intensive care patients in the Netherlands [17]. The registry collects data on the severity of illness from the first 24 hours of a patient's ICU admission, including the diagnosis, Glasgow Coma Scale (GCS), physiological and laboratory values needed to calculate severity of illness score such as the APACHE II [1,2], SAPS II [3] and APACHE IV [2,4] scores. In addition, NICE registers ICU and hospital LoS and mortality. To ensure that the data are of a high quality, the data are subjected to quality checks, onsite data quality audits take place and data collectors participate in training sessions.

We obtained permission from the secretary of the NICE board, Dr. D.W. de Lange, email: info@stichting-nice.nl, to use data from the NICE registry at the time of the study. The NICE board assesses each application to use the data on the feasibility of the analysis and whether or not the confidentiality of patients and ICUs will be protected. To protect confidentiality, raw data from ICUs is never provided to third parties. For the analyses described in this paper, we used an anonymized dataset. The use of anonymized data does not require informed consent in the Netherlands. The data are officially registered in accordance with the Dutch Personal Data Protection Act.

The data in this study was obtained from all medical and unplanned surgical admissions between January 1st 2011 and December 31st 2011 to 83 ICUs, representing more than 90% of all ICUs in the Netherlands. Of the ICUs, 52 (63%) were general, 25 (30%) teaching and 6 (7%) university-affiliated hospitals. We applied the APACHE IV exclusion criteria [2] and excluded patients younger than 16 on admission to the ICU; with ICU LoS shorter than four hours; with hospital LoS longer than 365 days; with unknown hospital discharge date; who died before ICU admission; readmissions; coming from another ICU; with unknown ICU admission type; or with unknown diagnosis, burns or following a transplant. In addition, we excluded patients, who were discharged to another ICU, as their observed ICU LoS was truncated, and patients with missing values for model covariates.

Definition of length of stay

We defined ICU LoS as the period between ICU admission date and time and ICU discharge date and time. We rounded ICU LoS to the nearest number of whole hours to enable us to perform Poisson and negative binomial regression. We present the results of the validation of our models in days, with decimals representing fractional days.

Regression methods

We used eight regression methods to predict ICU LoS: 1) OLS regression on untransformed ICU LoS, 2) OLS regression on ICU LoS truncated at 30 days; 3) OLS regression on log-transformed ICU LoS; 4) a GLM with a Gaussian distribution and a logarithmic link function; 5) Poisson regression; 6) negative binomial regression; and 7) Gamma regression with a logarithmic link function; 8) CPH regression. In addition, we predicted LoS using the APACHE IV model in its original form and recalibrated on our data [18]. When predicting ICU LoS using an OLS regression model, we replaced negative values with zeros, since ICU LoS is always positive. We present the details of the statistical background of these methods in text S1.

Survival status

We developed the prognostic models once using data from all patients and once using data from ICU survivors and ICU non-survivors separately. We defined survivors and non-survivors by their survival status at discharge from the ICU.

Variable selection

We initially included a set of patient characteristics, presented in Table S1, previously shown to be associated with ICU LoS [1,2,5,19] in each of the models. The models were subsequently simplified using stepwise backward selection with the Akaike Information Criterion. We compared univariate regression models, in which we included age and APACHE IV physiology score (APS) as continuous covariates and as natural regression splines [20] with two to ten degrees of freedom. As a result of these analyses, we included age and APS in further models using natural regression splines with three degrees of freedom.

Cyclical terms

For survivors of ICU treatment, patient discharge often takes place at set times during the day, which leads to a multimodal distribution of observed ICU LoS, with a period of one day. However, predictions could be biased when predicting ICU LoS using regression methods, which typically assume a unimodal distribution. Hence, we also developed models with cyclical terms for discharge time as covariates [16]. These cyclical terms are presented in more detail in text S2.

Overall, we applied eight (three OLS models, four GLMs, one CPH model) different regression methods, with and without cyclical terms to the entire dataset and to separate datasets for survivors and non-survivors. Hence, in total we developed 32 regression models and calculated predictive performance for all patients using these 32 models and the original and recalibrated APACHE IV models.

Performance assessment

To evaluate each model's ability to predict ICU LoS, we examined four measures of predictive performance based on differences between predicted and observed ICU LoS. These were: 1) squared Pearson correlation coefficient (R^2) [21]; 2) root mean squared prediction error (RMSPE); 3) mean absolute

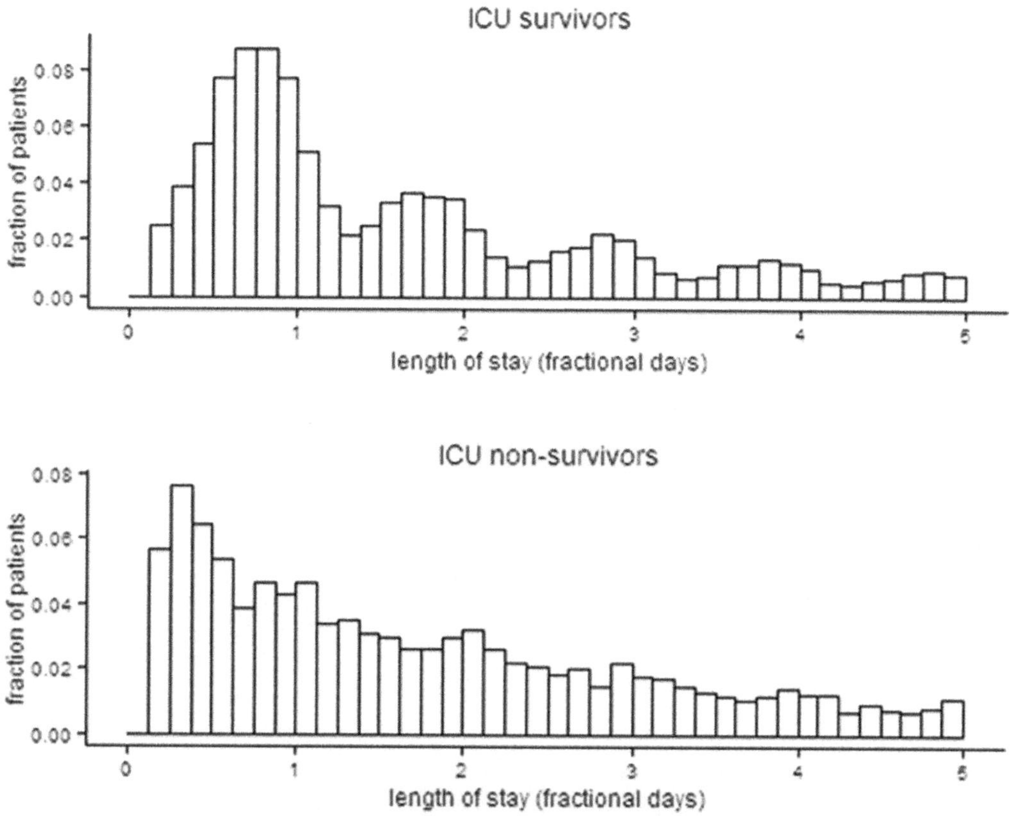

Figure 1. Distribution of ICU LoS for survivors and non-survivors.

prediction error (MAPE); 4) prediction bias [9,15]. We describe these measures in more depth in text S3.

The R^2 is the fraction of variance in observed ICU LoS that is explained by a model. It ranges from 0 to 1, where higher values correspond to better predictions. The RMSPE represents the mean residual, or unexplained, standard error of predictions obtained using a model. Because of the extreme skewedness of the distribution of ICU LoS, the RMSPE increases quickly if a long LoS are erroneously predicted to be short or vice versa. In other words, a single mistake by the model may dominate the RMSPE. Therefore, we also present the MAPE, which does not have this limitation. Finally we assess whether a model's predictions systematically deviate from observed LoS values, using the prediction bias. For RMSPE, MAPE and prediction bias, lower values correspond to better.

We assessed the performance of the models on the original sample, using resampling [22] with 100 bootstrap samples to correct for optimistic bias. The optimistic bias of a model was estimated by calculating the mean and standard deviation of differences in model performance measures between the model developed on the original sample and developed on each bootstrap sample. The optimistic bias, for each performance measure, was added to the performances of the model developed on the original sample. The standard error of the optimistic bias was used to calculate the 95%-confidence interval of the performances. The proportional hazards assumption was not verified for CPH models that were developed on bootstrap samples. We considered a difference in performance between two models to be statistically significant if the bootstrap 95%-confidence interval of the difference in their performance did not contain zero. The 95%-confidence interval was calculated, taking the mean and standard deviation of the differences in performance between to models calculated for each bootstrap iteration.

Since the models we developed may perform differently for patients with a ICU LoS shorter or longer than four days and for patients with different main APACHE IV admission diagnosis categories, we estimated the performance for all patients and for these subgroups of patients separately.

Since the distribution of LoS is positively skewed and models for ICU LoS have differing capacity to predict this type of data, we not only estimated the performance of the models all patients, but also for the subgroups of patients with ICU LoS smaller than four days and greater than or equal to four days. This is roughly the 75% percentile of the ICU LoS distribution. Further, univariate analyses were performed to calculate R^2 for the different patient characteristics to evaluate the contribution to the model. Finally, performance was calculated for the different main categories of the APACHE IV admission diagnosis, to investigate the performance for different diagnostic groups.

All statistical analyses were performed using R statistical software version 2.15.1 [23].

Results

Data

In 2011, data from 33,732 patients with medical or unplanned surgical ICU admissions satisfying APACHE IV inclusion criteria were recorded in the NICE database. Of these, 627 (3.2%) were subsequently discharged to an ICU in another hospital, eight (0.0%) had missing values for gender and 430 (2.4%) had missing values for GCS and were excluded. Hence, we included 32,667

Table 1. Demographics of ICU admissions included in the analysis, for ICU survivors and ICU non-survivors separately (n = 32,667).

	ICU survivors	ICU non-survivors
Number of ICU admissions	28,280	4,387
ICU LoS in days, median (25%–75%)	1.7 (0.8–4.0)	2.3 (0.9–6.0)
ICU LoS in days, mean (sd)	4.0 (7.6)	5.6 (9.8)
Age in year, mean (sd)	60.7 (18.0)	68.6 (14.1)
Male (count %)	15,651 (55.1)	2,502 (57.0)
Admission type (count (%))		
Medical	20,903 (75.2)	3,537 (81.4)
Urgent surgery	7,377 (24.8)	850 (18.6)
APACHE IV APS, median (25%–75%)	44 (28–63)	95 (70–119)
Ventilation first 24 hours of ICU admission (count (%))	12,199 (42.2)	3,712 (84.5)
One or more chronic diagnoses (count (%))	19,463 (62.9)	4,137 (94.3)
One or more diagnoses at admission (<24 h) (count (%))	7,557 (26.9)	2,788 (63.8)
Confirmed infection (count (%))	5,922 (21.2)	1,302 (29.9)
Use of vasoactive drugs (count (%))	8,435 (29.5)	3,128 (71.5)
Lowest GCS first 24 hours, median (25%–75%)	15 (13–15)	6 (3–15)
Non-operative APACHE IV diagnosis category (count (%))		
Cardiovascular	5,932 (20.98)	1,740 (39.66)
Gastro-intestinal	1,630 (5.76)	244 (5.56)
Genito-uritary	705 (2.49)	52 (1.19)
Hematological	233 (0.81)	48 (1.09)
Metabolic	866 (3.06)	26 (0.59)
Musculoskeletal/skin	99 (0.35)	8 (0.18)
Neurological	4,214 (14.90)	408 (9.30
Respiratory	6,005 (21.23)	914 (20.83
Transplantation	7(0.02)	0 (0.00)
Trauma	1,209 (4.28)	97 (2.21)
Post-operative APACHE IV diagnosis category (count (%))		
Cardiovascular	2,248 (7.95)	378(8.62)
Gastro-intestinal	2,684 (9.49)	268 (6.11)
Genito-uritary	427 (1.51)	4 (0.09)
Hematological	4 (0.01)	0 (0.00)
Metabolic	12 (0.04)	0 (0.00)
Musculoskeletal/skin	324 (1.15)	9 (0.21)
Neurological	581 (2.05)	108 (2.46)
Respiratory	217 (0.77)	13 (0.30)
Transplantation	92 (0.33)	0 (0.00)
Trauma	795 (2.81)	70 (1.60)

LoS = Length of Stay, sd = standard deviation, GCS = Glasgow Coma scale.

patients in this study, of whom 28,280 (86.7%) were ICU survivors and 4,387 (13.3%) were ICU non-survivors.

Figure 1 shows the distribution of observed ICU LoS for the first five days of ICU admission for survivors and non-survivors. The distribution of ICU LoS was right skewed with a median of 1.7 (interquartile range (IQR) 0.8 to 4.0) days and a mean of 4.0 (standard deviation 7.6) days for survivors and a median and of 2.3 (IQR 0.9 to 6.0) days and a mean of 5.6 (standard deviation 9.8) days for non-survivors. For survivors the distribution of ICU LoS was multimodal.

Table 1 presents the demographics of the ICU survivors and non-survivors included in this study. Differences between survivors and non-survivors were tested using t-tests and χ^2-tests and found to be statistically significant (gender $p = 0.017$, all other variables $p<0.001$). In Table S1, we summarize the patient characteristics, which remained in the models after stepwise backward selection of variables.

For several patient characteristics, we found opposite associations with ICU LoS for survivors and non-survivors in all models. For instance, chronic dialysis resulted in a larger expected ICU LoS for non-survivors (OLS regression coefficient 1.91, (95% confidence interval −0.06 to 3.89) and a smaller expected ICU LoS for survivors (OLS regression coefficient −1.20, 95% confidence interval −1.97 to −0.44. The proportional hazards

Table 2. Estimated performance of regression models, when using all patients for model construction and model validation, but no cyclical terms.

	No cyclical terms included			
	R^2	Root mean squared prediction error (RMSPE)	Mean absolute prediction error (MAPE)	BIAS
OLS regression LoS	0.143	7.324	3.571	0.030
	(0.129 to 0.156)	(6.966 to 7.683)	(3.505 to 3.637)	(−0.051 to 0.112)
OLS regression LoS truncated at 30 days	0.208	5.150	3.099	0.015
	(0.2001 to 0.215)	(5.061 to 5.239)	(3.053 to 3.144)	(−0.044 to 0.074)
OLS regression log(LoS)	0.149	7.665	3.004	−1.850
	(0.132 to 0.166)	(7.302 to 8.029)	(2.928 to 3.080)	(−1.932 to −1.768)
GLM: Gaussian	0.154	7.279	3.431	−0.015
	(0.136 to 0.171)	(6.919 to7.640)	(3.366 to 3.496)	(−0.095 to 0.065)
GLM:Poisson	0.154	7.276	3.433	0.007
	(0.137 to 0.171)	(6.916 to 7.635)	(3.368 to 3.498)	(−0.073 to 0.086)
GLM: negative binomial	0.148	7.304	3.445	0.019
	(0.132 to 0.163)	(6.947 to 7.662)	(3.379 to 3.511)	(−0.061 to 0.100)
GLM: Gamma	0.147	7.306	3.446	0.020
	(0.132 to 0.163)	(6.948 to 7.663)	(3.380 to 3.512)	(−0.060 to 0.100)
Cox PH regression	0.088	8.739	3.927	−2.993
	(0.080 to 0.095)	(8.395 to 9.084)	(3.841 to 4.013)	(−3.083 to −2.903)
APACHE IV (original) LoS truncated at 30 days	0.163	5.546	4.103	1.640
	(0.156 to 0.169)	(5.470 to 5.621)	(4.063 to 4.144)	(1.579 to 1.700)
APACHE IV (recalibrated) LoS truncated at 30 days	0.169	5.291	3.375	0.366
	(0.162 to 0.175)	(5.204 to 5.379)	(3.331 to 3.420)	(0.305 to 0.427)

Confidence intervals were obtained with bootstrap sampling.
LoS = Length of Stay, OLS = Ordinary Least Square, GLM = General Linear Model.

assumption was met for each of the CPH models that were developed on the entire dataset.

Comparison of different regression methods

We present the estimates of predictive performance obtained from the bootstrap procedure in Table 2. We obtained values of R^2 between 0.088 and 0.208, of RMSPE between 5.150 and 8.739 days, of MAPE between 3.004 and 3.927 days and of prediction bias between −2.993 and 0.030 days.

The model predicting ICU LoS truncated at 30 days had the best performance. When considering R^2, RMSPE and MAPE, the performance of the APACHE IV model is better than the models we developed. However, the prediction bias is more than one day for this model. Of the models which did not truncate LoS, the predictions made by the Poisson model and the Gaussian GLM had the largest values of R^2 and smallest values of the RMSPE, and predictions made by the Poisson model had the smallest prediction bias, although the differences were not statistically significant. The values of R^2 were significantly smaller and values for RMSPE, MAPE and prediction bias were significantly larger for CPH regression, compared to the values for the other models. Predictions with OLS regression had a large prediction bias and RMSPE, but small MAPE. The prediction bias for CPH regression and OLS regression of log-transformed LoS was negative, implying that these models systematically underestimate ICU LoS. We found a relatively large bias when using OLS regression on the log-transformed ICU LoS and comparing back-transformed predictions with observed ICU LoS. This bias is caused by the fact that we replaced negative predictions by zero and inflated when predicted values are back-transformed to the original scale.

We performed univariate GLM Poisson analyses to calculate R^2 for each of the patient characteristics. The largest values for R^2 were for mechanical ventilation in the first 24 hours of ICU stay (0.078), APS (0.067) and vasoactive medication (0.058).

We present the mean and standard deviation of the observed and predicted ICU LoS using the GLM Poisson model for a selection of common ICU diagnoses for ICU survivors and non-survivors in Table 3. Based on the R^2 values, the models performed well for the categories operative metabolic, operative genito-uritary and non-operative trauma and poorly for post-operative neurological, post-operative musculoskeletal/skin and non-operative neurological.

Performance of separate models for survivors and non-survivors

Table 4 presents the estimated performance of separate models developed for survivors and non-survivors. In general, the performance of these models was better than the models for all patients. For survivors, the values for R^2 were between 0.103 and

Table 3. Observed and predicted ICU LoS (median (IQR)), for ICU survivors and ICU non-survivors.

APACHE IV diagnosis	ICU survivors		ICU non-survivors	
	Observed	**Predicted**	**Observed**	**Predicted**
Non-operative				
Cardiovascular	1.98 (0.95 to 4.31)	2.13 (1.09 to 4.04)	2.23 (0.93 to 4.72)	2.10 (1.48 to 3.04)
Gastro-intestinal	1.21 (0.74 to 2.77)	1.25 (0.92 to 2.08)	1.54 (0.72 to 4.38)	1.97 (1.25 to 2.74)
Genito-uritary	1.85 (0.88 to 3.53)	1.69 (1.19 to 2.71)	2.13 (1.04 to 5.46)	2.83 (1.85 to 3.81)
Metabolic	1.15 (0.75 to 2.04)	1.15 (0.90 to 1.54)	2.07 (0.85 to 5.89)	2.41 (1.63 to 3.43)
Musculoskeletal/skin	1.57 (0.71 to 3.27)	1.51 (0.99 to 2.48)	4.58 (1.51 to 8.23)	4.04 (2.66 to 5.47)
Neurological	0.91 (0.57 to 1.94)	0.97 (0.73 to 1.63)	1.28 (0.70 to 3.35)	1.42 (1.07 to 2.09)
Respiratory	2.59 (1.05 to 5.83)	2.54 (1.61 to 4.16)	3.73 (1.14 to 9.39)	3.69 (2.42 to 4.93)
Trauma	1.31 (0.70 to 2.91)	1.30 (1.05 to 2.22)	1.53 (0.44 to 8.02)	1.93 (1.42 to 2.79)
Post-operative				
Cardiovascular	2.31 (0.89 to 6.21)	2.69 (1.70 to 4.03)	2.53 (1.17 to 8.70)	3.49 (2.06 to 4.83)
Gastro-intestinal	1.62 (0.74 to 3.85)	1.75 (1.05 to 3.04)	2.23 (0.89 to 8.39)	3.08 (1.88 to 4.14)
Genito-uritary	0.79 (0.52 to 1.39)	0.78 (0.56 to 1.25)	4.07 (0.29 to 7.91)	1.38 (1.23 to 1.73)
Metabolic[1]	1.29 (0.84 to 2.26)	1.42 (0.94 to 1.54)		
Musculoskeletal/skin	0.90 (0.67 to 2.03)	1.05 (0.77 to 1.92)	4.16 (1.60 to 8.43)	3.08 (2.17 to 4.77)
Neurological	1.77 (0.89 to 5.57)	2.50 (1.35 to 3.70)	3.23 (1.20 to 5.56)	2.51 (1.99 to 3.81)
Respiratory	0.99 (0.72 to 3.51)	1.44 (0.97 to 1.99)	3.35 (3.15 to 5.78)	3.80 (3.02 to 4.67)
Trauma	1.26 (0.71 to 3.88)	1.57 (1.02 to 2.69)	2.45 (0.90 to 10.04)	2.49 (2.13 to 4.09)
Post- and non-operative				
Hematological[2]	1.19 (0.69 to 3.05)	1.42 (0.95 to 2.34)	4.83 (1.49 to 9.89)	4.37 (2.46 to 5.69)
Transplantation[3]	1.76 (1.10 to 2.85)	1.95 (1.34 to 2.43)		

Predictions were obtained using the Poisson model, constructed using all patients, but no cyclical terms.
[1]*There were no non-survivors in the APACHE IV diagnose categories metabolic and transplantation.*
[2]*Post- and non-operative hematological patients were combined because of the low number of post-operative hematological patients.*
[3]*Post- and non-operative patients were combined because of the low number of non-operative patients with complications after transplantation.*

0.266, for RMSPE between 4.786 and 8.401 days, for MAPE between 2.701 and 3.754 and for the bias between −2.742 and 0.025 days. For non-survivors, the values of R^2 were between 0.069 and 0.129, of RMSPE between 6.405 and 11.060, of MAPE between 4.325 and 5.165 and of the bias between −4.567 and 0.020 days.

Generally speaking, the models for ICU survivors performed better than the models for ICU non-survivors. Furthermore, as before, the best results for R^2 and the RMSPE were obtained with GLMs, in particular the Gaussian GLM and the Poisson model, but the Gaussian model resulted in a relatively large prediction bias. The predictions obtained from the CPH model and OLS model of log transformed ICU LoS exhibited a large prediction bias.

Cyclical terms

Table 5 shows the results we obtained when we included the cyclical terms for discharge time in the models. In general, the values of R^2 and prediction bias were higher and the values of the RMSPE, the MAPE and the bias were smaller when we included the cyclical terms.

Performance for patients with short and long ICU LoS

Table 6 presents the predictive performance of each of the regression models, separately for patients with an ICU LoS less or more than four days. The models are the same as those presented in Table 1 in that they were developed using data from all patients and without cyclical terms for discharge time.

For patients ICU LoS of less than four days, we obtained the best predictions using CPH regression; OLS regression on LoS truncated at 30 days and OLS regression of log-transformed ICU LoS. These models had better results for R^2, RMSPE, MAPE and prediction bias, than the other models. For patients with an ICU LoS of longer than four days, we obtained the best values for R^2 the Poisson model. For these patients, we obtained the worst values of R^2, RMSPE, MAPE and prediction bias from CPH regression and OLS regression on log-transformed LoS. When separate models were developed for survivors and non-survivors separately, see respectively Table S2 and S3 and when cyclical terms were included for discharge time, this gave similar findings, see Table S4.

Discussion

In this study, we compared regression methods for predicting LoS for unplanned ICU admissions on a large registry dataset. As expected, the distribution of ICU LoS in our dataset was extremely skewed to the right. In addition, the ICU mortality among the patients in our dataset was substantial (12%), and ICU LoS was generally longer for survivors than non-survivors. Furthermore, there were considerable differences in observed ICU LoS for different APACHE IV diagnoses.

Table 4. Estimated performance of regression models, when constructing models using ICU survivors and ICU non-survivors separately, but no cyclical terms.

	Survivors				non-survivors			
	R^2	Root mean squared prediction error (RMSPE)	Mean absolute prediction error (MAPE)	BIAS	R^2	Root mean squared prediction error (RMSPE)	Mean absolute prediction error (MAPE)	BIAS
OLS regression LoS	0.184	6.868	3.238	0.025	0.091	9.446	5.165	0.020
	(0.166 to 0.203)	(6.418 to 7.318)	(3.159 to 3.317)	(−0.059 to 0.109)	(0.074 to 0.109)	(8.687 to 10.205)	(4.941 to 5.389)	(−0.245 to 0.285)
OLS regression LoS truncated at 30 days	0.266	4.786	2.816	0.013	0.129	6.405	4.325	0.008
	(0.256 to 0.276)	(4.684 to 4.887)	(2.768 to 2.864)	(−0.042 to 0.069)	(0.109 to 0.149)	(6.178 to 6.632)	(4.195 to 4.455)	(−0.169 to 0.184)
OLS regression log (LoS)	0.196	7.135	2.701	−1.584	0.094	9.969	4.369	−2.892
	(0.174 to 0.217)	(6.675 to 7.596)	(2.619 to 2.783)	(−1.669 to − 1.499)	(0.074 to 0.113)	(9.136 to 10.801)	(4.112 to 4.627)	(−3.161 to 2.623)
GLM: Gaussian	0.202	6.797	3.063	−0.033	0.094	9.470	5.027	−0.130
	(0.179 to 0.224)	(6.348 to 7.246)	(2.985 to 3.141)	(−0.115 to 0.050)	(0.059 to 0.128)	(8.742 to 10.199)	(4.800 to 5.255)	(−0.389 to 0.129)
GLM: Poisson	0.202	6.793	3.061	−0.007	0.098	9.412	5.062	−0.006
	(0.180 to 0.224)	(6.341 to 7.245)	(2.983 to 3.139)	(−0.090 to 0.075)	(0.072 to 0.124)	(8.666 to 10.158)	(4.837 to 5.287)	(−0.261 to 0.249)
GLM: negative binomial	0.196	6.821	3.068	−0.010	0.097	9.418	5.063	0.003
	(0.175 to 0.216)	(6.370 to 7.272)	(2.989 to 3.146)	(−0.092 to 0.073)	(0.077 to 0.117)	(8.665 to 10.172)	(4.837 to 5.288)	(−0.253 to 0.260)
GLM: Gamma	0.196	6.821	3.068	−0.010	0.097	9.422	5.066	0.004
	(0.175 to 0.216)	(6.371 to 7.272)	(2.990 to 3.146)	(−0.092 to 0.073)	(0.077 to 0.117)	(8.668 to 10.176)	(4.840 to 5.292)	(−0.252 to 0.261)
Cox PH regression	0.103	8.401	3.754	−2.742	0.069	11.060	5.137	−4.567
	(0.093 to 0.113)	(7.975 to 8.827)	(3.662 to 3.847)	(−2.838 to − 2.647)	(0.059 to 0.080)	(10.227 to 11.893)	(4.848 to 5.426)	(−4.861 to − 4.272)

Confidence intervals were obtained using bootstrap sampling.
LoS = Length of Stay, OLS = Ordinary Least Square, GLM = General Linear Model.

Table 5. Estimated performance of regression models, when constructing models using all patients and cyclical terms.

	Cyclical terms included			
	R^2	Root mean squared prediction error (RMSPE)	Mean absolute prediction error (MAPE)	BIAS
OLS regression (LoS)	0.144	7.317	3.566	0.034
	(0.131 to 0.157)	(6.958 to 7.675)	(3.500 to 3.631)	(−0.048 to 0.115)
OLS regression LoS truncated at 30 days	0.210	5.141	3.093	0.018
	(0.203 to 0.218)	(5.053 to 5.229)	(3.049 to 3.138)	(−0.041 to 0.078)
OLS regression log(LoS)	0.150	7.647	2.991	−1.827
	(0.135 to 0.164)	(7.283 to 8.012)	(2.916 to 3.067)	(−1.909 to −1.745)
GLM: Gaussian	0.156	7.270	3.424	−0.018
	(0.138 to 0.174)	(6.909 to 7.632)	(3.360 to 3.489)	(−0.098 to 0.061)
GLM: Poisson	0.157	7.264	3.424	0.007
	(0.141 to 0.173)	(6.905 to 7.623)	(3.359 to 3.489)	(−0.073 to 0.086)
GLM: negative binomial	0.151	7.288	3.435	0.017
	(0.137 to 0.165)	(6.925 to 7.651)	(3.369 to 3.501)	(−0.063 to 0.098)
GLM: Gamma	0.151	7.286	3.436	0.017
	(0.137 to 0.165)	(6.908 to 7.664)	(3.369 to 3.502)	(−0.063 to 0.097)
Cox PH regression	0.086	8.743	3.939	−2.985
	(0.079 to 0.094)	(8.399 to 9.087)	(3.853 to 4.024)	(−3.075 to −2.895)

Confidence intervals were obtained with bootstrap sampling.
LoS = Length of Stay, OLS = Ordinary Least Square, GLM = General Linear Model.

The predictive performance of all of our models was disappointing, with an R^2 at most around 20% and a RMSPE of more than seven days. Even in absolute terms, our predictions were, on average, three days different from the observed ICU LoS. Given that more than half of the patients had an ICU LoS of less than two days, it is fair to say that these predictions are not particularly useful. The differences in predictive performance between the models were generally small. Overall, the Poisson model and Gaussian GLM performed somewhat better than the other models, while CPH regression and OLS regression of log-transformed ICU LoS were superior for patients with an ICU LoS of less than four days. The models generally performed better for ICU survivors than for non-survivors. Because patients are often discharged at set times during the day, we hypothesized that the inclusion of cyclical terms for discharge times would improve the performance of the models. However, the performance only improved marginally after we included these terms.

ICU discharge decisions often do not only depend on a patient's recovery, but on organizational circumstances such as availability of beds on the general ward and the need to free up ICU beds for other patients. These organizational circumstances depend on structural factors related to the ICU and the hospital. We have deliberately chosen not to include ICU and hospital level covariates in our models, because we wished to investigate the feasibility of predicting ICU LoS for future use in tools to compare ICUs [24].

Previously researchers have used regression models to predict ICU LoS, but they have generally not critically appraised and compared the performance of different models [6,9,11–13,25]. The APACHE IV model for predicting ICU LoS uses OLS regression on ICU LoS truncated at 30 days. We have shown (Table 4) that this model leads to biased results for patients admitted to the ICU for less than four days, but performs better for patients with ICU LoS longer than four days, perhaps due to truncation. Other researchers have used CPH regression to predict ICU LoS following cardiac surgery and have found that their models were able to discriminate between shorter and longer treatment durations, but were unsuitable for predictions in individual patients [25]. Researchers examining hospital LoS following CABG surgery found that the model assumptions for linear regression were not satisfied for LoS or log transformed LoS and conclude that the use of GLMs with a logarithmic link function should be considered for this type of data [15]. Another study compared twelve methods to estimate ICU LoS using a cohort of patients in Australian and New Zealand [27]. These researchers compared OLS regression on log-transformed ICU LoS; GLMs with a log-link function (distributions Poisson, gamma, negative binomial and inverse-Gaussian); linear mixed models; skew-normal; skew-t models; extended estimating equations and a finite mixture model. They obtained values for R^2 between 0.17 and 0.22 and found that linear mixed models and OLS regression on log-transformed LoS performed best.

Because ICU LoS is right skewed, OLS regression is theoretically not a good choice. Researchers have suggested truncating observed ICU LoS, to improve the performance of OLS regression [6,9,11–13]. In this study, we used OLS regression on ICU LoS truncated at 30 days (Table 2). However, when comparing ICU LoS among hospitals, truncation of ICU LoS can be unfair because there may be substantial differences in the values that were truncated and the largest improvements in efficiency can probably be achieved in patients with the longest ICU LoS.

The predictive performance of separate models for survivors and non-survivors was higher than for combined models. This may be caused by differences in the signs of regression coefficients between survivors and non-survivors. Factors that aggravate illness severity tend to increase the length of stay for survivors and shorten it for non-survivors. Nevertheless, a fundamental draw-

Table 6. Performance measures using all patients for model prediction, but not including cyclical terms as covariate separated, for patients with length of stay smaller than the 75% percentile and larger or equal than the 75% percentile for validation.

	ICU LoS smaller than 75% percentile				ICU LoS larger or equal to the 75% percentile			
	R^2	Root mean squared prediction error (RMSPE)	Mean absolute prediction error (MAPE)	BIAS	R^2	Root mean squared prediction error (RMSPE)	Mean absolute prediction error (MAPE)	BIAS
OLS regression LoS	0.124	3.208	2.391	2.012	0.038	13.578	7.129	−5.945
	(0.114 to 0.134)	(3.164 to 3.252)	(2.364 to 2.418)	(1.980 to 2.045)	(0.024 to 0.052)	(12.800 to 14.355)	(6.873 to 7.385)	(−6.245 to −5.645)
OLS regression LoS truncated at 30 days	0.130	2.826	2.124	1.709	0.063	9.078	6.037	−5.273
	(0.121 to 0.139)	(2.798 to 2.854)	(2.101 to 2.147)	(1.740 to 1.798)	(0.053 to 0.073)	(8.874 to 9.282)	(5.868 to 6.206)	(−5.482 to −5.063)
OLS regression log(LoS)	0.132	1.429	1.010	0.497	0.033	15.157	9.015	−8.924
	(0.120 to 0.144)	(1.393 to 1.465)	(0.995 to 1.025)	(0.476 to 0.517)	(0.020 to 0.046)	(14.417 to 15.896)	(8.717 to 9.313)	(−9.230 to −8.618)
GLM: Gaussian	0.112	3.122	2.137	1.903	0.040	13.540	7.333	−5.798
	(0.102 to 0.121)	(3.068 to 3.176)	(2.107 to 2.166)	(1.870 to 1.936)	(0.024 to 0.057)	(12.763 to 14.317)	(7.086 to 7.581)	(−6.090 to −5.506)
GLM: Poisson	0.109	3.119	2.147	1.938	0.044	13.357	7.273	−5.769
	(0.100 to 0.119)	(3.065 to 3.172)	(2.118 to 2.176)	(1.905 to 1.971)	(0.029 to 0.058)	(12.705 to 14.008)	(7.031 to 7.516)	(−6.051 to −5.487)
GLM: negative binomial	0.106	3.175	2.156	1.952	0.041	13.378	7.294	−5.759
	(0.097 to 0.115)	(3.121 to 3.229)	(2.126 to 2.186)	(1.919 to 1.985)	(0.028 to 0.054)	(12.727 to 14.030)	(7.050 to 7.538)	(−6.045 to −5.474)
GLM: Gamma	0.106	3.177	2.157	1.952	0.038	13.559	7.330	−5.803
	(0.097 to 0.116)	(3.123 to 3.231)	(2.128 to 2.187)	(1.919 to 1.985)	(0.024 to 0.052)	(12.786 to 14.331)	(7.079 to 7.580)	(−6.099 to −5.507)
Cox (PH) regression	0.135	1.593	1.269	−0.023	0.020	17.261	11.903	−11.903
	(0.127 to 0.143)	(1.569 to 1.617)	(1.251 to 1.286)	(−0.051 to 0.006)	(0.011 to 0.028)	(16.565 to 17.957)	(11.589 to 12.218)	(−12.218 to −11.589)
APACHE IV (original) LoS truncated at 30 days	0.094	4.079	3.636	3.601	0.053	8.551	5.506	−4.245
	(0.087 to 0.102)	(4.051 to 4.107)	(3.608 to 3.664)	(3.572 to 3.630)	(0.044 to 0.062)	(8.353 to 8.749)	(5.351 to 5.661)	(−4.452 to −4.037)
APACHE IV (recalibrated) LoS truncated at 30 days	0.096	3.176	2.499	2.202	0.053	9.042	6.003	−5.142
	(0.088 to 0.104)	(3.145 to 3.207)	(2.473 to 2.526)	(2.168 to 2.235)	(0.044 to 0.062)	(8.837 to 9.246)	(5.833 to 6.174)	(−5.348 to −4.937)

LoS = Length of Stay, OLS = Ordinary Least Square, GLM = General Linear Model.

back is that some hospitals may achieve shorter average ICU LoS because their mortality rates are higher, which again would make the comparison unfair. Furthermore, this could explain partly the poor performance of the models.

Compared to previously published studies, our work stands out because we applied resampling methods to compare eight types of models constructed using advanced modelling methods, such as regression splines and cyclical terms, and we based our study on a large multi-center dataset. Furthermore, we used cyclic terms of time of discharge as a way to model center effects in models with patients variables only. This approach has not been used to predict ICU LoS previously. Yet our work also has a number of limitations. First, we did not evaluate modern prediction methods from the field of statistical learning, such as ensemble [26] and kernel methods [27]. As a result, we have not explored all methods for predicting ICU LoS, which could be done in future research. Second, we had no information on how the logistic policies vary between the ICUs included in our study. For example, some ICUs usually discharged patients in the morning, while others do this in the afternoon. Thirdly, for this study we did not include any interaction terms in our models. Developing a model to predict ICU LoS may require more accurate analyses on the role of interaction terms in the model. Fourth, we did not include predictions of LoS for elective surgery patients in this study. Patients undergoing unplanned ICU-admission differ considerably from those undergoing elective surgery and often have a protocolized ICU LoS. Hence, we choose not to develop a single model for patients with planned and unplanned ICU admissions. Fitfth, interestingly, many patients in our cohort of unplanned ICU-admissions had a very short LoS on the ICU. Of our patients 25% had an ICU LoS shorter than 0.8 days. This group of patients included both medical and unplanned surgical patients and many different reasons for ICU admission were present, such as monitoring during endoscopic procedures and monitoring after overdose of sedatives. Some patients only required short ICU treatment for respiratory failure, e.g. pulmonary edema well responding to administration of diuretics. Also, LoS could be very short in patients who died within the first hours after ICU admission. We do not expect that the shorter LoS in our population influences our conclusions regarding the preferred regression model for length of stay as the shape of the LoS distribution in other ICU populations is comparable. Sixth, the performance of the CPH models may have been underestimated, because we did not verify the proportional hazards assumption for models developed within the bootstrap procedure. However, we believe that violations of this assumption were unlikely, as it was satisfied for all models that were developed on the entire dataset.

Our findings have implications for the use of patient level predictions of ICU LoS. We believe that currently available models for ICU LoS, are unsuitable for use in quality indicators and that further research is needed to develop models of ICU LoS. A relatively small group of patients determines the variation in ICU LoS, but it is extremely difficult to identify these patients. We are not sure whether observed differences in ICU LoS are due to variations in the quality of care. Therefore we advise against using currently available models for ICU LoS in unplanned ICU admissions as input for policy development or evaluation [6,9].

Conclusions

It is difficult to predict ICU LoS for patients with unplanned admissions using patient characteristics at ICU admission time only, even with sophisticated statistical modelling methods. Although the differences were small, GLMs with a logarithmic link function predicted ICU LoS slightly better than other models for untransformed ICU LoS. For patients with ICU LoS shorter than four days, CPH regression and OLS regression of log-transformed LoS were superior. All models performed only marginally better when we included cyclical terms for discharge time. Models developed using survivors and non-survivors separately performed better than models developed on data for all patients. We conclude that currently available models for ICU LoS are not suitable for predicting individual patient data and should not be used as an indicator for ICU quality or efficiency or as tools to develop policies around unplanned ICU admissions.

Supporting Information

Table S1 Variables included in the regression models after performing stepwise backward selection of variables.

Table S2 Performance measures using ICU survivors for model prediction, but not including cyclical terms as covariate separated, for patients with length of stay smaller than the 75% percentile and larger or equal than the 75% percentile for validation.

Table S3 Performance measures using ICU non-survivors for model prediction, but not including cyclical terms as covariate separated, for patients with length of stay smaller than the 75% percentile and larger or equal than the 75% percentile for validation.

Table S4 Performance measures using all patients for model prediction and cyclical terms as covariate separated, for patients with length of stay smaller than the 75% percentile and larger or equal than the 75% percentile for validation.

Dataset S1 Description of patient characteristics used to perform the analyses.

Text S1 Statistical regression methods.

Text S2 Cyclical terms included as covariate in the models.

Text S3 Performance assessment of the models developed.

Acknowledgments

We acknowledge all participating ICUs of the National Intensive Care Registry for contributing patient level data. We thank R. Holman PhD for carefully reviewing this manuscript.

Author Contributions

Analyzed the data: IV. Wrote the paper: IV NDK EDJ NP.

Reference

1. Knaus WA, Draper EA, Wagner DP, Zimmerman JE (1985) APACHE II: a severity of disease classification system. Crit Care Med 13 (10): 818–29.
2. Zimmerman JE, Kramer AA, McNair DS, Malila FM (2006) Acute Physiology and Chronic Health Evaluation (APACHE) IV: hospital mortality assessment for today's critically ill patients. Crit Care Med 34 (5): 1297–310.
3. Le Gall JR, Lemeshow S, Saulnier F (1993) A new Simplified Acute Physiology Score (SAPS II) based on a European/North American multicenter study. JAMA 270 (24): 2957–63.
4. Zimmerman JE, Kramer AA (2008) Outcome prediction in critical care: the Acute Physiology and Chronic Health Evaluation models. Curr Opin Crit Care 14 (5): 491–7.
5. Vasilevskis EE, Kuzniewicz MW, Cason BA, Lane RK, Dean ML, et al. (2009) Mortality probability model III and simplified acute physiology score II: assessing their value in predicting length of stay and comparison to APACHE IV. Chest 136 (1): 89–101.
6. Zimmerman JE, Kramer AA, McNair DS, Malila FM, Shaffer VL (2006) Intensive care unit length of stay: Benchmarking based on Acute Physiology and Chronic Health Evaluation (APACHE) IV. Crit Care Med 34 (10): 2517–29.
7. Becker RB, Zimmerman JE, Knaus WA, Wagner DP, Seneff MG, et al. (1995) The use of APACHE III to evaluate ICU length of stay, resource use, and mortality after coronary artery by-pass surgery. J Cardiovasc Surg (Torino) 36 (1): 1–11.
8. Woods AW, MacKirdy FN, Livingston BM, Norrie J, Howie JC (2000) Evaluation of predicted and actual length of stay in 22 Scottish intensive care units using the APACHE III system. Acute Physiology and Chronic Health Evaluation. Anaesthesia 55 (11): 1058–65.
9. Moran JL, Bristow P, Solomon PJ, George C, Hart GK (2008) Mortality and length-of-stay outcomes, 1993–2003, in the binational Australian and New Zealand intensive care adult patient database. Crit Care Med 36 (1): 46–61.
10. Niskanen M, Reinikainen M, Pettila V (2009) Case-mix-adjusted length of stay and mortality in 23 Finnish ICUs. Intensive Care Med 35 (6): 1060–7.
11. Rapoport J, Teres D, Zhao Y, Lemeshow S (2003) Length of stay data as a guide to hospital economic performance for ICU patients. Med Care 41 (3): 386–97.
12. Al Tehewy M, El Houssinie M, El Ezz NA, Abdelkhalik M, El Damaty S (2010) Developing severity adjusted quality measures for intensive care units. Int J Health Care Qual Assur 23 (3): 277–86.
13. Nathanson BH, Higgins TL, Teres D, Copes WS, Kramer A, et al. (2007) A revised method to assess intensive care unit clinical performance and resource utilization. Crit Care Med 35 (8): 1853–62.
14. Manning WG, Mullahy J (2001) Estimating log models: to transform or not to transform? J Health Econ 20 (4): 461–94.
15. Austin PC, Rothwell DM, Tu JV (2002) A Comparison of Statistical Modeling Strategies for Analyzing Length of Stay after CABG Surgery. Health Services and Outcomes Research Methodology, 3 (2): 107–33.
16. Stolwijk AM, Straatman H, Zielhuis GA (1999) Studying seasonality by using sine and cosine functions in regression analysis. J Epidemiol Community Health 53 (4): 235–8.
17. Dutch National Intensive Care Evaluation (NICE) foundation (2014) Available: http://www.stichting-nice.nl.
18. Brinkman S, Bakhshi-Raiez F, Abu-Hanna A, de Jonge E, Bosman RJ, et al. (2011) External validation of Acute Physiology and Chronic Health Evaluation IV in Dutch intensive care units and comparison with Acute Physiology and Chronic Health Evaluation II and Simplified Acute Physiology Score II. J Crit Care 26 (1): 105–8.
19. Kramer AA, Zimmerman JE (2010) A predictive model for the early identification of patients at risk for a prolonged intensive care unit length of stay. BMC Med Inform Decis Mak 10: 27.
20. Hastie T, Tibshirani R, Friedman J (2001) Basic Expansions and Regularization. The Elements of Statistical Learning: Data Mining, Inference, and Prediction. p. 115–63.
21. Steyerberg EW (2009) Evaluation of Performance. Clinical Prediction models: A practical Approach to Development, Validation, and updating. Springer; p. 83–99.
22. Steyerberg EW (2009) Overfitting and Optimism in Prediction Models. Clinical Prediction models: A practical Approach to Development, Validation, and updating. Springer; p. 83–99.
23. R Foundation for Statistical Computing (2005) A Language and Environment for Statistical Computing [computer program]. Vienna, Austria: R Foundation for Statistical Computing.
24. Becker RB, Zimmerman JE (1996) ICU scoring systems allow prediction of patient outcomes and comparison of ICU performance. Crit Care Clin 12 (3): 503–14.
25. Widyastuti Y, Stenseth R, Wahba A, Pleym H, Videm V (2012) Length of intensive care unit stay following cardiac surgery: is it impossible to find a universal prediction model? Interactive Cardiovascular & Thoracic Surgery 15 (5): 825–32.
26. Zhou Z (2012) Ensemble Methods: Foundation and Algorithms. Chapman & Hall;
27. Shawe-Taylor J, Cristiano N (2004) Kernel Methods for Pattern Analysis. Cambridge University Press; 2004.

The Effect of Pylorus Removal on Delayed Gastric Emptying after Pancreaticoduodenectomy: A Meta-Analysis of 2,599 Patients

Wenming Wu[9], Xiafei Hong[9], Lilan Fu, Shanglong Liu, Lei You, Li Zhou, Yupei Zhao*

Department of General Surgery, Peking Union Medical College Hospital, Chinese Academy of Medical Sciences and Peking Union Medical College, Beijing, China

Abstract

Background: Delayed gastric emptying is a serious complication of pancreaticoduodenectomy. The effect of pylorus removal on delayed gastric emptying has not been well evaluated.

Study Design: We searched five databases (PubMed, EMBASE and the Cochrane Central Register of Controlled Trials, Scopus and Web of Science) up to July 2014. The meta-regression analysis was performed to evaluate any factors accountable for the heterogeneity. Publication bias was assessed by Egger's test, and corrected by Duval's trim and fill method. Subgroup analyses were conducted for different surgical techniques of pyloric removal. Other intraoperative and postoperative parameters were compared between two groups.

Results: We included 27 studies involving 2,599 patients, with a moderate-high heterogeneity for primary outcome ($I^2 = 63\%$). Meta-regression analysis showed that four variables primarily contributed to the heterogeneity, namely nasogastric tube intubation time, solid food start time, preoperative diabetes percentage and the number of patients in pylorus-preserving group. After excluding four studies, the remaining twenty-three studies showed reduced heterogeneity ($I^2 = 51\%$). Then we used Duval's trim and fill method to correct publication bias. The corrected MH odds ratio was 0.78 (95% CI: 0.52–1.17). A subgroup analysis showed that pylorus removal tends to reduce delayed gastric emptying incidence for subtotal stomach-preserving pancreaticoduodenectomy or pylorus-resecting pancreaticoduodenectomy, compared with pylorus-preserving group. However, standard Whipple procedure failed to show any significant reduction of DGE compared with pylorus-removal group. No significant differences were observed in terms of length of hospital stay, infection and pancreatic fistula; however, pylorus removal resulted in longer operation time, more blood loss and higher mortality.

Conclusion: The pylorus removal does not significantly reduce the overall incidence of delayed gastric emptying. Subtotal stomach-preserving pancreaticoduodenectomy or pylorus-resecting pancreaticoduodenectomy tends to reduce delayed gastric emptying incidence, but needs further validation.

Editor: Beicheng Sun, The First Affiliated Hospital of Nanjing Medical University, China

Funding: The authors have no support or funding to report.

Competing Interests: The authors have declared that no competing interests exist.

* Email: zhao8028@263.net

[9] These authors contributed equally to this work.

Introduction

Pancreaticoduodenectomy is an important surgical intervention for periampullary diseases. According to resection extent of pyloric region, pancreaticoduodenectomy uses either pylorus-preserving or pylorus-removing procedures. Specifically, pylorus-preserving pancreaticoduodenectomy (PPPD) preserves all of the stomach and part of the proximal duodenum [1,2]. On the contrary, pylorus-removing pancreaticoduodenectomy (PRPD) includes different surgical techniques, namely the standard Whipple procedure (SWP), subtotal stomach-preserving pancreaticoduodenectomy (SSPPD) and pylorus-resecting pancreaticoduodenectomy (PrPD). SWP usually resects the pylorus along with 30–40% of the distal stomach [3]. SSPPD and PrPD involve the resection of the pyloric ring together with 2–3 cm of the distal stomach and preserve the majority of the stomach [3,4].

Delayed gastric emptying (DGE) is a serious postoperative morbidity of pancreaticoduodenectomy. DGE may prolong hospital stay, compromise the quality of life, and impair long-term nutrition status. The International Study Group of Pancreatic Surgery (ISGPS) has proposed a grading system to catogorize different level of severity of DGE. ISGPS grade B/C DGE usually has more clinical impacts since it might change the postoperative clinical management. In additional, ISGPS grade C DGE are more frequently seen with other postoperative complications [5,6].

It is believed that postoperative pyloric dysfunction will predispose a patient to DGE. Pancreaticoduodenectomy may

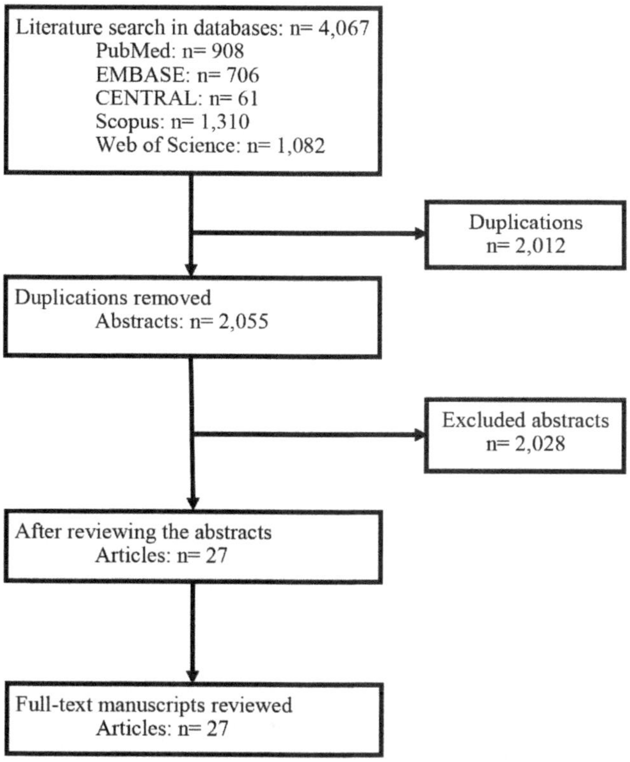

Figure 1. Flowchart of the literature search and studies inclusion. Abbreviations: CENTRAL, Cochrane Central Register of Controlled Trials.

cause pyloric dysfunction due to the devascularization and denervation of the pyloric region. Inadequate blood supply that leads to ischemic gastroparesis is one of the mechanisms that may cause DGE [7]. Pyloric denervation, such as vagal nerve injury, may cause pylorospasm and DGE [8]. The preservation of blood supply and innervation of the pyloric region or the dilatation of the pylorus may reduce the incidence of DGE [9,10].

Previously meta-analyses [11–13] have compared the PPPD with SWP, and one recent meta-analysis analyzed the intraoperative and postoperative outcomes of several randomized controlled trials (RCTs) [14]. As for DGE, all of the meta-analyses indicated a high heterogeneity among studies. In fact, many preoperative and postoperative factors might influence incidence of DGE, including preoperative diabetes, pancreatic fistula, postoperative complications, preoperative biliary drainage, and method of reconstruction. These variables may account for the observed heterogeneity across individual studies [15]. In addition, the variations in the surgical techniques, specifically the proportion of the stomach that is resected during PRPD, may be a confounding variable; therefore, further subgroup analyses are needed.

In this study, we systematically evaluated the following questions: 1) Whether pyloric ring removal reduces the overall incidence of DGE; 2) The factors that contribute to the overall heterogeneity among studies; and 3) Whether the variations in the surgical techniques (PrPD/SSPPD versus SWP) lead to different results with regard to the incidence of DGE.

Materials and Methods

Review Strategy and Quality Assessment

The review process was adhered to the Preferred Reporting Items for Systematic Reviews and Meta-Analyses statement [16]. The literature search strategy and eligibility criteria for inclusion and exclusion of studies and study outcomes were specified in advance to avoid bias. We searched PubMed, EMBASE, the Cochrane Central Register of Controlled Trials (CENTRAL), Scopus and Web of Science for studies published up until July 2014, without restrictions placed on the language or publication date. The search strategy was as follows:

PubMed: 'pancreaticoduodenectomy' AND ('pyloric' OR 'pylorus') (in Title/Abstract)

EMBASE: 'pancreaticoduodenectomy' AND ('pyloric' OR 'pylorus') (in Keywords with 'Map Term to Subject Heading')

CENTRAL and *Scopus*: 'pancreaticoduodenectomy' AND ('pyloric' OR 'pylorus') (in Title, Abstract, Keywords)

Web of Science: 'pancreaticoduodenectomy' AND ('pyloric' OR 'pylorus') (in Topic)

All abstracts were retrieved and reviewed independently by two authors according to the eligibility criteria (listed below). A third author supervised the review process and settled disagreements on the study inclusion. To determine the inconsistency between reviewers, an inter-reviewer reliability analysis was conducted using a kappa statistic. If a study was included, the full-text of the article was retrieved and the relevant data were extracted. If additional data were considered to be necessary, the reviewers would contact the authors of the original articles. We evaluated the quality and the risk of bias of nonrandomized studies using the Newcastle-Ottawa quality assessment tool [17].

Eligibility Criteria

Inclusion and exclusion criteria were pre-defined to avoid bias.

Inclusion criteria. (1) Studies had to feature a comparison between PRPD and PPPD; and (2) the sample size in each surgical procedure should be greater than 10 patients.

Exclusion criteria. (1) Only data from a single group of patients (either PRPD or PPPD) were reported; (2) the incidence of DGE was not reported; or (3) the article was published in the form of a case report, review article, letter to the editor, editorial or conference abstract.

Outcomes

Primary outcomes. (1) Incidence of DGE

Definition: An International Study Group of Pancreatic Surgery (ISGPS) grade of DGE B/C was calculated for studies that followed the scoring system of the ISGPS [6]. For those studies that did not use the ISGPS scoring system, the overall incidence of DGE was considered.

Secondary outcomes. (1) Blood loss, (2) operation time, (3) length of hospital stay, (4) mortality, (5) pancreatic fistula, and (6) infection.

Statistical Analysis

For the baseline characteristics, we applied the *Chi*-squared test for categorical variables and Student's t-test for continuous variables. The mean and standard deviation (S.D.) of the continuous variables were estimated using the median, range and the number of patients [18]. *P-values* less than 0.05 were considered statistically significant. With respect to the outcomes, data from the original articles were extracted and analyzed using the Review Manager 5.1 software (Cochrane Collaboration). The I^2 index was used as an indicator of the between-study

Table 1. Clinical characteristics of the included studies.

First author	Publi-cation year	Study design	Surgical techniques of PRPD group	DGE definition	Gender (M: F)			Age (Mean ± S.D.)		
					PRPD	PPPD	P value	PRPD	PPPD	P value
Akizuki [4]	2008	PNR	SSPPD	NGT ≥ POD 10 or Solid food ≥ POD 14	18, 12	20, 14	0.56	65±10	66±13	0.56
Di Carlo [21]	1999	PNR	SWP	NGT> POD 10 or Vomiting> POD 10	24, 15	46, 28	0.95	61.1±8.8	62.0±8.3	0.59
Duffy [22]	2003	Retro	SWP	NGT ≥ POD 7 or Oral Intake ≥ POD 7	14, 9	20. 12	1.00	67.3±9.3	67.3±14.0	1.00
Fujii [23]	2012	Retro	SSPPD SWP	ISGPS Grade B/C	74, 51	19, 14	1.00	63.7±7.3	63.8±12.0	0.95
Gao [24]	2007	Retro	SWP	NGT ≥ POD 10 or Solid food ≥ POD 14	64, 40	23, 19	0.57	58.2±11.9	58.4±14.5	0.93
Hackert [25]	2013	PNR	PrPD	ISGPS Grade B/C	22, 18	22, 18	1.00	65.0±10.0	65.0±10.0	1.00
Hayashibe [26]	2007	Retro	SSPPD	NGT ≥ POD 10 or Regular diet ≥ POD 14	8, 13	4, 8	0.70	64.3±9.5	60.9±8.5	0.40
Hoem [27]	2012	PNR	SWP		22, 16	24, 18	1.00	69.5±9.8	66.0±12.3	0.17
Horstmann [28]	2004	PNR	SWP	NGT> POD 7 or Regular diets> POD 14				62	59	
Jimenez [29]	2000	Retro	SWP	Oral intake> POD 14	16, 17	20, 19	1.00	50.0±15.5	45.0±15.8	0.18
Kawai [3]	2011	RCT	PrPD	ISGPS Grade B/C	38, 28	33, 31	0.60	67±9	68±9	0.58
Kurahara [30]	2010	Retro	SSPPD	ISGPS Grade B/C	38, 26	26, 22	0.58	66.8	66.4	0.24
Lin [31]	2005	RCT	SWP	NGT ≥ POD 10	13, 6	10, 4	1.00	66.7±9.5	64.5±8.5	0.50
Makhija [32]	2002	PNR	SWP	NGT> POD 7						
Matsumoto [19]	2014	RCT	SSPPD	ISGPS Grade B/C	35, 15	29, 21	0.30	67±9	66±10	0.81
Mosca [33]	1997	Retro	SWP	NGT> POD 14						
Nanashima [34]	2013	Retro	SSPPD	ISGPS Grade B/C	15, 12	21, 7	0.22	66±12	68±8	0.56
Paquet [35]	1998	RCT	SWP							
Patel [36]	1995	Retro	SWP	Oral fluids ≥7 POD	28, 24	6,9	0.39	63.0±15.0	61.3±13.6	0.70
Pirro [37]	2002	Retro	SWP	NGT> POD 7						
Roder [38]	1992	PNR	SWP		32, 30	28, 20	0.56	60.0±12.5	64.0±9.5	0.07
Seiler [39]	2005	RCT	SWP	NGT> POD 5	33, 33	36, 28	0.29	65.0±13.2	64.8±14.3	0.30
Srinarmwong [40]	2008	RCT	SWP	NGT ≥ POD 10 or Regular diet ≥ POD 90	8, 5	10, 4	0.69	62.5±5.8	62.2±6.6	0.93
Takahashi [41]	1999	Retro	SWP							
Tani [42]	2009	Retro	SWP	NGT ≥ POD 10 or Regular diet ≥ POD 14	11, 6	18, 20	0.26	65.0±12.6	69.3±8.8	0.15

Table 1. Cont.

First author	Publi-cation year	Study design	Surgical techniques of PRPD group	DGE definition	Gender (M: F)			Age (Mean ± S.D.)		
					PRPD	PPPD	P value	PRPD	PPPD	P value
Tran [43]	2004	RCT	SWP	NGT ≥ POD 10 or Regular diet ≥ POD 14	50, 37	58, 25	0.11	62.0±8.5	64.0±5.8	0.27
Van Berge Henegouwen [44]	1997	PNR	SWP	NGT ≥ POD 10 or Regular diet ≥ POD 14	55, 45	45, 55	0.20	58.8±9.0	62.0±10.0	0.10

Abbreviations: PRPD, pylorus-removing pancreaticoduodenectomy; PrPD, pylorus-resecting pancreaticoduodenectomy; SSPPD, subtotal stomach-preserving pancreaticoduodenectomy; SWP, Standard Whipple procedure; PNR, Prospective nonrandomized study. Retro, Retrospective Study; RCT, Randomized Controlled Trial; NGT, Nasogastric tube; POD, Postoperative day.

heterogeneity. We used meta-regression to identify potential variables causing the heterogeneity. The meta-regression analysis and Duval's trim and fill correction were conducted by Comprehensive Meta Analysis Version 2.2 (Biostat, Englewood, NJ, USA). For meta-regression analyses, the factors were predefined. All of the following factors were previously reported to influence the incidence of DGE and were thus used as variables: preoperative diabetes, pancreatic fistula, postoperative complications, preoperative biliary drainage, method of reconstruction, percentage of malignancies, DGE evaluation method, nasogastric tube (NGT) intubation and solid food start time for the conventional method, and the use of prokinetic medicine [15,19,20]. Other common variables that were also routinely included were publication year, study design, total patient number, patient number in PRPD group, patient number in PPPD group, blood loss, operation time and infection. Subgroup analyses were conducted to assess the different surgical techniques of PRPD.

Results

Literature Search

Our search strategy yielded 4,076 abstracts from the aforementioned five databases. After the exclusion of duplications, two reviewers independently reviewed 2,055 abstracts. In this step, case reports, review articles, letters to the editor, editorials and conference abstracts were excluded. Abstracts that did not compare PRPD with PPPD or that did not report the incidence of DGE were also excluded. Thus, twenty-seven original articles were included, and the full-text of the manuscripts were read and evaluated [3,4,19,21–44]. Finally, we included all twenty-seven studies for this systematic review and meta-analysis with an inter-reviewer reliability of kappa = 0.978 ($P<0.001$) (Figure 1).

2,599 patients were included (1,289 who underwent PRPD and 1,310 who underwent PPPD). The publication year ranged from 1992 to 2014. Seven studies were RCTs, eight studies were prospective nonrandomized studies, and another twelve studies were retrospective ones. Nineteen studies featured SWP as a procedure for the pyloric removal group; five studies used SSPPD, and two studies used PrPD. One study [23] featured both SSPPD and SWP as PRPD. The definition of DGE varied across the studies; therefore, we listed the detailed information for each in Table 1. The gender and age of patients in the two groups were not significantly different.

For nonrandomized studies, a modified table that included the key components of the Newcastle-Ottawa quality assessment tool was employed to assess the quality and the risk of publication bias [17,45]. The modified table focused on the representativeness, comparability, ascertainment of exposure and follow-up. The overall bias was also estimated at the end of the table (Table S1).

Primary Outcomes

The overall DGE incidence of PRPD to PPPD was not significantly different. First, we analyzed the effect of pylorus removal for all included studies. The I^2 index was 63%, which indicated that heterogeneity was moderate to high. We used meta-regression to explore the potential variables that might account for the heterogeneity. We used method of movement as the calculation method and considered a variable to be significant if the P value in 'Model' section was less than 0.05 (Table 2). Four variables showed statistical significance for the meta-regression, which were patient number in PPPD group, presence of

Table 2. Meta-regression for variables that influence the incidence of DGE.

Variables	Model		Residual	
	(Qmodel)	P value	(Qresid)	P value
Study Design (Randomized Versus Nonrandomized)	0.011	0.912	28.964	0.266
Surgery Type (SWP Versus SSPPD/PrPD)	3.320	0.068	30.248	0.215
Method of Reconstruction (Antecolic versus Retrocolic)	1.100	0.294	9.571	0.386
DGE Evaluation Method (Whether using ISGPS Grading System)	3.583	0.058	29.820	0.231
Prokinetic Medicine Usage (Whether routinely used)*	NA	NA	NA	NA
Total Patients Number	2.674	0.102	27.974	0.309
Patients Number in PRPD group	0.176	0.675	28.359	0.292
Patients Number in PPPD group	5.534	0.019	28.956	0.266
Publication Year	0.655	0.419	29.573	0.241
Operation Time	2.353	0.125	18.219	0.197
Blood Loss	0.126	0.722	17.224	0.244
Percentage of Malignancies	0.068	0.793	27.095	0.300
Pancreatic Fistula	2.018	0.155	28.096	0.256
Infection	0.013	0.908	25.957	0.302
Postoperative Complications	0.084	0.771	26.731	0.268
Preoperative Diabetes	10.271	0.001	4.861	0.431
Preoperative Biliary Drainage	0.087	0.767	3.364	0.339
NGT Intubation Period	4.104	0.043	7.442	0.490
Solid Food Start Time for Conventional Methods†	3.864	0.049	8.302	0.504

*Only one study reported the routine use of prokinetic medicine, and thus the meta-regression for this variable could not be conducted.
†Solid food start days were obtained from the original publications or from the authors. If this parameter was not available, the mean days solid food in the PPPD (the conventional method) group was used.
Abbreviations: PRPD, pylorus-removing pancreaticoduodenectomy; PrPD, pylorus-resecting pancreaticoduodenectomy; SSPPD, subtotal stomach-preserving pancreaticoduodenectomy; SWP, Standard Whipple procedure; NGT, Nasogastric tube.

preoperative diabetes, NGT intubation time and solid food start time. For each variable, we aimed to identify studies that might contribute to the heterogeneity. Two studies [26,34] featured a longer NGT intubation period and solid food start time. In detail, the NGT intubation time was over POD 11 and the solid food start time was over POD 15 for these two studies. One of them [34] also had a higher rate of preoperative diabetes, with 67.3% of total patients diagnosed of diabetes. We also sequentially removed studies with the smallest number of participants in PPPD group. Three studies [26,31,40] was removed, with PPPD patient number of 12, 14 and 14, respectively. Therefore, four studies [26,31,34,40] were removed from further analysis with a reduced heterogeneity ($I^2 = 51\%$).

The remaining 23 studies were included in the meta-analysis using a random-effect model. The MH odds ratio was 0.61 (95% CI: 0.41–0.88; $P<0.01$) (Figure 2A). However, publication bias was detected by Egger's test ($P = 0.05$). Then, Duval's trim and fill method was used to correct the result (Figure 2B). Six potential missing studies were replaced to the right of the mean odds ratio, which were illustrated as black dots. The MH odds ratio was 0.78 (95% CI: 0.52–1.17) after correction. Therefore, we concluded that the removal of the pylorus did not reduce the overall incidence of DGE.

Next, we wanted to evaluate whether different surgical techniques within the PRPD group would have different impacts on DGE. The PRPD group contained three different surgical techniques, namely SSPPD, PrPD and SWP. Two of them, SSPPD and PrPD, were similar, because both preserve the majority of the stomach. In contrast, SWP usually resects 20–40% of the stomach volume. Therefore, we conducted subgroup analyses of SWP, SSPPD, PrPD and SSPPD/PrPD, respectively.

The DGE incidence of SWP to PPPD was not significantly different. With respect to SWP, eighteen studies were included. The MH odds ratio was 0.64 (95% CI: 0.40–1.00; $P = 0.05$, random-effect model) with moderate heterogeneity ($I^2 = 57\%$) (Figure 3A). Although publication bias was not significant by Egger's test ($P = 0.069$), Duval's trim and fill method could replace four missing studies to the right of the mean odds ratio (Figure 3B). After correction, the MH odds ratio was 0.85 (95% CI: 0.53–1.38).

The DGE incidence of SSPPD to PPPD was significantly different. With respect to SSPPD, four studies were included. The MH odds ratio was 0.46 (95% CI: 0.25–0.83; $P = 0.01$, fixed-effect model) with little heterogeneity ($I^2 = 24\%$) (Figure 3C). No significant publication bias was detected by Egger's test ($P = 0.56$). The removal of the pylorus did reduce the incidence of DGE after SSPPD compared with PPPD.

The DGE incidence of PrPD to PPPD was significantly different. With respect to PrPD, only two studies were included. The MH odds ratio was 0.31 (95% CI: 0.11–0.91; $P = 0.03$, fixed-effect model) with little heterogeneity ($I^2 = 0\%$) (Figure 3D). Egger's test was not conducted due to the low number of included studies. The removal of the pylorus did reduce the incidence of DGE after PrPD compared with PPPD.

The DGE incidence of SSPPD/PrPD to PPPD was significantly different. With respect to SSPPD/PrPD, six

A

Study or Subgroup	PRPD Events	PRPD Total	PPPD Events	PPPD Total	Weight	Odds Ratio M-H, Random, 95% CI
Akizuki et al, 2008	3	30	3	34	3.3%	1.15 [0.21, 6.17]
Di Carlo et al, 1999	6	39	9	74	5.3%	1.31 [0.43, 4.00]
Duffy et al, 2003	3	23	7	32	3.9%	0.54 [0.12, 2.34]
Fujii et al, 2012	7	125	9	33	5.5%	0.16 [0.05, 0.47]
Gao et al, 2007	19	104	15	42	6.8%	0.40 [0.18, 0.90]
Hackert et al, 2013	3	40	9	40	4.2%	0.28 [0.07, 1.12]
Hoem et al, 2012	3	38	1	42	2.1%	3.51 [0.35, 35.32]
Horstmann et al, 2004	4	19	13	113	4.8%	2.05 [0.59, 7.12]
Jimenez et al, 2000	4	33	13	39	4.8%	0.28 [0.08, 0.95]
Kawai et al, 2011	2	66	5	64	3.3%	0.37 [0.07, 1.97]
Kurahara et al, 2010	9	64	10	48	5.9%	0.62 [0.23, 1.67]
Makhija et al, 2002	1	32	2	48	1.9%	0.74 [0.06, 8.54]
Matsumoto et al, 2014	5	50	10	50	5.1%	0.44 [0.14, 1.41]
Mosca et al, 1997	1	61	14	157	2.5%	0.17 [0.02, 1.32]
Paquet et al, 1998	1	23	6	17	2.2%	0.08 [0.01, 0.78]
Patel et al, 1995	21	52	9	15	5.1%	0.45 [0.14, 1.46]
Pirro et al, 2002	10	28	7	35	5.2%	2.22 [0.72, 6.90]
Roder et al, 1992	0	62	9	48	1.5%	0.03 [0.00, 0.59]
Seiler et al, 2005	30	66	20	64	7.3%	1.83 [0.90, 3.76]
Takahashi et al, 1999	1	54	1	22	1.5%	0.40 [0.02, 6.63]
Tani et al, 2009	1	17	10	38	2.4%	0.17 [0.02, 1.50]
Tran et al, 2004	18	83	19	87	7.2%	0.99 [0.48, 2.05]
Van Berge Henegouwen et al, 1997	34	100	37	100	8.0%	0.88 [0.49, 1.57]
Total (95% CI)		**1209**		**1242**	**100.0%**	**0.61 [0.41, 0.88]**
Total events	186		238			

Heterogeneity: $Tau^2 = 0.37$; $Chi^2 = 45.17$, df = 22 (P = 0.003); $I^2 = 51\%$
Test for overall effect: Z = 2.61 (P = 0.009)

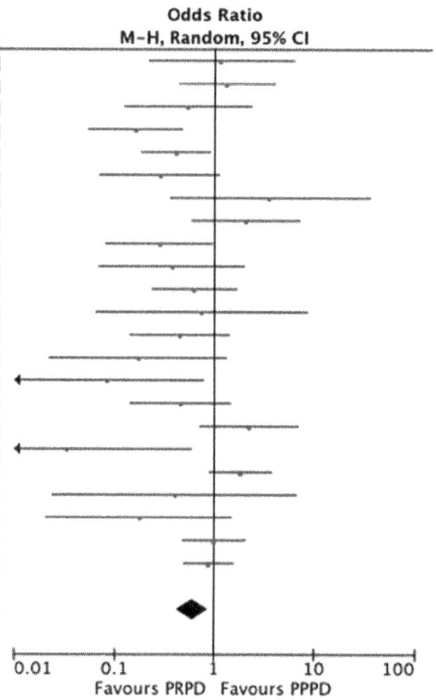

B

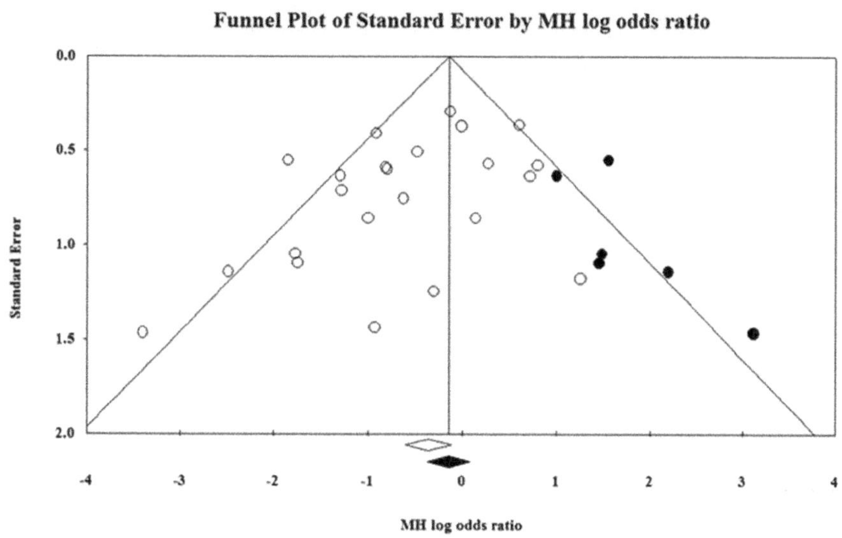

Figure 2. Delayed gastric emptying (DGE) incidence for overall studies. A. Meta-analysis of DGE of twenty-three studies. **B**. Funnel plot of Duval's trim and fill correction of DGE incidence for the twenty-three studies. Included studies are illustrated as white dots. Potential missing studies are illustrate as black dots.

studies were included. The MH odds ratio was 0.41 (95% CI: 0.25–0.70; $P<0.01$, fixed-effect model) with little heterogeneity ($I^2 = 0\%$) (Figure 3E). No significant publication bias was detected by Egger's test ($P = 0.77$). The removal of the pylorus did reduce the incidence of DGE after SSPPD/PrPD compared with PPPD.

Secondary Outcomes

PRPD significantly increased blood loss (Figures S1), operation time (Figures S2) and mortality (Figures S4). Other parameters, including length of hospital stay (Figures S3), pancreatic fistula (Figures S5) and infection (Figures S6), were not significantly different between the PRPD and PPPD groups. Detailed information was summarized in Table 3.

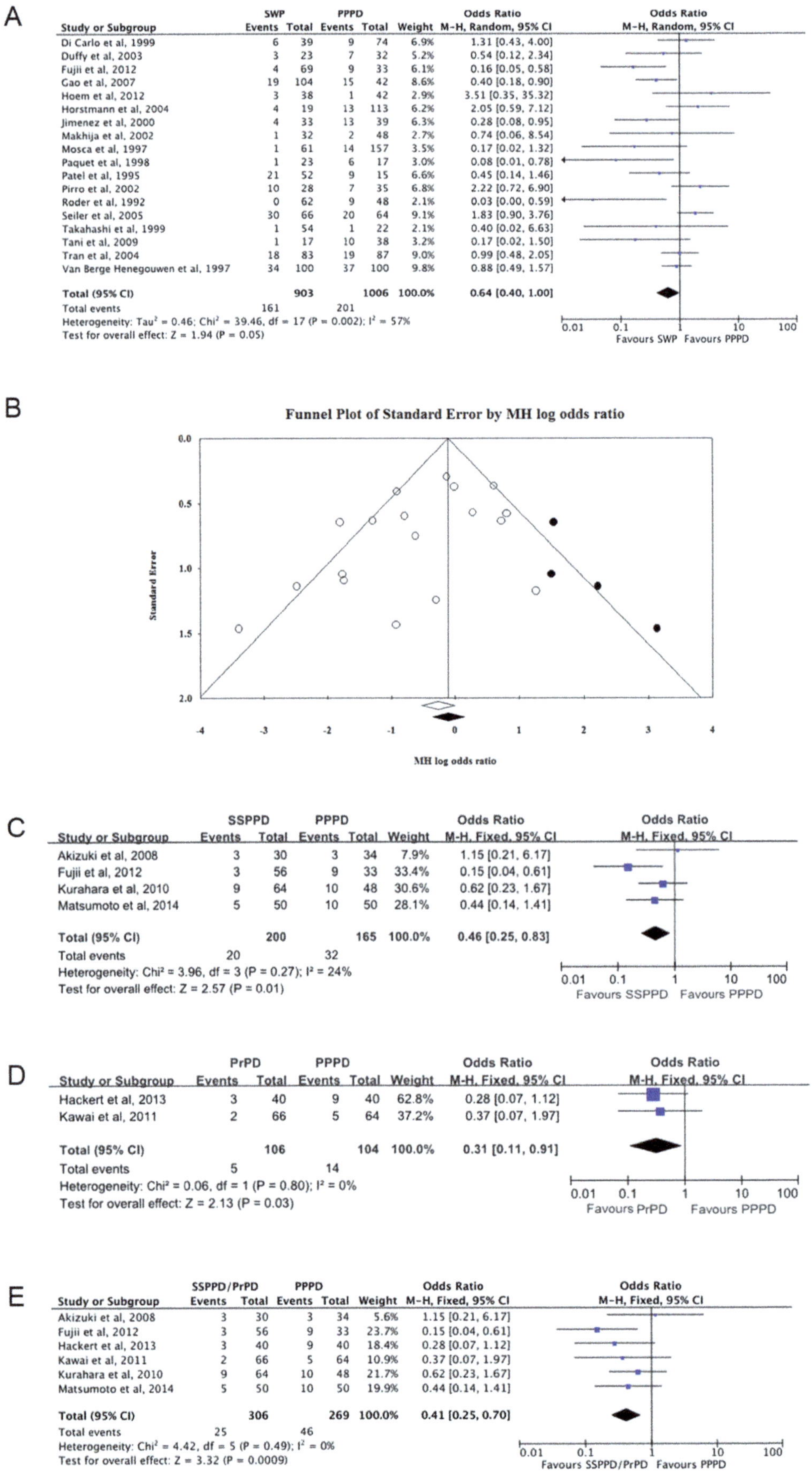
A
Study or Subgroup | SWP Events | SWP Total | PPPD Events | PPPD Total | Weight | Odds Ratio M-H, Random, 95% CI
Di Carlo et al, 1999 6 39 9 74 6.9% 1.31 [0.43, 4.00]
Duffy et al, 2003 3 23 7 32 5.2% 0.54 [0.12, 2.34]
Fujii et al, 2012 4 69 9 33 6.1% 0.16 [0.05, 0.58]
Gao et al, 2007 19 104 15 42 8.6% 0.40 [0.18, 0.90]
Hoem et al, 2012 3 38 1 42 2.9% 3.51 [0.35, 35.32]
Horstmann et al, 2004 4 19 13 113 6.2% 2.05 [0.59, 7.12]
Jimenez et al, 2000 4 33 13 39 6.3% 0.28 [0.08, 0.95]
Makhija et al, 2002 1 32 2 48 2.7% 0.74 [0.06, 8.54]
Mosca et al, 1997 1 61 14 157 3.5% 0.17 [0.02, 1.32]
Paquet et al, 1998 1 23 6 17 3.0% 0.08 [0.01, 0.78]
Patel et al, 1995 21 52 9 15 6.6% 0.45 [0.14, 1.46]
Pirro et al, 2002 10 28 7 35 6.8% 2.22 [0.72, 6.90]
Roder et al, 1992 0 62 9 48 2.1% 0.03 [0.00, 0.59]
Seiler et al, 2005 30 66 20 64 9.1% 1.83 [0.90, 3.76]
Takahashi et al, 1999 1 54 1 22 2.1% 0.40 [0.02, 6.63]
Tani et al, 2009 1 17 10 38 3.2% 0.17 [0.02, 1.50]
Tran et al, 2004 18 83 19 87 9.0% 0.99 [0.48, 2.05]
Van Berge Henegouwen et al, 1997 34 100 37 100 9.8% 0.88 [0.49, 1.57]
Total (95% CI) 903 1006 100.0% 0.64 [0.40, 1.00]
Total events 161 201
Heterogeneity: Tau² = 0.46; Chi² = 39.46, df = 17 (P = 0.002); I² = 57%
Test for overall effect: Z = 1.94 (P = 0.05)
Odds Ratio M-H, Random, 95% CI
0.01 0.1 1 10 100
Favours SWP Favours PPPD
B
Funnel Plot of Standard Error by MH log odds ratio
Standard Error
0.0 0.5 1.0 1.5 2.0
-4 -3 -2 -1 0 1 2 3 4
MH log odds ratio
C
Study or Subgroup | SSPPD Events | SSPPD Total | PPPD Events | PPPD Total | Weight | Odds Ratio M-H, Fixed, 95% CI
Akizuki et al, 2008 3 30 3 34 7.9% 1.15 [0.21, 6.17]
Fujii et al, 2012 3 56 9 33 33.4% 0.15 [0.04, 0.61]
Kurahara et al, 2010 9 64 10 48 30.6% 0.62 [0.23, 1.67]
Matsumoto et al, 2014 5 50 10 50 28.1% 0.44 [0.14, 1.41]
Total (95% CI) 200 165 100.0% 0.46 [0.25, 0.83]
Total events 20 32
Heterogeneity: Chi² = 3.96, df = 3 (P = 0.27); I² = 24%
Test for overall effect: Z = 2.57 (P = 0.01)
Odds Ratio M-H, Fixed, 95% CI
0.01 0.1 1 10 100
Favours SSPPD Favours PPPD
D
Study or Subgroup | PrPD Events | PrPD Total | PPPD Events | PPPD Total | Weight | Odds Ratio M-H, Fixed, 95% CI
Hackert et al, 2013 3 40 9 40 62.8% 0.28 [0.07, 1.12]
Kawai et al, 2011 2 66 5 64 37.2% 0.37 [0.07, 1.97]
Total (95% CI) 106 104 100.0% 0.31 [0.11, 0.91]
Total events 5 14
Heterogeneity: Chi² = 0.06, df = 1 (P = 0.80); I² = 0%
Test for overall effect: Z = 2.13 (P = 0.03)
Odds Ratio M-H, Fixed, 95% CI
0.01 0.1 1 10 100
Favours PrPD Favours PPPD
E
Study or Subgroup | SSPPD/PrPD Events | SSPPD/PrPD Total | PPPD Events | PPPD Total | Weight | Odds Ratio M-H, Fixed, 95% CI
Akizuki et al, 2008 3 30 3 34 5.6% 1.15 [0.21, 6.17]
Fujii et al, 2012 3 56 9 33 23.7% 0.15 [0.04, 0.61]
Hackert et al, 2013 3 40 9 40 18.4% 0.28 [0.07, 1.12]
Kawai et al, 2011 2 66 5 64 10.9% 0.37 [0.07, 1.97]
Kurahara et al, 2010 9 64 10 48 21.7% 0.62 [0.23, 1.67]
Matsumoto et al, 2014 5 50 10 50 19.9% 0.44 [0.14, 1.41]
Total (95% CI) 306 269 100.0% 0.41 [0.25, 0.70]
Total events 25 46
Heterogeneity: Chi² = 4.42, df = 5 (P = 0.49); I² = 0%
Test for overall effect: Z = 3.32 (P = 0.0009)
Odds Ratio M-H, Fixed, 95% CI
0.01 0.1 1 10 100
Favours SSPPD/PrPD Favours PPPD

Figure 3. Subgroup analyses for delayed gastric emptying (DGE) incidence. A. Subgroup analysis of DGE for patients with SWP. **B**. Funnel plot of Duval's trim and fill correction of DGE incidence for the SWP studies. Included studies are illustrated as white dots. Potential missing studies are illustrate as black dots. **C**. Subgroup analysis of DGE for patients with SSPPD. **D**. Subgroup analysis of DGE for patients with PrPD. **E**. Subgroup analysis of DGE for patients with SSPPD/PrPD.

Discussion

DGE prolongs the hospitalization and the quality of life of patients. The removal of the pylorus is believed to influence the incidence of DGE, because postoperative pyloric dysfunction could occur secondary to devascularization and denervation [7,8,46]. Whether the removal of additional area of the pylorus during PPPD reduces the incidence of DGE has been investigated by several studies and is a matter of debate. It is necessary to realize that DGE is affected by various confounding factors, such as the route of reconstruction, prokinetic drug usage and the postoperative recovery program [3,47,48]. Different studies may not be consistent with respect to these factors, which would increase heterogeneity across studies. In contrast, a single study may suffer from an inadequate number of patients needed to reach adequate statistical power. Therefore, it is critical to identify the major confounding factors that would explain the heterogeneity. The subsequent analysis would be possible and meaningful after the exclusion of studies most accountable for the heterogeneity.

We first tested the heterogeneity concerning the incidence of DGE, which was moderate-high. To explore the potential variables, we conducted meta-regression analyses for the list of nineteen variables. Four of them showed statistical significance for the meta-regression. A longer solid food start time or NGT intubation time was associated with a greater reduction of DGE in the RPPD, compared with the PPPD group. In fact, the solid food start time was an important indicator of postoperative management. Balzano et al reported that the incidence of DGE would reduce for fast-track recovery program compared with the conventional method after pancreaticoduodenectomy [48]. Therefore, whether an additional resection of the pylorus could reduce the incidence of DGE should be evaluated within studies with a similar solid food start time and NGT intubation time. Another confounding factor, preoperative diabetes, has also been reported as a risk factor for DGE by a recent meta-analysis [15]. As for the number of patients in PPPD group, we sequentially excluded studies with the smallest patient number. When we excluded the studies with fewer than 15 patients, the patient number was no longer significantly contributed to the overall heterogeneity of DGE. In summary, four studies were excluded after meta-regression analysis, and a 12% reduction of I^2 index was achieved by the exclusion. A meta-analysis of the remaining 23 studies showed no significantly difference whether or not the pylorus was removed.

Next, we were interested in the different surgical techniques within the PRPD group. The major difference lay in the resected proportion of the stomach. The SSPPD and PrPD procedures only involve the resection of a relatively small portion of the pyloric stomach compared with SWP. SSPPD and PrPD are intended to preserve the pooling ability of the stomach [4]. Because DGE is closely related to stomach function, different surgical techniques in the PRPD group should be analyzed separately. A subgroup analysis showed that SSPPD, PrPD and SSPPD/PrPD, but not SWP, reduced the incidence of DGE. We interpreted the results in the following ways: 1) Preservation of the majority of stomach during the resection of the pylorus may help reduce the incidence of DGE; and 2) Because the SSPPD group only had four studies, PrPD group only contained only two studies, these results should be interpreted with cautions. More studies are needed to validate the results.

As for secondary outcomes, PRPD tended to involve a longer operation time, more blood loss and a higher mortality rate. However, the length of hospital stay was not significantly different. Similarly, the incidence of pancreatic fistula and infection was not significantly different between the two groups.

We acknowledged that our meta-analysis has several limitations. First, only four and two studies in SSPPD and PrPD group, respectively; therefore, the conclusion that removal of additional portions of the pylorus would significantly reduce the incidence of DGE after SSPPD or PrPD needs to be validated by more well-designed, prospective randomized studies with adequate patient sample sizes. Second, studies included in this meta-analysis were more non-RCTs than RCTs; therefore, cautions should be taken when interpreting the results from the analysis. We expect better designed studies to address whether or not SSPPD or PrPD will truly reduce DGE incidence.

In conclusion, this meta-analysis shows that pylorus removal doesn't reduce the overall incidence of DGE, compared with pylorus-preservation procedure. Subgroup analysis shows that pylorus removal may reduce the incidence of DGE when patients undergo SSPPD or PrPD. However, pylorus removal doesn't

Table 3. Outcomes of blood loss, operation time, and length of hospital stay, mortality, pancreatic fistula and infection after PRPD versus PPPD.

Outcomes	No. Patients	No. Studies	Risk Difference/Mean Difference (95% CI)	P value	I^2 index
Blood Loss	1417	16	273 (129, 418)	<0.01	67%
Operation Time	1408	16	35.6 (17.3, 53.9)	<0.01	75%
Length of Hospital Stay	1262	13	0.05 (−1.74, 1.85)	0.95	43%
Mortality	2487	26	0.02 (0.00, 0.03)	0.02	0%
Pancreatic Fistula	2467	26	0.00 (−0.03, 0.03)	0.96	41%
Infection	2229	24	0.01 (−0.01, 0.04)	0.29	0%

Abbreviations: PRPD, pylorus-removing pancreaticoduodenectomy; PPPD, pylorus-preserving pancreaticoduodenectomy.

significantly reduce the incidence of DGE when patients undergo SWP.

Supporting Information

Figure S1 Forest plot of blood loss for included studies. Blood loss is significant more in PRPD than PPPD. Abbreviations: PRPD, pylorus-removing pancreaticoduodenectomy; PPPD, pylorus-preserving pancreaticoduodenectomy.

Figure S2 Forest plot of operation time for included studies. Operation time is significant longer in PRPD than PPPD.Abbreviations: PRPD, pylorus-removing pancreaticoduodenectomy; PPPD, pylorus-preserving pancreaticoduodenectomy.

Figure S3 Forest plot of length of hospital stay for included studies. There is no significant difference between PRPD and PPPD.Abbreviations: PRPD, pylorus-removing pancreaticoduodenectomy; PPPD, pylorus-preserving pancreaticoduodenectomy.

Figure S4 Forest plot of mortality for included studies. Mortality incidence is significant higher in PRPD than PPPD.Abbreviations: PRPD, pylorus-removing pancreaticoduodenectomy; PPPD, pylorus-preserving pancreaticoduodenectomy.

Figure S5 Forest plot of pancreatic fistula for included studies. There is no significant difference between PRPD and PPPD.Abbreviations: PRPD, pylorus-removing pancreaticoduodenectomy; PPPD, pylorus-preserving pancreaticoduodenectomy.

Figure S6 Forest plot of infection for included studies. There is no significant difference between PRPD and PPPD.Abbreviations: PRPD, pylorus-removing pancreaticoduodenectomy; PPPD, pylorus-preserving pancreaticoduodenectomy.

Table S1 Study quality assessment and the risk of publication bias by Newcastle-Ottawa quality tool for non-randomized studies.

Checklist S1 PRISMA checklist for this meta-analysis.

Acknowledgments

The authors thank Prof. Thilo Hackert, Department of Surgery, University of Heidelberg, Germany, for his kindly help in providing original data for this meta-analysis.

Author Contributions

Conceived and designed the experiments: WW XH LF YZ. Performed the experiments: WW XH LF SL LY LZ. Analyzed the data: WW XH LF SL LY LZ. Contributed reagents/materials/analysis tools: WW XH LF SL LY LZ. Wrote the paper: WW XH LF.

References

1. Traverso L, Longmire W Jr (1978) Preservation of the pylorus in pancreaticoduodenectomy. Surgery, gynecology & obstetrics 146: 959–962.
2. Watson K (1944) Carcinoma of ampulla of vater successful radical resection. British Journal of Surgery 31: 368–373.
3. Kawai M, Tani M, Hirono S, Miyazawa M, Shimizu A, et al. (2011) Pylorus ring resection reduces delayed gastric emptying in patients undergoing pancreatoduodenectomy: a prospective, randomized, controlled trial of pylorus-resecting versus pylorus-preserving pancreatoduodenectomy. Ann Surg 253: 495–501.
4. Akizuki E, Kimura Y, Nobuoka T, Imamura M, Nishidate T, et al. (2008) Prospective nonrandomized comparison between pylorus-preserving and subtotal stomach-preserving pancreaticoduodenectomy from the perspectives of DGE occurrence and postoperative digestive functions. J Gastrointest Surg 12: 1185–1192.
5. Schafer M, Mullhaupt B, Clavien PA (2002) Evidence-based pancreatic head resection for pancreatic cancer and chronic pancreatitis. Ann Surg 236: 137–148.
6. Wente MN, Bassi C, Dervenis C, Fingerhut A, Gouma DJ, et al. (2007) Delayed gastric emptying (DGE) after pancreatic surgery: a suggested definition by the International Study Group of Pancreatic Surgery (ISGPS). Surgery 142: 761–768.
7. Liberski SM, Koch KL, Atnip RG, Stern RM (1990) Ischemic gastroparesis: resolution after revascularization. Gastroenterology 99: 252–257.
8. Kim DK, Hindenburg AA, Sharma SK, Suk CH, Gress FG, et al. (2005) Is pylorospasm a cause of delayed gastric emptying after pylorus-preserving pancreaticoduodenectomy? Ann Surg Oncol 12: 222–227.
9. Gauvin JM, Sarmiento JM, Sarr MG (2003) Pylorus-preserving pancreaticoduodenectomy with complete preservation of the pyloroduodenal blood supply and innervation. Arch Surg 138: 1261–1263.
10. Fischer CP, Hong JC (2006) Method of pyloric reconstruction and impact upon delayed gastric emptying and hospital stay after pylorus-preserving pancreaticoduodenectomy. J Gastrointest Surg 10: 215–219.
11. Karanicolas PJ, Davies E, Kunz R, Briel M, Koka HP, et al. (2007) The pylorus: take it or leave it? Systematic review and meta-analysis of pylorus-preserving versus standard whipple pancreaticoduodenectomy for pancreatic or periampullary cancer. Ann Surg Oncol 14: 1825–1834.
12. Iqbal N, Lovegrove RE, Tilney HS, Abraham AT, Bhattacharya S, et al. (2008) A comparison of pancreaticoduodenectomy with pylorus preserving pancreaticoduodenectomy: a meta-analysis of 2822 patients. Eur J Surg Oncol 34: 1237–1245.
13. Diener Markus K, Fitzmaurice C, Schwarzer G, Seiler Christoph M, Antes G, et al. (2011) Pylorus-preserving pancreaticoduodenectomy (pp Whipple) versus pancreaticoduodenectomy (classic Whipple) for surgical treatment of periampullary and pancreatic carcinoma. Cochrane Database of Systematic Reviews: John Wiley & Sons, Ltd.
14. Yang C, Wu H-S, Chen X-L, Wang C-Y, Gou S-M, et al. (2014) Pylorus-Preserving Versus Pylorus-Resecting Pancreaticoduodenectomy for Periampullary and Pancreatic Carcinoma: A Meta-Analysis. PloS one 9: e90316.
15. Qu H, Sun GR, Zhou SQ, He QS (2013) Clinical risk factors of delayed gastric emptying in patients after pancreaticoduodenectomy: a systematic review and meta-analysis. Eur J Surg Oncol 39: 213–223.
16. Liberati A, Altman DG, Tetzlaff J, Mulrow C, Gotzsche PC, et al. (2009) The PRISMA statement for reporting systematic reviews and meta-analyses of studies that evaluate healthcare interventions: explanation and elaboration. BMJ 339: b2700.
17. Wells GA, Shea B, O'Connell D, Peterson J, Welch V, et al. (2000) The Newcastle-Ottawa Scale (NOS) for assessing the quality of nonrandomised studies in meta-analyses. Available: http://www.ohri.ca/programs/clinical_epidemiology/oxford.htm/. Accessed March 2014.
18. Hozo SP, Djulbegovic B, Hozo I (2005) Estimating the mean and variance from the median, range, and the size of a sample. BMC Med Res Methodol 5: 13.
19. Matsumoto I, Shinzeki M, Asari S, Goto T, Shirakawa S, et al. (2014) A prospective randomized comparison between pylorus- and subtotal stomach-preserving pancreatoduodenectomy on postoperative delayed gastric emptying occurrence and long-term nutritional status. J Surg Oncol 109: 690–696.
20. Sato G, Ishizaki Y, Yoshimoto J, Sugo H, Imamura H, et al. (2014) Factors influencing clinically significant delayed gastric emptying after subtotal stomach-preserving pancreatoduodenectomy. World J Surg 38: 968–975.
21. Di Carlo V, Zerbi A, Balzano G, Corso V (1999) Pylorus-preserving pancreaticoduodenectomy versus conventional whipple operation. World J Surg 23: 920–925.
22. Duffy JP, Hines OJ, Liu JH, Ko CY, Cortina G, et al. (2003) Improved survival for adenocarcinoma of the ampulla of Vater: Fifty-five consecutive resections. Archives of Surgery 138: 941–950.
23. Fujii T, Kanda M, Kodera Y, Nagai S, Sahin TT, et al. (2012) Preservation of the pyloric ring has little value in surgery for pancreatic head cancer: a comparative study comparing three surgical procedures. Ann Surg Oncol 19: 176–183.
24. Gao HQ, Yang YM, Zhuang Y, Wang WM, Wu WH, et al. (2007) [Influencing factor analysis of delayed gastric emptying after pylorus-preserving pancreaticoduodenectomy]. Zhonghua Wai Ke Za Zhi 45: 1048–1051.
25. Hackert T, Hinz U, Hartwig W, Strobel O, Fritz S, et al. (2013) Pylorus resection in partial pancreaticoduodenectomy: impact on delayed gastric emptying. Am J Surg 206: 296–299.

26. Hayashibe A, Kameyama M, Shinbo M, Makimoto S (2007) The surgical procedure and clinical results of subtotal stomach preserving pancreaticoduodenectomy (SSPPD) in comparison with pylorus preserving pancreaticoduodenectomy (PPPD). J Surg Oncol 95: 106–109.
27. Hoem D, Viste A (2012) Improving survival following surgery for pancreatic ductal adenocarcinoma–a ten-year experience. Eur J Surg Oncol 38: 245–251.
28. Horstmann O, Markus PM, Ghadimi MB, Becker H (2004) Pylorus preservation has no impact on delayed gastric emptying after pancreatic head resection. Pancreas 28: 69–74.
29. Jimenez RE, Fernandez-del Castillo C, Rattner DW, Chang Y, Warshaw AL (2000) Outcome of pancreaticoduodenectomy with pylorus preservation or with antrectomy in the treatment of chronic pancreatitis. Ann Surg 231: 293–300.
30. Kurahara H, Takao S, Shinchi H, Mataki Y, Maemura K, et al. (2010) Subtotal stomach-preserving pancreaticoduodenectomy (SSPPD) prevents postoperative delayed gastric emptying. J Surg Oncol 102: 615–619.
31. Lin PW, Shan YS, Lin YJ, Hung CJ (2005) Pancreaticoduodenectomy for pancreatic head cancer: PPPD versus Whipple procedure. Hepatogastroenterology 52: 1601–1604.
32. Makhija R, Tsai P, Kingsnorth A (2002) Pylorus-preserving pancreatoduodenectomy with Billroth I type reconstruction: a viable option for pancreatic head resection. J Hepatobiliary Pancreat Surg 9: 614–619.
33. Mosca F, Giulianotti PC, Balestracci T, Di Candio G, Pietrabissa A, et al. (1997) Long-term survival in pancreatic cancer: pylorus-preserving versus Whipple pancreatoduodenectomy. Surgery 122: 553–566.
34. Nanashima A, Abo T, Sumida Y, Tobinaga S, Nonaka T, et al. (2013) Comparison of results between pylorus-preserving pancreaticoduodenectomy and subtotal stomach-preserving pancreaticoduodenectomy: report at a single cancer institute. Hepatogastroenterology 60: 1182–1188.
35. Paquet KJ (1998) Comparison of Whipple's pancreaticoduodenectomy with the pylorus-preserving pancreaticoduodenectomy - a prospectively controlled, randomized long-term trial. Chirurgische Gastroenterologie 14: 54–58.
36. Patel AG, Toyama MT, Kusske AM, Alexander P, Ashley SW, et al. (1995) Pylorus-preserving Whipple resection for pancreatic cancer. Is it any better? Arch Surg 130: 838–842; discussion 842–833.
37. Pirro N, Sielezneff I, Cesari J, Consentino B, Gregoire R, et al. (2002) Pancreaticoduodenectomy for adenocarcinoma of the head of pancreas: does the pylorus-preserving change morbidity and prognosis? Annales De Chirurgie 127: 95–100.
38. Roder JD, Stein HJ, Huttl W, Siewert JR (1992) Pylorus-preserving versus standard pancreatico-duodenectomy: an analysis of 110 pancreatic and periampullary carcinomas. Br J Surg 79: 152–155.
39. Seiler CA, Wagner M, Bachmann T, Redaelli CA, Schmied B, et al. (2005) Randomized clinical trial of pylorus-preserving duodenopancreatectomy versus classical Whipple resection-long term results. Br J Surg 92: 547–556.
40. Srinarmwong C, Luechakiettisak P, Prasitvilai W (2008) Standard whipple's operation versus pylorus preserving pancreaticoduodenectomy: a randomized controlled trial study. J Med Assoc Thai 91: 693–698.
41. Takahashi S, Aiura K, Saitou J, Hayatsu S, Hoshimoto S, et al. (1999) PpPD and PD for advanced carcinoma of the head of the pancreas. Japanese Journal of Gastroenterological Surgery 32: 2427–2431.
42. Tani M, Kawai M, Hirono S, Ina S, Miyazawa M, et al. (2009) Pylorus-preserving pancreaticoduodenectomy versus conventional pancreaticoduodenectomy for pancreatic adenocarcinoma. Surg Today 39: 219–224.
43. Tran KTC, Smeenk HG, van Eijck CHJ, Kazemier G, Hop WC, et al. (2004) Pylorus preserving pancreaticoduodenectomy versus standard Whipple procedure - A prospective, randomized, multicenter analysis of 170 patients with pancreatic and periampullary tumors. Annals of Surgery 240: 738–745.
44. van Berge Henegouwen MI, van Gulik TM, DeWit LT, Allema JH, Rauws EA, et al. (1997) Delayed gastric emptying after standard pancreaticoduodenectomy versus pylorus-preserving pancreaticoduodenectomy: an analysis of 200 consecutive patients. J Am Coll Surg 185: 373–379.
45. Yin Z, Fan X, Ye H, Yin D, Wang J (2013) Short- and long-term outcomes after laparoscopic and open hepatectomy for hepatocellular carcinoma: a global systematic review and meta-analysis. Ann Surg Oncol 20: 1203–1215.
46. Kurosaki I, Hatakeyama K (2005) Preservation of the left gastric vein in delayed gastric emptying after pylorus-preserving pancreaticoduodenectomy. J Gastrointest Surg 9: 846–852.
47. Ohwada S, Satoh Y, Kawate S, Yamada T, Kawamura O, et al. (2001) Low-dose erythromycin reduces delayed gastric emptying and improves gastric motility after Billroth I pylorus-preserving pancreaticoduodenectomy. Ann Surg 234: 668–674.
48. Balzano G, Zerbi A, Braga M, Rocchetti S, Beneduce AA, et al. (2008) Fast-track recovery programme after pancreatico- duodenectomy reduces delayed gastric emptying. Br J Surg 95: 1387–1393.

Risk of Hospitalization for Community Acquired Pneumonia with Renin-Angiotensin Blockade in Elderly Patients: A Population-Based Study

Sachin Shah[1], Eric McArthur[3], Alexandra Farag[1], Michael Nartey[1], Jamie L. Fleet[1], Greg A. Knoll[4], S. Joseph Kim[5], Amit X. Garg[1,2,3], Arsh K. Jain[1,2,3]*

1 Division of Nephrology, Department of Medicine, Western University, London, Ontario, Canada, **2** Department of Epidemiology and Biostatistics, Western University, London, Ontario, Canada, **3** Institute for Clinical Evaluative Sciences, London, Ontario, Canada, **4** Division of Nephrology, Kidney Research Centre, Ottawa Hospital Research Institute, University of Ottawa, Ottawa, Ontario, Canada, **5** Division of Nephrology, Toronto General Hospital, University Health Network, University of Toronto, Toronto, Ontario, Canada

Abstract

Objective: To characterize the 90-day risk of hospitalization with pneumonia among patients treated with different anti-hypertensive drug classes.

Design: Population based cohort study using five linked databases.

Participants: Individuals over the age of 65 who filled a new outpatient prescription for one of four anti-hypertensive medications: ACE inhibitors (n = 86 775), ARBs (n = 33 953), calcium channel blockers (CCB, n = 34 240), beta blockers (BB, n = 35 331) and thiazide diuretics (n = 64 186).

Primary Outcome: Hospitalization with pneumonia within 90 days of a qualifying prescription. We adjusted for ten *a priori* selected covariates, including age, sex, diabetes and number of visits to a family doctor.

Results: Baseline characteristics of the groups were relatively well matched, except for age, sex, diabetes and frequency of family doctor visits. 128 of the 86 775 patients (0.15%) initiated on an ACE inhibitor and 43 of the 33953 patients (0.13%) of patients initiated on an ARB were hospitalized with pneumonia in the subsequent 90 days. 135 of 64 186 patients (0.21%) initiated on a thiazide, 112 of 35 331 patients (.32%) initiated on a BB, and 89 of 34 240 (0.26%) patients initiated on a CCB achieved the primary outcome. Compared to calcium channel blockers, ACE inhibitors (adjusted OR 0.61, 95% CI 0.46 to 0.81) and ARBs (adjusted OR 0.52, 95% CI 0.36 to 0.76) were associated with a lower risk of pneumonia. No benefit was seen with thiazides (adjusted OR 0.87, 95% CI 0.66 to 1.14) or beta blockers (adjusted OR 1.21, 95% CI 0.91 to 1.60).

Conclusion: Initiating medications that block the renin angiotensin system, compared to other anti-hypertensive medications, is associated with a small absolute reduction in the 90 day risk of hospitalization with pneumonia.

Editor: Ryuichi Morishita, Osaka University Graduate School of Medicine, Japan

Funding: This project was conducted at the Institute for Clinical Evaluative Sciences (ICES) Western Site. ICES is funded by an annual grant from the Ontario Ministry of Health and Long-term Care. ICES@Western is funded by an operating grant from the Academic Medical Organization of Southwestern Ontario. Dr. Jain receives unrestricted grant support from the Academic Medical Organization of Southwestern Ontario. The opinions, results and conclusions reported in this paper are those of the authors and are independent of the funding sources. The funders had no role in study design, data collection and analysis, decision to publish, or preparation of the manuscript.

Competing Interests: The authors have declared that no competing interests exist.

* Email: arsh.jain@lhsc.on.ca

Introduction

Community-acquired pneumonia (CAP) is commonly encountered in clinical practice and its incidence increases with age [1,2]. It is the eighth leading cause of death in Canada and the United States and the leading cause of infection-related hospitalization [3]. Following hospitalization for pneumonia, 30-day mortality rates have been reported as high as 23% [3]. This significant clinical burden has prompted attempts to identify strategies that may reduce the incidence of CAP. Specifically, there is a growing body of literature demonstrating a reduced incidence of pneumonia in patients treated with angiotensin converting enzyme (ACE) inhibitors [4–8]. While not fully understood, the proposed mechanism by which ACE inhibitors may protect against pneumonia is related to improvement in both cough and swallowing reflexes, an effect thought to be mediated through increased levels of substance P and bradykinins [9–14].

Recently, a meta-analysis of randomized and non-randomized studies demonstrated a reduced risk of pneumonia in ACE inhibitor users [6]. No benefit was seen with ARBs, which is consistent with the proposed mechanism, as this class of medication does not affect substance P and bradykinin levels [15]. However, rather interestingly, there was a trend towards a reduced risk of pneumonia with ARBs when only randomized trials were considered (odds ratio (OR) for pneumonia 0.9, 95% confidence interval (CI) 0.79 to 1.01).

Given these heterogeneous results, we conducted the current study to characterize the 90-day risk for hospitalization with pneumonia in a large population of older adults initiated on ACE inhibitors, ARBs, beta blockers (BB) or thiazides in a routine outpatient care setting. We compared these patients to a similar group of older adults prescribed a calcium-channel blocker (CCB). We hypothesized that a reduction in the incidence of pneumonia would be seen with both ACE inhibitors and ARBs when compared to the CCBs, but no benefit would be seen with thiazides or BBs.

Methods

Ethics

We conducted this study according to a prespecified protocol that was approved by the Research Ethics Board at Sunnybrook Health Sciences Centre (Toronto, Ontario, Canada).

Study Design and Setting

We conducted a population-based retrospective cohort study using health administrative data from Ontario, Canada. Ontario is Canada's most populous province with approximately 13 million residents who receive universal access to hospital and physician services (Statistics Canada). Ontario's 1.8 million residents over the age of 65 years also receive prescription drug coverage.

Data Sources

We used five linked databases housed at the Institute for Clinical Evaluative Sciences to conduct this study. We ascertained vital statistics from the Registered Persons Database (RPDB). The RPDB records the demographic information for people issued a provincial health card. We used the Ontario Drug Benefits (ODB) database to ascertain prescription drug exposure, including the independent variables and drug-related baseline characteristics. The ODB records prescription drug use for patients over the age of 65 years (a universal benefit) and has an error rate of <1% [16]. We identified admissions to hospital and baseline characteristics using the Canadian Institute for Health Information Discharge Abstract Database (CIHI-DAD). The CIHI-DAD records hospital admissions and related diagnostic and procedural information. For similar information relating to emergency department admissions, we used the National Ambulatory Care Reporting System (NACRS) database. We used the Ontario Health Insurance Plan (OHIP) database to ascertain information relating to physician services.

Patients

We restricted enrollment to patients over the age of 65 years who, between June 1, 2003 and December 31, 2011, filled a prescription for any of five drug classes: ACE inhibitor, ARB, CCB, BB or thiazide. We chose to use a new user design with 90 day outcomes in order to reduce the incidence of intervening health events that may have biased patient outcome. We excluded all individuals who, in the prior 180 days, were taking any type of anti-hypertensive, diuretic or anti-arrhythmic. In order to compare mutually exclusive groups, we excluded patients who had filled a prescription for more than one study drug class on the day the new prescription was filled. To help further limit confounding by indication, we excluded any conditions that may dictate use of one study drug over the other. These exclusions were baseline evidence of coronary artery disease or congestive heart failure or chronic kidney disease. All comorbidities were assessed in the five years preceding the qualifying prescription, except for chronic kidney disease (one year). Finally, to further reduce the risk of recent health events influencing prescription choice we excluded patients who were admitted to hospital in the 90 days preceding the qualifying prescription date, or visited an emergency department in the 30 days preceding the qualifying prescription date.

Outcomes

All outcomes were assessed in the 90 days after initiation of one of the study drugs (ACE inhibitor, ARB, BB, thiazide or CCB). We chose 90 day outcomes for two reasons. First, the short duration of follow-up was felt to help mitigate against the risk of contamination (such as crossing-over from one study drug class to another or adding in a different study drug). Second, prescriptions covered by the provincial drug plan are prescribed at no more than 100-day intervals. We assessed the rates of contamination directly by looking at how many patients in each study group received an alternate study drug during follow-up.

Primary outcome: Admission to hospital with pneumonia. We defined the primary outcome of hospital admission with pneumonia as any admission with a J12-J18 or P23 International Classification of Diseases, 10th revision (ICD-10) diagnostic code in any of the CIHI-DAD's diagnostic fields. In patients greater than 65 years of age who are in a hospitalized setting, similar codes have been shown to be extremely accurate in identifying cases of pneumonia (sensitivity and specificity about 98% and 97%, respectively).

In a sensitivity analysis, we restricted our primary outcome to patients whose primary reason for admission was pneumonia. We achieved this by using one of the aforementioned diagnostic codes, but restricting to the "admitdx" field only in the CIHI-DAD.

Sub-group analysis: Diabetes. Given the increased risk of pneumonia with diabetes and the possibility that these patients would not be equally distributed among the groups, we performed a sub-group analysis of patients with and without diabetes. We assessed for any effect modification of diabetes on the association of anti-hypertensive medication type and our primary outcome. Diabetics were identified as any patient who filled a prescription for a medication used to treat diabetes (insulin or oral hypoglycemic) in the 180 days preceding the qualifying prescription.

Tracer Outcome: Hospitalization with cholecystitis. We tested the specificity of our findings by determining each group's risk of cholecystitis, an outcome we did not expect to be influenced by the choice of anti-hypertensive medication. We defined cholecystitis as any admission 90 days following the prescription date with the ICD-10 diagnosis code K8000, K8001, K8010, K8011, K8040, K8041, K81 found in any of the CIHI-DAD's diagnostic fields. We also used provider claim diagnosis codes 574 and 575 submitted by healthcare providers.

Statistical methods

We compared the prevalence of baseline characteristics between the medication groups (ACE, ARB, thiazides, BB and CCB) using standardized differences with CCB acting as the referent group. This metric describes differences between group means as a proportion of the pooled standard deviation. Larger values

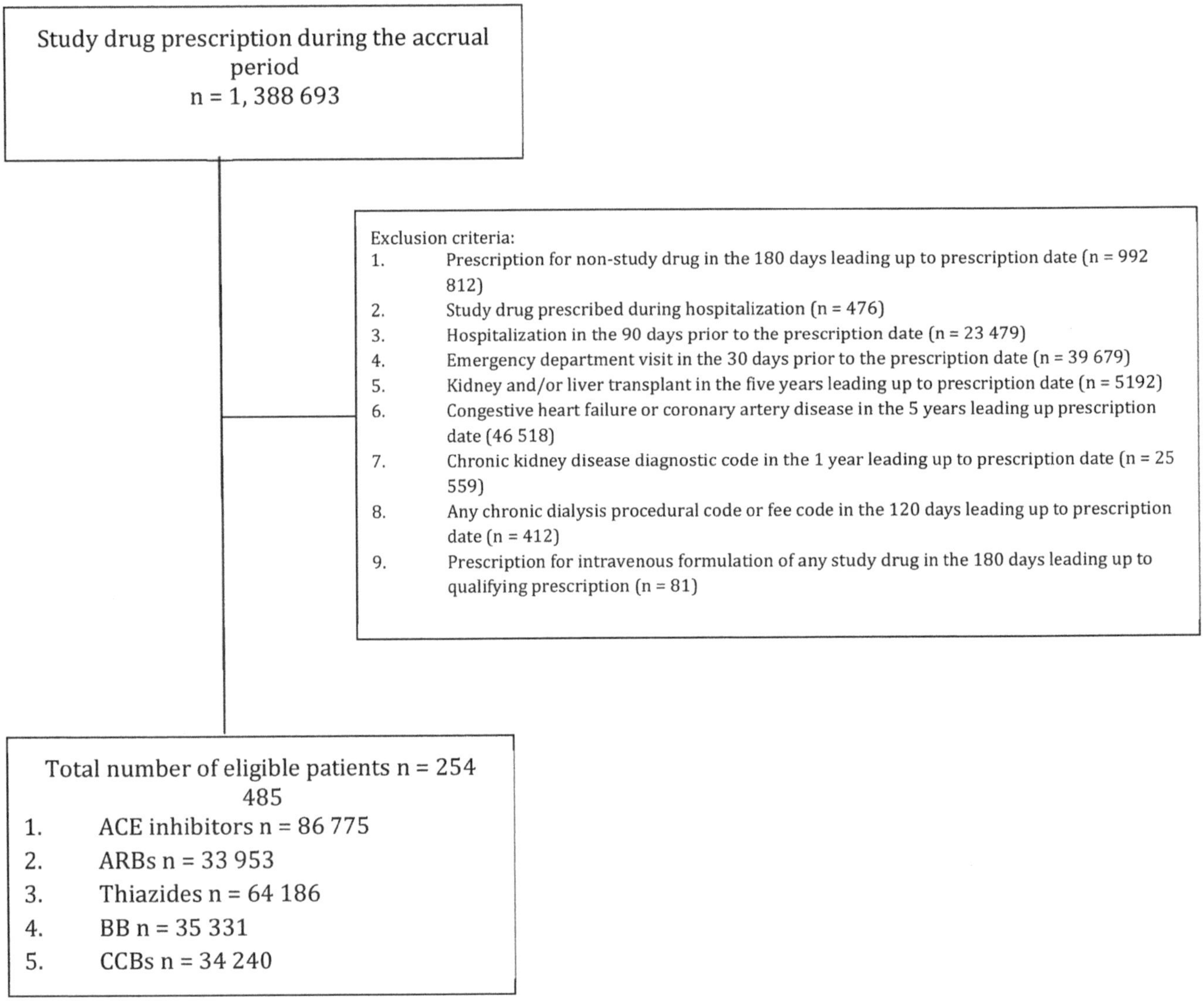

Figure 1. Flow diagram for the construction of our cohort.

indicate larger differences and those greater than 10% are considered meaningful [17,18].

The administrative datasets at the Institute for Clinical Evaluative Sciences allowed for essentially 100% follow-up on all patients during the 90-day risk period. We used a multivariable logistic regression model to adjust for the following ten covariates selected *a priori*: age, sex, number of different visits to a family doctor in the one year preceding the prescription date, Charlson Co-morbidity Index Score, chronic liver disease, pneumonia, chronic lung disease (including asthma and COPD), stroke, diabetes mellitus, and dementia. Baseline characteristics were assessed in the five years preceding the qualifying prescription. We conducted all analysis with SAS 9.2 (SAS Institute Incorporated, Cary, North Carolina, USA, 2008). A two-sided P value of <0.05 was considered statistically significant.

Results

Figure 1 shows the steps of cohort assembly. Over the study period, we identified 254 485 patients who met enrollment criteria, of whom 86 775 (34.0%) filled a prescription for an ACE inhibitor, 33 953 (13.3%) for an ARB, 34 240 (13.5%) for a CCB, 35 331 for a BB (13.9%), and 64 186 (25.2%) for a thiazide (Table 1). Mean age was 73.4 years. Total person-years follow-up for the entire cohort was 53 916.

Table 1 shows the distribution of baseline characteristics across anti-hypertensive agent groups. Of the 10 baseline characteristics analyzed, six baseline characteristics were similarly distributed across the two groups, with standardized differences less than 0.1. However, women were more likely to receive a thiazide followed by a CCB and then an ACE inhibitor. Patients receiving an ACE inhibitor or ARB were slightly younger than those receiving a thiazide or CCB. Patients on an ACE inhibitor, ARB or thiazide were more likely to have seen a family doctor three or more times in the year leading up to the prescription date. Patients receiving a BB were more likely to have been prescribed a greater number of individual drugs in the year leading up to the index. Patients with diabetes were more likely to be on an ACE inhibitor or ARB compared to a CCB, and were more likely to be on a CCB compared to a thiazide.

Table 1. Baseline characteristics by study drug class use.

Variable		ACE		ARB		THIAZIDE		Beta Blocker		CCB		Standardized Differences[1] (ACE vs CCB)	Standardized Differences[1] (ARB vs CCB)	Standardized Differences[1] (THI vs CCB)	Standardized Differences[1] BB vs CCB)
Total Patients	**N**	**86775**		**33953**		**64186**		**35331**		**34240**					
Female	**N**	44988	51.84%	19181	56.49%	43742	68.15%	21411	60.60%	20617	60.21%	0.17	0.08	0.17	0.01
Age	**Mean (or Median)**	73.01		72.66		73.93		73.46		73.91		0.15	0.20	0.00	0.07
	SD (or IQR)	5.94		5.82		6.46		6.4		6.46					
	65–69.9	30802	35.50%	12951	38.14%	20200	31.47%	12329	34.90%	10769	31.45%	0.09	0.14	0.00	0.07
	70–74.9	25914	29.86%	9974	29.38%	18009	28.06%	9648	27.31%	9703	28.34%	0.03	0.02	0.01	0.02
	75–79.9	16868	19.44%	6339	18.67%	13035	20.31%	6849	19.39%	6855	20.02%	0.01	0.03	0.01	0.02
	80–84.9	8914	10.27%	3229	9.51%	8182	12.75%	4149	11.74%	4394	12.83%	0.08	0.11	0.00	0.03
	85–89.9	3263	3.76%	1124	3.31%	3465	5.40%	1721	4.87%	1806	5.27%	0.07	0.10	0.01	0.02
	≥90	1014	1.17%	336	0.99%	1295	2.02%	635	1.80%	713	2.08%	0.07	0.09	0.00	0.02
Visits to Primary Care Providers	**Mean (or Median)**	9.85		9.71		9.44		10.76		9.54		0.03	0.02	0.01	0.11
	SD (or IQR)	9.42		8.51		9.51		11.5		9.79					
	0	5185	5.98%	2193	6.46%	4354	6.78%	2453	6.94%	3364	9.82%	0.14	0.12	0.11	0.10
	1–2	9410	10.84%	3618	10.66%	7751	12.08%	3953	11.19%	4483	13.09%	0.07	0.08	0.03	0.06
	≥3	72180	83.18%	28142	82.89%	52081	81.14%	28925	81.87%	26393	77.08%	0.15	0.15	0.10	0.12
Charlson Comorbidity Index Score	**0**	76352	87.99%	30950	91.16%	58654	91.38%	31570	89.35%	31251	91.27%	0.11	0.00	0.00	0.06
	1	4909	5.66%	1303	3.84%	2192	3.42%	1484	4.20%	1252	3.66%	0.10	0.01	0.01	0.03
	2	3892	4.49%	1265	3.73%	2512	3.91%	1597	4.52%	1259	3.68%	0.04	0.00	0.01	0.04
	≥3	1622	1.87%	435	1.28%	828	1.29%	680	1.92%	478	1.40%	0.04	0.01	0.01	0.04
Comorbid conditions[2]	**Chronic Liver Disease**	2195	2.53%	1031	3.04%	1349	2.10%	1018	2.88%	939	2.74%	0.01	0.02	0.04	0.01
	Diabetes Mellitus	22190	25.57%	4760	14.02%	2189	3.41%	2405	6.81%	2117	6.18%	0.55	0.26	0.13	0.03
	≥1 Pneumonia in previous 5 years	696	0.80%	196	0.58%	526	0.82%	389	1.10%	284	0.83%	0.00	0.03	0.00	0.03

Table 1. Cont.

Variable		ACE		ARB		THIAZIDE		Beta Blocker		CCB		Standardized Differences[1] (ACE vs CCB)	Standardized Differences[1] (ARB vs CCB)	Standardized Differences[1] (THI vs CCB)	Standardized Differences[1] BB vs CCB)
Total Patients	N	86775		33953		64186		35331		34240					
	COPD and/or chronic lung disease and/ or asthma	14377	16.57%	6020	17.73%	11254	17.53%	5332	15.09%	6101	17.82%	0.03	0.00	0.01	0.07
	Stroke	495	0.57%	91	0.27%	241	0.38%	272	0.77%	131	0.38%	0.03	0.02	0.00	0.05
	Dementia	3910	4.51%	1178	3.47%	3260	5.08%	2085	5.90%	1534	4.48%	0.00	0.05	0.03	0.06

Abbreviations: SD, standard deviation; n, number; ACE, angiotensin converting enzyme; ARB, angiotensin receptor blocker; CCB, calcium channel blocker; BB, beta blocker.
[1]The standardized difference is the difference between group means expressed as a proportion of that characteristic's pooled standard deviation. It is less sensitive to sample size than hypothesis testing. Standardized differences greater than 0.1 are considered significant.
[2]Comorbidities were identified using administrative codes in the five years preceding the qualifying anti-hypertensive prescription.date, chronic lung disease, stroke, dementia.

Primary Outcome

Results of the primary outcome are presented in Table 2. Those prescribed a CCB were used as the referent group. A total of 128 patients (0.15%) initiated on an ACE inhibitor and 43 patients (0.13%) initiated on an ARB were hospitalized with pneumonia in the subsequent 90 days. In contrast, 135 patients (0.21%) initiated on a thiazide, 112 (0.32%) of patients initiated on a BB, and 89 patients (0.26%) initiated on a CCB achieved the primary outcome. Prescription for ACE inhibitors was associated with a lower risk of hospital admission with pneumonia (adjusted OR 0.61, 95% CI0.46 to 0.81). A similar benefit was seen with ARBs (adjusted OR 0.52, 95% CI 0.36 to 0.76). In contrast, no benefit was seen with thiazides (adjusted OR 0.87, 95% CI 0.66 to 1.14) or BB (adjusted OR 1.21, 95% CI 0.91 to 1.60).

In our sensitivity analysis, with a more conservative definition of pneumonia, the results were similar (table 3).

Table 4 shows the contamination rates of each study group. Contamination with another study drug occurred 15–20% of the time. Of note, Thiazides, BBs, and CCBs were most commonly contaminated by a drug from either the ACE inhibitor or ARB drug class.

Sub-group Analysis

There was no evidence that the presence or absence of diabetes modified the association between anti-hypertensive type and 90-day hospitalization with pneumonia (p-value for interaction >.08 for each medication class). In patients without diabetes mellitus, a benefit on pneumonia rates was seen with both ACE inhibitors (adjusted OR 0.67, 95% CI 0.50 to.89) and ARBs (adjusted OR 0.49, 95% CI 0.32 to 0.75). In patients with diabetes (14.3% of the cohort), the benefit was consistent for those patients on ACE inhibitors (adjusted OR 0.29, 95% CI 0.13 to 0.65). No significant benefit was seen with ARBs (adjusted OR 0.61, 95% CI 0.27 to 1.74), recognizing that the number of events was small (ARB group n = 11 and CCB (referent) group n = 8).

Tracer Outcome

Using CCB as the referent group, the risk of hospital admission for cholecystitis was not significantly different for patients on ACE inhibitors (adjusted OR 0.94, 95% CI 0.75 to 1.17), ARBs (adjusted OR 0.91, 95% CI 0.69 to 1.19), BBs (adjusted OR 1.10, 95% CI 0.84 to 1.40), or thiazides (adjusted OR 0.80, 95% CI 0.63 to 1.02).

Discussion

In this population-based cohort study, we observed adult patients who were initiated on an ACE inhibitor, ARB, BB or thiazide in the outpatient setting and compared them to patients who were started on CCBs. We followed these patients for hospitalization with pneumonia within 90 days of filling their prescription. Similar to previous studies, we observed a significant reduction in pneumonia rates in patients prescribed an ACE inhibitor. In contrast to previous studies, we found that this protective effect also extended to ARBs. No such benefit was seen when thiazides and BBs were compared to CCBs.

Our study adds to the growing body of literature surrounding ACE inhibitor use and its potential to curb the incidence of pneumonia. The magnitude of benefit for ACE inhibitors was consistent with previously published reports, and in particular, a recent meta-analysis (adjusted OR 0.61 in our study vs. adjusted OR 0.66 in the meta-analysis) [6]. Interestingly, in our study both ACE inhibitors and ARBs had a fairly robust benefit with a similar adjusted OR (0.52 with ARBs). The latter is quite intriguing given

Table 2. Association between antihypertensive use and hospital admissions for pneumonia.

	Number of events, n (%)	Relative Risk [95% CI]	
		Unadjusted	Adjusted*
ACE inhibitor	128 (0.15%)	0.57 [0.43, 0.74]	0.61 [0.46, 0.81]
ARB	43 (0.13%)	0.49 [0.34, 0.70]	0.52 [0.36, 0.76]
Thiazide	135 (0.21%)	0.81 [0.62, 1.06]	0.87 [0.66, 1.14]
BB	112 (0.32%)	1.22 (0.92, 1.61)	1.21 (0.91, 1.60)
CCB	89 (0.26%)	1.00	1.00

Abbreviations: CI, confidence interval; ACE, angiotensin converting enzyme; ARB, angiotensin receptor blocker; CCB, calcium channel blocker; BB, beta blocker. For each analysis, patients prescribed calcium channel blockers were the referent group.

* Adjustment was by multivariable logistic regression modeling with the following variables: age, sex, primary care provider visits, Charlson comorbidity index score, chronic liver failure, pneumonia in the 5 years leading up to prescription date, chronic lung disease, stroke, dementia, diabetes.

the meta-analysis described above, which failed to show a reduction in the incidence of pneumonia with ARBs. As already noted, there was a discrepancy between the randomized and the two observational studies included in the meta-analysis [20,21], and when only randomized studies were analyzed, there was a trend towards benefit with ARBs.

There are multiple potential reasons for the discrepancy between our results and the previous observational studies assessing ARB use. Etminan et al. [19] examined patients with coronary artery disease exclusively. Further, only about three percent of the cases and controls studied were taking ACE inhibitors or ARBs. Mukamal et al. [20] analyzed patients based on the anti-hypertensive drug class for which they held the longest prescription. However, patients could be on several study drug classes. As such, the benefit of ACE inhibitor and/or ARB use may have been masked as patients taking these drugs may have also been included in the control group. Lastly, both studies failed to demonstrate a protective role for ACE Inhibitors on pneumonia related hospitalization rates. As the protective effect of ACE inhibitors have been demonstrated in multiple populations, results of these two observational studies should be assessed with caution. Likely, there are issues with study design or residual confounding that have affected these studies.

There are several reasons why we are confident in our study's findings. First, the lack of benefit with thiazides and BBs provides evidence that the benefit seen is related solely to RAS blocking agents. As already mentioned, the magnitude of benefit with both ACE inhibitors and ARBs were quite similar, and in the case of ACE inhibitors, was consistent with a recent meta-analysis. It is worth mentioning that the rates of contamination were relatively small. However, given that thiazides, CCBs and BBs were most commonly contaminated RAS blocking agents, we would expect these intervening events to bias towards the null hypothesis, further bolstering our findings. Finally, our tracer outcome of cholecystitis showed no significant signal, also suggesting that residual confounding was not exerting a strong influence on our results.

Limitations

Our study has some important limitations. As with all observational studies, the exposures we studied were not randomly assigned. While the groups were well balanced on most covariates the risk of residual confounding cannot be ruled out.

Both ACE inhibitors and ARBs reduced the incidence of pneumonia related hospitalization. The relative risk reduction for both agents was impressive, however, the absolute risk reduction and event rate were quite small. While notable, we do not feel that this negates the findings of our study given the short duration of follow-up of our study.

The population studied here was highly selected and several conditions considered to be risk factors for pneumonia were excluded. While cohort restriction is a powerful method for controlling for confounding [21], and this helped reduce indication bias, it may have implications on the generalizability

Table 3. Association between antihypertensive use and hospital admissions for pneumonia using 'admit diagnosis' only (sensitivity analysis).

	Number of events, n (%)	Relative Risk [95% CI]	
		Unadjusted	Adjusted
ACE inhibitor	105 (0.12%)	0.56 [0.42, 0.75]	0.60 [0.44, 0.82]
ARB	33 (0.10%)	0.45 [0.30, 0.68]	0.50 [0.33, 0.77]
Thiazide	109 (0.17%)	0.79 [0.58, 1.06]	0.84 [0.62, 1.13]
BB	84 (0.24%)	1.1 (0.81, 1.50)	1.23 (0.82, 1.54)
CCB	74 (0.22%)	1.00	1.00

Abbreviations: CI, confidence interval; ACE, angiotensin converting enzyme; ARB, angiotensin receptor blocker; CCB, calcium channel blocker; BB, beta blocker. For each analysis, patients prescribed calcium channel blockers were the referent group. Adjustment was by multivariable logistic regression modeling with the following variables: age, sex, primary care provider visits, Charlson comorbidity index score, chronic liver failure, pneumonia in the 5 years leading up to prescription date, chronic lung disease, stroke, dementia, diabetes.

Table 4. Rates of contamination with non-index study drugs.

Index Study Drug	ACE		ARB		THI		BB		CCB	
	n	%	n	%	n	%	n	%	n	%
Contamination with any non-index study drug during follow-up	14720	17%	5000	15%	13448	21%	5319	15%	6904	20%
Contamination with any ACE inhibitor during follow-up	N/A	N/A	560	2%	8100	13%	2214	6%	2996	9%
Contamination with any ARB during follow-up	4308	5%	N/A	N/A	1901	3%	894	3%	1381	4%
Contamination with any thiazide during follow-up	6183	7%	2313	7%	N/A	N/A	1647	5%	2645	8%
Contamination with any BB during follow-up	2193	3%	858	3%	1875	3%	N/A	N/A	1409	4%
Contamination with any CCB during follow-up	4187	5%	2165	6%	3620	6%	1717	5%	N/A	N/A

Abbreviations: CI, confidence interval; ACE, angiotensin converting enzyme; ARB, angiotensin receptor blocker; CCB, calcium channel blocker; BB, beta blocker.

of our results. However, the main comorbidities excluded in our study (i.e. patients with congestive heart failure, coronary artery disease and chronic kidney disease) leave little flexibility in the choice of anti-hypertensive medication prescribed by physicians, and RAS blockade is typically indicated. For example, in patients with congestive heart failure, existing evidence would dictate the use of RAS blocking medications to reduce morbidity and mortality. The impact of RAS blocking agents on the incidence of pneumonia is unlikely to significantly bias a prescriber's choice in such situations, given their known benefits on cardiovascular health in the heart failure population [22]. In contrast, in our selected population, where clinicians are faced with clinical equipoise, our findings may support use of RAS blocking agents over other classes of anti-hypertensives. It should be noted that while several comorbidities were excluded, a large portion of our cohort were diabetic. As diabetes is a risk factor for the development of pneumonia, and diabetic patients may preferentially be prescribed RAS blocking agents for blood pressure management, we felt that the inclusion of this group would bias towards the null hypothesis if at all. Interestingly, diabetic status did not impact the results of the primary outcome in our subgroup analysis.

Finally, there is a paucity of literature surrounding the biologic rationale for a reduction in the incidence of pneumonia with both ACE inhibitors and ARBs. While benefit from ACE inhibitors has been thought to be due to increased substance p and bradykinin levels, these levels are unaffected by ARBs [15]. As such, there must be a second, mutually exclusive rationale for the benefit observed with ARBs, or, an alternative explanation for both ACE inhibitors and ARBs. One plausible explanation is a reduction in the inflammatory response seen with both ACE inhibitors and ARBs [23–25]. Specifically, by reducing the inflammatory response, ACE inhibitors and ARBs may reduce the severity of pneumonia, thereby preventing pneumonia related hospitalization. Our study did not capture the incidence of pneumonia as a whole, only those severe enough to require hospitalization. Some would argue that this is the most important outcome given its association with morbidity and mortality [3].

Conclusions

Initiation of a medication which blocks the renin angiotensin system, compared to other anti-hypertensive medications, is associated with a small 90-day reduction in the absolute risk of hospitalization with pneumonia. The magnitude of benefit seems to be similar between both ACE inhibitors and ARBs. When faced with clinical equipoise, such as in a population similar to the one studied here, physicians may preferentially prescribe one of these medications over other anti-hypertensives to help combat the morbidity associated with pneumonia. Further studies to corroborate our findings and identify potential mechanisms for this benefit are required.

Acknowledgments

We thank Brogan Inc, Ottawa, for use of its Drug Product and Therapeutic Class Database.

Author Contributions

Conceived and designed the experiments: SS AKJ AXG SJK GAK. Performed the experiments: EM. Analyzed the data: EM. Contributed reagents/materials/analysis tools: SS AKJ AXG SJK GAK EM MN AF JF. Wrote the paper: SS AKJ EM.

References

1. Marrie TJ (2000) Community-acquired pneumonia in the elderly. Clin Infect Dis 31: 1066–1078. Available: http://cid.oxfordjournals.org/content/31/4/1066.full. Accessed 2013 Jun 18.
2. Almirall J, Bolíbar I, Balanzó X, González CA (1999) Risk factors for community-acquired pneumonia in adults: a population-based case-control study. Eur Respir J 13: 349–355. Available: http://www.ncbi.nlm.nih.gov/pubmed/10065680.
3. Asadi L, Sligl WI, Eurich DT, Colmers IN, Tjosvold L, et al. (2012) Macrolide-based regimens and mortality in hospitalized patients with community-acquired pneumonia: a systematic review and meta-analysis. Clin Infect Dis 55: 371–380. Available: http://cid.oxfordjournals.org/content/55/3/371.full. Accessed 2013 May 27.
4. Ohkubo T, Chapman N, Neal B, Woodward M, Omae T, et al. (2004) Effects of an angiotensin-converting enzyme inhibitor-based regimen on pneumonia risk. Am J Respir Crit Care Med 169: 1041–1045. Available: http://www.ncbi.nlm.nih.gov/pubmed/14990394. Accessed 2013 Jun 18.
5. Sekizawa K, Matsui T, Nakagawa T, Nakayama K, Sasaki H (1998) ACE inhibitors and pneumonia. Lancet 352: 1069. Available: http://www.thelancet.com/journals/lancet/article/PIIS0140-6736(05)60114-6/fulltext. Accessed 2013 Jun 18.
6. Caldeira D, Alarcão J, Vaz-Carneiro A, Costa J (2012) Risk of pneumonia associated with use of angiotensin converting enzyme inhibitors and angiotensin receptor blockers: systematic review and meta-analysis. BMJ 345: e4260. Available: http://www.pubmedcentral.nih.gov/articlerender.fcgi?artid=3394697&tool=pmcentrez&rendertype=abstract. Accessed 2013 Jun 18.
7. Okaishi K (1999) Reduction of risk of pneumonia associated with use of angiotensin I converting enzyme inhibitors in elderly inpatients. Am J Hypertens 12: 778–783. Available: http://ajh.oxfordjournals.org/content/12/8/778.full. Accessed 2013 Jun 18.
8. Vinogradova Y, Hippisley-Cox J, Coupland C (2009) Identification of new risk factors for pneumonia: population-based case-control study. Br J Gen Pract 59: e329–38. Available: http://www.pubmedcentral.nih.gov/articlerender.fcgi?artid=2751937&tool=pmcentrez&rendertype=abstract. Accessed 2013 Jun 18.
9. Marik PE (2003) Aspiration Pneumonia and Dysphagia in the Elderly. Chest 124: 328–336. Available: http://journal.publications.chestnet.org/article.aspx?articleid=1081684&issueno=1&ijkey=c0cffa346c3a07901d8ab29aaad13ef71c3bc905&keytype2=tf_ipsecsha. Accessed 2013 May 23.
10. Israili ZH (1992) Cough and Angioneurotic Edema Associated with Angiotensin-Converting Enzyme Inhibitor Therapy: A Review of the Literature and Pathophysiology. Ann Intern Med 117: 234. Available: http://annals.org/article.aspx?articleid=705706. Accessed 2013 Jun 18.
11. Tomaki M, Ichinose M, Miura M, Hirayama Y, Kageyama N, et al. (1996) Angiotensin converting enzyme (ACE) inhibitor-induced cough and substance P. Thorax 51: 199–201. Available: http://thorax.bmj.com/content/51/2/199.abstract. Accessed 18 June 2013.
12. Nakayama K, Sekizawa K, Sasaki H (1998) ACE inhibitor and swallowing reflex. Chest 113: 1425. Available: http://www.ncbi.nlm.nih.gov/pubmed/9596334. Accessed 2013 Jun 18.
13. Morice AH, Lowry R, Brown MJ, Higenbottam T (1987) Angiotensin-converting enzyme and the cough reflex. Lancet 2: 1116–1118. Available: http://www.ncbi.nlm.nih.gov/pubmed/2890021. Accessed 2013 Jun 18.
14. Fox AJ, Lalloo UG, Belvisi MG, Bernareggi M, Chung KF, et al. (1996) Bradykinin-evoked sensitization of airway sensory nerves: a mechanism for ACE-inhibitor cough. Nat Med 2: 814–817. Available: http://www.ncbi.nlm.nih.gov/pubmed/8673930. Accessed 2013 Jun 18.
15. Arai T, Yasuda Y, Takaya T, Toshima S, Kashiki Y, et al. (2001) Angiotensin-converting enzyme inhibitors, angiotensin-II receptor antagonists, and pneumonia in elderly hypertensive patients with stroke. Chest 119: 660–661. Available: http://www.ncbi.nlm.nih.gov/pubmed/11171758. Accessed 2013 Jun 19.
16. Levy AR, O'Brien BJ, Sellors C, Grootendorst P, Willison D (2003) Coding accuracy of administrative drug claims in the Ontario Drug Benefit database. Can J Clin Pharmacol 10: 67–71. Available: http://www.ncbi.nlm.nih.gov/pubmed/12879144. Accessed 2013 Jun 19.
17. Austin PC (2009) Using the Standardized Difference to Compare the Prevalence of a Binary Variable Between Two Groups in Observational Research. Commun Stat - Simul Comput 38: 1228–1234. Available: http://dx.doi.org/10.1080/03610910902859574. Accessed 2013 Jun 19.
18. Mamdani M, Sykora K, Li P, Normand S-LT, Streiner DL, et al. (2005) Reader's guide to critical appraisal of cohort studies: 2. Assessing potential for confounding. BMJ 330: 960–962. Available: http://www.bmj.com/content/330/7497/960. Accessed 2013 Jun 7.
19. Etminan M, Zhang B, Fitzgerald M, Brophy JM (2006) Do angiotensin-converting enzyme inhibitors or angiotensin II receptor blockers decrease the risk of hospitalization secondary to community-acquired pneumonia? A nested case-control study. Pharmacotherapy 26: 479–482. Available: http://www.ncbi.nlm.nih.gov/pubmed/16553505. Accessed 2013 Jun 19.
20. Mukamal KJ, Ghimire S, Pandey R, O'Meara ES, Gautam S (2010) Antihypertensive medications and risk of community-acquired pneumonia. J Hypertens 28: 401–405. Available: http://www.ncbi.nlm.nih.gov/pubmed/20051911. Accessed 2013 Jun 19.
21. Joffe MM, Colditz GA (1998) Restriction as a method for reducing bias in the estimation of direct effects. Stat Med 17: 2233–2249. Available: http://www.ncbi.nlm.nih.gov/pubmed/9802181. Accessed 2013 Jun 10.
22. Yusuf S, Sleight P, Pogue J, Bosch J, Davies R, et al. (2000) Effects of an angiotensin-converting-enzyme inhibitor, ramipril, on cardiovascular events in high-risk patients. The Heart Outcomes Prevention Evaluation Study Investigators. N Engl J Med 342: 145–153. Available: http://www.ncbi.nlm.nih.gov/pubmed/10639539. Accessed 2013 May 22.
23. Hagiwara S, Iwasaka H, Matumoto S, Hidaka S, Noguchi T (2009) Effects of an angiotensin-converting enzyme inhibitor on the inflammatory response in in vivo and in vitro models. Crit Care Med 37: 626–633. Available: http://www.ncbi.nlm.nih.gov/pubmed/19114890. Accessed 2013 Jun 19.
24. Gonzalez NC, Allen J, Schmidt EJ, Casillan AJ, Orth T, et al. (2007) Role of the renin-angiotensin system in the systemic microvascular inflammation of alveolar hypoxia. Am J Physiol Heart Circ Physiol 292: H2285–94. Available: http://www.ncbi.nlm.nih.gov/pubmed/17208999. Accessed 2013 Jun 19.
25. Nahmod KA, Nahmod VE, Szvalb AD (2013) Potential Mechanisms of AT1 Receptor Blockers on Reducing Pneumonia-Related Mortality. Clin Infect Dis 56: 1193–1194. Available: http://cid.oxfordjournals.org/content/56/8/1193.full. Accessed 2013 Jun 19.

18

Early Prediction of Intensive Care Unit–Acquired Weakness Using Easily Available Parameters: A Prospective Observational Study

Luuk Wieske[1,2,3]*, Esther Witteveen[1,3], Camiel Verhamme[2], Daniela S. Dettling-Ihnenfeldt[4], Marike van der Schaaf[4], Marcus J. Schultz[1,3], Ivo N. van Schaik[2], Janneke Horn[1]

1 Department of Intensive Care Medicine, Academic Medical Center, Amsterdam, the Netherlands, **2** Department of Neurology, Academic Medical Center, Amsterdam, the Netherlands, **3** Laboratory of Experimental Anesthesiology and Intensive Care (L•E•I•C•A), Academic Medical Center, Amsterdam, the Netherlands, **4** Department of Rehabilitation, Academic Medical Center, Amsterdam, the Netherlands

Abstract

Introduction: An early diagnosis of Intensive Care Unit–acquired weakness (ICU–AW) using muscle strength assessment is not possible in most critically ill patients. We hypothesized that development of ICU–AW can be predicted reliably two days after ICU admission, using patient characteristics, early available clinical parameters, laboratory results and use of medication as parameters.

Methods: Newly admitted ICU patients mechanically ventilated ≥2 days were included in this prospective observational cohort study. Manual muscle strength was measured according to the Medical Research Council (MRC) scale, when patients were awake and attentive. ICU–AW was defined as an average MRC score <4. A prediction model was developed by selecting predictors from an a-priori defined set of candidate predictors, based on known risk factors. Discriminative performance of the prediction model was evaluated, validated internally and compared to the APACHE IV and SOFA score.

Results: Of 212 included patients, 103 developed ICU–AW. Highest lactate levels, treatment with any aminoglycoside in the first two days after admission and age were selected as predictors. The area under the receiver operating characteristic curve of the prediction model was 0.71 after internal validation. The new prediction model improved discrimination compared to the APACHE IV and the SOFA score.

Conclusion: The new early prediction model for ICU–AW using a set of 3 easily available parameters has fair discriminative performance. This model needs external validation.

Editor: Jorge I. F. Salluh, D'or Institute of Research and Education, Brazil

Funding: The authors received no specific funding for this work. Dr. L. Wieske is supported by a personal grant (ZonMw–AGIKO grant [project number 40-00703-98-11636]) from the Netherlands Organization for Health Research and Development. The funders had no role in study design, data collection and analysis, decision to publish, or preparation of the manuscript.

Competing Interests: The authors of this manuscript have the following competing interests: Prof. I.N. van Schaik received departmental honoraria for serving on scientific advisory boards and a steering committee for CSL-Behring. The other authors declare that they have no competing interests.

* Email: L.Wieske@amc.uva.nl

Introduction

Intensive Care Unit–acquired weakness (ICU–AW) is a frequent and debilitating neuromuscular complication of critical illness. [1,2] Development of ICU-AW is associated with increased mortality and short- and long term morbidity. [3–5] Currently, no specific treatments for ICU-AW exist. For future treatments to be successful, timing may be of importance. The first signs of ICU-AW can be found starting from day 2 after admission when decreased excitability of muscle and nerve can be observed. [6,7] Initiation of treatment at this moment may be more effective because the observed abnormalities may still be reversible. [8,9] Such early treatment would require an early diagnosis of ICU-AW. At present, the diagnosis of ICU–AW is based on clinical examination using manual muscle strength assessment. [1] In most critically ill patients, manual muscle strength assessment is not possible early in the disease course due to impaired consciousness or attentiveness. [10] A solution to this diagnostic delay may be to quantify the risk that a patient will develop ICU–AW using a prediction model early after ICU admission.

ICU–AW is associated with several risk factors, including sepsis, the presence of multiple organ dysfunction syndrome (MODS) and severity of illness. [11] Prediction of ICU–AW on the basis of these risk factors is scarcely studied. A combination of the Acute Physiology and Chronic Health Evaluation (APACHE) score and presence of the Systemic Inflammatory Response Syndrome

(SIRS) could identify patients at high risk for development of ICU-AW, although the predictive performance was not reported. [12] A cumulative Sequential Organ Failure Assessment (SOFA) score of the first week of ICU admission also has predictive value but this approach does not allow early prediction [13].

We hypothesized that early prediction of ICU–AW is possible and reliable. To investigate this, we built a prediction model based on previously identified risk factors for ICU–AW. The predictive performance of the model was compared to those of the APACHE IV scores and the SOFA score.

Methods

Design and ethical approval

We performed a prospective observational cohort study using the STARD guidelines. [14] The institutional review board of the Academic Medical Center, Amsterdam, The Netherlands, decided (decision notice W13_080#13.17.0100) that data for this study could be collected and analyzed without written informed consent of the patient and specifically approved the use of that data for this study because no additional procedures were performed and therefore this study did not fulfill the criteria for medical research stated in the Dutch 'Law on medical research'.

Study setting

The study was performed in a 30 beds tertiary mixed medical-surgical ICU of the Academic Medical Center in the Netherlands. In this ICU, several standards of care are applied including glucose control between 90 mg/dl and 144 mg/dl. Sedation is stopped as soon possible. Norepinephrine is the first line vasopressor drug and corticosteroids (100 mg of hydrocortisone intravenously 3 times daily) are given in refractory septic shock. All patients receive early rehabilitation.

In– and exclusion criteria

Consecutive, newly admitted ICU patients, mechanically ventilated for ≥2 days, were included. We excluded patients who had a neuromuscular disorder (e.g. Guillain-Barré syndrome), stroke, out-of-hospital cardiac arrest or spinal injury as reason for ICU admission. In addition, we excluded patients with a poor pre-hospital functional status (modified Rankin scale ≥4 [15]) and patients with pre-existing spinal injury.

Strength assessment (reference standard)

Physical therapists, blinded for all other parameters, assessed muscle strength when patients were alert (Richmond Agitation and Sedation Scale between −1 and 1 [16]) and attentive (able to follow verbal commands using arms or eye-lids). When patients are alert and attentive, muscle strength can be reliably assessed using the MRC score. [17] MRC scores were assessed bilaterally in 6 pre-specified muscle groups: wrist dorsiflexors, elbow flexors, shoulder abductors, hip flexors, knee extensors and ankle dorsiflexors. MRC scores of muscle groups were summated and divided by the number of muscle groups that could be tested to obtain an average MRC score. When a muscle group could not be assessed, no value was imputed. ICU–AW was diagnosed when weakness had developed after ICU admission, was symmetric and the average MRC score was <4 [1].

Candidate predictors

Candidate predictors were based on risk factors for ICU-AW identified through a literature search (see material S1). We extracted risk factors that were easily available in the first two days after ICU admission and had a univariate association, in at least one study. To improve suitability for prediction, some of the extracted risk factors were redefined into candidate predictors with more clear definitions. Candidate predictors regarding medical history and the presence of suspected sepsis were scored during ICU admission; all others were obtained from the electronic patient record after ICU discharge. Candidate predictors were collected blinded for the reference standard.

Additional data collected

The following additional clinical characteristics were collected: the Acute Physiology and Chronic Health Evaluation IV (APACHE IV) score and the maximal Sequential Organ Failure Assessment (SOFA) score during the first two days after ICU admission. Also, data on the number of days with mechanical ventilation, length of stay in the ICU and ICU mortality were collected.

Sample size

We assumed that ICU–AW would occur in 50% of patients [11] and that 5 patients with ICU–AW needed to be included per candidate predictor. We defined a set of 20 candidate predictors, so 200 patients were needed.

Statistical analysis

Candidate predictors with right-tailed distributions were logarithmically transformed. Predictors for the model were selected from candidate predictors using two steps. First, using a bootstrapped backward selection process, candidate predictors included in ≥50% of the bootstrap samples (N:1000; $p<0.5$ for inclusion) were selected. [18,19] Next, the selected candidate predictors were consecutively entered in a logistic regression model and only those candidate predictors that led to a discriminatory increase in model fit were retained. Candidate predictors were entered in descending order of inclusion frequency in bootstrap samples. For every addition, the change in Akaike Information Criterion (AIC) between models was compared. [20] An AIC change >–2 between additions was interpreted as non-discriminatory and the candidate predictors included before that addition were selected as predictors.

Next, we constructed a model with these predictors. Discriminative performance was analyzed using the area under the Receiver Operating Characteristic (AUC–ROC) curve and internally validated using bootstrapping (N:1000). We defined AUC-ROC values between 0.90–1 as excellent, 0.80–0.90 as good, 0.70–0.80 as fair, 0.60–0.70 as poor and <0.60 as failed. Odds ratios were adjusted using the calibration slope after internal validation. [18] Calibration was assessed graphically and using goodness of fit (Hosmer–Lemeshow test).

Performance of the new prediction model was compared to the APACHE IV score and maximal SOFA score in the first two ICU days using continuous net reclassification improvement (cNRI), which is a measure of discrimination resembling the AUC-ROC but more sensitive to change [21].

Finally, we performed two sensitivity analyses; we investigated discrimination of the prediction model for more severe ICU-AW (ICU-AW defined using a lower cut-off, i.e. an average MRC<3). Second, we investigated the influence of missing data by repeating predictor selection and model discrimination analyses on data sets in which missing data was imputed using multivariate imputation by chained equations (10 iterations of 10 imputations). [22] For the imputation model, all 20 candidate predictors as well as the presence of ICU-AW were used. Imputed values were checked for validity.

Mean values are presented with standard deviation (±SD), median values with interquartile range (IQR) and proportions with percentages and total numbers. Differences between proportions were assessed using chi-square test. Differences between normally distributed variables were assessed using Welch's t-test; differences between non-normally distributed continuous variables were assessed using Wilcoxon rank-sum test. Analyses were done using R (version: 2.15.2).

Results

Patients

Figure 1 displays the flow chart. Patients were screened from January 2011 until December 2012. Muscle strength could be assessed in 212 patients. Of those patients, 103 patients (49%) were diagnosed with ICU–AW. Table 1 shows patient and admission characteristics.

Candidate predictors

The literature search identified two systematic reviews on risk factors for ICU-AW. [11,23] Three additional recently published cohort studies were found. [24–26] We extracted 17 risk factors (see material S1) and redefined some of the risk factors so that they were suitable as candidate predictors (see figure S1). Three extra candidate predictors that have never been investigated but are likely to be of importance in ICU-AW were added, i.e. presence of pre-existing polyneuropathy, presence of risk factors for polyneuropathy and systemic corticosteroid use prior to ICU admission. All 20 candidate predictors are displayed in table 2; table S1 displays descriptions and definitions.

Predictor selection

Table 2 gives an overview of the distributions of the different candidate predictors for patients who did or did not develop ICU–AW. Because of the low number of patients with a pre–existing polyneuropathy, this candidate predictor was excluded from predictor selection. After backward selection, highest lactate, treatment with any aminoglycoside, age and lowest ionized Ca^{2+} were included in ≥50% of bootstrap samples (table 2). After consecutive addition of these candidate predictors into a logistic regression model, addition of lowest ionized Ca^{2+} did not result in discriminatory change in AIC (table 3). Therefore, highest lactate, treatment with any aminoglycoside and age were selected as predictors.

Prediction model

Table 3 shows the multivariate odds ratios for the 3 predictors, both unadjusted and adjusted for overfitting. The AUC–ROC of the prediction model was 0.72 (95%-CI: 0.65–0.79; panel A figure 2) and decreased to 0.71 after interval validation. The model showed good calibration (panel B of figure 2) without evidence for lack of fit. A spreadsheet calculator based on the prediction model is provided as material S2.

Comparison with APACHE IV and SOFA scores

The AUC-ROC of the maximal SOFA score in the first two ICU days for prediction of ICU-AW was 0.64 (95%-CI: 0.57–0.72); the AUC-ROC of the APACHE IV score was 0.66 (95%-CI: 0.58–0.73). Discrimination improved when using the new prediction model, both when compared to the maximal SOFA score in the first two ICU days and APACHE IV score (cNRI: 34% (95%-CI: 6 to 62) and 48% (95%-CI: 20 to 75), respectively).

Sensitivity analyses

For prediction of more severe ICU–AW (severe ICU-AW defined as an average MRC score <3; 64 of 212 patients met this definition), discriminative performance of the prediction model was not different (AUC-ROC: 0.72).

Highest lactate levels were missing in 17 patients; no other parameters had missing values. When repeating the backward selection process on data sets with missing lactate levels imputed, the same candidate predictors had a selection frequency of ≥50% and no additional candidate predictors were identified. Furthermore, based on change in AIC, addition of lowest ionized Ca^{2+} was non-discriminatory in all the imputation models. The discriminative performance of the prediction model was not different (averaged AUC–ROC after internal validation: 0.71) in the imputed data sets.

Table 1. Patient and admission characteristics.

	ICU-AW (N:103)	no ICU-AW (N:109)	p-value
age, mean ± SD	63±15	59±16	0.08
females, n (%)	52 (50)	40 (37)	0.06
reason for admission: planned surgical, n (%)	18 (17)	26 (24)	
reason for admission: emergency surgical, n (%)	28 (27)	21 (19)	0.29
reason for admission: medical, n (%)	57 (55)	62 (57)	
APACHE IV score, mean ± SD (3 missing)	89±25	74±28	<0.01
maximal SOFA score in first two days, mean ± SD	11±3	9±3	<0.01
average MRC score, median (IQR)	2.5 (1.3 to 3.2)	4.8 (4 to 5)	n.a.
day of MRC assessment after ICU admission, median (IQR)	9 (6–16)	7 (5–9)	<0.01
days with MV, median days (IQR)	13 (6 to 22)	6 (4 to 8)	<0.01
LOS ICU, median days (IQR)	16 (9 to 28)	8 (6 to 11)	<0.01
ICU mortality, n (%)	35 (34)	10 (9)	<0.01

ICU-AW: Intensive Care Unit – acquired weakness; LOS ICU: length of stay in the intensive care unit; APACHE IV: Acute Physiology and Chronic Health Evaluation IV; SOFA: Sequential Organ Failure Assessment; MV: mechanical ventilation; MRC: Medical Research Council; n.a.: not applicable.

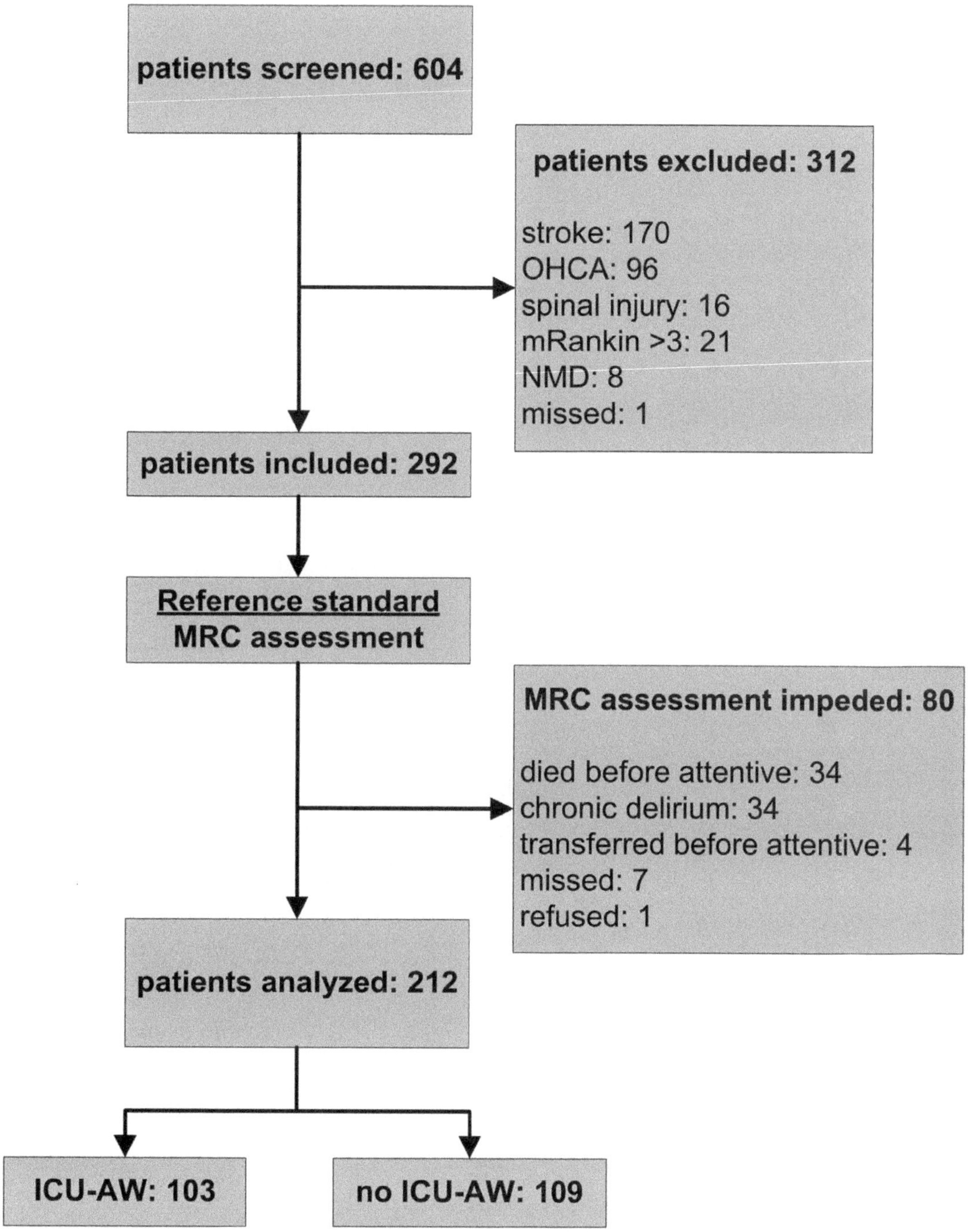

Figure 1. Study flowchart. ICU-AW: Intensive Care Unit – acquired weakness; OHCA: out-of hospital cardiac arrest; mRankin: modified Rankin score; NMD: neuromuscular disorder; MRC: muscle strength as assessed with Medical Research Council scale.

Discussion

After the first two days of stay in the ICU, development of ICU-AW can be predicted using highest lactate levels, treatment with any aminoglycoside and age as predictors. Discriminative performance of the prediction model was fair.

Comparison with previous studies

This is the first prediction model that has been developed specifically for early prediction of ICU-AW. When compared to previously identified predictors for ICU-AW, i.e. the APACHE and SOFA scores, the new prediction model had better discriminative performance [12,13].

Other, more technically demanding, methods for early prediction of ICU-AW have also been investigated. Weber-Carstens et al studied early electrophysiological testing and found a sensitivity of 83% and specificity of 89% for direct muscle stimulation. [27] This is indicative of a better discriminative performance than our prediction model, but electrophysiological studies in general, and direct muscle stimulation in particular, are technically demanding

Table 2. Candidate predictors for development of prediction model for early prediction of Intensive Care Unit – acquired weakness.

candidate predictors*	distribution		p-value	selection percentage in bootstrap samples
	ICU-AW (N:103)	no ICU-AW (N:109)		
patient characteristics				
females, n (%)	52 (50)	40 (37)	0.06	37.1
age, mean ± SD	63±15	59±16	0.08	57.6
risk factor for a polyneuropathy in medical history, n (%)	35 (34)	40 (37)	0.79	13.4
pre-existing polyneuropathy prior to ICU admission, n (%)	3 (3)	1 (1)	0.57	n.a.
systemic corticosteroid use prior to ICU admission, n (%)	7 (7)	9 (8)	0.89	10.7
clinical parameters				
suspected sepsis, n (%)	78 (76)	70 (64)	0.09	14.7
unplanned admission, n (%)	85 (83)	83 (76)	0.33	10.9
presence of shock, n (%)	75 (73)	67 (61)	0.11	24.6
RASS score, median (IQR)	-3 (-5 to −1)	-2 (-3 to 0)	<0.01	48.2
laboratory parameters				
average urine production, median ml/h (IQR)	70 (20 to 122)	102 (64 to 134)	<0.01	14.4
highest glucose, mean mg/dl ± SD	243.8±78.5	220.5±67.3	0.02	38.5
lowest glucose, mean mg/dl ± SD	85.8±22.3	89.6±25.8	0.25	22.2
lowest pH, mean ± SD	7.21±0.1	7.25±0.1	0.02	17.3
lowest P/F ratio, median (IQR)	186 (127 to 245)	178 (134 to 246)	0.98	27.9
lowest platelet count, median $\times 10^9$/L (IQR)	103 (45 to 151)	127 (85 to 197)	0.01	21.0
highest lactate, median mmol/L (IQR; 17 missing)	4.5 (3.0 to 7.0)	2.8 (1.7 to 4.8)	<0.01	89.5‡
lowest ionized Ca^{2+}, mean mmol/L ± SD	0.97±0.11	0.98±0.13	0.53	51.6
medication				
treatment with any corticosteroid, n (%)	81 (79)	63 (58)	<0.01	33.9
repeated treatment with any neuromuscular blocker§, n (%)	17 (17)	18 (17)	1.00	20.3
treatment with any aminoglycoside, n (%)	51 (50)	30 (28)	<0.01	80.4

*all clinical, laboratory and medication parameters were scored using information from the first two ICU days, except for the RASS score which was scored around two days after ICU admission;
‡logarithmically transformed;
§more than one administration of any neuromuscular blocker.
ICU-AW: Intensive Care Unit – acquired weakness; RASS: Richmond Agitation and Sedation Scale; n.a.: not applicable.
Table displaying distributions and differences between patients with and without Intensive Care Unit – acquired weakness for the candidate predictors. In the final column selection percentages of the candidate predictors in bootstrap samples based on backward selection are presented.

and are not widely available in ICUs. [1] Diagnostic potential of other methods for an early diagnosis of ICU-AW, like ultrasound or biological markers, has been scarcely studied [1,28,29].

Biological plausibility of the prediction model

Several hypotheses have been proposed that provide biological plausibility for the predictors that have been included in our model. Bolton proposed that tissue hypoxia caused by impaired microcirculation, for which lactate levels are a marker, is involved in pathogenesis of ICU-AW. [30,31] Aminoglycosides may be involved in ICU-AW because they can impair neuromuscular transmission and because of their neurotoxicity. [30,32] With aging, there is an accumulating burden of (neuromuscular) co-morbidities, a physiological loss of skeletal muscle mass and a decrease in mobility; all of which could lead to an increased susceptibility to develop ICU-AW. [33] All of these hypotheses remain speculative since none have been investigated properly.

We would like to emphasize that a good discriminatory performance of a predictor does not mean that this predictor also plays a (important) role in the pathogenesis of ICU-AW.

Table 3. Construction of prediction model.

candidate predictors	selection percentage in bootstrap samples	change in AIC	multivariate OR (95%-CI)	adjusted multivariate OR†
highest lactate‡ (17 missing)	89.5	n.a.	2.18 (1.39 to 3.43)	2.08
treatment with any aminoglycoside	80.4	−5.8	2.75 (1.44 to 5.26)	2.59
age	57.6	−2.8	1.02 (1.00 to 1.04)	1.02
lowest ionized Ca^{2+}	51.6	−1.6	not included	n.a.

‡logarithmically transformed.
†adjusted for overfitting using a shrinkage factor (i.e. calibration slope) of 0.94 obtained after internal validation.
n.a.: not applicable; AIC: Akaike Information Criterion; OR: odds ratio; CI: confidence interval.
Candidate predictors that were included in ≥50% of bootstrap samples (table 2) were entered consecutively into a logistic regression model starting with the most selected candidate predictor. For every subsequent step, the change in Akaike Information Criterion (AIC) was compared and candidate predictors were only included in the prediction model if addition resulted in a change in AIC<−2. In the final columns unadjusted and adjusted multivariate odds ratio's for predictors included in the prediction model are presented.

Prediction model analyses do not require multivariate analyses to assess an independent association between a variable and the outcome, from which a causal relation may be inferred. [34] For prediction, only the discriminatory performance is important. Sepsis for example was not selected although it is a well-known risk factor for ICU-AW because it was not discriminatory in our population as it was highly prevalent in both patients with and without ICU-AW.

Strengths and limitations

Strengths of this study are the inclusion of a diagnostically relevant population and the use of easily available predictors. Our study also has limitations. First, the number of candidate predictors was larger than the general rule of thumb of 1 candidate predictor for 10 events. [34] Although our candidate predictors were based on previously identified risk factors, this does not necessarily mean that these parameters are also good predictors. We expected that not all candidate predictors would have predictive value and therefore decided to include more candidate predictors than is recommended. To reduce the subsequent risk of overfitting, we performed a bootstrapped backward selection process, followed by an additional selection step based on model fit. The prediction model we developed and evaluated was adequately powered, with 1 predictor per 33 events and a modest degree of overfitting evident after internal validation. Second, we chose a liberal p-value for inclusion in the prediction model to prevent erroneous elimination of "true" predictors. [18] This may however increase the risk of including "noise" predictors. Finally, we chose not to include composite candidate predictors, like existing severity of illness or organ failures scores (for example APACHE or SOFA). These existing scores contain several variables that are not associated with ICU-AW or include variables that we already included. Therefore, adding these scores as a whole would have led to the inclusion of variables twice or variables with no discriminatory value. A large and inefficient dataset would have been needed to feed the model. Our goal was to only add simple candidate predictors with a unique discrim-

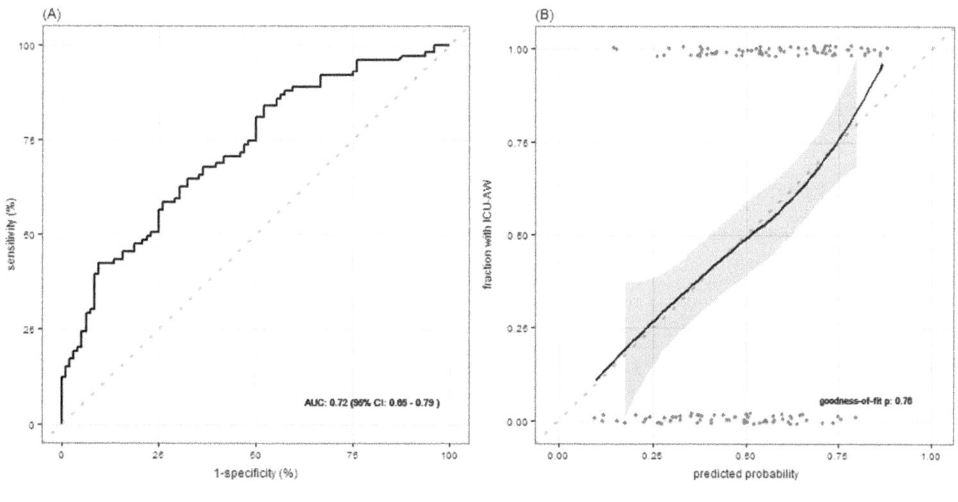

Figure 2. Model performance for early prediction of Intensive Care Unit - acquired weakness. Panel A shows the receiver operating characteristic (ROC) curve assessing discrimination of the prediction model. Panel B shows model calibration assessed with a fitted curve based on loess regression with 95% confidence interval (perfect model calibration is illustrated by the dotted line). Goodness-of-fit assessed with the Hosmer–Lemeshow test is shown. Grey points represent predicted probabilities for individual patients. AUC: area under the receiver operating characteristic curve; CI: confidence interval; ICU-AW: Intensive Care Unit - acquired weakness.

inatory value in order to keep the data set necessary as small and efficient as possible.

Framework for future studies

The ability to predict ICU-AW early after ICU admission and circumvent this limitation of muscle strength assessment as a diagnostic method can be an important step in critical care and research. Our study indicates that this prediction model, using easily available predictors, may be an option to achieve this. However, we did not investigate external validity, which is mandatory to ascertain the true discriminative performance of a prediction model. [35] It will be important to externally validate this prediction model in a multicenter setting to maximize generalizability. The discriminative performance after external validation, possibly recalibrated and updated with new predictors in future, will determine the true value of this model and whether or not it can be used in the clinic.

If the model is found to be reliable enough for clinical application it may be used to improve prognostication and to guide patient management. Also, prediction may be used to start therapies early, before structural damage to nerves and muscles has occurred, which is thought to possibly increase treatment effects. [10] Currently, no high quality evidence is available supporting an intervention for ICU-AW but some prospects exist. Early mobilization, starting when patients are still sedated, may be effective for preventing ICU-AW. [36] Early administration of intravenous immunoglobulins did not prevent ICU-AW. [37] Other pharmacological options, like melatonin, oxytocin, levetiracetam, indomethacin and leupeptin, have only been investigated in animals models. [38–40] Clinical research is needed to confirm these observations and to find new therapeutic options.

Conclusion

Early prediction of ICU–AW is possible using a set of 3 easily available predictors. Discriminative performance of the prediction model seems fair but needs external validation.

Supporting Information

Figure S1 Redefining of relevant risk factors into candidate predictors.

Table S1 Descriptions and definitions for candidate predictors.

Material S1 Supporting text concerning selection of candidate predictors.

Material S2 Spreadsheet calculator.

Material S3 Data set.

Acknowledgments

This research was performed within the framework of CTMM, the Center for Translational Molecular Medicine (www.ctmm.nl), project MARS (grant 04I-201).

Author Contributions

Conceived and designed the experiments: LW EW CV MJS INvS JH. Performed the experiments: LW EW DSD-I MvdS. Analyzed the data: LW EW CV DSD-I MvdS MJS INvS JH. Contributed to the writing of the manuscript: LW EW CV DSD-I MvdS MJS INvS JH.

References

1. Stevens RD, Marshall SA, Cornblath DR, Hoke A, Needham DM, et al. (2009) A framework for diagnosing and classifying intensive care unit-acquired weakness. Crit Care Med 37: S299–308.
2. Latronico N, Bolton CF (2011) Critical illness polyneuropathy and myopathy: a major cause of muscle weakness and paralysis. Lancet Neurol 10: 931–941.
3. Latronico N, Shehu I, Seghelini E (2005) Neuromuscular sequelae of critical illness. Curr Opin Crit Care 11: 381–390.
4. Ali NA, O'Brien JM, Hoffmann SP, Phillips G, Garland A, et al. (2008) Acquired weakness, handgrip strength, and mortality in critically ill patients. Am J Respir Crit Care Med 178: 261–268.
5. Sharshar T, Bastuji-Garin S, Stevens RD, Durand M-C, Malissin I, et al. (2009) Presence and severity of intensive care unit-acquired paresis at time of awakening are associated with increased intensive care unit and hospital mortality. Crit Care Med 37: 3047–3053.
6. Khan J, Harrison TB, Rich MM, Moss M (2006) Early development of critical illness myopathy and neuropathy in patients with severe sepsis. Neurology 67: 1421–1425.
7. Tennilä A, Salmi T, Pettilä V, Roine RO, Varpula T, et al. (2000) Early signs of critical illness polyneuropathy in ICU patients with systemic inflammatory response syndrome or sepsis. Intensive Care Med 26: 1360–1363.
8. Latronico N, Shehu I, Guarneri B (2009) Use of electrophysiologic testing. Crit Care Med 37: S316–S320.
9. Novak KR, Nardelli P, Cope TC, Filatov G, Glass JD, et al. (2009) Inactivation of sodium channels underlies reversible neuropathy during critical illness in rats. J Clin Invest 119: 1150–1158.
10. Hough CL, Lieu BK, Caldwell ES (2011) Manual muscle strength testing of critically ill patients: feasibility and interobserver agreement. Crit Care 15: R43.
11. Stevens RD, Dowdy DW, Michaels RK, Mendez-Tellez PA, Pronovost PJ, et al. (2007) Neuromuscular dysfunction acquired in critical illness: a systematic review. Intensive Care Med 33: 1876–1891.
12. De Letter MA, Schmitz PI, Visser LH, Verheul FA, Schellens RL, et al. (2001) Risk factors for the development of polyneuropathy and myopathy in critically ill patients. Crit Care Med 29: 2281–2286.
13. Bednarík J, Vondracek P, Dusek L, Moravcova E, Cundrle I (2005) Risk factors for critical illness polyneuromyopathy. J Neurol 252: 343–351.
14. Bossuyt PM, Reitsma JB, Bruns DE, Gatsonis CA, Glasziou PP, et al. (2003) The STARD statement for reporting studies of diagnostic accuracy: explanation and elaboration. The Standards for Reporting of Diagnostic Accuracy Group. Ann Intern Med 44: 639–650.
15. Van Swieten JC, Koudstaal PJ, Visser MC, Schouten HJ, van Gijn J (1988) Interobserver agreement for the assessment of handicap in stroke patients. Stroke 19: 604–607.
16. Sessler CN, Gosnell MS, Grap MJ, Brophy GM, O'Neal PV, et al. (2002) The Richmond Agitation-Sedation Scale: validity and reliability in adult intensive care unit patients. Am J Respir Crit Care Med 166: 1338–1344.
17. Vanpee G, Hermans G, Segers J, Gosselink R (2014) Assessment of limb muscle strength in critically ill patients: a systematic review. Crit Care Med 42: 701–711.
18. Steyerberg EW, Eijkemans MJ, Harrell FE, Habbema JD (2001) Prognostic modeling with logistic regression analysis: in search of a sensible strategy in small data sets. Med Decis Making 21: 45–56.
19. Brunelli A, Rocco G (2006) Internal validation of risk models in lung resection surgery: bootstrap versus training-and-test sampling. J Thorac Cardiovasc Surg 131: 1243–1247.
20. Akaike H (1974) A new look at the statistical model identification. Autom Control IEEE Trans 19: 716–723.
21. Pencina MJ, D'Agostino Ralph B S, Steyerberg EW (2010) Extensions of net reclassification improvement calculations to measure usefulness of new biomarkers. Stat Med 30: 11–21.
22. Heymans MW, van Buuren S, Knol DL, van Mechelen W, de Vet HCW (2007) Variable selection under multiple imputation using the bootstrap in a prognostic study. BMC Med Res Methodol 7: 33.
23. De Jonghe B, Cook D, Sharshar T, Lefaucheur J-P, Carlet J, et al. (1998) Acquired neuromuscular disorders in critically ill patients: a systematic review. Groupe de Reflexion et d'Etude sur les Neuromyopathies En Reanimation. Intensive Care Med 24: 1242–1250.
24. Nanas S, Kritikos K, Angelopoulos E, Siafaka A, Tsikriki S, et al. (2008) Predisposing factors for critical illness polyneuromyopathy in a multidisciplinary intensive care unit. Acta Neurol Scand 118: 175–181.

25. Weber-Carstens S, Deja M, Koch S, Spranger J, Bubser F, et al. (2010) Risk factors in critical illness myopathy during the early course of critical illness: a prospective observational study. Crit Care 14: R119.
26. Anastasopoulos D, Kefaliakos A, Michalopoulos A (2011) Is plasma calcium concentration implicated in the development of critical illness polyneuropathy and myopathy? Crit Care 15: R247.
27. Weber-Carstens S, Koch S, Spuler S, Spies CD, Bubser F, et al. (2009) Nonexcitable muscle membrane predicts intensive care unit-acquired paresis in mechanically ventilated, sedated patients. Crit Care Med 37: 2632–2637.
28. Cartwright MS, Kwayisi G, Griffin LP, Sarwal A, Walker FO, et al. (2013) Quantitative neuromuscular ultrasound in the intensive care unit. Muscle Nerve 47: 255–259.
29. Grimm A, Teschner U, Porzelius C, Ludewig K, Zielske J, et al. (2013) Muscle ultrasound for early assessment of critical illness neuromyopathy in severe sepsis. Crit Care 17: R227.
30. Bolton CF (2005) Neuromuscular manifestations of critical illness. Muscle Nerve 32: 140–163.
31. Marshall JC (2001) Inflammation, coagulopathy, and the pathogenesis of multiple organ dysfunction syndrome. Crit Care Med 29: S99–106.
32. Maramattom BV, Wijdicks EFM (2006) Acute neuromuscular weakness in the intensive care unit. Crit Care Med 34: 2835–2841.
33. Puthucheary Z, Montgomery H, Moxham J, Harridge S, Hart N (2010) Structure to function: muscle failure in critically ill patients. J Physiol 588: 4641–4648.
34. Moons KGM, Kengne AP, Woodward M, Royston P, Vergouwe Y, et al. (2012) Risk prediction models: I. Development, internal validation, and assessing the incremental value of a new (bio)marker. Heart 98: 683–690.
35. Moons KGM, Kengne AP, Grobbee DE, Royston P, Vergouwe Y, et al. (2012) Risk prediction models: II. External validation, model updating, and impact assessment. Heart 98: 691–698.
36. Hermans G, De Jonghe B, Bruyninckx F, Van den Berghe G (2014) Interventions for preventing critical illness polyneuropathy and critical illness myopathy. Cochrane database Syst Rev 1: CD006832.
37. Brunner R, Rinner W, Haberler C, Kitzberger R, Sycha T, et al. (2013) Early treatment with IgM-enriched intravenous immunoglobulin does not mitigate critical illness polyneuropathy and/or myopathy in patients with multiple organ failure and SIRS/sepsis: a prospective, randomized, placebo-controlled, double-blinded trial. Crit Care 17: R213.
38. Ruff RL, Secrist D (1984) Inhibitors of prostaglandin synthesis or cathepsin B prevent muscle wasting due to sepsis in the rat. J Clin Invest 73: 1483–1486.
39. Erbaş O, Yeniel AÖ, Akdemir A, Ergenoğlu AM, Yilmaz M, et al. (2013) The beneficial effects of levetiracetam on polyneuropathy in the early stage of sepsis in rats: electrophysiological and biochemical evidence. J Invest Surg 26: 312–318.
40. Erbaş O, Ergenoglu AM, Akdemir A, Yeniel AÖ, Taskiran D (2013) Comparison of melatonin and oxytocin in the prevention of critical illness polyneuropathy in rats with experimentally induced sepsis. J Surg Res 183: 313–320.

Residual Viremia Is Preceding Viral Blips and Persistent Low-Level Viremia in Treated HIV-1 Patients

Laura Marije Hofstra[1], Tania Mudrikova[2], Arjen J. Stam[1], Sigrid Otto[3], Kiki Tesselaar[3], Monique Nijhuis[1], Annemarie M. J. Wensing[1]*

1 Department of Medical Microbiology, Virology, University Medical Center Utrecht, Utrecht, the Netherlands, **2** Department of Internal Medicine and Infectious Diseases, University Medical Center Utrecht, Utrecht, the Netherlands, **3** Laboratory of Translational Immunology, University Medical Center Utrecht, Utrecht, the Netherlands

Abstract

Background: It has been suggested that low-level viremia or blips in HIV-infected patients on antiretroviral treatment are related to assay variation and/or increased sensitivity of new commercial assays. The 50-copy cut-off for virologic failure is, therefore, under debate.

Methods: Treated patients with low-level viremia (persistent viral loads (VL) of 50–1000 copies/mL, group A, N = 16) or a blip (single detectable VL, group B, N = 77) were compared to a control group (consistently suppressed viremia since start therapy (<50 copies/mL), N = 79). Residual viremia (detectable viral RNA <50 copies/ml) in the year preceding the first VL above 50 copies/mL (T0) was determined using Roche Cobas-Amplicor v1.5 or CAP-CTM v2.0. Subsequent virologic failure (2 consecutive VLs>500 or 1 VL>1000 copies/mL that was not followed by a VL<50 copies/mL; median follow up 34 months) was assessed.

Results: Significantly more patients in groups A and B had residual viremia in the year preceding T0 compared to controls (50% and 19% vs 3% respectively; p<0.001). Residual viremia was associated with development of low-level viremia or blips (OR 10.9 (95% CI 2.9–40.6)). Subsequent virologic failure was seen more often in group A (3/16) and B (2/77) than in the control group (0/79).

Conclusion: Residual viremia is associated with development of blips and low-level viremia. Virologic failure occurred more often in patients with low-level viremia. These results suggest that low-level viremia results from viral production/replication rather than only assay variation.

Editor: Cecilio López-Galíndez, Centro Nacional de Microbiología - Instituto de Salud Carlos III, Spain

Funding: This work was supported in part by The Netherlands Organisation for Scientific Research (NWO) VIDI (91796349). The funders had no role in study design, data collection and analysis, decision to publish, or preparation of the manuscript. Funding did not cover all expenses; additional costs were covered internal.

Competing Interests: The authors have declared that no competing interests exist.

* Email: a.m.j.wensing@umcutrecht.nl

Introduction

Combination antiretroviral therapy (cART) suppresses HIV replication, resulting in a decline of the plasma viral load (VL). The goal of cART historically followed the limit of detection of the assay used to measure HIV RNA levels. Currently in clinical practice the cut-off of 50 copies per milliliter is used [1,2] but after the introduction of new commercial assays with increased sensitivity and a limit of detection below 50 copies/mL this cut-off has become subject of debate.

Viremia below 50 copies/mL is often referred to as residual viremia. After initiation of cART the VL usually declines below the established cut-off of 50 copies within 3–6 months and continues to decline further within the first year. In clinical practice, a substantial number of patients achieve maximal suppression. In these patients the assay cannot detect any signal, referred to as target not detected (TND). However, in a selection of patients on cART persistent or transient residual viremia below the cut-off of 50 copies/mL is observed [3,4]. It is a matter of longstanding debate whether residual viremia is a result of virus production by latently infected cells or is caused by ongoing viral replication despite therapy with the risk of selection of resistance. Therefore its clinical relevance remains uncertain. In a cross sectional analysis of patients on cART, Doyle *et al* showed that residual viremia enhances the chance of viral rebound (viremia above 50 copies/mL) and therefore suggested that the goal of cART may need to be revised to a lower cut-off than 50 copies/mL [5].

Viral rebound can be either transient (a single viral load above 50 copies/mL), generally referred to as viral blip, or persistent (continuous detectable viral load between 50 and 1000 copies/mL) which is called low-level viremia. As for residual viremia, there is

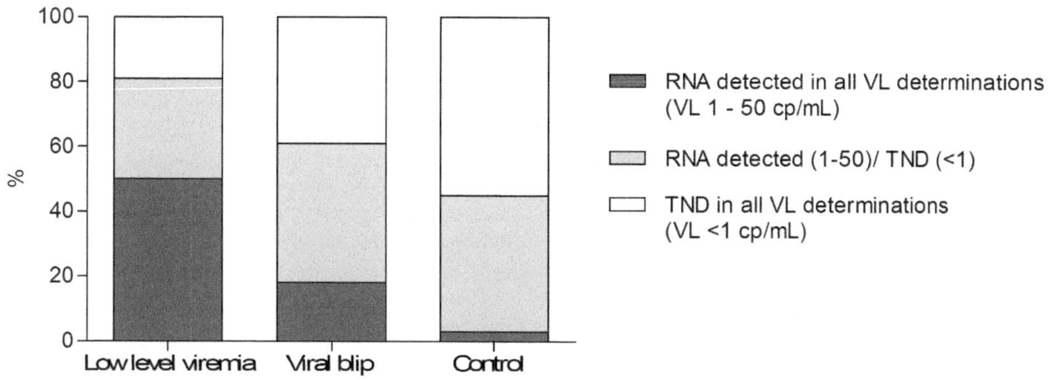

Figure 1. Methods. A = patients with low-level viremia; B = patients with a single viral blip; C = patients with continuously suppressed viremia; T0 = first detectable viral load for patients of group A and B. Analysis of viral loads in year preceding T0 to determine level of residual viremia. Follow up to determine rate of subsequent virologic failure.

vivid discussion regarding the source and clinical relevance of viral blips and low-level viremia.

After introduction of the Roche Cobas Taqman assay, which has a limit of detection of 20 copies/mL and a higher rate of detectability than the former Roche Amplicor assay [6], physicians worldwide observed an increase in the frequency of blips [7,8]. This mounted the idea that this was a result of assay variation and/or increased sensitivity rather than virus production or replication [9,10]. Based on these discussions the DHHS Guidelines for use of antiretroviral agents raised the definition of virologic failure to a confirmed viral load above 200 copies/mL, assigning most cases of apparent viremia to isolated blips or assay variability with no increased risk of virologic failure [11].

This proposed cut-off of 200 copies/mL is not based on extensive clinical data. Several studies have looked in to the risk of virologic failure after viral rebound, but data on viral rebound between 50 and 200 copies/mL is limited. A large observational cohort of patients on cART recently showed that even low-level viremia between 50 and 199 copies/mL was associated with increased risk of virologic failure [12]. Furthermore, it was recently shown that levels of activated (CD3+ HLA-DR+) T cells predicted the occurrence of viral blips, suggesting viral rebound may reflect viral production from activated immune cells instead of assay variation [13]. An association between immune activation and a modest increased risk of a subsequent blip was also observed using CD38/HLA-DR expression on CD8+ T cells [14].

To investigate the relevance of blips and low-level viremia, we compared patients with and without blips and low-level viremia from our clinical center: we determined the presence of residual viremia in the year preceding viral rebound, assessed a possible role for immune activation and studied rates of subsequent virologic failure.

Methods

Ethical statement

Patients were included from the observational AIDS Therapy Evaluation in the Netherlands (ATHENA) cohort, which follows HIV-positive patients who are registered in one of the designated treatment centers in the Netherlands. Patients can opt-out after being informed on the purpose of data collection by their treating physician. Patients who have decided not to opt out are anonymously recorded in a central database.

Patients

Adult HIV-infected patients who had a first detectable VL (T0) in the period April 2009– August 2010 were identified retrospectively from our outpatient clinic (University Medical Center Utrecht) to allow two years of follow-up. Patients treated with cART for more than 1 year who achieved at least 2 consecutive VL<50 copies/mL were included. Patients who had documented treatment interruption were excluded. Patients were grouped according to their VL pattern (figure 1). Group A included patients with repeatedly consecutive detectable VL (e.g. T0 was followed by more samples with a detectable VL, with a maximum plasma viral load of 1000 copies/mL; thus considered to have low-level viremia) and group B included patients with a single detectable VL (e.g. T0 was followed by a sample with an undetectable VL without a change in treatment; which we considered a viral blip). Both groups were compared to a control group of randomly selected adult HIV-infected patients who also were treated with cART for at least 1 year and did not experience detectable viremia after achieving viral suppression. For these patients, T0 was defined as the VL determination closest to the mean date of T0 in group A and B, allowing analysis of a similar timeframe.

Data collection

Clinical data were retrieved from the local Athena database. To determine the role of residual viremia, a longitudinal analysis of VL results below 50 copies/mL in the year preceding T0 was performed. VL monitoring was performed on EDTA plasma samples using Roche Cobas Taqman v2.0. Part of the VL determinations in the year preceding T0 were performed with the Roche Cobas Amplicor v1.5 assay, which was a similar percentage among groups. The result of the VL determination was either RNA detected (e.g. a VL between 1 and 50 copies/mL, residual viremia) or target not detected (TND, e.g. no signal in the PCR, zero viremia). We determined the percentage of patients who had in the year preceding T0 (1) RNA detected at all determinations, (2) TND at all determinations or (3) RNA detected in some determinations and TND in others.

Follow-up

All patients were followed up from T0 for at least 24 months to determine whether virologic failure or a subsequent episode of detectable viremia occurred. Virologic failure was defined as two consecutive VLs >500 copies/mL or a VL exceeding 1000 copies/mL that was not followed by a VL<50 copies/mL on the same regimen. A secondary outcome was a subsequent episode of detectable viremia (VL>50 copies/mL). Patients with low-level viremia first had to achieve a VL<50 copies/mL before they were classified as having a subsequent episode of detectable viremia. Population genotypic analysis was performed if requested by treating physician. Resistance-associated mutations were defined according to the IAS-USA mutation list [15].

Immune activation markers

In a random subset of patients, stored samples of T0 were analyzed for levels of immune activation markers. The concentration of soluble markers CD14 and CXCL9 was measured using ELISAs. All samples were assayed on the same plate.

Statistical analysis

Baseline clinical laboratory and treatment characteristics were compared between group A, B and control group using chi-squared, one way ANOVA and Kruskal-Wallis tests. A logistic regression model was used to identify factors that were associated with the occurrence of blips and low-level viremia. Residual viremia in the year preceding T0 and the duration of treatment were included in the multivariable analysis, as well as all other factors with a p value <0.2 in univariable analysis. Factors with a p value<0.05 in multivariable analysis were considered to be associated with blips and low-level viremia. Standard Kaplan-Meier estimation and log-rank comparisons were used to evaluate time to virologic failure and time to detectable viremia. Due to a very low number of events Cox regression models for assessing factors associated with virologic failure could not be used. All of the statistical tests were two sided at the 5% level and performed with SPSS software (version 20.0).

Results

In total, 93 eligible patients were identified and included in the study group; 16 patients with low-level viremia (group A) and 77 patients with a viral blip (group B). For group A, the maximum level of low-level viremia was 50–200 copies/mL for 10 patients, 200–500 copies/mL for 4 patients and 500–1000 copies/mL for 2 patients. For group B, 53 patients had a blip between 50 and 200 copies/mL, 14 patients between 200–500 copies/mL and 10 patients >500 copies/mL. 79 patients were assigned to the control group. In all groups, the majority was male, of European origin with a mean age around 45 years (table 1). No differences in CD4 count at presentation were observed. There was a trend towards shorter duration of cART and more PI-based regimens in group A, compared to group B and the control group.

We analyzed the presence of residual viremia in the year preceding T0 (figure 2). In all three groups the number of viral load determinations with a result below 50 copies/mL was comparable, with a median number of samples of 2 in group A (range: 2–5), 3 in group B (range 2–6) and 3 in the control group (range 2–5). Significantly more patients in group A and B (50% and 19%) had residual viremia in all VL determinations in the year preceding T0, compared to the control group (3%; p< 0.0005). The majority of patients (55%) in the control group had no RNA detected (target not detected =TND) in all VL determinations. Patients with continuous residual viremia had a significantly shorter treatment duration compared to patients with continuous TND (mean 41 vs. 83 months, p<0.001).

Correlates of detectable viremia were determined with use of a logistic regression model (table 2). In univariable analysis, heterosexual transmission route, PI-based regimen and detected residual viremia in the preceding year showed an increased odds ratio for developing detectable viremia and were included in multivariable analysis. Only residual viremia in the preceding year was associated with the development of detectable viremia in multivariable analysis (OR 10.9 (95% CI 2.9–40.6)).

In general, patients attend the outpatient clinic every 3–6 months, as was observed in patients of the control group (table 1, time to next visit: 97% 3 months or more). In contrast, the majority of patients in group A and B returned within the first 2 months after detectable viremia, before the regular scheduled visit.

Patients were followed for a median of 34 months to determine the occurrence of virologic failure or a new episode of detectable viremia. Seven patients (3 of group B; 4 of control group) were lost to follow up. Virologic failure was observed in 3 patients of group A, 2 patients of group B and in none of the control group patients (figure 3). In the five patients with virologic failure, the first detectable viral load (T0) varied between 117 and 567 copies/mL. Considering the secondary outcome, detectable viremia was significantly more often seen in patients who previously had a viral blip or low-level viremia than in patients who had a sustained suppressed viral load. In the control group only 3 patients developed a first viral blip to levels below 200 copies/mL; all others maintained a suppressed VL.

In group A, all 3 patients with virologic failure were on a PI-based regimen. In one patient, adherence counseling without a change in therapy was sufficient to suppress the VL. For the other two, virologic suppression followed after a switch in therapy which was guided by drug resistance testing. Selection of multiple major PI and RT drug resistance mutations was observed in one of them. In 7 patients from group A without virologic failure resistance testing did not reveal resistance mutations relevant to the used regimen. Maintenance of the same regimen (6 PI-based, 1 NNRTI-based) – with an increased dosing of the boosted PI in 1 patient – resulted in sustained virologic suppression in five patients. Two patients switched therapy from an NNRTI-based to a PI-based regimen without guidance of a resistance test which was followed by virologic suppression in 1 patient.

In group B, two patients experienced virologic failure. Resistance testing did not reveal selection of new relevant major resistance mutations. Suppression on the same regimen (1 NNRTI-based, 1 PI-based) was achieved in both after adherence counseling. Resistance testing was also performed in three patients without virologic failure (2 NNRTI-based, 1 PI-based regimen) and did not show selection of resistance. One patient of group B developed an episode of low-level viremia after the initial blip and reached virologic suppression following a switch from an NNRTI to a PI-based regimen.

To investigate a possible relation between immune activation and the occurrence of viral rebound, two soluble immune activation markers at T0 were studied in a random subset of patients (group A n = 15; group B n = 33; control group n = 30). A trend towards higher CXCL9 levels in patients with low-level viremia (mean 130,98 pg/mL) or a viral blip (mean 119,21) compared to patients with a consistently suppressed VL (mean 93,62 pg/mL; p 0.098). There was no difference in soluble CD14 levels among groups (Figure 4). We did not observe a relation between the levels of CXCL9 or soluble CD14 and plasma HIV RNA, nor with the duration of therapy.

Discussion

Low-level viremia and viral blips are frequently seen in clinical practice. We observed that an unexpected detectable viral load generates uncertainty among clinicians and patients resulting in a

Table 1. Baseline characteristics of the study population.

Characteristic	Study group		Control group	P
	Group A (LLV)	Group B (blip)		
N	16	77	79	
Age – yr	45±11	46±9	45±11	0.77
Male sex	11 (69)	61 (79)	61 (77)	0.66
Origin				0.84
European	11 (69)	51 (66)	56 (71)	
Sub Saharan African	3 (19)	17 (22)	15 (19)	
Other	2 (12)	9 (12)	8 (10)	
Route of transmission				0.21
MSM	9 (56)	31 (40)	31 (39)	
Heterosexual	5 (31)	33 (43)	25 (32)	
Other	2 (12)	13 (17)	23 (29)	
Duration of known HIV infection – months	83±52	116±75	104±63	0.33
Baseline CD4 count – median (Q1, Q3)	285 (109, 460)	266 (89, 443)	308 (146, 471)	0.85
Baseline log viral load – median (Q1, Q3)	5.1 (3.9, 6.3)	5.3 (4.8, 5.8)	5.2 (4.7, 5.7)	0.56
Duration of cART – months	47±39	72±50	74±50	0.06
cART regimen				0.10
NNRTI based	5 (31)	36 (47)	48 (61)	
PI based	11 (69)	37 (48)	29 (37)	
Time to next visit				<0.001
1–2 months	9 (56)	47 (61)	2 (3)	
3 months or more	7 (44)	30 (39)	77 (98)	

visit to the outpatient clinic ahead of the regular schedule. There is extensive debate whether these patients have an increased risk of virologic failure. Guidelines of DHHS raised the cut-off of virologic failure to 200 copies/mL and stated that patients with isolated blips do not need a change in treatment, whereas for patients with low-level viremia below 200 copies/ml there is no consensus regarding clinical management [11]. Other guidelines continue to use a cut-off of 50 copies/mL for virologic failure [1,2].

In our cohort, patients with low-level viremia had a higher risk of virologic failure. This corresponds with all five previous studies on this issue [12,16–19] of which four used the cut-off of 50 copies/mL to define low-level viremia [16–19]. The most recent large observational study distinguished subgroups based on the level of viremia (50–199, 200–499 and 500–999 copies/mL) and

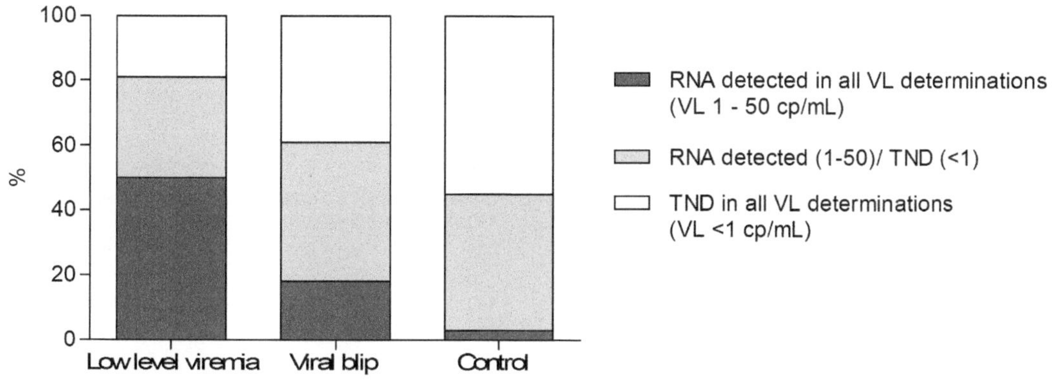

Figure 2. Longitudinal analysis of viral load results in preceding year. Low-level viremia is often preceded by positive VL results; in 50% of these patients HIV-1 RNA was detected in all VL determinations in the preceding year, compared to only 3% of patients with a sustained suppressed VL (p<.0001).

Table 2. Logistic Regression Analysis of correlates of detectable viremia>50 copies/mL at T0, multivariable analysis.

	Univariable analysis		Multivariable analysis	
	OR (95% CI)	**P value**	**OR (95% CI)**	**P value**
Age	1.01 (0.98–1.04)	0.51	-	-
Sex				
Female	1.00 (reference)			
Male	0.99 (0.48–2.02)	0.98	-	-
Origin				
European	1.00 (reference)			
Sub Saharan African	1.20 (0.56–2.58)	0.63	-	-
Other	1.24 (0.47–3.31)	0.67	-	-
Transmission route				
MSM	1.00 (reference)		1.00 (reference)	
Hetero	1.18 (0.59–2.35)	0.64	1.38 (0.66–2.85)	0.39
Other	0.51 (0.23–1.13)	0.10	0.48 (0.20–1.12)	0.09
Known HIV infection	1.01 (0.66–1.54)	0.98	-	-
Baseline (log) CD4 count	0.97 (0.77–1.22)	0.78	-	-
Baseline (log) viral load	0.96 (0.67–1.37)	0.82	-	-
Duration cART	0.83 (0.56–1.24)	0.37	1.25 (0.79–1.98)	0.35
Regimen				
PI based	1.00 (reference)		1.00 (reference)	
NNRTI based	0.52 (0.28–0.96)	0.04	0.64 (0.33–1.26)	0.21
Other	1.21 (0.21–7.02)	0.83	1.36 (0.22–8.55)	0.82
Residual viremia				
Always TND	1.00 (reference)		1.00 (reference)	
TND/+	1.50 (0.78–2.88)	0.22	1.74 (0.89–3.42)	0.11
Always +	9.56 (2.63–34.67)	0.001	10.90 (2.93–40.57)	<0.0005

reported an increased risk of virologic failure in all subgroups. Although the risk was highest in patients with viremia between 500–999 copies/mL, patients with low-level viremia between 50 and 200 copies/mL still showed a 2-fold higher risk of failure [12]. In our cohort, two of three patients with virologic failure had low-level viremia between 50 and 200 copies/mL, supporting this observation.

Resistance testing was only performed on request of the physician. Selection of resistance was observed in only 1 of 9 patients, at a VL around 500 copies/mL. Eight out of nine patients were using a boosted PI-based regimen, which may explain the limited selection of resistance as boosted PIs have a high intrinsic genetic barrier for resistance. Previous studies did show selection of resistance, including PI resistance, in a subset of patients with low-level viremia, even at VLs up to 200 copies/mL [20,21]. The presence of resistance mutations during low-level viremia has been shown to be associated with risk of failure, suggesting that resistance testing has added value in these cases [22,23]. In a Spanish cohort it was shown that optimization of therapy after resistance testing in patients with low-level viremia resulted in viral suppression below 50 copies/mL in 90% of patients after 1 year [24].

Regarding viral blips, a number of studies have been performed leading to different conclusions. We observed a much lower risk of virologic failure in patients with viral blips compared to patients with low-level viremia. This is in line with nine studies that did not report an increased risk of virologic failure in patients with blips [17,19,25–31]. As in our cohort, these studies defined a viral blip as a viral load above 50 copies/mL. In contrast, four studies did find an increased risk of virologic failure in patients with viral blips [16,32–34], of which three used a definition of a VL exceeding 400 or 500 copies/mL. A recent study in therapy-naïve patients that distinguished on the level of viral blips (50–199, 200–499 and >500 copies/mL) only reported an increased risk of failure in patients with a blip that exceeded 500 copies/mL [34]. Thus the results of current available literature suggests the height of the blip may be important, explaining why previous literature not taking the viral load into account seemed to be conflicting on this issue.

The nature of blips and low-level viremia is subject of debate and it has been suggested that it is a result of increased sensitivity or assay variation. However, several studies have demonstrated an association between residual viremia measured at a single time point and the risk of viral rebound, using several assays, including ultrasensitive assays and Taqman assay v.2.0 [5,35–37]. Studies that failed to show such an association either had a relatively small sample size or had a rare development of rebound overall [38,39]. Our cohort is the first that assessed residual viremia in longitudinal samples preceding the viral blip or low-level viremia. We observed that most patients with low-level viremia had residual viremia throughout the preceding year, while more than half of patients in the control group continuously had no detectable viremia. We observed this difference, although to a lesser extent, also for patients who experienced blips. Of interest, the presence of

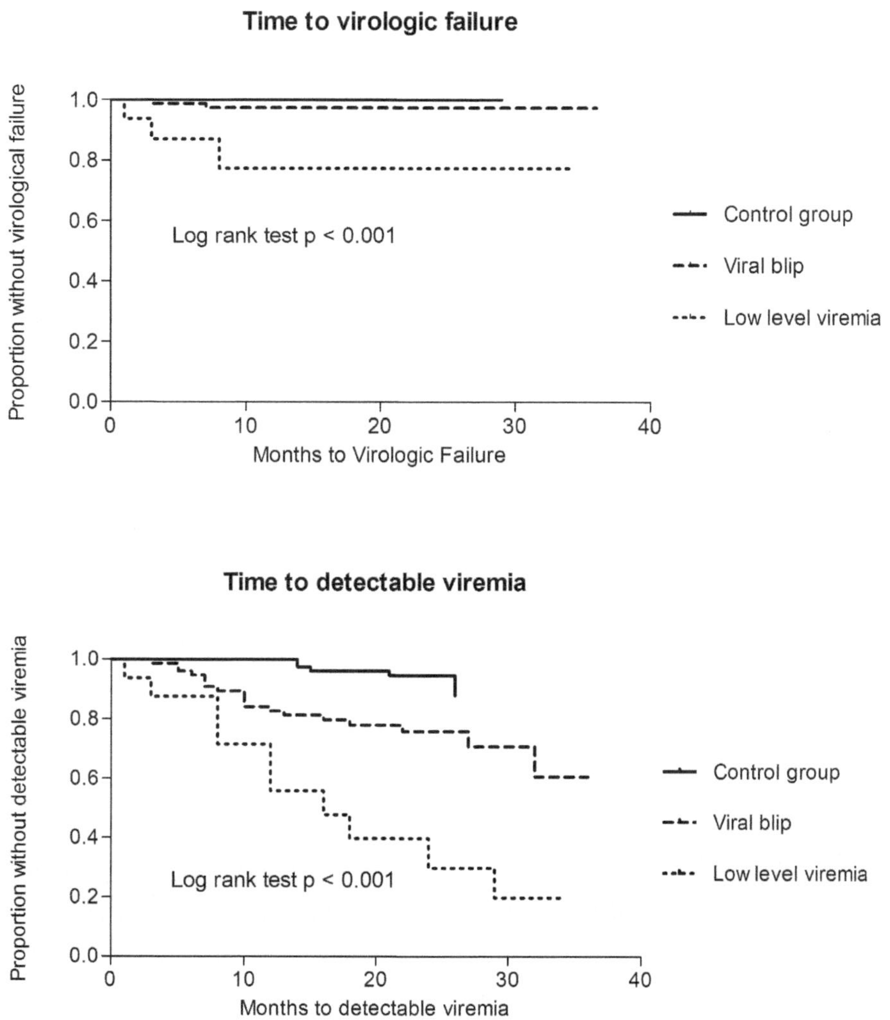

Figure 3. Kaplan-Meier plot of time to virologic failure (VL>1000 cp/mL) and of time to detectable viremia (≥50 cp/mL).

residual viremia was related to the duration of therapy, which has also been shown as a relevant factor in other studies [5,35,37].

The association between residual viremia and blips or low-level viremia on one hand and the duration of therapy on the other hand, suggests that we are detecting a biologically relevant

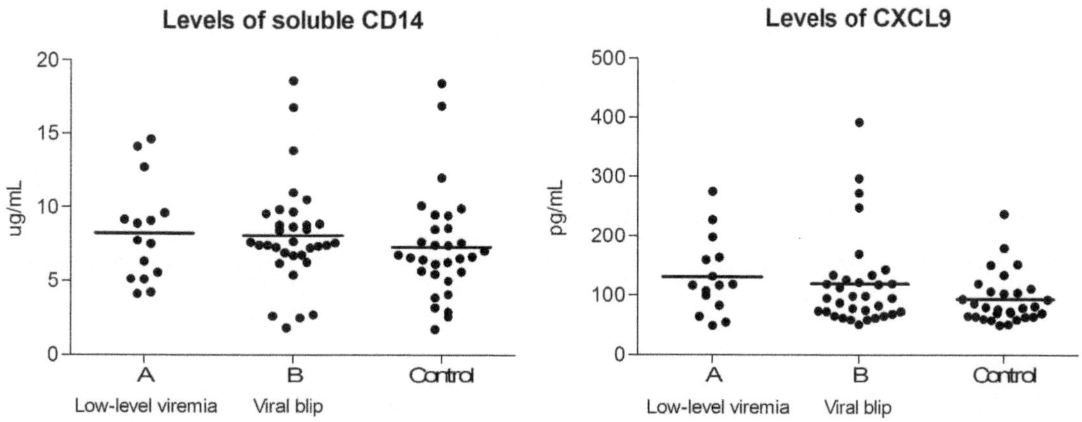

Figure 4. Levels of immune activation markers at T0. Lines indicate mean values. No significant difference in levels of soluble CD14 among the groups (p 0.489). There is a trend towards higher levels of CXCL9 in patients with low-level viremia and viral blips than in patients with continuously suppressed viremia (p 0.098).

phenomenon. With the use of assays with single-copy sensitivity it has been shown that the viral load, after initial decline below 50 copies/mL, continues to decay slowly [3]. Therefore, it is plausible to expect that patients in the first years of therapy more often have residual viremia and are more likely to experience viral blips or low-level viremia. Whether this is a result of virus production or replication remains uncertain and it is not unlikely that both processes coexist. We compared levels of immune activation markers CXCL9 and soluble CD14 and observed slightly higher levels of CXCL9 in patients with low-level viremia. Prospective longitudinal studies are necessary to look further into the possible role of immune activation in residual viremia, viral blips and low-level viremia.

We observed low rates of virologic failure in our cohort. A relevant factor is the active switching of therapy in some patients before virologic failure could occur, which is an inevitable limitation of the retrospective nature of the study. The retrospective design enables selection of all patients who had low-level viremia and viral blips in our clinic. Although the sample size was relatively small, which is reflected in the large confidence intervals in our logistic regression analysis, all values in the interval support the conclusion that residual viremia is associated with the development of low level viremia and viral blips. Based on our results we cannot assess how often patients with residual viremia would develop low-level viremia or viral blips, but it has been shown previously that 10 to 40% of patients with residual viremia will have a rebound above 50 copies/mL [5].

Clinical management of blips and low-level viremia remains a complex issue, as it is difficult to distinguish viral production from viral replication with subsequent risk of selection of resistance. In some cases blips and low-level viremia represents viral production that is irrelevant for long-term virological outcome. Current available observational evidence indicates that patients with blips exceeding 500 copies/mL and patients with persistent viral loads above 50 copies/mL have a higher risk of virologic failure. In these patients it is more likely that viral replication occurred with subsequent risk of selection of drug resistant variants, and therefore a regimen switch after assessing present drug resistance should be highly considered.

Acknowledgments

Parts of this work was previously presented by L.M.H. at the 13th European AIDS Conference, Belgrade, Serbia in 2011 and was published as abstract PS12/4.

Author Contributions

Conceived and designed the experiments: LMH TM KT MN AMJW. Performed the experiments: LMH AJS SO. Analyzed the data: LMH TM AJS SO KT MN AMJW. Contributed to the writing of the manuscript: LMH TM AJS KT MN AMJW.

References

1. Thompson MA, Aberg JA, Hoy JF, Telenti A, Benson C, et al. (2012) Antiretroviral treatment of adult HIV infection: 2012 recommendations of the International Antiviral Society-USA panel. Jama 308: 387–402.
2. European AIDS Clinical Society (2013) EACS Guidelines.
3. Palmer S, Maldarelli F, Wiegand A, Bernstein B, Hanna GJ, et al. (2008) Low-level viremia persists for at least 7 years in patients on suppressive antiretroviral therapy. Proceedings of the National Academy of Sciences of the United States of America 105: 3879–3884.
4. Maldarelli F, Palmer S, King MS, Wiegand A, Polis MA, et al. (2007) ART suppresses plasma HIV-1 RNA to a stable set point predicted by pretherapy viremia. PLoS Pathogens 3: 484–488.
5. Doyle T, Smith C, Vitiello P, Cambiano V, Johnson M, et al. (2012) Plasma HIV-1 RNA detection below 50 copies/ml and risk of virologic rebound in patients receiving highly active antiretroviral therapy. Clin Infect Dis 54: 724–732.
6. Swenson LC, Cobb B, Geretti AM, Harrigan PR, Poljak M, et al. (2014) Comparative performances of HIV-1 RNA load assays at low viral load levels: results of an international collaboration. J Clin Microbiol 52: 517–523.
7. Lima V, Harrigan R, Montaner JS (2009) Increased reporting of detectable plasma HIV-1 RNA levels at the critical threshold of 50 copies per milliliter with the Taqman assay in comparison to the Amplicor assay. J Acquir Immune Defic Syndr 51: 3–6.
8. Smit E, Bhattacharya S, Osman H, Taylor S (2009) Increased frequency of HIV-1 viral load blip rate observed after switching from roche cobas amplicor to cobas taqman assay. Journal of Acquired Immune Deficiency Syndromes 51: 364–365.
9. Nettles RE, Kieffer TL, Kwon P, Monie D, Han Y, et al. (2005) Intermittent HIV-1 viremia (Blips) and drug resistance in patients receiving HAART. Jama 293: 817–829.
10. Lee PK, Kieffer TL, Siliciano RF, Nettles RE (2006) HIV-1 viral load blips are of limited clinical significance. J Antimicrob Chemother 57: 803–805.
11. Panel on Antiretroviral Guidelines for Adults and Adolescents (2012) Guidelines for the use of antiretroviral agents in HIV-1-infected adults and adolescents. Department of Health and Human Services.
12. Laprise C, de Pokomandy A, Baril JG, Dufresne S, Trottier H (2013) Virologic Failure Following Persistent Low-level Viremia in a Cohort of HIV-Positive Patients: Results From 12 Years of Observation. Clin Infect Dis.
13. Zoufaly A, Kiepe J, Hertling S, Hufner A, Degen O, et al. (2014) Immune activation despite suppressive highly active antiretroviral therapy is associated with higher risk of viral blips in HIV-1-infected individuals. HIV Med.
14. Taiwo B, Hunt PW, Gandhi RT, Ellingson A, McKenna M, et al. (2013) CD8+ T-cell activation in HIV-1-infected patients experiencing transient low-level viremia during antiretroviral therapy. Journal of Acquired Immune Deficiency Syndromes 63: 101–104.
15. Johnson VA, Calvez V, Gunthard HF, Paredes R, Pillay D, et al. (2011) 2011 update of the drug resistance mutations in HIV-1. Top Antivir Med 19: 156–164.
16. Greub G, Cozzi-Lepri A, Ledergerber B, Staszewski S, Perrin L, et al. (2002) Intermittent and sustained low-level HIV viral rebound in patients receiving potent antiretroviral therapy. Aids 16: 1967–1969.
17. Raboud JM, Rae S, Woods R, Harris M, Montaner JS (2002) Consecutive rebounds in plasma viral load are associated with virological failure at 52 weeks among HIV-infected patients. Aids 16: 1627–1632.
18. Sungkanuparph S, Groger RK, Overton ET, Fraser VJ, Powderly WG (2006) Persistent low-level viraemia and virological failure in HIV-1-infected patients treated with highly active antiretroviral therapy. HIV Med 7: 437–441.
19. Geretti AM, Smith C, Haberl A, Garcia-Diaz A, Nebbia G, et al. (2008) Determinants of virological failure after successful viral load suppression in first-line highly active antiretroviral therapy. Antivir Ther 13: 927–936.
20. Delaugerre C, Gallien S, Flandre P, Mathez D, Amarsy R, et al. (2012) Impact of low-level-viremia on HIV-1 drug-resistance evolution among antiretroviral treated-patients. PLoS One 7: e36673.
21. Taiwo B, Gallien S, Aga E, Ribaudo H, Haubrich R, et al. (2011) Antiretroviral drug resistance in HIV-1-infected patients experiencing persistent low-level viremia during first-line therapy. J Infect Dis 204: 515–520.
22. Swenson LC, Min JE, Woods CK, Cai E, Li JZ, et al. (2014) HIV drug resistance detected during low-level viraemia is associated with subsequent virologic failure. AIDS.
23. Gonzalez-Serna A, Min JE, Woods C, Chan D, Lima VD, et al. (2014) Performance of HIV-1 Drug Resistance Testing at Low-Level Viremia and Its Ability to Predict Future Virologic Outcomes and Viral Evolution in Treatment-Naive Individuals. Clin Infect Dis 58: 1165–1173.
24. McConnell MJ, Mier-Mota J, Flor-Parra F, Martinez-Fernandez FJ, Lopez-Cortes LF, et al. (2011) Improved viral suppression after treatment optimization in HIV-infected patients with persistent low-level Viremia. Journal of Acquired Immune Deficiency Syndromes 58: 446–449.
25. Havlir DV, Bassett R, Levitan D, Gilbert P, Tebas P, et al. (2001) Prevalence and predictive value of intermittent viremia with combination hiv therapy. Jama 286: 171–179.
26. Mira JA, Macias J, Nogales C, Fernandez-Rivera J, Garcia-Garcia JA, et al. (2002) Transient rebounds of low-level viraemia among HIV-infected patients under HAART are not associated with virological or immunological failure. Antiviral Therapy 7: 251–256.
27. Sklar PA, Ward DJ, Baker RK, Wood KC, Gafoor Z, et al. (2002) Prevalence and clinical correlates of HIV viremia ('blips') in patients with previous suppression below the limits of quantification. AIDS 16: 2035–2041.
28. Sungkanuparph S, Overton ET, Seyfried W, Groger RK, Fraser VJ, et al. (2005) Intermittent episodes of detectable HIV viremia in patients receiving nonnucleoside reverse-transcriptase inhibitor-based or protease inhibitor-based highly active antiretroviral therapy regimens are equivalent in incidence and prognosis. Clinical Infectious Diseases 41: 1326–1332.
29. Podsadecki TJ, Vrijens BC, Tousset EP, Rode RA, Hanna GJ (2007) Decreased adherence to antiretroviral therapy observed prior to transient human immunodeficiency virus type 1 viremia. J Infect Dis 196: 1773–1778.

30. Martinez V, Marcelin AG, Morini JP, Deleuze J, Krivine A, et al. (2005) HIV-1 intermittent viraemia in patients treated by non-nucleoside reverse transcriptase inhibitor-based regimen. Aids 19: 1065–1069.
31. Ibrahim KY, Recordon-Pinson P, Malvy D, Fleury H, Segurado AC (2012) Intermittent HIV-1 viremia (Blips) and virological failure in a cohort of people living with HIV from Sao Paulo, Brazil. AIDS Patient Care and STDs 26: 512–515.
32. Easterbrook PJ, Ives N, Waters A, Mullen J, O'Shea S, et al. (2002) The natural history and clinical significance of intermittent viraemia in patients with initial viral suppression to <400 copies/ml. Aids 16: 1521–1527.
33. Masquelier B, Pereira E, Peytavin G, Descamps D, Reynes J, et al. (2005) Intermittent viremia during first-line, protease inhibitors-containing therapy: significance and relationship with drug resistance. J Clin Virol 33: 75–78.
34. Grennan JT, Loutfy MR, Su D, Harrigan PR, Cooper C, et al. (2012) Magnitude of virologic blips is associated with a higher risk for virologic rebound in HIV-infected individuals: a recurrent events analysis. J Infect Dis 205: 1230–1238.
35. Maggiolo F, Callegaro A, Cologni G, Bernardini C, Velenti D, et al. (2012) Ultrasensitive Assessment of Residual Low-Level HIV Viremia in HAART-Treated Patients and Risk of Virological Failure. J Acquir Immune Defic Syndr 60: 473–482.
36. Alvarez Estevez M, Chueca Porcuna N, Guillot Suay V, Pena Monge A, Garcia Garcia F, et al. (2013) Quantification of viral loads lower than 50 copies per milliliter by use of the Cobas AmpliPrep/Cobas TaqMan HIV-1 test, version 2.0, can predict the likelihood of subsequent virological rebound to >50 copies per milliliter. J Clin Microbiol 51: 1555–1557.
37. Pugliese P, Delpierre C, Cuzin L, Poizot-Martin I, Rey D, et al. (2013) An undetectable polymerase chain reaction signal in routine HIV plasma viral load monitoring is associated with better virological outcomes in patients receiving highly active antiretroviral therapy. HIV Medicine 14: 509–515.
38. Gianotti N, Galli L, Racca S, Salpietro S, Cossarini F, et al. (2011) Residual viraemia does not influence 1 year virological rebound in HIV-infected patients with HIV RNA persistently below 50 copies/mL. J Antimicrob Chemother 67: 213–217.
39. Charpentier C, Landman R, Laouenan C, Joly V, Hamet G, et al. (2012) Persistent low-level HIV-1 RNA between 20 and 50 copies/ML in antiretroviral-treated patients: Associated factors and virological outcome. Journal of Antimicrobial Chemotherapy 67: 2231–2235.

Hospital Admission following Induced Abortion in Eastern Highlands Province, Papua New Guinea – A Descriptive Study

Lisa M. Vallely[1]*, Primrose Homiehombo[2], Angela Kelly-Hanku[2,3], Antonia Kumbia[4], Glen D. L. Mola[5], Andrea Whittaker[6]

1 Sexual and Reproductive Health Unit, Papua New Guinea Institute of Medical Research, Alotau, Milne Bay Province, Papua New Guinea, **2** Sexual and Reproductive Health Unit, Papua New Guinea Institute of Medical Research, Goroka, Eastern Highlands Province, Papua New Guinea, **3** International HIV Research Group, School of Public Health and Community Medicine, University of New South Wales, Sydney, Australia, **4** Division of Obstetrics and Gynaecology, Eastern Highlands Provincial Hospital, Goroka, Eastern Highlands Province, Papua New Guinea, **5** School of Medicine and Health Sciences, University of Papua New Guinea, Port Moresby, Papua New Guinea, **6** School of Social Sciences, Monash University, Victoria, Australia

Abstract

Background: In Papua New Guinea abortion is restricted under the Criminal Code Act. While safe abortions should available in certain situations, frequently they are not available to the majority of women. Sepsis from unsafe abortion is a leading cause of maternal mortality. Our findings form part of a wider, mixed methods study designed to identify complications requiring hospital treatment for post abortion care and to explore the circumstances surrounding unsafe abortion.

Methods: Through a six month prospective study we identified all women presenting to the Eastern Highlands Provincial Hospital following spontaneous and induced abortions. We undertook semi-structured interviews with women and reviewed individual case notes, extracting demographic and clinical information.

Findings: Case notes were reviewed for 56% (67/119) of women presenting for post abortion care. At least 24% (28/119) of these admissions were due to induced abortion. Women presenting following induced abortions were significantly more likely to be younger, single, in education at the time of the abortion and report that the baby was unplanned and unwanted, compared to those reporting spontaneous abortion. Obtained illegally, misoprostol was the method most frequently used to end the pregnancy. Physical and mechanical means and traditional herbs were also widely reported.

Conclusion: In a country with a low contraceptive prevalence rate and high unmet need for family planning, all reproductive age women need access to contraceptive information and services to avoid, postpone or space pregnancies. In the absence of this, women are resorting to unsafe means to end an unwanted pregnancy, putting their lives at risk and putting an increased strain on an already struggling health system. Women in this setting need access to safe, effective means of abortion.

Editor: Virginia J. Vitzthum, Indiana University, United States of America

Funding: This study was supported by through AusAID PNG funding for sexual and reproductive health research at the PNGIMR and Marie Stopes PNG. The funders had no role in study design, data collection and analysis, decision to publish, or preparation of the manuscript.

Competing Interests: The authors have declared that no competing interests exist.

* Email: lmvallely@yahoo.com

Introduction

Of the 44 million abortions that took place globally in 2008 nearly half were considered unsafe [1]. An important distinction between a safe and an unsafe abortion is that a safe induced abortion has few health consequences for the woman whereas an unsafe induced abortion can pose a significant health threat to them, in terms of both morbidity and mortality [2,3]. Forty per cent of women seeking induced abortion live in countries where it is legally restricted. But even where induced abortion is legal, access to such services is often poor [4]. The majority of unsafe abortions that take place every year occur in developing countries [5], frequently undertaken by individuals without the necessary skills to perform the procedure; alternatively they may be self-induced. The circumstances and environment in which unsafe abortion is performed may be aggravated by unhygienic conditions and interventions or incorrect administration of medication [5].

Unsafe, induced abortion procedures may involve the ingestion of harmful substances and physical means such as insertion of a foreign object or substance through the cervix and into the uterus, or external force, such as squeezing the abdomen [5–7]. More recently, it is suggested that the increasing availability and use of the E1 prostaglandin analogue, misoprostol, is replacing many of these risky methods of unsafe abortion [6,8,9]. It has been suggested that in developing countries, even when used incorrectly, severe complications and maternal deaths are lower with the use of misoprostol when compared to physical means of unsafe abortion [10,11].

Over the past few decades there has been a decline in maternal mortality [12] however, mortality from unsafe induced abortion has remained the same, accounting for approximately 15% of all maternal deaths [12]. The majority of maternal deaths attributable to unsafe abortion occur in developing countries, frequently linked to lack of access to care during an emergency [5]. In addition to maternal deaths many more women suffer both short and long term health consequences [1], including haemorrhage, sepsis and infertility [6].

Whether legal or not, induced abortion is a sensitive topic and induced abortion is frequently stigmatized [1]. While this stigma may be perceived, or experienced, for those seeking both abortion and post abortion care, stigma is also reported in relation to service delivery and at the policy level [13,14]. In countries where induced abortion is restricted or inaccessible due, for example, to legal socio-cultural or geographical barriers, seeking information on incidence, practices and outcomes is difficult. When abortion occurs in clandestine situations, it may not be reported or may be declared as a spontaneous abortion [1]. Using estimates of indirect methods, for example information relating to complications treated in hospital, studies on conditions of unsafe abortions and women's reports through health and population surveys can provide some information [1]. However, these data need to be reviewed with caution and it can be reasonable to assume that they are an underestimate. Women living in rural areas with poor access to hospitals, which tend to be situated in urban areas, are unlikely or unable to obtain care if they have an abortion complication [4]. In addition, many women may have unsafe abortions, but no complications and therefore not present for hospital level care and having no detectable encounter with the health system. Maternal deaths may also occur in the community setting and remain unrecognised or unreported as an abortion related death.

As well as the health consequences for the individual woman, consequences of unsafe abortion result in increased costs to health systems: use of hospital beds, blood supplies, medication, operating theatres, anaesthesia and medical specialists all stretch a resource poor situation [4,15]. Efforts to reduce unsafe abortion and to understand why and under what circumstances women resort to such abortions are crucial if maternal mortality due to unsafe abortion is to be reduced [16].

Papua New Guinea (PNG) has the highest maternal mortality ratio in the Oceania region and one of the highest in the world, with an estimated 594 maternal deaths per 100,000 live-births [12]. Sepsis due to unsafe abortion is reported as a leading cause of maternal mortality in PNG [17,18]. The country has a low contraceptive prevalence rate for modern methods of family planning among married women (24%) and a high unmet need for family planning (27%) [19–21].

In PNG the legal framework surrounding abortion is contained within the Criminal Code Act of 1974 [22], which reproduces the 1899 Criminal Code Act of Queensland, adopted as the law of the colony of British New Guinea. Since 1993, following a request from the PNG Department of Health to the State Solicitor, an induced abortion may be undertaken to save a woman's life and/or to preserve the woman's physical and mental health, and can be legally performed by trained providers in safe conditions, provided there is agreement by two medical officers. However, in reality safe, induced abortions are not available for the majority of women in PNG and induced abortion is not available in any public health facility in PNG [17]. Although in every urban setting a health practitioner (usually a doctor in private practice) is willing to safely induce abortion, fees at private clinics are too expensive for the majority of Papua New Guineans [17].

As with many aspects of maternal health in PNG, there is a paucity of research relating to unsafe abortion. Work undertaken in the early 1990s and in 2011 relating to sexual and reproductive health indicates that women do seek and undertake illegal, unsafe, often self-induced abortion to end an unwanted pregnancy [23,24]. To date no study has described women's experiences, including seeking care post abortion, clinical presentation and management at hospital.

The findings presented in this paper form part of a wider, mixed methods study. The overall aim of the study was to identify the types of complications that require hospital treatment as a result of spontaneous and induced abortion and to explore the reasons why and under what circumstances women resort to induced abortion. Through a qualitative component, we explored the reasons why women resort to unsafe abortion, the techniques used, the events leading to hospital admission and the decision making processes relating to both the abortion and seeking post abortion care. The qualitative data relating to the wider study is presented elsewhere [25,26]. In this paper we present demographic and clinical information for women presenting for hospital level care as a result of self-reported spontaneous and induced abortion. We describe the socio-cultural differences, clinical presentation and outcomes between the two groups of women. Timing and methods used for unsafe abortion are also described.

Methods

Ethics statement

This research was approved by the Medical Research Advisory Committee (MRAC 11.32) PNG in December 2011; the Institutional Review Board of the Papua New Guinea Institute of Medical Research (IRB 1201) in February 2012; and the University of Queensland Human Research Ethics Committee in Australia (LV080312) in March 2012. An amendment to protocol was approved in July 2012. Written consent was obtained from all those who participated in the semi structured interviews and case note review. To ensure anonymity all participants were assigned a unique study identity number.

Study site

Situated in the Highlands region of PNG, the Eastern Highlands Province has an estimated population of 540,000; the majority live in rural areas. The Eastern Highlands Provincial Hospital in Goroka is the referral hospital for the province. In 2012 there were a total of 1,186 gynaecology admissions at the hospital and an estimated 15 births a day. In 2009, a retrospective study undertaken at the hospital identified puerperal sepsis and abortion related sepsis as leading causes of maternal mortality [17]. At the same hospital a prospective study, undertaken in 2011, identified misoprostol as the most widely used means to induce an abortion [27].

Data collection

A prospective, mixed methods study of women presenting to the Eastern Highlands Provincial Hospital with complications following self-reported spontaneous and induced abortion was undertaken over a six month period. We sought to identify all women admitted to the hospital with suspected or confirmed abortion, including both spontaneous and induced abortion. All data collection was undertaken by one trained and experienced research midwife from the Papua New Guinea Institute of

Medical Research (PNGIMR) and overseen by the principle investigator for the study.

Between 28th May and 30th November 2012, daily review of available admission records, including ward admission books, was undertaken by the research midwife at the emergency department, out-patient department, well woman clinic and the obstetric and gynaecology ward. We sought to identify any woman admitted with a complication indicative that an abortion may have taken place, including spontaneous abortion, safe abortion and unsafe abortion. Inclusion criteria were women identified in the admission book or through clinical records as bleeding during pregnancy; reporting an induced, illegal abortion; reporting a spontaneous abortion; excessive vaginal bleeding; lower abdominal pain with vaginal discharge/bleeding; fever with vaginal bleeding/discharge; foreign body in uteri or pelvic injury. In line with the PNG National Department of Health guidelines, abortion was defined as vaginal bleeding before 20 weeks gestation or fetal weight of less than 500 grams.

Semi structured interviews

Semi structured interviews were introduced during the second month of data collection (27th July 2012), following an amendment to the original research protocol and ethics approval. Semi structured interviews were included to ensure all cases of unsafe abortion, not revealed as such at the time of admission or not identified on clinical examination, were identified. Following informed consent procedures, a semi structured interview guide (Figure S1) was used to conduct interviews with women meeting the inclusion criteria. We sought to identify women's reasons for seeking hospital level care, their reaction to the pregnancy and their feelings in relation to the pregnancy loss.

Case note review

Following identification of women through the admission book, or following the semi structured interview, women identified reporting as either a spontaneous or induced abortion were approached and informed consent procedures completed. For women providing consent a piloted study specific case note record form was used to identify basic socio-demographic information, reproductive and obstetric history, presenting complaints, time between onset of symptoms and seeking care, diagnosis and clinical management received.

Data management

All clinical data were entered into a study specific MS Access database by one member of the sexual and reproductive health team at the PNGIMR and was cleaned prior to analysis. All semi structured interviews were transcribed and translated by the research midwife. Transcripts were managed using NVivo 9 (QSR International Pty Ltd 2010), a qualitative data software programme.

Data analysis

Statistical analyses were conducted in Stata 12.1 (StataCorp LP, Texas, USA) to compare socio-demographic, behavioural and clinical outcomes among women reporting spontaneous and induced abortion. Due to the modest sample size of the study, it was not possible to conduct multivariate analysis to examine independent risk factors. Semi structured interviews were reviewed and discussed between the principle investigator and the research midwife to identify additional cases of induced abortion not identified through the hospital admission records. Transcripts were reviewed to identify information relating to induced abortions, including gestation at abortion and abortion method used.

Results

Over the six-month study period we identified 129 women who met the inclusion criteria. All women were identified through the ward admission book at the obstetric and gynaecology ward. Of these 129 women, 119 (92%) were identified as presenting with complications following a self-reported spontaneous or induced abortion (Figure 1). At least 24% (28/119) of all abortion related admissions were due to induced abortion.

Semi structured interviews

Semi structured interviews were undertaken with 44 women out of a possible 79 recruited after the amendment to protocol, therefore the proportion of those consenting to participate in the semi structured interviews was 57% (44/79). Of these 44 semi structured interviews, 23 (52%) were conducted among women reporting spontaneous abortion and 21 (48%) were among women reporting induced abortion (Figure 1).

As a result of conducting semi structured interviews five women not reporting any interference with their pregnancy during the hospital admission process disclosed to the research midwife that they had interfered with their pregnancy. Of these five women, three were suspected as induced based on clinical examination; the remaining two had no report of clinical evidence that an induced abortion had taken place. Because of their disclosure during the semi structured interview they are reported here as induced abortion. One woman, who disclosed to the doctor at the time of admission that she had induced her abortion, reported a spontaneous abortion during her semi-structured interview. Based on the clinical findings and her disclosure at admission, she remains classified for this study as an induced abortion.

Case note review

Case note review was undertaken for 56% (67/119) of all women identified. Case note review could not be undertaken for the remaining 46% (52/119) of women as consent was not obtained; 60% (31/52) were discharged home within 24 hours of admission (Figure 1). Of the 67 case notes reviewed, 39 (58%) women were identified as, or reported, a spontaneous abortion and 28 (42%) were identified as, or reported, an induced abortion (Figure 1). Seven women reporting induced abortion had their case notes reviewed before the introduction of the semi structured interviews.

Socio-demographic characteristics. Social and demographic details for all 67 women are shown in table 1. More than half of the women (35/67; 52%) were aged 15–24 years and were residing in Goroka district at the time of admission (35/67; 52%). Nearly three quarters (49/67; 73%) reported to be married. More than half of the women (41/67; 61%) were educated beyond grade seven and 15% (10/67) had received a tertiary or university level education; 25% (17/67) of women were a student (at either secondary school or university) at the time of admission. Compared to women who reported spontaneous abortion, those who had experienced induced abortion were significantly more likely to be aged 15–24 years (71% vs 39%, $p = 0.0078$); to be single (39% vs 3%, $p = 0.0001$); and were a student at time of admission to hospital (43% vs 13%, $p = 0.0053$).

Pregnancy history. Just over one third of women (25/67; 37%) had never given birth before; 27% (18/67) had given birth once in the past. More than half of the women (35/67; 52%) reported to be in their second trimester at the time of the abortion.

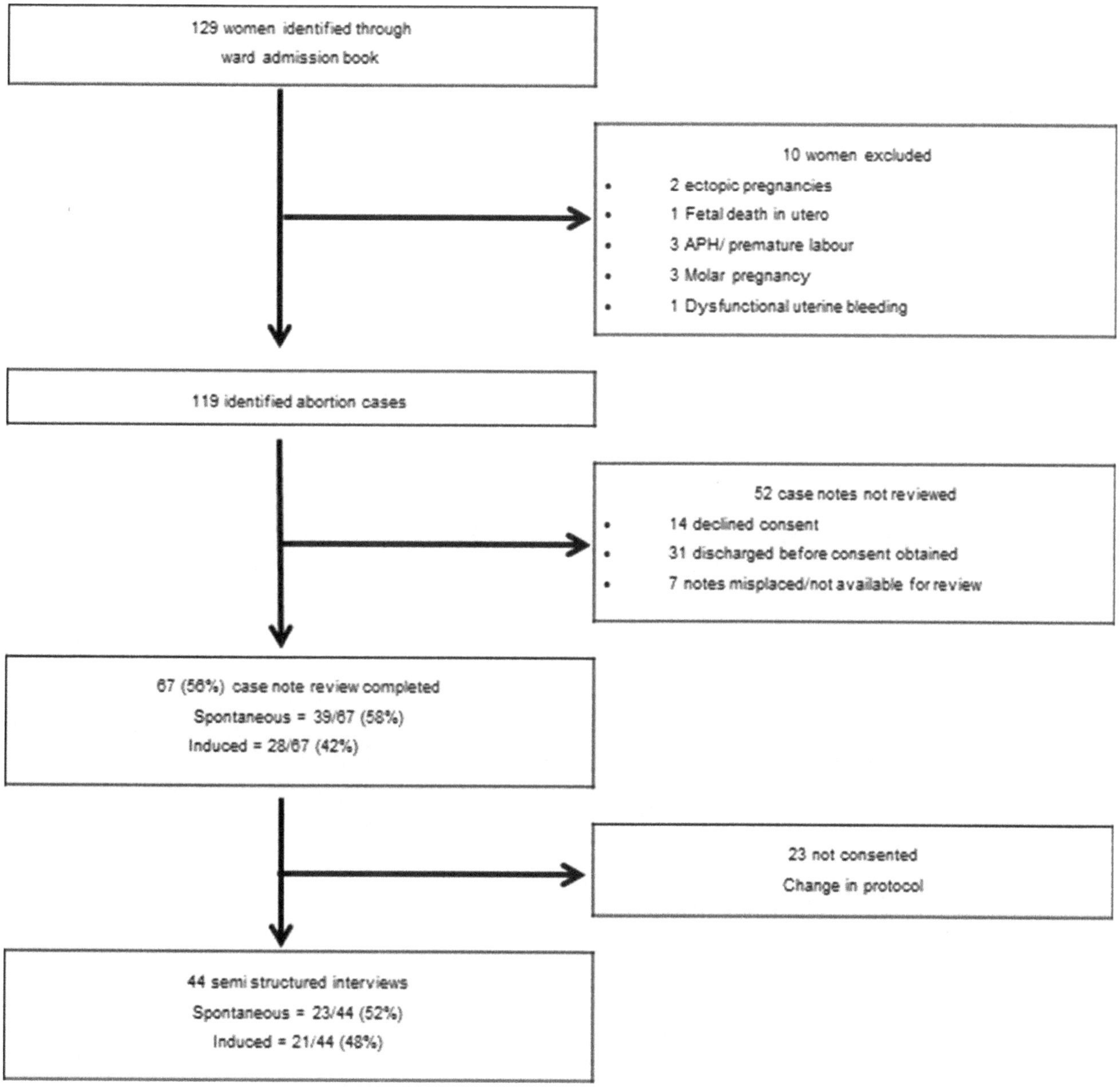

Figure 1. Identification of women admitted following spontaneous and induced abortion.

Almost half of the women (32/67; 48%) reported that the pregnancy had been planned; 28% (19/67) said that the pregnancy was unintended and not wanted (Table 2).

Parity and gestation at presentation to hospital was not significantly different between women reporting spontaneous abortion and those with induced abortion. Compared to women who reported spontaneous abortion, those who had experienced induced abortion were significantly more likely to report that the pregnancy was a mistake and the baby unwanted (64% vs 3%; $p < 0.0001$).

Clinical presentation. Duration of symptoms before presentation varied between presenting the same day as onset of symptoms, up to four weeks. Most women (47/67; 70%) presented between 0–5 days (Table 3). Vaginal bleeding with associated abdominal pain was the most widely reported presenting complaint, reported by 61% (41/67) of all women.

There was no significant difference between onset of symptoms and presentation between the two groups of women. Compared to women who reported spontaneous abortion, those who had experienced induced abortion were significantly more likely to present with bleeding, pain and fever (36% vs 5%; $p = 0.0013$). Women presenting following induced abortion were significantly more likely to present with signs of severe anaemia (27% vs 4%; $P = <0.001$). There was no significant difference between the two groups in terms of clinical signs of septic abortion (Table 3).

Clinical management. 97% (65/67) of women underwent a surgical procedure of whom 97% (63/65) had dilatation and curettage for retained products; two women had an exploratory laparotomy. Of the two who underwent laparotomy, one had inserted a stick into the vagina to induce an abortion three weeks earlier; she was found to have a pelvic abscess at laparotomy (Table 4). The other woman had a history of bleeding for two

Table 1. Social and demographic details : Case Note Review (n = 67).

		All women n = 67	Induced n = 28	Spontaneous n = 39	p-value
Age	15–24	35 (52%)	20 (71%)	15 (38%)	p = 0.0078
	25–34	26 (39%)	7 (25%)	19 (49%)	p = >0.05
	≥35	6 (9%)	1 (4%)	5 (13%)	p = >0.05
Marital status	Married	49 (73%)	13 (46%)	36 (92%)	p = >0.05
	Single	12 (18%)	11 (39%)	1 (3%)	p = 0.0001
	Separated	6 (9%)	4 (14%)	2 (5%)	p = >0.05
Province of birth	Eastern Highlands Province	51 (76%)	21 (75%)	30 (77%)	p = >0.05
	Other	15 (22%)	6 (21%)	9 (23%)	p = >0.05
	Not Known	1 (2%)	1 (4%)	0 (0%)	p = >0.05
Current address	Goroka district	35 (52%)	18 (64%)	17 (44%)	p = >0.05
	Other districts in Eastern Highlands	26 (39%)	9 (32%)	17 (44%)	p = >0.05
	Districts outside Eastern Highlands	6 (9%)	1 (4%)	5 (13%)	p = >0.05
Education level	University/tertiary	10 (15%)	4 (14%)	6 (15%)	p = >0.05
	Grade 11–12	6 (9%)	6 (21%)	0 (0%)	p = >0.05
	Grade 7–10	25 (32%)	8 (29%)	17 (44%)	p = >0.05
	Grade 4–6	12 (18%)	6 (21%)	6 (15%)	p = >0.05
	Grade 1–3	9 (13%)	3 (11%)	6 (15%)	p = >0.05
	No education	5 (7%)	1 (4%)	4 (10%)	p = >0.05
Employment	No paid job	4 (6%)	0 (0%)	4 (10%)	p = >0.05
	Subsistence farmer	26 (39%)	10 (36%)	16 (41%)	p = >0.05
	Housewife	10 (15%)	3 (11%)	7 (18%)	p = >0.05
	Teachers	2 (3%)	0 (0%)	2 (5%)	p = >0.05
	Student	17 (25%)	12 (43%)	5 (13%)	p = 0.0053
	Other paid work	8 (12%)	3 (11%)	5 (13%)	p = >0.05

weeks prior to presentation and despite evidence of inflamed cervix and drainage of a pelvic abscess was identified as a spontaneous abortion.

The majority of procedures were conducted by the obstetric registrar (53/66; 80%) or the senior obstetrician (11/66; 17%); the resident medical officer under took two procedures (Table 5). One woman received misoprostol for incomplete abortion and one woman required no intervention due to a complete abortion. Most women (64/67; 96%) received intravenous fluids, 61% (41/67) received blood or blood products. Those receiving blood or blood

Table 2. Obstetric History.

		All women	Induced	Spontaneous	p-value
		n = 67	n = 28	n = 39	
Parity	Nulliparous	25 (37%)	13 (46%)	12 (31%)	p = >0.05
	Para 1	18 (27%)	8 (29%)	10 (26%)	p = >0.05
	Para 2	9 (13%)	3 (11%)	6 (15%)	p = >0.05
	Para 3	9 (13%)	2 (7%)	7 (18%)	p = >0.05
	Para 4	3 (5%)	1 (4%)	2 (5%)	p = >0.05
	Para 5	3 (5%)	1 (4%)	2 (5%)	p = >0.05
Current pregnancy	Unplanned/unwanted	19 (28%)	18 (64%)	1 (3%)	p = <0.001
	Planned/wanted	32 (48%)	3 (11%)	29 (74%)	p = >0.05
	Unplanned/wanted	16 (24%)	7 (25%)	9 (23%)	p = >0.05
Reported gestation at admission	4–12 weeks	32 (48%)	11 (39%)	21 (54%)	p = >0.05
	13–20 weeks	32 (48%)	15 (54%)	17 (44%)	p = >0.05
	21–24 weeks	3 (4%)	2 (7%)	1 (3%)	p = >0.05

Table 3. Clinical presentation.

		All women	Induced	Spontaneous	p-value
		n=67	n=28	n=39	
Duration of symptoms before presenting	0–5 days	47 (70%)	17 (61%)	30 (77%)	p=>0.05
	6–10 days	11 (16%)	7 (25%)	4 (10%)	p=>0.05
	2–4 weeks	8 (12%)	4 (14%)	4 (10%)	p=>0.05
	Not known	1 (1%)	0 (0%)	1 (3%)	p=<0.001
Pale complexion	Any pale complexion	38 (57%)	15 (54%)	23 (59%)	p=>0.05
	Severe	5 (13%)	4 (27%)	1 (4%)	p=>0.05
	Moderate	20 (53%)	7 (47%)	13 (57%)	p=>0.05
	Mild	11 (29%)	4 (26%)	7 (30%)	p=>0.05
	Not specified	2 (5%)	0 (0%)	2 (9%)	p=>0.05
Presenting complaint	Just PV bleeding	10 (15%)	3 (11%)	7 (18%)	p=>0.05
	PV bleeding, abdominal pain	41 (61%)	13 (46%)	28 (72%)	p=>0.05
	PV bleeding, abdominal pain, fever	12 (5%)	10 (36%)	2 (5%)	p=0.0013
	Other	4 (6%)	2 (7%)	2 (5%)	p=>0.05
Signs of septic abortion		19 (28%)	11 (39%)	8 (21%)	p=>0.05

products were similar for both groups of women; 20 (49%) and 21 (51%) women respectively for induced and spontaneous cases.

Most women (41/67; 61%) stayed in hospital between for 3–4 days (Table 5). There were no significant differences relating to duration of hospital stay between the two groups of women.

Sixty three (94%) women received a method of family planning prior to discharge home of whom 62 received depo-provera; one opted for tubal ligation. Two women received family planning advice, one was referred onto a medical ward; family planning outcome was unknown for one woman.

There were no safe abortions undertaken at the hospital and no abortion related deaths recorded at the hospital during the six month study period.

Unsafe, induced abortions

Of the 119 women identified, 35 (29%) were identified through the ward admission book as having had an induced abortion. However, data is only presented for the 28 women consenting to case note review. Semi structured interview was undertaken with three quarters of these women (21/28; 75%). Most women (21/28; 75%) reported an induced abortion at the time of admission. Five women (5/28; 18%) had clinical signs that an induced abortion had taken place, although this was not disclosed at the time of admission; two of these women did disclose interference with the pregnancy during the semi structured interview. Two women (2/28; 7%) who disclosed during their semi structured interview that they had induced their abortion had no clinical signs that the abortion had been induced.

Table 4. Duration of hospital stay and management.

	All women	Induced	Spontaneous	p-value
	n=67	n=28	n=39	
Duration of hospital stay				
1–2 days	4 (6%)	1 (3.5%)	3 (8%)	P=>0.05
3–4 days	41 (61%)	18 (64%)	23 (59%)	P=>0.05
5–6 days	16 (24%)	6 (21%)	10 (26%)	P=>0.05
7–10 days	2 (3%)	1 (3.5%)	1 (2%)	P=>0.05
>10 days*	4 (6%)	2 (7%)	2 (5%)	P=>0.05
Management				
Dilatation and curretage	63 (94%)	26 (93%)	37 (95%)	P=>0.05
Exploratory laparotomy & drainage of pelvic abscess	2 (3%)	1 (3.5%)	1 (2.5%)	P=>0.05
Misoprostol	1 (1.5%)	1 (3.5%)	0	P=>0.05
Nil treatment	1 (1.5%)	0	1 (2.5%)	P=>0.05
Received blood or blood products	41 (61%)	20 (71%)	21 (54%)	P=>0.05

*2 women reporting spontaneous abortion stayed for 12 days; 2 women reporting induced abortion stayed for 20 & 21 days.

Table 5. Doctor providing management/treatment (NB Only 66/67 women had an intervention).

	All procedures n = 66	Dilatation & Curretage n = 63	Laparotomy n = 2	Misoprostol n = 1
Consultant obstetrician	11 (17%)	10 (16%)	1	0
Obstetric registrar	53 (80%)	51 (81%)	1	1
Resident Medical officer	2 (3%)	2 (3%)	0	0

Of all 28 induced cases identified, gestation at time of induction ranged between 7–24 weeks. More than half (17/28; 61%) took place in the second trimester, between 16–24 weeks gestation (Table 6).

Misoprostol was the most frequently reported method used to end pregnancy; 39% (11/28) of women reported using misoprostol. Both vaginal and oral routes of administration were mentioned with between two and five tablets taken (Table 6). Most women reported obtaining the misoprostol through a friend or relative working at a pharmacy; no women reported purchasing the misoprostol directly over the counter. Two women acquired the misoprostol through health care workers at hospitals outside of Goroka; another woman reported buying the misoprostol with a prescription which she had acquired through a health care worker at the hospital.

Six women (6/28; 21%) used physical means to end the pregnancy, including squeezing or tying a rope around the abdomen, excessive exercise, falling onto the abdomen, hard physical work and insertion of a stick into the vagina. The use of traditional herbs, a concoction frequently consisting of herbs, leaves and ginger which is boiled up and drunk resulting in vomiting and abdominal cramps was reported by three women (3/28; 11%). Two women reported that interference with the pregnancy had taken place through the use of witchcraft and evil spirits from another family member towards her (some areas of PNG have very strong cultural and spiritual belief relating to witchcraft, sorcery and evil spirits, especially in relation to understanding health and well-being). One woman reported receiving an injection from a health care worker at an undisclosed hospital. While she did not know what the injection was she stated that it was not a family planning injection. One woman mentioned that there had been some interference with the pregnancy due to physical violence from her husband and one described how she had drunk copious amount of strong instant coffee, bringing on vomiting and abdominal cramps (Table 6). None of the women reported trying or using more than one abortion method.

Discussion

At least 24% (28/119) of all abortion cases identified during the study period were due to induced abortion. Those identified as induced abortion were significantly more likely to be younger, single, in education at the time of the abortion, and reported that the pregnancy had been a mistake and was not wanted, compared to women reporting spontaneous abortion. Women presenting following an induced abortion were significantly more likely to present with abdominal pain, vaginal bleeding and fever, compared to those reporting a spontaneous abortion. They were also significantly more likely to be anaemic. Clinical management and outcome was similar for women in both groups with no significant differences in their management or duration of hospital stay.

Misoprostol to end an unwanted pregnancy is becoming increasingly used in both developed and developing countries [4,8] and has been previously reported in the setting for this study [27]. Table 7 outlines correct regimes for the use of misoprostol-only induced abortion. Although misoprostol used alone is a safe means of medically induced abortion, it is most often safe to do so when factors of gestation and correct dose are followed [3,28]. In the absence of adequate supervision from a skilled health worker

Table 6. Gestation and reported method of abortion.

	All induced abortions n = 28	Gestation at abortion 7–12 weeks n = 11	Gestation at abortion 16–24 weeks n = 17
Misoprostol	14 (50%)	8 (73%)	6 (35%)
PV misoprostol	*5 (36%)*	*2 (25%)*	*3 (50%)*
Oral misoprostol	*2 (14%)*	*2 (25%)*	-
PV & oral misoprostol	*4 (28%)*	*2 (25%)*	*2 (33%)*
Misoprostol, route unknown	*3 (21%)*	*2 (25%)*	*1 (17%)*
Physical means	6 (22%)	1 (9%)	5 (29%)
Traditional herbs	3 (11%)	1 (9%)	2 (12%)
Cultural beliefs/sorcery	2 (7%)	-	2 (12%)
Insertion of stick vaginally	1 (3%)	1 (9%)	-
Received injection from health care worker	1 (3%)	-	1 (6%)
Coffee	1 (3%)	-	1 (6%)

the situation becomes riskier [3,28]; and the use of sub optimal misoprostol regimes may result in several days of hospitalisation [29]. Of the 14 women identified in our study who used misoprostol, 12 followed incorrect regimes and six were in their second trimester of pregnancy. The only two women in our study who received a dose of misoprostol appropriate for their gestation received the misoprostol from hospital based health care workers. Both of these women were in their second trimester. Most of the women in our study who used misoprostol to induce their abortion were at risk of complications due to incorrect use of misoprostol, and second trimester abortion. What is unknown in this setting is whether women are accessing misoprostol earlier in their pregnancy, and using it correctly and more safely to end a first trimester abortion, therefore having no need to present for hospital level care.

Clinical management varied very little between the two groups of women and there was no different clinical management for managing induced abortion- whether women had used misoprostol or other means to end the pregnancy. National guidelines for incomplete abortion in PNG specify that incomplete abortion should be treated with either manual vacuum aspiration (MVA) or misoprostol [30]. Since its addition to the WHO essential drug list in 2011, misoprostol is available in all hospitals in PNG for use in managing incomplete abortions, induction of labour and prevention and treatment of postpartum haemorrhage. In this study only one woman was treated for incomplete abortion with misoprostol. The training and use of MVA techniques is still underway for many obstetricians in PNG, however dilatation and curettage is widely practiced, as identified in this study. Dilation and curettage requires trained, skilled health personnel, management that may consequently place an additional burden on a struggling workforce. MVA, when undertaken in the first trimester, is quicker and associated with less blood loss when compared to dilatation and curettage [31]. In addition, it may be carried out successfully by specifically trained nurses and midwives [32,33], thus reducing the clinical workload for doctors. Given the safety and effectiveness of both MVA and misoprostol in the first trimester [34,35] it is possible that some women presenting for post abortion care could be managed without the need of senior medical staff.

While grounds on which abortion can be legally performed has broadened in many developing countries, in countries where it remains illegal abortions frequently continue to take place in unsafe circumstances [36]. In many settings, the shift in legislative frameworks allowing for more legal abortions has resulted in a decline in the overall abortion rate, globally, however there has been little decline in unsafe abortions [37]. As with many developing countries, access to safe abortion in PNG is restricted due to the legal framework and lack of availability of safe abortion services through the government system. While a safe abortion should be available if a woman's physical or mental health is at risk, in reality safe abortions rarely take place, through government or non-government health services [17]. Safe abortions available through private clinics are restricted to the few practitioners in the urban settings offering the service at a cost unaffordable to most Papua New Guineans. As such, access to safe abortion in PNG remains unavailable and inaccessible to the vast majority, due not only to socio-cultural, geographical and financial constraints but also a lack of understanding relating to the legality of abortion, many women, and health care workers in PNG believe abortion to be "illegal" [26]. This situation is similar to other countries with restrictive abortion laws and availability of safe abortions almost exclusively restricted to those who can afford it [38]. Many of the factors inhibiting access to safe abortion services also play a role in women accessing health services for post abortion care, with many afraid of repercussions from health staff and the legal framework surrounding unsafe abortion practices [5,26,37].

Global estimates indicate that for every woman presenting to a health facility for management of complications following an unsafe abortion, several other women do not reach a health facility for post abortion care services [1]. Given the poor uptake of maternal health services generally in PNG, for example the supervised birth rate is 53% and the contraceptive prevalence rate is 24% [18], it is reasonable to assume that our study only highlights a small proportion of women undertaking an unsafe abortion, with many more women never reaching a health facility and therefore never part of any official statistics. Given the wide use of misoprostol among our study participants it is a possibility that some women accessed misoprostol resulting in a safe, albeit illegal abortion and therefore not requiring hospital level care. There is also the possibility that some unsafe abortions result in the death of the woman, perhaps never being recognised as a maternal mortality or reported as an abortion related death. There were no abortion-related maternal deaths recorded at the hospital during the study period. While abortion related maternal deaths have previously been reported from the same study setting, the ten deaths, from a total of 29 recorded over a three year and five month period were recorded as deaths relating to haemorrhage and abortion-related sepsis; only three were confirmed as abortion related [17].

Despite its limitations, this is the first study from PNG that has attempted to capture both spontaneous and induced abortions presenting for hospital level care, highlighting the clinical presentations and management of a vulnerable group of women. The data presented is from one hospital setting undertaken over a relatively short period of time. Despite our best efforts we were only able to review just over half of the case notes for women admitted following an abortion. Being unable to obtain informed

Table 7. Recommended guidelines for Misoprostol-only medical abortion [Source: WHO 2012].

Gestation	Recommended method
Pregnancies up to 12 weeks	800 mcg of misoprostol administered vaginally or sublingually.
(84 days)	Repeat at 3 hourly intervals, but for no longer than 12 hours.
Pregnancies of gestational age over 12 weeks (84 days)	400 mcg of misoprostol administered vaginally or sublingually.
	Repeat at 3 hours for up to five doses.
Pregnancies beyond 24 weeks	No specific dosing recommendations due to lack of clinical studies.
	But dose of misoprostol should be reduced, due to the greater sensitivity of the uterus to prostaglandins.

consent was due to a number of reasons, including restricted access to the ward, doctors ward rounds and theatre lists and women being discharged home within a short time frame. The early discharge home of some of the women may indicate that these particular women may have presented with less complicated morbidity; some may have presented earlier following onset of symptoms or may have been in the earlier stages of pregnancy. The use of semi structured interviews was included during the study as we felt we were missing some of the induced cases. Following this amendment to study design we identified just an additional two cases of induced abortion that would otherwise have been missed. Most women presenting following an induced abortion did report as such at the time of admission. Others were identified based on their history and clinical examination. However, it is possible that we missed other women presenting following induced abortion due to the limited number of case notes reviewed. This study was limited by the amount of data we were able to collect and we recognise that a larger study and sample size would have allowed us to more fully develop the findings and describe patterns and differences between the two groups of women. As this was a hospital based study, we captured only women seeking specialist medical care.

Aside from the limitations this study highlights the burden on the hospital and hospital staff for clinical management of all women presenting following both spontaneous and induced abortion. It is hoped that the findings will help assist with policy and planning, particularly in relation to management of incomplete abortion and to reproductive health services for women.

Conclusion

Our study only highlights the plight of women who present to hospital for post abortion care. As in many developing countries women in PNG are vulnerable to unplanned pregnancies and subsequently unsafe abortions. In a country with a low CPR and high unmet need for family planning, women of all ages need access to contraceptive information and services to avoid, postpone or space pregnancies. In the absence of this, women are resorting to unsafe means to end an unwanted pregnancy. In view of the proportion of women admitted to hospital following unsafe abortion, women need access to safe, effective means of abortion. In addition, the training of clinical staff in the use of MVA and misoprostol for incomplete abortions could reduce the burden on an already constrained health system. Knowledge of the legal framework on induced abortion in PNG needs to be improved in the community and among medical staff to improve access for those women eligible for a legal induced abortion. Improved access to safe abortion services together with the review of post abortion care services in PNG could help in reducing the burden of maternal mortality and morbidity from unsafe, induced abortions.

Acknowledgments

The authors thank the women who willingly shared their experiences of pregnancy loss. We also thank the staff at the gynaecology ward, especially the ward clerk and staff at the emergency department at EHP hospital for their support in helping to identify women admitted with pregnancy loss. This study was supported by Marie Stopes PNG.

Author Contributions

Analyzed the data: LV AKH. Wrote the paper: LV AKH GM AW. Responsible for the design of the study: LV AW AKH. Designed the case record form: LV GDLM. Designed the interview guides: LV PH AKH. Responsible for the overall coordination of the project: PH. Collected all clinical data: PH. Undertook all interviews: PH. Analysed all clinical data: LV AKH. Reviewed the semi structured interview transcripts: LV AKH. Led the writing of the manuscript: LV AKH. Reviewed the manuscript: AK GDLM AW.

References

1. Sedgh G, Singh S, Shah IH, Ahman E, Henshaw SK, et al. (2012) Induced abortion: incidence and trends worldwide from 1995 to 2008. Lancet 379: 625–632.
2. Singh S, Sedgh G, Hussain R (2010) Unintended pregnancy: worldwide levels, trends, and outcomes. Stud Fam Plann 41: 241–250.
3. WHO (2012) Safe abortion: technical and policy guideance for health systems. Geneva: World Health Organization.
4. Singh S (2006) Hospital admissions resulting from unsafe abortion: estimates from 13 developing countries. Lancet 368: 1887–1892.
5. WHO (2011) Unsafe Abortion: Global and Regional Estimates of the Incidence and its Associated Mortality in 2008. Geneva: WHO.
6. Grimes DA, Benson J, Singh S, Romero M, Ganatra B, et al. (2006) Unsafe abortion: the preventable pandemic. Lancet 368: 1908–1919.
7. Belton S, Whittaker A (2007) Kathy Pan, sticks and pummelling: Techniques used to induce abortion by Burmese women on the Thai border. Social Science & Medicine 65: 1512–1523.
8. Culwell KR, Hurwitz M (2013) Addressing barriers to safe abortion. International Journal of Gynecology and Obstetrics 121: S16–S19.
9. Winikoff B, Sheldon WR (2012) Abortion: what is the problem? Lancet 379: 594–596.
10. Sherris J, Bingham A, Burns MA, Girvin S, Westley E, et al. (2005) Misoprostol use in developing countries: results from a multicountry study. Int J Gynaecol Obstet 88: 76–81.
11. Harper CC (2007) Reducing maternal mortality due to elective abortion: potential impact of misoprostol in low-resource settings. International Journal of Gynecology and Obstetrics 98: 66–69.
12. Kassebaum NJ, Bertozzi-Villa A, Coggeshall MS, Shackelford KA, Steiner C, et al. (2014) Global, regional, and national levels and causes of maternal mortality during 1990–2013: a systematic analysis for the Global Burden of Disease Study 2013. Lancet; Doi:101016/s0140-6736(14)60696-6.
13. Levandowski BA, Kalilani-Phiri L, Kachale F, Awah P, Kangaude G, et al. (2012) Investigating social consequences of unwanted pregnancy and unsafe abortion in Malawi: The role of stigma. International Journal of Gynecology and Obstetrics 118: S167–S171.
14. Moore AM, Jagwe-Wadda G, Bankole A (2011) Men's attitudes about abortion in Uganda. Journal of Biosocial Science 43: 31–45.
15. Murray SF, Davies S, Phiri RK, Ahmed Y (2001) Tools for monitoring the effectiveness of district maternity referral systems. Health policy and planning 16: 353–361.
16. Kulczycki A (2009) Abortion and Postabortion care. In: Ehiri JE, editor. Maternal and Child Health: Global Challenges, Programs and Policies: Springer Science & Business Media 2009. 191–201.
17. Sanga K, de Costa C, Mola G (2010) A review of maternal deaths at Goroka General Hospital, Papua New Guinea 2005–2008. The Australian & New Zealand journal of obstetrics & gynaecology 50: 21–24.
18. NDoH-NHIS (2009) National Health Information Systems. National Department of Health, Papua New Guinea.
19. PNG-DHS (2009) Demographic Health Survey of Papua New Guinea 2006. National Statistics Office, Port Moresby.
20. NDoH-NHIS (2009) National Health Information System National Department of Health, Port Moresby, PNG.
21. UnitedNations (2013) Papua New Guinea Indicators. Available: http://unstats.un.org/unsd/pocketbook/PDF/2013/Papua%20New%20Guinea.
22. GoPNG (1974) Criminal Code Act 1974 Government of Papua New Guinea. pp. Ordinance No. 7 of 1902, revised 1974. Chapter 1262, parts 1225, 1226, 1280.
23. USAID NAC-PNG (2011) Behaviours, Knowledge, and exposure to interventions: Report from a behavioural surveillance survey, Port Moresby, Papua New Guinea. National AIDS council Papua New Guinea.
24. Jenkins C (1994) National Study of Sexual and Reproductive Knowledge and Behaviour in Papua New Guinea. Papua New Guinea Institute of Medical Research, Goroka, Papua New Guinea.

25. Vallely L, Homiehombo P, Kelly-Hanku A, Whittaker A (2014) Misoprostol, herbs, external force and spiritual beliefs: a qualitative study of unsafe abortion methods from Papua New Guinea. BMC RH (submitted March 2014).
26. Vallely LM, Homiehombo P, Kelly-Hanku A, Kumbia A, Mola GD, et al. (2013) Pregnancy Loss: a mixed methods study of spontaneous and induced abortion presenting to Eastern Highlands Provincial Hospital, Goroka, Papua New Guinea. Goroka: PNG Institute of Medical Research.
27. Asa I, De Costa C, Mola G (2012) A prospective survey of cases of complications of induced abortion presenting to Goroka hospital, Papua New Guinea. Australian and New Zealand Journal of Obstetrics and Gynaecology 52: 491–493.
28. Harris LH, Grossman D (2011) Confronting the challenge of unsafe second-trimester abortion. International Journal of Gynecology and Obstetrics 115: 77–79.
29. Basu JK, Basu D (2009) The management of failed second-trimester abortion Contraception 80: 170–173.
30. Mola G, editor (2010) Manual of standard management in obstetrics and gynaecology for doctors, Health Extension Officers and nurses in Papua New Guinea. 6th ed. Port Moresby.
31. Say L, Kulier R, Gulmezoglu M, Campana A (2005) Medical versus surgical methods for first trimester termination of pregnancy. Cochrane Database Syst Rev: Cd003037.
32. Jejeebhoy SJ, Kalyanwala S, Zavier AJF, Kumar R, Mundle S, et al. (2011) Can nurses perform manual vacuum aspiration (MVA) as safely and effectively as physicians? Evidence from India. Contraception 84: 615.
33. Kawonga M, Blanchard K, Cooper D, Cullingworth L, Dickson K, et al. (2008) Integrating medical abortion into safe abortion services: experience from three pilot sites in South Africa. J Fam Plann Reprod Health Care 34.
34. Dao B, Blum J, Thieba B, Raghavan S, Ouedraego M, et al. (2007) Is misoprostol a safe, effective and acceptable alternative to manual vacuum aspiration for postabortion care? Results from a randomised trial in Burkina Faso, West Africa. BJOG: An International Journal of Obstetrics & Gynaecology 114: 1368–1375.
35. Bique C, Usta M, Debora B, Chong E, Westheimer E, et al. (2007) Comparison of misoprostol and manual vacuum aspiration for the treatment of incomplete abortion. International journal of gynaecology and obstetrics 98: 222–226.
36. Guttmacher (2012) Facts on Induced Abortion Worldwide. Guttmacher Institute. Available: http://www.guttmacher.org/pubs/fb_IAW.pdf.
37. Sedgh G, Singh S, Shah IH, Hman E, Henshaw SK, et al. (2012) Induced abortion: Incidence and trends worldwide from 1995 to 2008. The Lancet 379: 625–632.
38. Singh S, Wulf D, Hussain R, Bankole A, Sedgh G (2009) Abortion worldwide: A decade of uneven progress. New York: Guttmacher Institute.

21

The Orthopaedic Trauma Patient Experience: A Qualitative Case Study of Orthopaedic Trauma Patients in Uganda

Nathan N. O'Hara[1]*, Rodney Mugarura[2], Gerard P. Slobogean[1], Maryse Bouchard[3]

1 Department of Orthopaedics, University of British Columbia, Vancouver, British Columbia, Canada, **2** Department of Orthopaedics, Makerere University, Kampala, Uganda, **3** Department of Orthopaedics, Seattle Children's Hospital, Seattle, Washington, United States of America

Abstract

The disability adjusted life years (DALYs) associated with injuries have increased by 34% from 1990 to 2010, making it the 10th leading cause of disability worldwide, with most of the burden affecting low-income countries. Although disability from injuries is often preventable, limited access to essential surgical services contributes to these increasing DALY rates. Similar to many other low- and middle-income countries (LMIC), Uganda is plagued by a growing volume of traumatic injuries. The aim of this study is to explore the orthopaedic trauma patient's experience in accessing medical care in Uganda and what affects the injury might have on the socioeconomic status for the patient and their dependents. We also evaluate the factors that impact an individual's ability to access an appropriate treatment facility for their traumatic injury. Semi-structured interviews were conducted with patients 18 year of age or older admitted with a fractured tibia or femur at Mulago National Referral Hospital in Kampala, Uganda. As limited literature exists on the socioeconomic impacts of disability from trauma, we designed a descriptive qualitative case study, using thematic analysis, to extract unique information for which little has been previously been documented. This methodology is subject to less bias than other qualitative methods as it imposes fewer preconceptions. Data analysis of the patient interviews (n = 35) produced over one hundred codes, nine sub-themes and three overarching themes. The three overarching categories revealed by the data were: 1) the importance of social supports; 2) the impact of and on economic resources; and 3) navigating the healthcare system. Limited resources to fund the treatment of orthopaedic trauma patients in Uganda leads to reliance of patients on their friends, family, and hospital connections, and a tremendous economic burden that falls on the patient and their dependents.

Editor: Raghavan Raju, Georgia Regents University, United States of America

Funding: This study was funded by the Uganda Sustainable Trauma Orthopaedic Program. The funders had no role in study design, data collection and analysis, decision to publish, or preparation of the manuscript.

Competing Interests: The authors have declared that no competing interests exist.

* Email: nathan.ohara@vch.ca

Introduction

The disability adjusted life years (DALYs) associated with injuries have increased by 34% from 1990 to 2010, making it the 10th leading cause of disability worldwide, with most of the burden affecting low-income countries [1]. Although disability from injuries is often preventable, limited access to essential surgical services contributes to the increasing DALY rates [2,3].

Similar to many other low- and middle-income countries (LMIC), Uganda is plagued by a growing volume of traumatic injuries. An estimated 50% of injuries in the country are due to road traffic collisions [4,5]. Long bone fractures (femur and tibia) are the most common, non-fatal orthopaedic injuries accounting for over 15% of hospital admissions [6]. With timely and effective treatment of these injuries, a patient could expect a favourable recovery with minimal disability, as is seen and expected in high-income countries (HIC). However, scarce resources within the Ugandan and LMIC health systems leave many injured patients untreated or inadequately treated causing significant long-term disability.

Studies have highlighted the disproportionate prevalence and burden of orthopaedic trauma in males aged 18 to 45 [5,7,8]. What has less frequently been reported is that these males are often the sole breadwinners for a family of dependents. The health of this demographic is vital to the economic growth of a LMIC in both the short- and long-term [9]. In addition, this demographic is at higher risk of sustaining an injury. Increased labour participation, particularly in urban areas, put individuals at greater risk of road traffic accidents as they commonly commute on less safe means of transportation (small motorcycle taxis) [10].

Effective treatment of an injury is contingent upon timely admission to an appropriately resourced healthcare facility, and the capacity for that health facility to provide adequate treatment ultimately preventing disability. The pertinent provision of care enables people to fully recover and therefore stay economically productive, support their dependents and contribute to the economic growth of the country.

The findings presented represent one aspect of a study to qualify and quantify the socio-economic impact of orthopaedic trauma in Uganda. The aim of this branch of the study is to explore the orthopaedic trauma patient's experience in accessing medical care in Uganda and what affects the injury might have on the socioeconomic status of the patient and their dependents. We also evaluate the factors that impact an individual's ability to access an appropriate treatment facility for their traumatic injury.

Methods

A descriptive qualitative case study was undertaken at Mulago National Referral Hospital in Kampala, Uganda. Data were collected through semi-structured interviews with patients 18 year of age or older admitted with a fractured tibia or femur. Patients with isolated lower extremity long bone fractures were selected, as it is well known that these injuries can cause significant disability; while mortality rates are lower than intracranial or poly-trauma [11]. Multi-trauma and head injury patients, were not only less likely to survive, but also less likely to be able to participate in the study. All patients who met the eligibility criteria during the study period were included in the sample. None of the patients who met the eligibility criteria refused to participant in the study.

Two authors conducted the interviews: NNO (male), a research manager with previous qualitative research experience and training, and RM (male), a clinical research fellow in orthopaedics with experience working and training in the Ugandan health system. Relationships between interviewers and patients were not established prior to the interviews. All interviews were semi-structured and conducted with the support of a local medical intern (female) who assisted as a translator. Each participant was only interviewed once and responses were recorded with a tablet survey tool (*QuickTap Survey, TabbleDaddle Inc., Toronto, Canada*) and augmented with interviewer notes. The patients were introduced to the interviewers and provided with a basic background on the study and the training of the researchers prior to the interviews. Written informed consent was obtained from all participants prior to the participation in the interview process. Interviews were conducted on the patient wards. Each interview lasted approximately 30 minutes. Family members of the patient were occasionally present during the interview. The interview questions were adapted from the 2009/10 National Panel Survey and augmented with clinical expertise from authorship group [12]. Data saturation was not discussed with the participants and interview transcripts or study findings were not presented to the patients for additional comments. Research ethics approval for this study was obtained from the University of British Columbia Clinical Research Ethics Board and the Mulago Research Ethics Committee. This study was conducted in compliance with the guidelines of the Helsinki Declaration.

As limited literature exists on the socioeconomic impact of disability from trauma, we designed a descriptive qualitative case study, using thematic analysis, to extract unique information for which little has been previously documented [13,14,15]. This methodology is subject to less bias than other qualitative methods as it imposes fewer preconceptions [16]. Data collected from the interviews was independently coded by two of the authors (NNO and MB). Initial inductive analysis discovered emergent themes and patterns in the data. Through authorship consensus, themes were condensed into overarching categories that represented and accurately explained the data set. Quotations used in the discussion were not identified to preserve confidentiality. Nvivo 9 Software was used to help facilitate management and analysis of the qualitative data.

Results

Thirty-five interviews were conducted with patients who were admitted with a tibia or femur fracture to Mulago National Referral Hospital in Kampala, Uganda between September 30, 2013 and October 11, 2013. **Table 1** summarizes the characteristics of the study sample. Participants were predominantly male (86%) with a mean age of 42.7 years (SD = 17.5). Eighty-three percent of the participants were working at the time of injury but only 14% of the participants had a formal contract with their employer. 74% were the main breadwinner for their household supporting an average of 5.7 dependents. The median annual income for the study participants was $1200 (IQR: $276 - $4040). Most of the participants were injured by motor vehicles (80%), 69% arrived within 24 hours of their injury but only 23% of the admitted patients received treatment within two weeks of their injury. (A complete summary of all patient data is available in the **Table S1**.)

Data analysis produced over one hundred codes, nine sub-themes and three overarching themes. A matrix of dominant and important themes can be found in **Table 2**. The three overarching categories revealed by the data were: 1) the importance of social supports; 2) the impact of and on economic resources; and 3) navigating the healthcare system (**Figure 1**). Sub-themes discovered within the importance of social supports were support of family and friends and the presence of difficult social situations. The impact of and on economic resources themes were distilled into three sub-themes: personal income, benefits of income and barriers to income. Transportation to hospital, personal factors affecting healthcare and impact of income on care received were the sub-themes derived from navigating the healthcare system, the third overarching theme. (A complete summary of all codes and their frequencies is available in the **Table S2**.).

Discussion

In Uganda, like many other LMICs, an individual's socioeconomic status has a profound impact on their ability to access the healthcare system and to receive timely treatment for an injury [10]. There are many potential barriers to hospital admission and treatment for injured patients in Uganda. Our findings identified common barriers to hospital admission such as lack of available funds for transportation and the patient's proximity to an appropriately equipped health facility. Interestingly, these impediments are often different from the patient's expressed barriers to treatment, which include limited social support and a lack of social contacts working within health system.

Social Supports

Qualitative analysis highlighted two dominant themes associated with the social supports of injured patients: 1) the support of friends and family and 2) the presence of difficult social situations. Traumatic injuries were found to not only have a substantial impact on the patient but also on their family and friends. 83% of the patients in the study were working at the time of injury, often supporting a spouse, children and siblings. Following the injury, which rendered most patients unable to work, many patients were unable to pay the school fees of their children. Furthermore, surgical wards have limited nursing care. Injured patients had to rely on those dependents for hygiene and feeding. One elderly patient noted his son would have to support all of his medical costs. The presence of difficult social situations emerged during the analysis as a second sub-theme. Patients spoke of the struggle

Table 1. Characteristics of study sample.

Characteristics		N	%
Gender			
	Male	**30**	86
Age			
	Mean =42.7 years (**SD**=17.5)		
Occupation			
	Business/Service	**13**	37
	Farmer	**7**	20
	Labourer	**6**	17
	Boda-Boda Driver*	**5**	14
	None	**4****	11
Annual Income			
	Median = $1200 USD, IQR = ($276 - $4040)		
Mechanism of Injury			
	Multi-vehicle trauma	**13**	37
	Pedestrian–vehicle trauma	**10**	29
	Single-vehicle trauma	**5**	14
	Fall from standing	**4**	11
	Gun shot wound	**2**	6
	Violence (non-gun)	**1**	3
Time from Injury to Admission			
	Less than 24 hrs	**24**	69
	24 – 48 hrs	**2**	6
	48-72 hrs	**1**	3
	3 – 10 days	**5**	14
	More than 10 days	**3**	9

(n=35).
*Boda-Bodas are motorcycles used to taxi people.
** 3 of 4 of these participants were aged ≥64 years.

Table 2. Sample of codes and themes from interview data.

Line-by-line Code	Frequency of code
Supports children	21
Supports spouse	20
Direct admission to Mulago Hospital	18
Transfer to Mulago Hospital from another hospital	14
Children in school	12
No treatment at "other" hospital	12
Immediate transfer to hospital from injury site	11
Supports siblings	10
Waiting on ward for treatment/Delayed treatment	8
Makes decent/good money	7
Diploma/degree	7
Little money/income	5

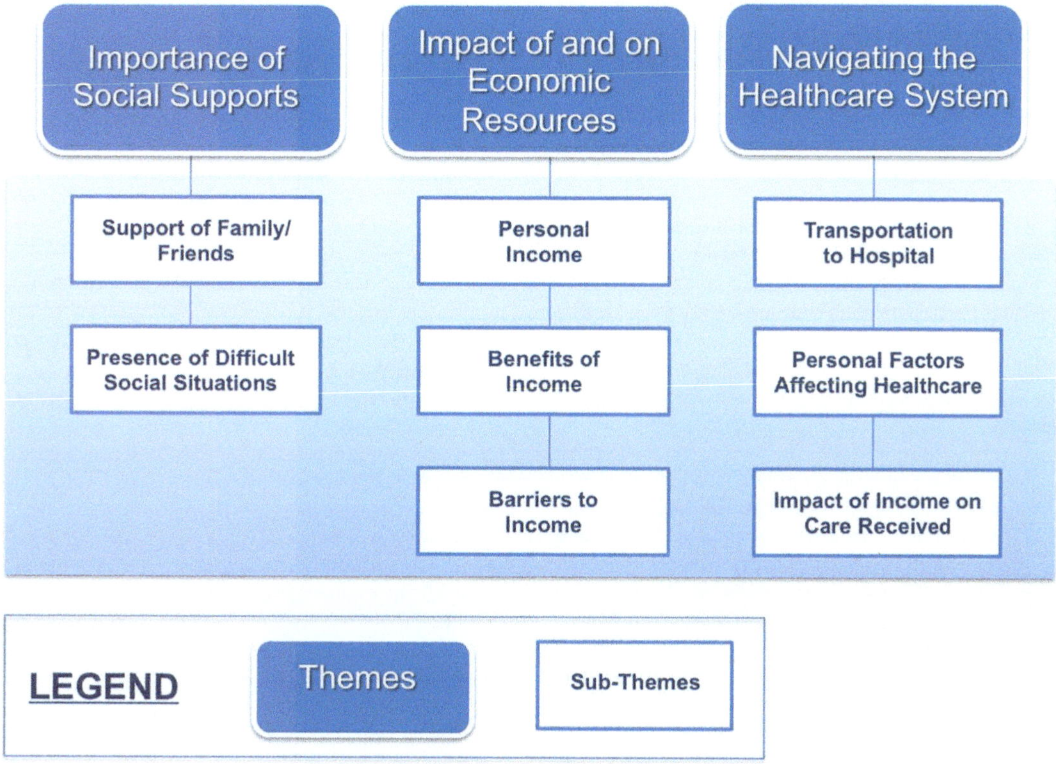

Figure 1. Themes and sub-themes derived from qualitative analysis.

associated with the death of a family member in the same traumatic event, the anxiety associated with struggling to support dependents during the time of injury, and burden of unrelated illness and mental health conditions.

Navigating Access to Care

Data analysis revealed important sub-themes relevant to navigating the Ugandan health system after a traumatic injury. A greater understanding of the relationship between minimal income and delays to hospital admission were discovered. One patient delayed travelling to the hospital for almost a month after a femur fracture due to concern about the cost of transport to the hospital in Kampala and the presumed cost of treatment. Some patients noted they had limited information on availability of appropriate health services. One patient waited two weeks for an orthopaedic consultant to visit a regional hospital and eventually voluntarily arranged to be transported to Kampala for a consultation. Other patients noted they would seek care based on the location of their family support network. A patient from Arua, a town in the northwest of the country, was given the option to be admitted in nearby Gulu (a 3-hour drive) or Kampala (a 8-hour drive). Even though Kampala was a farther, more expensive trip, the individual chose to travel to Kampala because they had family there.

Economic Burden of Catastrophic Injury

Of the 83% of study participants that were working at the time of injury, 74% were the main breadwinner for their household supporting an average of 5.7 dependents. One patient, a peasant farmer, supports his family by selling excess yield at the local market. His last sale of five months of effort provided the equivalent of $12 USD. Another patient was informally employed but unable to earn enough money to support his wife and three children, so he attempted to steal fuel to sell for extra income but was shot in the leg by an on-site security officer.

Economic activity in Uganda is largely derived from the informal sector. The informal sector of the economy refers all economic activities by workers that are not covered or insufficiently covered by formal arrangements [17]. Those employed in the informal sector are typically not privileged to forms of social insurance and pension. Wages are typically provided based on work completed and can be suspended frequently and without notice. A catastrophic injury to an individual who is informally employed, not only has a profound impact on the injured individual, but also greatly affects the dependents of that individual. Informal economies are pervasive in many low-income countries with potentially negative consequences. These consequences may include decreased competitiveness and growth, incomplete coverage of formal social programs, undermining social cohesion and law and order, and fiscal losses due to undeclared economic activity impeding the overall economic growth and impacting economic equality [18]. Participants in the informal economy do not have their income taxed directly. Therefore, increased economic productivity in this segment of the economy does not support the growth of public services such as government-funded health care. A strong formal economy fuels a social safety net that supports citizens through catastrophic events.

It is worth noting that even if a patient is admitted to a hospital shortly after injury, limited funding for the health system often requires them to buy the implant needed for their treatment. The costs of standard trauma implants for managing long bone fractures are high: a 10-hole plate and screw construct is $300

USD and a femoral intramedullary rod is $900 USD [19]. One patient commented that he has little chance of being able to buy the necessary implant for his treatment and will most likely have to be treated with traction, a sub-optimal method which renders a patient bed-ridden for months while the fracture heals.

Those patients with dependents routinely commented that their hospitalization and subsequent withdrawal from the workforce during recovery had a devastating affect on their dependents. Injured breadwinners were faced with difficult decisions on what treatment options they could afford balanced with the financial needs of their dependents. The patient often lacked the adequate savings to continuing paying for their children's school fees during their hospital stay, forcing them to withdraw from school at least temporarily.

Study Limitations

The study particants were interviewed within two weeks of admission. A greater understanding of socioeconomic issues related to a traumatic injury may be identified with a longer period of data collection. It is reasonable to assume that the longer a person waits on the wards without treatment, the greater their motivation to seek available economic resources to facilitate a faster treatment where they are admitted or transfer to a private hospital for more immediate treatment.

We acknowledge that the study is limited to those patients who were eventually admitted to the country's tertiary hospital. There are most likely many other patients that did not make it to the appropriate health facility or declined to seek treatment due to an inability to bear the costs of care. A complete analysis of the socio-economic effects on trauma patients would require the ability to interview all injured people, including those who have not been able to access appropriate medical care. Considering the inadequacy of emergency medical services in Uganda and the large number of smaller medical facilities and clinics, identifying all patients would be difficult. We therefore consider our smaller, focused study sample to be a good primary index and investigation into the barriers to care and impacts of injury.

Suggestions for Further Research

This field of research would benefit from further insight into the long-term socio-economic implications of traumatic injuries. Evaluating if these patients return to the same level of economic productivity, if they maintain the same socio-economic status post-injury and the impact of these injuries on their dependents would be valuable information for policy makers. There are many potential factors that will contribute to a patient's recovery. For instance, one patient noted that his brothers have good jobs and will be able to support him while he recovers. This seemed like an unfortunately rare circumstance among this patient population.

An increased awareness of the factors that lead to the timely and effective treatment of orthopaedic injuries in low-income countries will enable government and policy makers to create effective interventions for improving trauma care. We have found that a strong social support system for the patient, the ability of the patient to understand and navigate the health system, and the impact of an injured breadwinner on that individual and their dependents, are crucial elements in determining whether an injured patient will receive timely, appropriate care.

Conclusion

The appreciation of the association between traumatic injuries and their implications for economic growth should lead to improved resource allocation for both prevention and treatment these injuries. Improved mechanisms to fund the management of treating trauma patients (government funding, availability of loans, access to insurance) would potentially alleviate the present reliance of patients on their friends, family, and hospital connections, and diminish the economic burden that falls on the patient and their dependents.

Supporting Information

Table S1 Data Set Characteristics.

Table S2 Code Frequencies.

Table S3 Qualitative Interview Questions.

Table S4 COREQ Checklist.

Acknowledgments

We thank Dr. Tito Beyeza, Dr. Piotr Blachut and Dr. Peter O'Brien for valuable insight and support.

Author Contributions

Conceived and designed the experiments: NNO RM GPS. Performed the experiments: NNO RM. Analyzed the data: NNO MB RM GPS. Contributed reagents/materials/analysis tools: NNO MB GPS RM. Wrote the paper: NNO MB GPS RM.

References

1. Murray CJ, Vos T, Lozano R, Naghavi M, Flaxman AD, et al. (2012) Disability-adjusted life years (DALYs) for 291 diseases and injuries in 21 regions, 1990–2010: a systematic analysis for the Global Burden of Disease Study 2010. Lancet 380(9859): 2197-2223.
2. Weiser TG, Regenbogen SE, Thompson KD, Haynes AB, Lipsitz SR, et al. (2008) An estimation of the global volume of surgery: a modelling strategy based on available data. Lancet 372(9633): 139–144.
3. Grimes CE, Bowman KG, Dodgion CM, Lavy CBD (2011) Systematic review of barriers to surgical care in low-income and middle-income countries. World J Surg 35(5): 941–950.
4. Demyttenaere SV, Nansamba C, Nganwa A, Mutto M, Lett R, et al. (2009) Injury in Kampala, Uganda: 6 years later. Can J Surg 52(5): E146-150.
5. Hsia RY, Ozgediz D, Mutto M, Jayaraman S, Kyamanywa P, et al. (2010) Epidemiology of injuries presenting to the national hospital in Kampala, Uganda: implications for research and policy. Int J Emerg Med 3(3): 165-172.
6. Mock C, Cherian MN (2008) The global burden of musculoskeletal injuries: challenges and solutions. Clin Orthop Relat Res 466(10): 2306-2316.
7. Kobusingye OC, Guwatudde D, Owor G, Lett RR (2002) Citywide trauma experience in Kampala, Uganda: a call for intervention. Inj Prev 8(2): 133-136.
8. Galukande M, Jombwe J, Fualal J, Gakwaya A (2009) Boda-boda injuries a health problem and a Burden of Disease in Uganda: A tertiary Hospital survey. East Central Afr J Surg 14(2): 33-37.
9. Bloom DE, Canning D, Sevilla J (2004) The effect of health on economic growth: a production function approach. World Dev 32(1): 1-13.
10. Nantulya VM, Reich MR (2002) The neglected epidemic: road traffic injuries in developing countries. Br Med J 324(7346): 1139.
11. Begg S, Tomijima N, Vos T, Mathers CD (2003) Global burden of injury in the year 2000: an overview of methods. Geneva: WHO.
12. The World Bank (2011) Uganda 2011/12 national panel survey. Available: http://econ.worldbank.org/WBSITE/EXTERNAL/EXTDEC/EXTRESEARCH/EXTLSMS/0, contentMDK:23511127~menuPK:4196952~pagePK:64168445~piPK:64168309~theSitePK:3358997~isCURL:Y,00.html. Accessed 10 June 2014.
13. Keen J, Packwood T (1995) Case study evaluation. Br Med J 311(7002): 444.
14. Fereday J, Muir-Cochrane E (2006) Demonstrating rigor using thematic analysis: A hybrid approach of inductive and deductive coding and theme development. Int J Qual Methods 5(1): 80-92.
15. Braun V, Clarke V (2006) Using thematic analysis in psychology. Qual Res Psychol 3(2): 77-101.

16. Sandelowski M (1991) Telling stories: Narrative approaches in qualitative research. J Nurs Scholarsh 23(3): 161-166.
17. International Labour Organization (2012) Resource guide on the informal economy. Available: http://www.ilo.int/public/english/support/lib/resource/subject/informal.htm. Accessed 10 May 2014.
18. The World Bank (2013) Workers in the informal economy. Available: http://web.worldbank.org/WBSITE/EXTERNAL/TOPICS/EXTSOCIALPROTECTION/EXTLM/0, contentMDK:20224904~menuPK:584866~pagePK:148956~piPK:216618~theSitePK:390615,00.html. Accessed 25 May 2014.
19. Bouchard M (2011) Responding to the global injury burden by improving access to orthopaedic medical devices: A qualitative case study of orthopaedic services in Uganda. M.Sc. Thesis, The University of Toronto. Available: https://tspace.library.utoronto.ca/bitstream/1807/30520/6/Bouchard_Maryse_201111_MSc_Thesis.pdf. Accessed 10 June 2014.

Results from an Audit Feedback Strategy for Chronic Obstructive Pulmonary Disease In-Hospital Care: A Joint Analysis from the AUDIPOC and European COPD Audit Studies

Jose Luis Lopez-Campos[1,2*], M. Isabel Asensio-Cruz[1], Ady Castro-Acosta[2,3], Carmen Calero[1,2], Francisco Pozo-Rodriguez[2,3], on behalf of the AUDIPOC and the European COPD Audit studies[¶]

1 Unidad Médico-Quirúrgica de Enfermedades Respiratorias, Instituto de Biomedicina de Sevilla (IBiS), Hospital Universitario Virgen del Rocio/Universidad de Sevilla, Sevilla, Spain, **2** Centro de Investigación Biomédica en Red de Enfermedades Respiratorias (CIBERES), Instituto de Salud Carlos III, Madrid, Spain, **3** Hospital 12 de Octubre, Instituto de Investigación i+12, Madrid, Spain

Abstract

Background: Clinical audits have emerged as a potential tool to summarize the clinical performance of healthcare over a specified period of time. However, the effectiveness of audit and feedback has shown inconsistent results and the impact of audit and feedback on clinical performance has not been evaluated for COPD exacerbations. In the present study, we analyzed the results of two consecutive nationwide clinical audits performed in Spain to evaluate both the in-hospital clinical care provided and the feedback strategy.

Methods: The present study is an analysis of two clinical audits performed in Spain that evaluated the clinical care provided to COPD patients who were admitted to the hospital for a COPD exacerbation. The first audit was performed from November–December 2008. The feedback strategy consisted of personalized reports for each participant center, the presentation and discussion of the results at regional, national and international meetings and the creation of health-care quality standards for COPD. The second audit was part of a European study during January and February 2011. The impact of the feedback strategy was evaluated in term of clinical care provided and in-hospital survival.

Results: A total of 94 centers participated in the two audits, recruiting 8,143 admissions (audit 1:3,493 and audit 2:4,650). The initially provided clinical care was reasonably acceptable even though there was considerable variability. Several diagnostic and therapeutic procedures improved in the second audit. Although the differences were significant, the degree of improvement was small to moderate. We found no impact on in-hospital mortality.

Conclusions: The present study describes COPD hospital care in Spanish hospitals and evaluates the impact of peer-benchmarked, individually written and group-oral feedback strategy on the clinical outcomes for treating COPD exacerbations. It describes small to moderate improvements in the clinical care provided to COPD patients with no impact on in-hospital mortality.

Editor: James D. Chalmers, University of Dundee, United Kingdom

Funding: AUDIPOC study was funded by Fondo de Investigación Sanitaria, Spanish Ministry of Health, project numbers PI07/90129, PI07/90309, PI07/90486, PI07/90503, PI07/90516, PI07/90721, PI08/90129, PI08/90578, PI08/90251, PI08/90529, PI08/90129, PI07/90403, PI08/90447, PI08/90457, PI08/90486, and PI08/90550. The European COPD audit was funded by the European Respiratory Society. The funders had no role in study design, data collection and analysis, decision to publish, or preparation of the manuscript.

Competing Interests: The authors have declared that no competing interests exist.

* Email: lcampos@separ.es

¶ Membership of the AUDIPOC and the European COPD Audit studies is provided in File S1.

Introduction

The existence of a gap between the healthcare that patients actually receive and the guidelines for that healthcare is now well acknowledged [1]. The variations in clinical practice establish a complex interplay of different factors that impact the resulting outcomes in ways that cannot be explained solely by patient characteristics [2]. In this scenario, clinical audits have emerged as a potential tool to summarize the clinical performance of healthcare over a specified period of time. The aim of a clinical audit is to provide health professionals with information that they can use to assess and adjust their performance [3], improving the clinical care provided to patients and the clinical outcomes. Accordingly, the information obtained in an audit should be used to improve care, and several pathways for this aim have been described [4].

In this context, feedback from the audited information constitutes a key step to improve clinical practice [5]. A key question is how successful audit and feedback are in motivating health professionals to modify their clinical practice. To date, several systematic reviews have assessed the effectiveness of audit and feedback with inconsistent results [6,7]. A recent Cochrane systematic review concluded that audit and feedback generally lead to small, but potentially important, improvements in health care that depend on both the baseline performance and how the feedback is provided [8]. Accordingly, the impact of audit and feedback should be monitored by auditing clinical practices after implementing an intervention [3]; however, it should be acknowledged that the potential effect may also be influenced by the characteristics of the studied disease.

Chronic obstructive pulmonary disease (COPD) is a major and growing health problem [9]. Patients with COPD often suffer episodes of exacerbation during the course of their disease that often require hospitalization; these exacerbations are associated with significant mortality and morbidity [10,11] and are responsible for most of the social and economic burden of COPD [12]. Thus, the clinical care provided to patients who are admitted to the hospital for a COPD exacerbation should be carefully evaluated. However, the impact of audit and feedback on clinical performance has not been evaluated for COPD exacerbations.

In recent years, Spain had used an auditing process for COPD, named AUDIPOC, which has resulted in the completion of two major clinical audits in the country [13,14]. In the present study, we evaluated the results of two consecutive clinical audits performed in Spain to assess the clinical care provided to patients who were admitted to the hospital with a physician discharge diagnosis of a COPD exacerbation. The analysis will compare the performances in both audits to evaluate the components of the feedback approach that enhance COPD clinical performance.

Methods

The present study is an analysis of two clinical audits performed in Spain that evaluated the clinical care provided to COPD patients who were admitted to the hospital for a COPD exacerbation. Both audits had a similar methodology that has been extensively reported in previous publications [13,14]. Briefly, both studies were clinical audits with prospective case ascertainment of consecutive exacerbation hospital admissions and retrospective data gathering from medical records. All cases admitted to the hospital in any Department or Unit during a 2-month period with a discharge diagnosis of COPD exacerbation were included. The inclusion of a case in the audit was finally decided upon discharge if the diagnosis of COPD exacerbation was included in the discharge report as the cause of admission. The cases with a specific diagnosis that was different from a COPD exacerbation upon admission, including pulmonary edema, pneumonia, pulmonary embolism, pneumothorax, rib fractures, aspiration, pleural effusion or any other associated respiratory or non-respiratory condition, were excluded. The medical records of the included patients were reviewed, and the audit data were extracted. The survivals were followed-up for 90 days from hospitalization to evaluate their vital status and whether the patient had been readmitted. The participant investigators were asked to complete a resource and organization database recording the hospital and respiratory unit or department resources.

The first audit was conducted from November–December 2008, and 129 hospitals participated, recruiting 5,178 patients. The second audit was part of a European study in which 432 centers from 13 countries recruited 18,016 patients. In Spain, 94 hospitals participated and recruited a total of 5,271 cases during January–February 2011. For the purpose of the present study, we selected the centers that participated in both audits. Ninety-four centers were included in this analysis. Altogether, a total of 8,143 cases were included in both audits.

The recorded variables have been reported and included information on the patient characteristics (e.g., age and gender), disease characteristics (e.g., disease severity, clinical features and exacerbation), resources available (e.g., hospital structure, hospital materials and human resources) and clinical practice (e.g., the adopted diagnostic and therapeutic interventions and the adjustment to clinical guidelines). Adherence to the clinical practice guidelines was analyzed following the GOLD recommendations for exacerbation management, which were available at the time of each audit. An adequate use of mechanical ventilation or antibiotics was considered to be present when a patient with such prescriptions correctly received them or when a patient who did not have such prescriptions did not receive them accordingly.

After the first audit, feedback was planned in three different ways. First, a specific report was created for each participant center. In this report, the value of each recorded variable was presented for that center and benchmarked against the regional and national values. Second, the results of the audit were presented in the Spanish Society of Pneumology and Thoracic Surgery (SEPAR) annual congress and in the European Respiratory Society (ERS) annual meeting, and all investigators were invited to attend. Additionally, several smaller local meetings were planned during the next two years following the first audit to communicate the results. Notably, investigators were encouraged to organize meetings at the regional level to discuss the audit results, and several meetings were organized. Third, after the first audit, the SEPAR organized a working committee to create COPD healthcare quality standards, which were made available to all respiratory physicians [15]. All these initiatives were performed during 2009 and 2010, and the second audit was conducted in 2011. After the first audit, participants were not informed of an upcoming second audit.

In Spain, both audits were approved by the institutional review board of Hospital Universitario Virgen del Rocío (approval acta 07/2008 and 16/2010) and confirmed by each participating hospital [13,16]. Additionally, the hospital management director of each center authorized the audit and agreed not to inform the medical staff that the audit was being conducted so that their medical practice would not change. According to ethical regulations, all data were de-identified in the database by an audit number that was not related to the medical record number or to any personal data. There was no personal information in the database that could be used to identify the patient.

Statistical analysis

The statistical computations were performed with the Statistical Package for Social Sciences (SPSS, IBM Corporation, Somers, NY) version 18.0. Variables were characterized by the mean and standard deviation or the absolute and relative frequencies of their categories. For describing the centers, we calculated the inter-regional range (IRR), which indicates the region with the highest or lowest mean value for a particular variable. Inferential studies comparing both audits were analyzed with the unpaired Student's *t*-test (evaluating the variance equivalence with the Levene's test) or chi-squared test (with the Fisher's exact test, if required). Kaplan-Meier curves were constructed that evaluated in-hospital survival using the log-rank test to compare the in-hospital global mortality in both audits. The alpha error was set at 0.05.

Results

Ninety-four Spanish hospitals participated in both clinical audits. The main characteristics of the participant hospitals are summarized in table 1. The participating hospitals were largely public hospitals, with a high proportion being university/teaching hospitals and having a respiratory ward or team. The distribution of the participating hospitals among the different administrative regions is given in table S1 of the online supplement. All the regions in the country participated in this study.

A total of 8,143 admissions were analyzed from the two audits (audit 1: 3,493; audit 2: 4,650). The characteristics of the patients are summarized in table 2. The cases were mostly males in their eighth decade of life with a high proportion of active smokers. The number of patients with no information on their forced expiratory volume in one second (FEV_1) was 3,273, including 2,874 patients without spirometry and 399 patients with some spirometric information but no FEV_1. Altogether, the availability of the FEV_1 significantly improved in the second audit. The majority of these patients were considered to have severe or very severe disease. More than 40% of the patients had not been previously admitted, and this percentage increased significantly in the second audit. Although there were some statistical differences, the clinical presentation according to the three Anthonisen criteria was not clinically different between the audits.

The diagnostic procedures improved by the second audit (table 3). The proportion of cases with blood gas analysis significantly increased from 88.5 to 90.9%, and radiographies were also slightly more frequently performed in the second audit than in the first (99.5% vs. 97.2%). Although the increases were significant, they were not extremely different. The severity of the blood gas alterations was similar between the audits. An unexpected finding was the high proportion of consolidations in the radiographies for the second audit.

The therapeutic interventions before admission, during hospitalization and at discharge are summarized in table 4. Before admission, the number of administered treatments increased in the second audit, with a special emphasis on short-acting bronchodilators, long-acting muscarinic antagonists (LAMA) and systemic steroids. During admission, there were also some differences between the audits, but they were less striking. Notably, there was a significant decrease in systemic steroid use and a slight decrease in oxygen use in the second audit. The therapeutic recommendations at discharge were similar. Although the differences were significant, the percentages of each therapeutic option were not very dramatic.

The 10 recommendations evaluated according to the GOLD guidelines are summarized in table 5. The majority of these recommendations improved in the second audit. However, although the differences were significant, they were not very striking.

The survival curves for both audits are shown in figure 1. The in-hospital mortality was not different between the two audits. The first audit reported 164 (4.7%) deaths, and the second reported 202 (4.3%) deaths, and this difference was not significantly different. Accordingly, the median survival in the Kaplan-Meier analysis was not significantly prolonged in the second audit (56.7 days) compared with the first audit (64.6 days). The lengths of stay were very similar between the two audits, with 8.7 (7.8) days in audit 1 and 8.5 (7.3) days in audit 2 (not significantly different).

Discussion

The present study describes the state of COPD hospital care in Spanish hospitals and evaluates the impact of a feedback strategy on clinical care. After two consecutive audits, with feedback performed in between audits, we have observed some improvements in the clinical care provided to COPD patients. However, the majority of these improvements were small or moderate and did not impact the in-hospital mortality. This finding suggests that performing a clinical audit and providing the participant centers with the results according to our feedback strategy increased awareness and improved some aspects of COPD exacerbations, although there was no clear benefit on the outcomes.

Clinical audits have gained traction in healthcare systems as a way of obtaining information on the clinical care being provided. This information is of interest both for people funding healthcare, who want to ensure that the care they purchase is of the highest possible standard, and for patients who hope to receive safe and effective healthcare. However, despite evidence from many studies on audit and feedback, there is still limited information on how to use these data. A recent systematic review assessed the effectiveness of audit and feedback and reported an inconsistent picture; some evaluations obtained positive results, whereas others did not [8]. Interestingly, although previous studies suggest that audit and feedback may improve the performance of health care providers, the effects are generally moderate or small [17]. In our study, we also found moderate or small improvements in the clinical performance for COPD. Notably, audit and feedback measures are most likely to be beneficial when the existing practice is farthest away from what is desired and when the feedback is more intensive. However, the initial situation in our study was not far from the current guidelines; therefore, the feedback effect may be limited by a ceiling effect. The rationale for this limitation is most likely because clinical care for COPD exacerbations does not require complex interventions. Additionally, the recommendations for clinical care are closely followed in the medical community in our country, and the current guidelines are well known [18]. However, in this case, even small to moderate improvements in quality are worthwhile. COPD is a dramatic disease with a high prevalence [19], high in-hospital mortality and high readmission rate [16], and adequate clinical care can influence its outcome. Therefore, any effort to improve clinical care for these patients is worthwhile. Accordingly, some examples should be highlighted. The use of spirometry for diagnosis was improved in the second audit (table 2). Spirometry is a simple, non-invasive diagnostic procedure that is a necessary pillar for diagnosing COPD. In Spain, the use of spirometry has recently been evaluated, showing significant bottlenecks in primary and secondary care [20]. Thus, improvements in the use of spirometry will contribute to a better diagnosis and identification of these patients. In this regard, it is worth noting that 4.5% of patients in the first audit and 5.3% of those in the second audit did not show an obstructive pattern on spirometry. Therefore, such patients should not have been diagnosed with COPD and consequently COPD exacerbations. According to current guidelines, the diagnosis of COPD exacerbations should be solely based on clinical symptoms. However, such definition may be problematic and has been recently challenged [21]. Notably, in this study we were auditing the clinical care provided to patients deemed to have COPD exacerbations by the clinician in charge and thus treated accordingly. Arterial blood gas analysis was increased by 2.4%.

Table 1. General characteristics of the hospitals participating in both audits.

Variables	Mean	IRR	p value*
General characteristics			
Number of beds (n)	555.3	273–1073	0.049
Catchment population (inhabitants)	324.344	149.799–705.727	NS
University/teaching hospital (%)	62	0–100	NS
Public hospital (%)	98.7	66.7–100	NS
Hospital with intensive care unit (%)	89.9	50–100	0.020
Number of beds in intensive care unit (n)	15	4–26	NS
Spirometry available (%)	100	100–100	NS
Hospital with a respiratory ward (%)	78.5	50–100	NS
Hospital with a respiratory team (%)	96.2	75–100	NS
Material resources			
Respiratory outpatient clinic (%)	100	100–100	NS
COPD outpatient clinic (%)	59.5	0–100	NS
Specialty triage system (%)	8.9	0–100	0.039
Emergency department (%)	86.1	66.7–100	NS
Intermediate care unit (%)	30.4	0–100	NS
Number of beds in intermediate care unit (n)	7.8	4–30	NS
Offer non-invasive ventilation for acidosis (%)	96.2	66.7–100	NS
Offer invasive ventilation for acidosis (%)	81.0	50–100	NS
Human resources			
Chest physicians (n)	8.7	5–16	0.071
Chest physicians per 1000 beds (n)	17.3	1.2–27.2	0.001
Respiratory trainees (n)	3.6	1.25–7.5	0.025
Respiratory trainees per 100 beds (n)	5.9	2.4–26	<0.001
Physiotherapists (n)	1.4	0.25–3	<0.001
Physiotherapists per 1000 beds (n)	3.1	0.3–15.4	<0.001
Specialist nurses (n)	4.5	0–21.3	<0.001
Specialist nurses per 100 beds (n)	7.1	0–20.4	<0.001
Lung function technicians (n)	2.1	1.4–2.3	0.046
Lung function technicians per 1000 beds (n)	4.8	1.1–11.4	0.011
Hospital performance			
Admissions for any cause in the previous year (n)	62.802.5	25.142–154.244	0.044
Percentage of COPD admissions in the unit (%)	57.9	29–83	NS
Daily respiratory physician on call (%)	25.3	0–100	NS
Number of ward rounds (n)	1.5	1–3.1	NS
Percentage of patients seen by physiotherapist (%)	21.9	0–90	NS
Percentage of patients seen by respiratory physician (%)	54.6	30–95	NS
Capacity to perform NIMV on all eligible patients (%)	56.6	0–100	NS
Capacity to perform IMV on all eligible patients (%)	76.6	50–100	NS
Early discharge program (%)	20.3	0–100	<0.001
Percentage of patients in the early discharge program (%)	20.4	5–40	NS
Ability to care for long-term oxygen therapy patients (%)	97.5	66.7–100	NS
Ability to care for home-ventilated patients (%)	89.9	66.7–100	NS
Percentage of patients with rehabilitation (%)	29.7	10–100	0.021

Data are expressed as the mean or relative frequency according to the nature of the variable. IRR: Inter-regional range. NS: not significant.
*p value for the differences between the Spanish regions calculated by the ANOVA or chi-square test.

The performance of a blood gas analysis is one of the key diagnostic measures for evaluating the severity of an exacerbation in hospitals. In those centers that do not offer this procedure, the alternative is to use pulse-oximetry to evaluate oxygen saturation. However, this method does not measure the pH or $PaCO_2$, potentially leading to an incorrect assessment [22]. The use of

Table 2. Characteristics of the patients included in each audit.

	Audit 1 (n = 3,493)	Audit 2 (n = 4,650)	p value*
Age (years)	73.3 (10.05)	72.7 (10.6)	0.007
Males (n)	3,036 (86.9)	4,001 (86.0)	NS
Tobacco			
• Current smokers (n)	772 (22.1)	1,129 (24.3)	0.023
• Ex-smokers (n)	2,069 (59.2)	3,022 (65.0)	<0.001
• Never smokers (n)	151 (4.3)	211 (4.5)	NS
• Missing (n)	501 (14.3)	288 (6.2)	<0.001
Tobacco history (pack-years)	55.4 (29.6)	51.8 (32.6)	<0.001
Comorbidities (Charlson)	2.8 (1.8)	1.7 (1.7)	<0.001
Body mass index (kg/m^2)	27.6 (5.3)	27.7 (5.4)	NS
Spirometry: FEV$_1$ (%)	44.8 (17.0)	45.1 (16.4)	NS
GOLD spirometric assessment:			
• No information available	1,812 (51.9)	1,461 (31.4)	<0.001
• No obstruction	157 (4.5)	247 (5.3)	NS
• Mild (n)	50 (1.4)	74 (1.6)	NS
• Moderate (n)	422 (12.1)	887 (19.1)	<0.001
• Severe (n)	737 (21.1)	1,424 (30.6)	<0.001
• Very severe (n)	315 (9.0)	557 (12.0)	<0.001
First admission (n)	1,415 (40.5)	2,093 (45.0)	<0.001
Respiratory ward (n)	1,921 (55.5)	2,637 (56.7)	NS
Dyspnea increase (n)	3,328 (95.3)	4,431 (95.3)	NS
Sputum increase (n)	2,258 (64.6)	3,140 (67.5)	0.004
Sputum color change (n)	1,654 (47.4)	2,349 (50.5)	0.002

Data are expressed as the mean (standard deviation) or absolute (relative) frequencies. NS: not significant. FEV$_1$: forced expiratory volume in one second.
*Calculated using the unpaired Student's *t*-test or chi-square test.

Table 3. Diagnostic procedures performed during admission in each audit.

	Audit 1 (n = 3,493)	Audit 2 (n = 4,650)	p value*
Blood gas analysis performed (n)	3,091 (88.5)	4,227 (90.9)	<0.001
With oxygen (n)	621 (17.8)	1,181 (26.1)	<0.001
pH	7.39 (0.06)	7.39 (0.07)	NS
PaO_2 (mmHg)	58.9 (15.0)	60.1 (21.5)	0.007
$PaCO_2$ (mmHg)	48.5 (14.7)	48.5 (15.8)	NS
Bicarbonate (mEq/l)	28.7 (5.1)	28.6 (5.2)	NS
Acidosis (n)	549 (15.7)	737 (15.8)	0.002
Radiography performed (n)	3,396 (97.2)	4,627 (99.5)	<0.001
Consolidation (n)	12 (0.3)	384 (8.3)	<0.001
Interstitial (n)	20 (0.6)	152 (3.3)	<0.001
Neoplasm (n)	53 (1.5)	66 (1.4)	NS
Pleural effusion (n)	119 (3.4)	161 (3.5)	NS
Pneumothorax (n)	2 (0.1)	6 (0.1)	NS

Data are expressed as the mean (standard deviation) or absolute (relative) frequencies. NS: not significant. PaO_2: partial pressure of oxygen in arterial blood. $PaCO_2$: partial pressure of carbon dioxide in arterial blood.
*Calculated using the unpaired Student's *t*-test or chi-square test.

Table 4. Therapeutic interventions performed in both audits.

	Previous admission			During admission			At discharge		
	Audit 1 (n = 3,493)	Audit 2 (n = 4,650)	p value*	Audit 1 (n = 3,493)	Audit 2 (n = 4,650)	p value*	Audit 1 (n = 3,493)	Audit 2 (n = 4,650)	p value*
SABA (n)	1,227 (35.1)	2,183 (46.9)	<0.001	3,069 (87.9)	4,184 (90.0)	0.003	1,703 (48.8)	1,894 (40.7)	<0.001
SAMA (n)	587 (16.8)	1,022 (22.0)	<0.001	3,062 (87.7)	4,333 (93.2)	<0.001	780 (22.3)	834 (17.9)	<0.001
LABA alone (n)	186 (5.3)	265 (5.7)	<0.001	–	–	–	229 (6.6)	339 (7.3)	<0.001
LAMA (n)	1,286 (36.8)	2,446 (52.6)	<0.001	–	–	–	2,243 (64.2)	3,055 (65.7)	<0.001
ICS alone (n)	277 (7.9)	301 (6.5)	<0.001	448 (12.8)	844 (18.2)	<0.001	284 (8.1)	278 (6.0)	<0.001
ICS/LABA combination (n)	1,529 (43.8)	2,819 (60.6)	<0.001	–	–	–	2,584 (74.0)	3,487 (75.0)	<0.001
Methylxanthines (n)	235 (6.7)	412 (8.9)	<0.001	347 (9.9)	113 (2.4)	<0.001	336 (9.6)	417 (9.0)	<0.001
Systemic steroids (n)	415 (11.9)	771 (16.6)	<0.001	3,185 (91.2)	4,123 (88.7)	<0.001	2,407 (68.9)	2,908 (62.5)	<0.001
Antibiotics (n)	524 (15.0)	847 (18.2)	<0.001	3,129 (89.6)	4,309 (92.7)	<0.001	1,808 (51.8)	2,284 (49.1)	<0.001
Oxygen (n)	–	–	–	3,355 (97.4)	4,422 (96.5)	0.009	1,474 (42.2)	1,892 (40.7)	<0.001
Non-invasive ventilation (n)	–	–	–	353 (10.1)	555 (11.9)	<0.001	210 (6.0)	318 (6.8)	<0.001
Invasive ventilation (n)	–	–	–	28 (0.8)	80 (1.7)	<0.001	–	–	–

Data are expressed as the mean (standard deviation) or absolute (relative) frequencies. NS: not significant. SABA: Short-acting beta agonist, SAMA: short-acting muscarinic antagonist. LABA: long-acting beta agonist, LAMA: long-acting muscarinic antagonist, ICS: inhaled corticosteroid.

*Calculated using the unpaired Student's *t*-test or chi-square test. The figures for non-invasive ventilation at discharge refer to home mechanical ventilation. –: not applicable or not recorded.

Table 5. Adjustment to the GOLD guidelines.

	Audit 1 (n = 3,493)	Audit 2 (n = 4,650)	p value*
Spirometry performed	2,066 (59.1)	3,202 (68.9)	<0.001
Blood gas analysis performed	3,091 (88.5)	4,227 (90.9)	<0.001
Radiography performed	3,396 (97.2)	4,627 (99.5)	<0.001
Treatment with oxygen	3,355 (97.4)	4,422 (96.5)	0.009
Short-acting bronchodilator use	3,337 (95.5)	4,473 (96.2)	NS
No methylxanthine use	3,146 (90.1)	4,537 (97.6)	<0.001
Systemic steroids	3,185 (91.2)	4,123 (88.7)	<0.001
Adequate antibiotic use	1,930 (61.5)	2,782 (60.3)	NS
Adequate NIMV use	2,625 (85.1)	3,491 (85.6)	NS
Adequate IMV use	2,994 (97.1)	3,906 (95.8)	0.005

Data are expressed as the mean (standard deviation) or absolute (relative) frequencies. NS: not significant. NIMV: non-invasive mechanical ventilation. IMV: invasive mechanical ventilation.
*Calculated using the unpaired Student's *t*-test or chi-square test.

chest radiography is another diagnostic intervention that is needed to eliminate other potential accompanying conditions that may mimic or worsen the exacerbation. In this regard, there is an ongoing debate on the significance of the consolidation frequently found in these COPD patients [23]. Additionally, from a therapeutic standpoint, several positive changes were observed after the feedback strategy was implemented. Short-acting bronchodilators were more frequently used, and the use of methylxanthines, which are no longer recommended, was decreased. Interestingly, the use of systemic steroids was also decreased, which is an unexplained finding that will need to be addressed in the future. The adequate use of invasive mechanical ventilation will also need to be further explored. However, all of these measures had a negligible impact on in-hospital mortality or length of stay and several factors are deemed to play a role in determining such clinically relevant endpoints. One potential explanation for such a finding is the presence of a ceiling effect with a good starting position for the majority of the items. Previous studies have demonstrated the influence of the baseline performance on the potential improvement gained [24]. Another explanation may be related to the feedback strategy used. Although it seems intuitive that health care professionals will modify their clinical practice if they receive feedback that their clinical practice is inconsistent with those of their peers or the accepted guidelines, this outcome has not been consistently demonstrated. Although there is some controversy that feedback with peer comparison is either more or less effective than other initiatives [25,26], we provided feedback that was benchmarked against the peer average because providing this information may help participants understand the relative deviation of their own measures, which could improve patient outcomes.

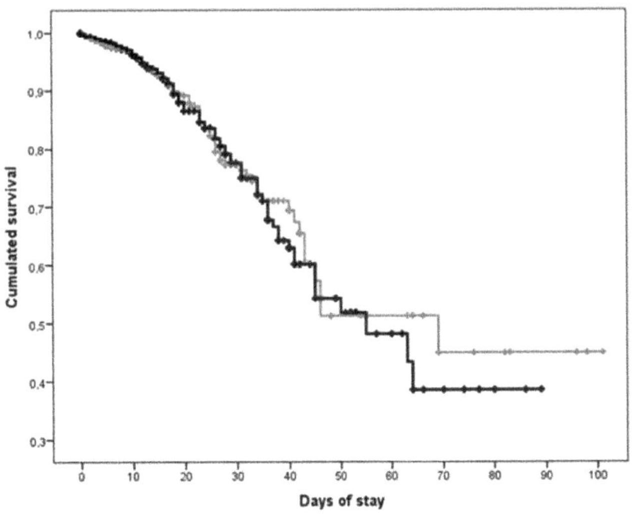

Figure 1. Kaplan-Meier curves comparing the in-hospital survival between the audits. The grey line represents the first audit. The black line represents the second audit.

Feedback can be delivered in different ways, and audit and feedback can be used as components of a multifaceted strategy to improve the quality of healthcare. In our study, we provided oral and written information at the individual level and oral information at the group level. Additionally, healthcare quality standards for COPD were constructed according to the experience with the first AUDIPOC audit [15]. Although this feedback strategy informs the participants of the audit results, alternative feedback strategies may result in different outcomes. For example, there are care bundles, including several evidence-based practices, that should be delivered to all patients to guarantee a set of minimum requirements for clinical care and several initiatives for COPD have been implemented [27,28].

Some limitations must be considered when interpreting our results. Within each region, the participating hospitals volunteered. Therefore, although all regions were sampled, there was no attempt at representative sampling. As a consequence, the hospitals involved in the study were different in organizational terms and there was a certain degree of variability concerning the available resources (Table 1). However, the participating centers were identical for both audits. Additionally, the investigators were the same for the majority of the involved centers. We therefore believe that the potential impact of structural differences between the first and the second audits should be minimal. Another limitation is the considerably high number of investigators who recorded the information using different information sources, as is intrinsically associated with audits.

In summary, our study evaluated the impact of a peer-benchmarked, individually written and group-oral feedback strategy on the clinical outcomes for treating COPD exacerbations. The results of our study suggest that performing a clinical audit and providing the participant centers with the results according to our feedback strategy increased awareness and improved some aspects of COPD exacerbation treatment. Accordingly, other feedback strategies may yield different results. Although we did not observe a clear benefit in the clinical outcomes, several aspects of the diagnostic and therapeutic clinical care provided to the COPD patients admitted to hospitals seemed to improve, which, in turn, may reduce the gap between the healthcare that patients receive and the guidelines for that care.

Supporting Information

Table S1 Percentual distribution of the cases included in both audits according to the region within the country.

File S1 Membership of the AUDIPOC and the European COPD Audit studies.

Acknowledgments

The authors are thankful to Enzo Emanuele, MD, PhD (Living Research s.a.s., Robbio, Italy) for his expert editorial assistance.

Author Contributions

Analyzed the data: JLLC MIAC CC. Contributed to the writing of the manuscript: JLLC ACA FPR.

References

1. Asch SM, Kerr EA, Keesey J, Adams JL, Setodji CM, et al. (2006) Who is at greatest risk for receiving poor-quality health care? N Engl J Med 354: 1147–1156.
2. Agabiti N, Belleudi V, Davoli M, Forastiere F, Faustini A, et al. (2010) Profiling hospital performance to monitor the quality of care: the case of COPD. Eur Respir J 35: 1031–1038.
3. Flottorp SA (2010) Using audit and feedback to health professionals to improve the quality and safety of health care. Copenhagen European Observatory on Health Systems and Policies: WHO. regional office for Europe; IX, 42 p.
4. Berwick DM, James B, Coye MJ (2003) Connections between quality measurement and improvement. Med Care 41: I30–38.
5. Mugford M, Banfield P, O'Hanlon M (1991) Effects of feedback of information on clinical practice: a review. Bmj 303: 398–402.
6. Stone EG, Morton SC, Hulscher ME, Maglione MA, Roth EA, et al. (2002) Interventions that increase use of adult immunization and cancer screening services: a meta-analysis. Ann Intern Med 136: 641–651.
7. van der Veer SN, de Keizer NF, Ravelli AC, Tenkink S, Jager KJ (2010) Improving quality of care. A systematic review on how medical registries provide information feedback to health care providers. Int J Med Inform 79: 305–323.
8. Ivers N, Jamtvedt G, Flottorp S, Young JM, Odgaard-Jensen J, et al. (2012) Audit and feedback: effects on professional practice and healthcare outcomes. Cochrane Database Syst Rev 6: Cd000259.
9. Lopez-Campos JL, Ruiz-Ramos M, Soriano JB (2014) Mortality trends in chronic obstructive pulmonary disease in Europe, 1994–2010: a joinpoint regression analysis. Lancet Respir Med 2: 54–62.
10. Miravitlles M, Ferrer M, Pont A, Zalacain R, Alvarez-Sala JL, et al. (2004) Effect of exacerbations on quality of life in patients with chronic obstructive pulmonary disease: a 2 year follow up study. Thorax 59: 387–395.
11. Soler-Cataluna JJ, Martinez-Garcia MA, Roman Sanchez P, Salcedo E, Navarro M, et al. (2005) Severe acute exacerbations and mortality in patients with chronic obstructive pulmonary disease. Thorax 60: 925–931.
12. Dalal AA, Shah M, D'Souza AO, Rane P (2011) Costs of COPD exacerbations in the emergency department and inpatient setting. Respir Med 105: 454–460.
13. Pozo-Rodriguez F, Alvarez CJ, Castro-Acosta A, Melero Moreno C, Capelastegui A, et al. (2010) [Clinical audit of patients admitted to hospital in Spain due to exacerbation of COPD (AUDIPOC study): method and organisation]. Arch Bronconeumol 46: 349–357.
14. Lopez-Campos JL, Hartl S, Pozo-Rodriguez F, Roberts CM, European CAt (2013) European COPD Audit: design, organisation of work and methodology. Eur Respir J 41: 270–276.
15. Soler-Cataluna JJ, Calle M, Cosio BG, Marin JM, Monso E, et al. (2009) [Health-care quality standards in chronic obstructive pulmonary disease]. Arch Bronconeumol 45: 196–203.
16. Pozo-Rodriguez F, Lopez-Campos JL, Alvarez-Martinez CJ, Castro-Acosta A, Aguero R, et al. (2012) Clinical audit of COPD patients requiring hospital admissions in Spain: AUDIPOC study. PLoS One 7: e42156.
17. Lilford RJ, Brown CA, Nicholl J (2007) Use of process measures to monitor the quality of clinical practice. Bmj 335: 648–650.
18. Miravitlles M, Soler-Cataluna JJ, Calle M, Molina J, Almagro P, et al. (2014) Spanish guideline for COPD (GesEPOC). Update 2014. Arch Bronconeumol 50 Suppl 1: 1–16.
19. Miravitlles M, Soriano JB, Garcia-Rio F, Munoz L, Duran-Tauleria E, et al. (2009) Prevalence of COPD in Spain: impact of undiagnosed COPD on quality of life and daily life activities. Thorax 64: 863–868.
20. Lopez-Campos JL, Soriano JB, Calle M, Encuesta de Espirometria en Espana P (2013) A comprehensive, national survey of spirometry in Spain: current bottlenecks and future directions in primary and secondary care. Chest 144: 601–609.
21. Lopez-Campos JL, Calero C, Lopez-Ramirez C. Exacerbations or complications? Redefining the concepts in COPD. Int J Clin Pract 2014 (in press).
22. Tsai CL, Ginde AA, Blanc PG, Camargo CA (2009) Improved care of acute exacerbation of chronic obstructive pulmonary disease in two academic emergency departments. Int J Emerg Med 2: 111–116.
23. Roberts CM, Lopez-Campos JL, Pozo-Rodriguez F, Hartl S, European CAt (2013) European hospital adherence to GOLD recommendations for chronic obstructive pulmonary disease (COPD) exacerbation admissions. Thorax 68: 1169–1171.
24. Ivers NM, Grimshaw JM, Jamtvedt G, Flottorp S, O'Brien MA, et al. (2014) Growing Literature, Stagnant Science? Systematic Review, Meta-Regression and Cumulative Analysis of Audit and Feedback Interventions in Health Care. J Gen Intern Med.
25. Kiefe CI, Allison JJ, Williams OD, Person SD, Weaver MT, et al. (2001) Improving quality improvement using achievable benchmarks for physician feedback: a randomized controlled trial. Jama 285: 2871–2879.
26. Sondergaard J, Andersen M, Stovring H, Kragstrup J (2003) Mailed prescriber feedback in addition to a clinical guideline has no impact: a randomised, controlled trial. Scand J Prim Health Care 21: 47–51.
27. Hopkinson NS, Englebretsen C, Cooley N, Kennie K, Lim M, et al. (2012) Designing and implementing a COPD discharge care bundle. Thorax 67: 90–92.
28. McCarthy C, Brennan JR, Brown L, Donaghy D, Jones P, et al. (2013) Use of a care bundle in the emergency department for acute exacerbations of chronic obstructive pulmonary disease: a feasibility study. Int J Chron Obstruct Pulmon Dis 8: 605–611.

ICU-Onset *Clostridium difficile* Infection in a University Hospital in China: A Prospective Cohort Study

Xiaohui Wang[1,2], Lin Cai[3], Rujia Yu[1,2], Wenzhi Huang[4], Zhiyong Zong[1,2,4]*

1 Center of Infectious Diseases, West China Hospital, Sichuan University, Chengdu, China, **2** Division of Infectious Diseases, State Key Laboratory of Biotherapy, Chengdu, China, **3** Department of Intensive Care Unit, West China Hospital, Sichuan University, Chengdu, China, **4** Department of Infection Control, West China Hospital, Sichuan University, Chengdu, China

Abstract

A prospective study was conducted to investigate the incidence, clinical profiles and outcome of ICU-onset CDI in a 50-bed medical ICU at a university hospital in China. Stools were collected from patients who developed ICU-onset diarrhea and was screened for *tcdA* (toxin A gene) and *tcdB* (toxin B gene) by PCR. CDI cases were compared with the ICU-onset non-CDI diarrhea cases for demographics, comorbidities, potential risk factors, major laboratory findings and outcomes. Stool samples from CDI cases were subjected to *C. difficile* culture and *C. difficile* isolates were screened for *tcdA*, *tcdB* and the binary toxin genes (*cdtA* and *cdtB*) using multiplex PCR. Strain typing of toxigenic *C. difficile* isolates was performed using multilocus sequence typing. There were 1,277 patients in the ICU during the study period and 124 (9.7%) developed ICU-onset diarrhea, of which 31 patients had CDI. The incidence of ICU-onset CDI was 25.2 cases per 10,000 ICU days. ICU-onset CDI cases had similar features with ICU-onset non-CDI diarrhea cases including the use of proton pump inhibitors and antibacterial agents. The crude mortality rate of ICU-onset CDI was 22.6%, but the attributable mortality rate of ICU-onset CDI was only 3.2% here. Toxigenic *C. difficile* isolates were recovered from 28 out of the 31 patients with CDI. *cdtA* and *cdtB* were found in two strains. Seventeen STs including 11 new STs were identified. All of the 11 new STs were single-locus variants of known STs and the 17 STs identified here could be clustered into 3 clades. The incidence of ICU-onset CDI here is similar to those in Europe and North America, suggesting that CDI is likely to be a common problem in China. Toxigenic *C. difficile* here belonged to a variety of STs, which may represent a significant clonal expansion rather than the true clonal diversity.

Editor: Andrew McDowell, University of Ulster, United Kingdom

Funding: The work was supported by the Technology support program of Sichuan provincial Science and Technology Agency, China (project no. 2011FZ0111). The funder had no role in study design, data collection and analysis, decision to publish, or preparation of the manuscript.

Competing Interests: The authors have declared that no competing interests exist.

* Email: zongzhiy@scu.edu.cn

Introduction

Clostridium difficile, a Gram-positive spore-forming anaerobic bacterium, is the leading cause of nosocomial diarrhea in industrialized countries [1,2]. Clinical manifestations of *C. difficile* infection (CDI) ranged from mild diarrhea to pseudomembranous colitis and the use of antibacterial agents is the major risk factor for the development of CDI [3]. Although CDI has been well recognized in Europe and North America [1,4], little is known about the prevalence of CDI and the clonal relatedness of *C. difficile* isolates in China [5]. This may be due to the lack of awareness and the absence of laboratory capacity to detect this nosocomial pathogen in most hospitals in China.

Patients in intensive care units (ICU) commonly received intensified antibacterial therapy and may therefore develop CDI. Furthermore, ICU patients may have a poor outcome when they developed CDI as they usually had comorbidities [6]. Surprisingly, studies on the incidence and outcome of CDI cases in ICU are scarce [6]. Available studies are typically retrospective and therefore might underestimate the incidence.

Material and Methods

Prospective cohort study

A prospective study was conducted to investigate the incidence, clinical profiles and outcome of ICU-onset CDI and to determine the clonal relatedness of ICU-onset toxigenic *C. difficile* isolates in a 50-bed medical ICU at West China Hospital, Sichuan University, Chengdu, southwest China, during a period of 35 weeks between May 2012 and January 2013.

Stools were collected from patients who developed ICU-onset diarrhea, which was defined as three or more loose stools per day for at least one day occurring within their stay in ICU. Diarrhea occurred during the stay in hospital but in an unit other than ICU was not considered as ICU-onset. The diarrhea in all of these patients occurred later than 48 hours after admission to the hospital and therefore were considered nosocomial. Total DNA of stool samples was prepared using the Stool DNA Kit (OMEGA, Norcross, GA) and was screened for the pathogenicity locus operon (Paloc) genes, *tcdA* (toxin A gene) and *tcdB* (toxin B gene) by PCR as described previously [7]. Of note, PCR for *tcdA* could yield 369-bp or 110-bp amplicons and samples with 110-bp amplicons were defined as negative for *tcdA* [7]. Patients with diarrhea who had a stool sample tested positive to either *tcdA* or *tcdB* were CDI cases.

Patients with ICU-onset diarrhea were tracked during the whole period of their stay in the hospital by the study team. The medical records of these patients were retrieved to compare CDI cases with the remaining ICU-onset non-CDI diarrhea cases from which stool DNA was negative to both *tcdA* and *tcdB* for demographics, comorbidities, potential risk factors, major laboratory findings and outcomes (Table 1). Whether CDI was an attributable cause, a contributing cause, or unrelated to the cause of death was judged by two physicians independently for each death based on the conclusion whether the patients would die or not if they did not have CDI. In the case of a disagreement, a consensus was reached after discussion.

Culture and strain typing

Stool samples from CDI cases that were positive to either *tcdA* or *tcdB* by PCR were treated with absolute ethanol, streaked onto cefoxitin cycloserine fructose agar (CCFA; OXOID, Basingstoke, UK) plates and incubated at 37°C for 72 hours. Colonies with the characteristic odor were subjected to Gram stain and multiplex PCR for detecting the presence of *tpi* (encoding triose phosphate isomerase of *C. difficile*), *tcdA*, *tcdB* and the binary toxin genes, *cdtA* and *cdtB*, as described previously [7,8]. *C. difficile* strains that were positive to either *tcdA* or *tcdB* were toxigenic strains.

Multilocus sequence typing (MLST) was performed for the toxigenic *C. difficile* strains as described previously [9]. For the three CDI patients where no toxigenic *C. difficile* was recovered from stool, total stool DNA was directly used for *C. difficile* MLST [9]. eBURST (version 3, http://eburst.mlst.net/) was used to assign sequence types (STs) to clonal complexes (CCs), which were defined as those sharing identical alleles at six of seven loci and were named after the predicted founder ST. STs of *C. difficile* were also clustered into clades by phylogenetic analysis using the concatenated sequences of the seven loci of MLST as described previously [9].

Statistical analysis

Statistical analysis was performed using SPSS version 18.0 (SPSS Inc., Chicago, IL). Differences in proportions were compared using a chi-squared test, while differences in median values were examined using a Mann-Whitney U test. The difference in LOS in ICU, which is in normal distribution, was examined using a Student's *t*-test.

Ethics statement

This study was approved by the Ethics Committee of West China Hospital and the need of patient consents was waived by the Ethics Committee.

Results, Discussion, and Conclusions

During the study period, there were 1,277 patients in the ICU and 124 (9.7%) developed ICU-onset diarrhea, of which 24 had a stool sample that tested positive for *tcdA* and *tcdB* (A+B+) and 7 had a sample positive for *tcdB* only (A-B+). Therefore, a total of 31 patients had CDI, accounting for 2.4% of the ICU patient population and 25.0% of those with ICU-onset diarrhea. The incidence of ICU-onset CDI was 25.2 cases per 10,000 ICU days, which is close to the 32 cases per 10,000 ICU days found in a medical ICU in the USA [10]. The ICU-onset CDI rate (2.4%) in this study is slightly lower than that in two UK ICUs (one medical-surgical and one trauma) [11] (3.3%, 62/185) but is significantly higher than rates found in multiple medical or medical-surgical ICUs in France (0.9%, 47/5260) [12] and in six medical-surgical ICUs in Canada (1.5%, 236/15314) [13]. Variations in the incidence and rate of ICU-onset CDI in different studies may be due to the type and location of ICUs and local infection control practices.

To identify risk factors for developing CDI and to demonstrate whether CDI was associated with poorer outcomes, CDI cases had commonly been compared with non-CDI cases in a few previous studies, e.g. [14–16]. However, most non-CDI cases had no diarrhea. Therefore, risk factors and outcome features identified for CDI through such comparisons are unlikely specific for CDI but may simply reflect for diarrhea as a whole. To overcome the shortcoming, for the 124 patients with ICU-onset diarrhea in this study, CDI cases (n = 31) were compared with the remaining 93 ICU-onset non-CDI diarrhea cases with characteristics listed in Table 1. Among 31 ICU-onset CDI cases, 13 (41.9%) were 65-year-old or above, 20 (64.5%) had at least one comorbidity and all received at least one antibacterial agent, most (28/31, 90.3%) of which were carbapenems or compounds containing β-lactamase inhibitors, within one month prior to the onset of CDI (Table 1). The interval between admission to ICU and onset of CDI ranged from 3 to 72 days (median 11 days). Overall, ICU-onset CDI cases features were similar to ICU-onset non-CDI diarrhea cases, except that non-CDI cases were associated with higher creatine levels and patients receiving aztreonam were more likely to develop CDI (Table 1). The differences between CDI and non-CDI diarrhea cases warrant further investigation. Of note, the use of proton pump inhibitors (PPIs) has been identified as a risk factor for developing CDI by comparing CDI and non-CDI cases in a few reports, e.g. [16]. However, here most cases with non-CDI nosocomial diarrhea also received PPIs prior to the onset of diarrhea (Table 1) and therefore the use of PPIs might not be a risk factor specific for the acquisition of CDI but rather a risk factor for developing nosocomial diarrhea. Similarly, age>65 years, using antibacterial agents, receiving chemotherapy and an indwelling nasogastric tube, which have all been well recognized as risk factors for developing CDI [14–16], might actually be risk factors for developing nosocomial diarrhea regardless of the etiology.

No patients with ICU-onset CDI needed renal dialysis or underwent colectomy but seven such patients died during their stay in hospital, corresponding to a crude mortality rate of 22.6%, which is consistent with crude mortality rates of ICU-onset CDI of 21.5% to 36.7% in several studies in Europe and North America [12,17]. Previous studies have not demonstrated the association of CDI with a higher hospital mortality rate [12,17]. However, here the crude mortality rate of ICU-onset CDI cases was higher than the overall mortality rate (16.4%) of all ICU patients during the same period but was similar to that (28.0%) of ICU-onset non-CDI diarrhea cases. This suggests that nosocomial diarrhea as a whole, rather than CDI specifically, was associated with a higher mortality rate in ICU.

Among the seven patients who died, CDI was considered the attributable cause for one and a contributing cause for another two. Correspondingly, the attributable mortality rate of ICU-onset CDI was 3.2% (1/31) here. Previous studies have demonstrated that attributable mortality rates of CDI ranged from 5.5% to 6.9% for all patients (including non-ICU patients) but reach as high as 16.7% in outbreaks [6]. The reason for a lower attributable mortality rate here remains unclear but may be due to the lack of an objective method to determine the attributable cause of death or the fact that the number of cases may be too low here.

Toxigenic *C. difficile* isolates were recovered from 28 out of the 31 patients with CDI, including 22 A+B+ and 6 A−B+ strains

Table 1. Features and outcomes of ICU-onset CDI and non-CDI diarrhea.

Feature[a]	**ICU-onset CDI (n = 31)**	**ICU-onset non-CDI diarrhea (n = 93)**	***P* value**
Age (years-old), mean±IQR	59.00±35.00	69.00±30.00	0.204
No. of cases ≥ 65-years-old	13 (41.9%)	39 (41.4%)	1.000
Sex, male/female	25/6	57/36	0.049
Diabetes	2 (6.5%)	20 (21.5%)	0.057
Malignancy	5 (16.1%)	15 (16.1%)	1.000
COPD	4 (12.9%)	15 (16.1%)	0.886
Pancreatitis	1 (3.2%)	13 (13.9%)	0.190
Renal failure	2 (6.5%)	20 (21.5%)	0.057
Liver failure	6 (19.3%)	8 (8.6%)	0.190
Nasogastric tube	30 (96.8%)	80 (86.0%)	0.190
APACHE II score on ICU admission median±IQR	21.00±14.00	23.00±12.50	0.072
SOFA score on ICU admission median±IQR	10.00±4.00	11.00±4.00	0.132
Charlson comorbidity index, median±IQR	4.00±5.00	5.00±4.00	0.429
Use of antibacterials[b] (%)	31 (100%)	90 (96.8%)	0.572
β-lactams/β-lactamase inhibitors	21 (67.74%)	78 (83.87%)	0.053
Carbapenems	14 (45.16%)	40 (43.01%)	0.834
1st cephalosporins	2 (6.45%)	1 (1.08%)	0.154
2nd-generation cephalosporins	0	2 (2.15%)	1.000
3rd-generation cephalosporins	3 (9.68%)	6 (6.45%)	0.842
4th-generation cephalosporins	1 (3.23%)	0	0.250
Aztreonam	3 (9.68%)	0	0.014
Cephamycins	2 (6.45%)	5 (5.38%)	1.000
Fluoroquinones	7 (22.58%)	21(22.58%)	1.000
Vancomycin	3 (9.68%)	14 (15.05%)	0.651
Clindamycin	0	1 (1.08%)	1.000
SMZ-TMP	0	1 (1.08%)	1.000
Tetracyclines	1 (3.23%)	2 (2.15%)	1.000
Linezolid	1 (3.23%)	2 (2.15%)	1.000
No. of antibacterials[b], median (range)	2 (1–5)	2 (0–7)	
Receiving chemotherapy (%)	4 (12.90%)	9 (9.68%)	0.866
Receiving any GAS (%)	28 (90.32)	85 (91.40%)	1.000
PPI	28 (90.32%)	83 (89.25%)	1.000
Histamine-2 receptor antagonists	0	2 (2.15%)	1.000
Maximum WBC [c], median±IQR	10.08±8.76	10.27±8.49	0.390
Maximum Temperature (°C) [c], median±IQR	38.00±1.60	38.10±1.55	0.970
Maximum creatine [c], median±IQR	63.00±74.00	124.00±184.40	0.000
LOS in hospital (days), median±IQR	28.00±35.00	33.00±35.50	0.956
LOS in ICU (days), mean±SD	31.74±43.21	23.25±20.06	0.298
LOS before onset (days), median±IQR	11.00±12.00	8.00±14.00	0.068
Death in hospital (mortality rate)	7 (22.6%)	(28%)	0.557

[a]IQR, interquartile range, for data that did not fit a normal distribution; SD, standard deviation, for data with a normal distribution.
[b]Used within 1 month prior to onset of diarrhea. None of patients with CDI or non-CDI diarrhea received aminoglycosides or macrolides.
[c]Collected on the day of onset or two days before.

(Table 2). Of note, A−B+ strains are relatively common in China, accounting for 17–34% of all toxigenic strains [18,19]. *cdtA* and *cdtB* were found in only two A+B+ strains (2/31, 6.5%). Binary toxin genes have been detected in 23% of toxigenic *C. difficile* in Europe [4]. In contrast, strains carrying binary toxin genes remain very rare in China [18] with two found in this study.

A total of 17 STs, including 11 new STs, were assigned for the 28 isolates (16 STs) and the three stool DNA samples (three STs; Table 2). This appears to suggest a remarkable clonal diversity in a single unit during a relative short period. However, all of the 11 new STs were single-locus variants of known STs. most of which were also found here (Figure 1). In addition, the 17 STs identified here belonged to 4 CCs and could be clustered into 3 clades

Table 2. The STs and toxin gene carriage of *C. difficile* strains.

ST[a]	Allele profile[b]	Ribotype[c]	CC	Clade[d]	Toxin A	Toxin B	Binary toxin	No. of strains
ST2	1-1-2-1-5-3-1	014/020	28	1/HA1	+	+	−	1
ST3	1-1-2-1-1-1-1	001	28	1/HA1	+	+	−	5
ST8	1-1-2-6-1-5-1	002	28	1/HA1	+	+	−	1
ST35	2-5-8-1-1-3-6	046	28	1/HA1	+	+	−	4
ST37	3-7-3-8-6-9-11	017	37	4/A-B+	−	+	−	3
ST54	1-4-7-1-1-3-3	012	28	1/HA1	+	+	−	4
ST208	2-7-8-1-1-3-6		28	1/HA1	+	+	−	1
ST209	1-6-4-7-2-8-11		5	3/HA2	+	+	+	2
ST210	1-1-2-1-1-1-11		28	1/HA1	+	+	−	1
ST211	2-5-8-1-1-3-11		28	1/HA1	+	+	−	1
ST212	1-4-7-1-1-3-6		28	1/HA1	+	+	−	1
ST213	1-11-6-6-1-12-6		99	1/HA1	+	+	−	1
ST214	1-1-2-1-5-3-12		28	1/HA1	+	+	−	1
ST215	3-7-3-8-6-9-29		37	4/A−B+	−	+	−	1
ST216	3-7-3-8-6-9-6		37	4/A−B+	−	+	−	1
ST218	2-5-8-1-1-3-1		28	1/HA1	+	+	−	1
ST219	3-7-3-1-6-9-11		37	4/A-B+	−	+	−	2

[a]Underlined STs include results from directly typing the stool DNA from three CDI patients with no recovery of *C. difficile*.
[b]Alleles are *adk-atpA-dxr-glyA-recA-sodA-tpi*.
[c]Ribotype is predicted and those for new STs are not available.
[d]Names of clades are from reference [9].

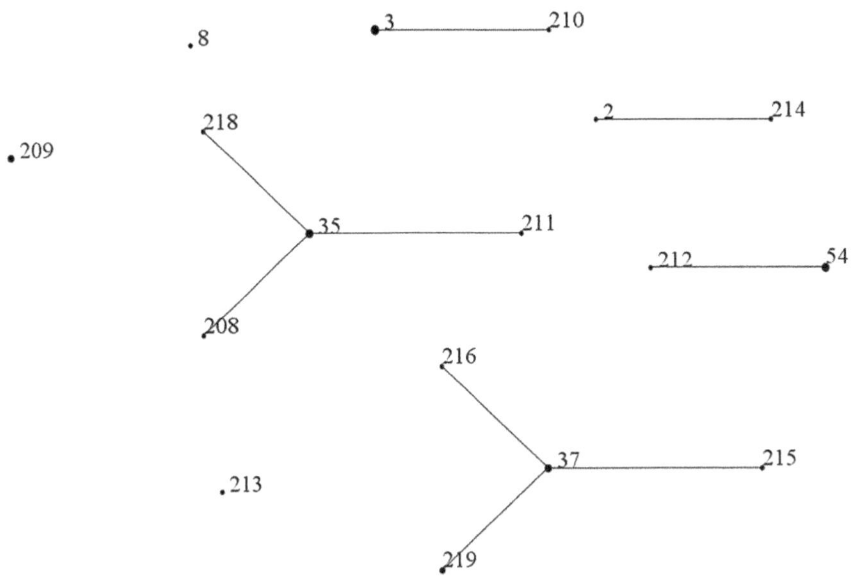

Figure 1. The relatedness of the STs seen in this study. The relatedness of STs were established using eBURST. ST209 and ST213 are a single-locus variant of ST5 and ST99, respectively.

(Table 2). The diversity of toxigenic *C. difficile* in this 50-bed unit is therefore largely a reflection of a significant clonal expansion. ST3 (n = 5), ST35 (n = 4) and ST54 (n = 3) were the most common types among A+B+ strains, while A−B+ strains belonged to ST37 or its single-locus variants. This is consistent with the findings in a university hospital in Zhejiang province, China [18]. In contrast, ST35, ST37 and ST54 were rarely identified in a large European survey [4], though ST2 (ribotype 014/020) and ST3 (ribotype 001) have also been found to be prevalent. Of note, ST1 (PCR ribotype 027), a hypervirulent type widely distributed in Europe and North America, and ST11 (ribotype 078), a type associated with community-acquired CDI commonly found in Europe, were not detected in this study. In China, only one strain of ribotype 027 and one strain of ribotype of 078 have been reported up to now [20,21].

There are several limitations of our study. First, this is a single center study, which may not represent the whole situation in China. Second, the patients were not followed after discharge from the hospital and therefore the long term outcomes and the recurrence of CDI among these cases remain unknown. Third, the number of CDI cases is limited here. Multi-center large-scale studies on CDI in ICUs are warranted.

In conclusion, to our knowledge, this is the first report of the incidence and outcome of ICU-onset CDI in China. The incidence of ICU-onset CDI in our unit is similar to those in Europe and North America in non-outbreaks settings, suggesting that CDI is likely to be a common problem in China and large-scale multi-center studies are required to reveal the burden of CDI in China. There is an urgent need to raise awareness of this disease among healthcare workers in China. Toxigenic *C. difficile* in the studied ICU belonged to a variety of STs, which is likely to represent a significant clonal expansion rather than the true clonal diversity.

Acknowledgments

We are grateful to Wenjing Wu, Shichao Zhu, Jingwen Li, Xuelian Liao and Xiaoke Zhang for their assistance in collecting clinical data and to Tianyu Hu and Tao Chen for their technical assistance. We also thank Sally Partridge and Andrew Ginn from the Centre of Infectious Diseases and Microbiology, Westmead Hospital, The University of Sydney, Australia, for their critical reading.

Author Contributions

Conceived and designed the experiments: XW ZZ. Performed the experiments: XW LC RY. Analyzed the data: XW WH ZZ. Wrote the paper: XW ZZ.

References

1. Freeman J, Bauer MP, Baines SD, Corver J, Fawley WN, et al. (2010) The changing epidemiology of *Clostridium difficile* infections. Clin Microbiol Rev 23: 529–549.
2. Rupnik M, Wilcox MH, Gerding DN (2009) *Clostridium difficile* infection: new developments in epidemiology and pathogenesis. Nat Rev Microbiol 7: 526–536.
3. Bartlett JG, Gerding DN (2008) Clinical recognition and diagnosis of *Clostridium difficile* infection. Clin Infect Dis 46 Suppl 1: S12–18.
4. Bauer MP, Notermans DW, van Benthem BH, Brazier JS, Wilcox MH, et al. (2011) *Clostridium difficile* infection in Europe: a hospital-based survey. Lancet 377: 63–73.
5. Jin K, Wang S, Huang Z, Lu S (2010) *Clostridium difficile* infections in China. J Biomed Res 24: 411–416.
6. Bobo LD, Dubberke ER, Kollef M (2011) *Clostridium difficile* in the ICU: the struggle continues. Chest 140: 1643–1653.
7. Lemee L, Dhalluin A, Testelin S, Mattrat MA, Maillard K, et al. (2004) Multiplex PCR targeting *tpi* (triose phosphate isomerase), *tcdA* (Toxin A), and *tcdB* (Toxin B) genes for toxigenic culture of *Clostridium difficile*. J Clin Microbiol 42: 5710–5714.
8. Persson S, Torpdahl M, Olsen KE (2008) New multiplex PCR method for the detection of *Clostridium difficile* toxin A (*tcdA*) and toxin B (*tcdB*) and the binary toxin (*cdtA/cdtB*) genes applied to a Danish strain collection. Clin Microbiol Infect 14: 1057–1064.
9. Griffiths D, Fawley W, Kachrimanidou M, Bowden R, Crook DW, et al. (2010) Multilocus sequence typing of *Clostridium difficile*. J Clin Microbiol 48: 770–778.
10. Lawrence SJ, Puzniak LA, Shadel BN, Gillespie KN, Kollef MH, et al. (2007) *Clostridium difficile* in the intensive care unit: epidemiology, costs, and colonization pressure. Infect Control Hosp Epidemiol 28: 123–130.

11. Ang CW, Heyes G, Morrison P, Carr B (2008) The acquisition and outcome of ICU-acquired *Clostridium difficile* infection in a single centre in the UK. J Infect 57: 435–440.
12. Zahar JR, Schwebel C, Adrie C, Garrouste-Orgeas M, Francais A, et al. (2012) Outcome of ICU patients with *Clostridium difficile* infection. Crit Care 16: R215.
13. Dodek PM, Norena M, Ayas NT, Romney M, Wong H (2013) Length of stay and mortality due to *Clostridium difficile* infection acquired in the intensive care unit. J Crit Care 28: 335–340.
14. Miller M, Gravel D, Mulvey M, Taylor G, Boyd D, et al. (2010) Health care-associated *Clostridium difficile* infection in Canada: patient age and infecting strain type are highly predictive of severe outcome and mortality. Clin Infect Dis 50: 194–201.
15. Morrison RH, Hall NS, Said M, Rice T, Groff H, et al. (2011) Risk factors associated with complications and mortality in patients with *Clostridium difficile* infection. Clin Infect Dis 53: 1173–1178.
16. Loo VG, Bourgault AM, Poirier L, Lamothe F, Michaud S, et al. (2011) Host and pathogen factors for *Clostridium difficile* infection and colonization. N Engl J Med 365: 1693–1703.
17. Micek ST, Schramm G, Morrow L, Frazee E, Personett H, et al. (2013) *Clostridium difficile* infection: a multicenter study of epidemiology and outcomes in mechanically ventilated patients. Crit Care Med 41: 1968–1975.
18. Chen YB, Gu SL, Wei ZQ, Shen P, Kong HS, et al. (2013) Molecular epidemiology of *Clostridium difficile* in a tertiary hospital of China. J Med Microbiol.
19. Yan Q, Zhang J, Chen C, Zhou H, Du P, et al. (2013) Multilocus sequence typing (MLST) analysis of 104 *Clostridium difficile* strains isolated from China. Epidemiol Infect 141: 195–199.
20. Wang P, Zhou Y, Wang Z, Xie S, Chen Y, et al. (2014) Identification of Clostridium difficile Ribotype 027 for the First Time in Mainland China. Infect Control Hosp Epidemiol 35: 95–98.
21. Huang H, Wu T, Zhu D, Wu J, Wang M, et al. (2011) Study on resistance of 188 *Clostridium difficile* clinical isolates Chin J Infect Chemother 11: 1–5.

Delirium, Sedation and Analgesia in the Intensive Care Unit

Alawi Luetz[1]ⓢ, Felix Balzer[1]ⓢ, Finn M. Radtke[1], Christina Jones[2], Giuseppe Citerio[3], Bernhard Walder[4], Bjoern Weiss[1], Klaus-Dieter Wernecke[5], Claudia Spies[1]*

1 Department of Anesthesiology and Intensive Care Medicine, Campus Charité Mitte and Campus Virchow-Klinikum, Charité – Universitätsmedizin Berlin, Berlin, Germany, **2** Whiston Hospital, Critical Care Unit, Prescot, Liverpool, United Kingdom, **3** Hospital San Gerardo, Department of Emergency Medicine, Monza, Italy, **4** Service d'Anesthesiologie, Hôpitaux Universitaires de Genève, Geneva, Switzerland, **5** Sostana GmbH, Berlin, Germany

Abstract

Analgesia, sedation and delirium management are important parts of intensive care treatment as they are relevant for patients' clinical and functional long-term outcome. Previous surveys showed that despite this fact implementation rates are still low. The primary aim of the prospective, observational multicenter study was to investigate the implementation rate of delirium monitoring among intensivists. Secondly, current practice concerning analgesia and sedation monitoring as well as treatment strategies for patients with delirium were assesed. In addition, this study compares perceived and actual practice regarding delirium, sedation and analgesia management. Data were obtained with a two-part, anonymous survey, containing general data from intensive care units in a first part and data referring to individual patients in a second part. Questionnaires from 101 hospitals (part 1) and 868 patients (part 2) were included in data analysis. Fifty-six percent of the intensive care units reported to monitor for delirium in clinical routine. Fourty-four percent reported the use of a validated delirium score. In this respect, the survey suggests an increasing use of delirium assessment tools compared to previous surveys. Nevertheless, part two of the survey revealed that in actual practice 73% of included patients were not monitored with a validated score. Furthermore, we observed a trend towards moderate or deep sedation which is contradicting to guideline-recommendations. Every fifth patient was suffering from pain. The implementation rate of adequate pain-assessment tools for mechanically ventilated and sedated patients was low (30%). In conclusion, further efforts are necessary to implement guideline recommendations into clinical practice. The study was registered (ClinicalTrials.gov identifier: NCT01278524) and approved by the ethical committee.

Editor: Marianna Mazza, Catholic University of Sacred Heart of Rome, Italy

Funding: The authors have no funding or support to report.

Competing Interests: Statistical analysis has been supervised by Professor Klaus-Dieter Wernecke, PhD, former head of the Institute of Medical Biometry at Charit Universitaetsmedizin Berlin and owner of Sostana GmbH.

* Email: claudia.spies@charite.de

ⓢ These authors contributed equally to this work.

Introduction

The management of pain, sedation and delirium has a significant impact on patients' clinical and functional long-term outcome.

Delirium affects up to 82% of the critically ill patients and is associated with long-term cognitive impairment [1] and a 3-fold increase of 6-month mortality [2]. Studies revealed that intensive care unit (ICU) delirium is underrecognized by intensivists and nurses in daily routine care [3]. Using a validated assessment tool significantly improves the ability of physicians [4] and nurses [5] to identify ICU delirium.

Sedation practice predicts long-term mortality in critically ill patients [6] and requires monitoring to define adequate targets and control the effect of applied sedatives.

Pain is the major stressor for critically ill patients [7] and chronic pain is a severe complication that was reported by 44% of patients 6 months to 1 year after ICU discharge [8]. Assessment for pain in mechanically ventilated patients is independently associated with improved outcome [9].

On a national as well as international level, societies of critical and intensive care medicine have taken efforts such as supporting the development of guidelines [10–12] and offering simulation- as well as online-training tools to drive attention on analgesia, sedation and delirium management. Nevertheless, previous national and international surveys demonstrated a low implementation of these screening tools into clinical practice: e.g., a survey conducted on 1384 ICU practitioners in North America revealed that more than half of them (59%) assessed their patients for delirium but only 20% used a valid delirium assessment tool [13].

The primary aim of this prospective, observational multicenter study was to investigate the implementation rate of delirium monitoring among intensivists. Secondly, we assessed the current practice of analgesia and sedation monitoring as well as treatment strategies for delirium. Finally, this study compares perceived and actual practice regarding delirium, sedation and analgesia management.

Results

Part one - Hospital and ICU data

The first questionnaire ("part one") yielded 101 complete forms that were included in the data analysis. Five hundred and fifyt-six forms were either not submitted or not completed (figure 1). Characteristics of the ICUs that participated in the survey are presented in detail in table 1. The median of patients per physician was 4 (3–6), and the median number of patients per registered nurse was 2 (1–2). The median number of beds per ICU was 12 (8–18).

Fifty-six percent (n = 56) of all ICUs reported some kind of screening for symptoms of delirium (table 2). Fourty-four percent (n = 44) used a validated delirium screening tool. The most frequently used score was the Confusion Assessment Method for the ICU (CAM-ICU) (n = 37, 84%) followed by the Intensive Care Delirium Screening Checklist (ICDSC) (n = 3, 7%), the Nursing Delirium Screening Scale (Nu-DESC) (n = 2, 5%), the Delirium Detection Score (DDS) (n = 1, 2%) and the Diagnostic and Statistical Manual of Mental Disorders, Version IV (n = 1, 2%).

Routine sedation monitoring was implemented in 88% (n = 89) of the ICUs (table 2). The most frequently used tool was the Richmond Agitation Sedation Scale (RASS) (n = 48, 54%). The Ramsay Sedation Scale was used by 27% (n = 24) and the Sedation Agitation Scale (SAS) by 6% (n = 5) of the participating ICUs. Thirteen percent (n = 12) of the respondents performed sedation monitoring without the use of a sedation score. Thirty-nine percent (n = 39) of the ICUs performed daily spontaneous breathing trials (SBT) and 44% (n = 44) conducted daily spontaneous awakening trials (SAT). The implementation rate of a daily, paired SBT and SAT was 34% (n = 34).

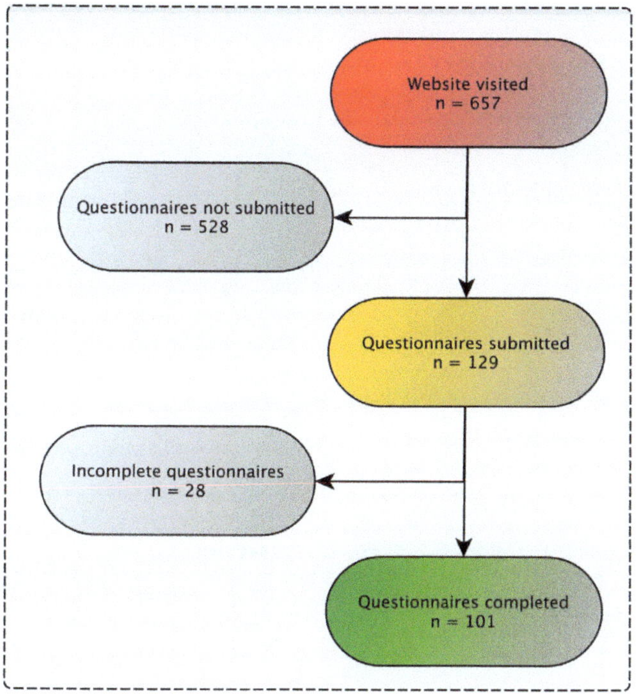

Figure 1. Consort diagram for questionnaire part one. This part of the survey gathered general information about the participating hospitals as well as (non-)pharmacological strategies for the management of analgesia, delirium and sedation.

Eighty percent (n = 81) of the ICUs did routinely monitor for pain (table 2). Ninety-three percent (n = 72) of them used a validated tool for pain assessment. Thirty percent (n = 24) made use of an instrument which was validated for deeply sedated and mechanically ventilated patients. The most frequently used pain score was the Visual Analogue Scale (VAS) (63%, n = 45) followed by the Numeric Rating Scale (NRS) (57%, n = 41).

Almost all ICUs (98%) treated delirious patients with specific pharmacological agents. Antipsychotics (APDs) were the most frequently used agents (99%, n = 98). Eighty-two percent (n = 81) of the ICUs used benzodiazepines (BDZs) as a part of their treatment regime table 3.

ICUs which performed routine delirium monitoring with a validated tool had implemented validated scores for analgesia (6%, n = 3), for sedation (14%, n = 6) or for sedation and analgesia (79%, n = 35). ICUs which did not screen for delirium with validated scores, used sedation scores (21%, n = 12), pain scores (16%, n = 9), sedation and pain scores (42%, n = 24) or neither sedation or pain scores (21%, n = 12) (figure 2).

Part two - Patients Data

In the second part of the survey ("part-two"), respondents of the first part were asked to enter patient specific data in a 32-item questionnaire.

One thousand and four questionnaires were submitted out of which 868 were fully completed and included in data analysis (figure 3). We summarized the charactaristics of patients in table 4.

The median time frame between ICU admission of patients and the day of study was 6 days (2–15). Respondents reported that 48% (n = 417) of the patients were monitored for symptoms of delirium; using a validated score in 27% (n = 234). Taking all patients into account that were evaluated with a validated delirium score, delirium prevalence was 44% (n = 103).

Fourty-three percent of patients (n = 369) were monitored with a validated sedation and pain score: 74% of them were were moderately or deeply sedated (RASS <-2/Ramsay>2/SAS <4) and 22% (n = 110) experienced significant pain levels (table 5).

Discussion

Our data reveal an implementation rate of delirium assessment with a validated score of 44% which is to our knowledge the highest rate documented so far. However, "part two" of the survey revealed that only 27% of the patients were in fact monitored with a validated score.

Data from previous national and international surveys reported implementation rates between 2% and 34% [14–16]. Most of them were surveys on a national level. In-line with recently published surveys, more than half of the ICUs which participated in our survey belonged to a university hospital (table 1). Results of previous surveys indicate that routine delirium monitoring is more often performed in university hospitals than in small teaching or regional public hospitals [17]. This was confirmed by our data as 54% of the university hospitals used validated delirium scores compared to 29% of the non-academic hospitals. Furthermore, we observed that 11% of the respondents assessed for delirious

Table 1. Characteristics of participating intensive care units.

Characteristics	n (%)
Type of hospital	
University	56 (55)
Teaching	31 (31)
Other	14 (14)
Type of intensive care unit	
Surgical	26 (26)
Medical	5 (5)
Mixed	69 (69)
Equipped for invasive mechanical ventilation	
All beds	75 (74)
Some beds	24 (24)
No beds	2 (2)
Estimated mean intensive care unit length of stay	
1–3 days	14 (14)
3–7 days	68 (67)
>8 days	15 (15)
No answer	4 (4)

symptoms without using a validated score. Literature suggests that delirium diagnosis due to clinical impression results in a high rate of failure or delayed detection [3].

In "part two" of the survey, we observed a one-day-prevalence of delirium of 44% which is consistent with previous reports [18]. Almost all of the ICUs (98%) stated that they treat delirious patients with specific pharmacological agents. Surprisingly, even ICUs that had not implemented some kind of delirium monitoring prescribed drugs for symptoms that maybe related to delirium. A national survey conducted by Gonçalves and colleagues revealed that delirium was the most frequent reason for sedation and midazolam was the most frequently used sedative [19]. There is increasing evidence that BZDs are a major risk factor for transitioning to delirium [20]. However, the majority of intensivists responded using BZDs for treatment of delirium.

In 2004 merely 8% of the ICUs in Germany monitored sedation with a validated score [21]. ICUs from our survey reported to use validated screening-instruments to assess sedation depth in 77% of the cases. The fact that only 43% of the patients were monitored regarding their sedation depth in actual practice emphasizes that structured training programs might be required to increase implementation rate [22].

If sedation is required, the coordination of a daily awakening and breathing trial has been shown to be an effective procedure to reduce mortality in ICU patients [23]. Thirty-four percent of the ICUs had implemented a paired SBT and SAT. These data reveal the necessity for improvement - especially regarding the implementation of evidence based sedation protocols.

From the patients' perspective, pain is the major stressors during critical illness [7,24]. Results from previous studies in the field of pain management drew the conclusion that using specific instruments for assessment, significantly improved outcome in critically ill patients. [9,25]. In our survey, eighty percent of respondents reported to routinely monitor for pain. Compared with results from previous surveys that showed implementation rates from 21% in general ICUs [26] up to 60% in European burn centers [15], our results indicate increasing awareness regarding pain assessment. A multicenter prospective observational study conducted in 2004/2005 revealed that specific pain scores were used in 28% of patients. Looking at our results of patient survey data, the use of pain scores drops to 43%. It is noteworthy that

Table 2. Frequencies of analgesia, delirium and sedation monitoring in participating intensive care units.

Frequency	Analgesia	Delirium	Sedation
	n (%)	n (%)	n (%)
≤8 hours	50 (49)	30 (30)	79 (78)
>8 hours	9 (9)	13 (13)	5 (5)
Daily	1 (1)	13 (13)	5 (5)
As needed	21 (21)	0 (0)	0 (0)
Never	20 (20)	45 (44)	12 (12)

Reported frequencies include validated as well as non-validated methods.

Table 3. Pharmacological treatment strategies for delirium as applied by the participating intensive care units.

Drug type	n (%)
Exclusively APDs	6 (6)
Exclusively BDZs	1 (1)
APDs and BDZs	18 (18)
APDs and Other*	12 (12)
APDs, BDZs and Other*	62 (61)
No answer	2 (2)

APDs, antipsychotics (e.g. haloperidol). BDZs, benzodiazepines. *α2 adrenergic agonist, selective serotonin re-uptake inhibitors.

70% of the ICUs did not use any assessment tool, specifically developed for assessing pain in sedated patients (e.g. Behavioural Pain Scale). Hence, sedated patients are at higher risk of suffering from insufficient analgesia.

This survey contributes to our knowledge about the management of analgesia, sedation and delirium in clinical practice. Until now, there are only two studies that have been conducted on an international level [15,27]. Furthermore, this study is the first to report about delirium, sedation and analgesia in a general ICU population, taking into account differences between perceived and actual practice.

Nevertheless, limitations are inherent to surveys. We would expect a responder bias regarding the participants of this study. It is more likely that colleagues who are interested in delirium, sedation and analgesia participated in the survey. Taking this into account, it seems interesting that we found notable discrepancies between guideline recommendations and current practice. Considering the above mentioned responder bias, this observed gap may be even larger in reality. Further studies are necessary to evaluate this realtionship.

Despite an extensive preparation (technical support, email reminders etc.), a sixth of all webpage visitors completed the questionnaire.

Regional differences regarding the management of analgesia, delirium and sedation were not assessed.

The results of our survey indicate that awareness concerning a systematic management of delirium, sedation and analgesia and patient outcome is increasing. However, our data also show that the implementation of these measures in daily routine lacks behind. In our opinion, intelligent and sustainable implementation strategies are of key importance in order to transfer guideline recommendations to practise. The discrepancy between observed practice and perceived practice is significant and shows a wide gap between what we think we do and what we really do. Further studies will be necessary to assess and evaluate implementation strategies and improve clinical practice.

Materials and Methods

This prospective, observational multicenter study (ethical approval No EA1/16- 5/10) was supported by the European Critical Care Research Network (ECCRN). The study was registered through Clinicaltrials.gov (identifier: NCT01278524) and approved by the data protection officer of the Charité - Universitaetsmedizin Berlin, Germany.

For collecting data, we developed two structured, web-based anonymous questionnaires in English (electronic case report file =

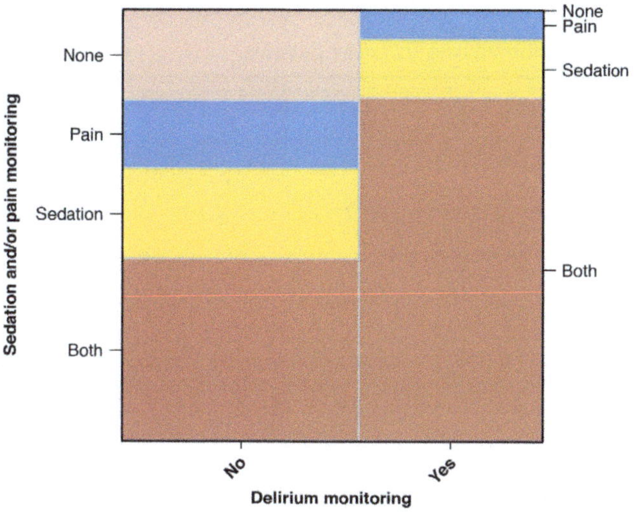

Figure 2. Monitoring of sedation, analgesia and delirium with validated scores. Mosaic plot: The areas of the mosaic tiles are proportional to the observed frequency of groups. Both, sedation and pain monitoring. None, no sedation and no pain monitoring.

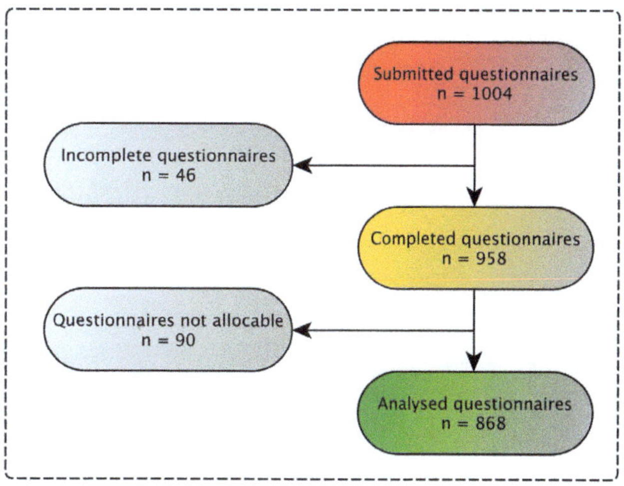

Figure 3. Consort diagram for questionnaire part 2. This part of the survey gathered actual practice on analgesia, delirium and sedation management among included patients. Not allocable = there was either no allocable token for questionnaire part one or most of the data were entered incorrectly (e.g. RASS = 10, BPS = −2).

Table 4. Demographic and clinical characteristics of included patients.

Characteristics (n = 868)	n (%)
Demographics	
Age, years	64 [51–73]*
Male	532 (61)
IMV	482 (56)
Type of admission	
Elective	238 (27)
Emergency	630 (73)
Reason for admission	
Surgical	378 (44)
Medical	440 (50)
Trauma	50 (6)

*Continuous variables are presented as medians with interquartile range [25th to 75th]. IMV, invasive mechanical ventilation.

eCRF) using the server based software LimeSurvey (Version 1.82+). The first questionnaire ("part one") contained 31 questions and was designed to gather general information about the participating hospital as well as (non-)pharmacological strategies for the management of analgesia, sedation and delirium (Appendix S1). In the second part, respondents were asked to enter patient specific data in a 32-item questionnaire. We asked to complete this questionnaire for each patient treated on the ICU during the 24 hour study period (January 25, 2011) (Appendix S2). In order to link hospital data of part one with patient related data of part two and keeping the survey anonymous, a token was generated for each participant: with opening the study website (www.improve-icu.com), users were presented a unique randomly generated numeric code. This code had to be entered at the beginning of each questionnaire. This numeric code allowed the allocation of the different questionnaires to one participating hospital.

We promoted the survey six months before it was carried out: Repeated email invitations were sent to all members of the European Society of Intensive Care Medicine (ESICM). Technical support was given by email and a telephone hotline on the day of study. Participants could access and complete the online questionnaires within one week. In addition to the online survey, participants were given the possibility to download a printable version of the survey and submit it by fax. Data from the printed and online questionnaires were merged in a database and exported to a worksheet for further statistical analysis.

Patients with a NRS or VRS or VAS of >4 or a BPS of >5 were considered to have relevant pain. Patients with a RASS <−2 or Ramsay >2 or SAS <4 werde considered to be moderately or deeply sedated.

Statistical Analysis: Exploratory data analysis were accomplished for all study variables. Discrete variables are expressed as counts (percentage) and continuous variables as medians with interquartile range (25th to 75th). Numerical calculations were performed with IBM SPSS Statistics Version 19 and Aabel 3.0.6, Gigawiz Ltd. Co.

Table 5. Methods and results of analgesia, delirium and sedation monitoring among included patients.

Symptom/Syndrome (n = 868)	n (%)
Analgesia	
No monitoring	499 (57)
Relevant pain*	110 (22)
Delirium	
No monitoring	451 (52.0)
Monitoring without score	183 (21.1)
Monitoring with score	234 (26.9)
Positive	103 (44.0)
Negative	131 (56.0)
Sedation	
No monitoring	499 (57)
Moderate to deep sedation**	273 (74)

Methods and results of monitoring that was actually performed in included patients (questionnaire part two). *NRS or VRS or VAS>4 or BPS>5. **RASS <−2 or Ramsay >2 or SAS <4. CAM-ICU, Confusion Assessment Method for the Intensive Care Unit. DDS, Delirium Detection Score. ICDSC, Intensive Care Delirium Screening Checklist.

Supporting Information

Appendix S1 First questionnaire ("part 1").

Appendix S2 Second questionnaire ("part 2").

Acknowledgments

We are very grateful to Sebastian Fueger for helping us collecting the data. Many thanks to Subhash Arora, Cori Gruetter, Anne Berit Guttormsen, Matthias Hänggi, Luis Sanchez Hurtado, Jesús Caballero López, Jesús López-Herce, Flavio E. Nacul, Joel Starkopf, Chris Subbe, Alessia Vargiolu and all ESICM members who participated in this survey. Furthermore we want to thank the European Critical Care Research Network of the European Society of Intensive Care Medicine for supporting this study.

Alawi Luetz is participant in the Charité Clinical Scientist Program funded by the Charité - Universitätsmedizin Berlin and the Berlin Institute of Health.

Author Contributions

Conceived and designed the experiments: AL FB FMR CJ GC B. Weiss CS. Performed the experiments: AL FB FMR CS. Analyzed the data: AL FB FMR CJ GC B. Walder B. Weiss KDW CS. Contributed reagents/materials/analysis tools: AL FB KDW CS. Wrote the paper: AL FB FMR CJ GC B. Walder B. Weiss KDW CS.

References

1. Pandharipande PP, Girard TD, Jackson JC, Morandi A, Thompson JL, et al. (2013) Long-term cognitive impairment after critical illness. N Engl J Med 369: 1306–16.
2. Ely EW, Shintani A, Truman B, Speroff T, Gordon SM, et al. (2004) Delirium as a predictor of mortality in mechanically ventilated patients in the intensive care unit. JAMA 291: 1753–62.
3. Spronk PE, Riekerk B, Hofhuis J, Rommes JH (2009) Occurrence of delirium is severely underestimated in the icu during daily care. Intensive Care Med 35: 1276–80.
4. Devlin JW, Fong JJ, Schumaker G, O'Connor H, Ruthazer R, et al. (2007) Use of a validated delirium assessment tool improves the ability of physicians to identify delirium in medical intensive care unit patients. Crit Care Med 35: 2721–4; quiz 2725.
5. Devlin JW, Marquis F, Riker RR, Robbins T, Garpestad E, et al. (2008) Combined didactic and scenario-based education improves the ability of intensive care unit staff to recognize delirium at the bedside. Crit Care 12: R19.
6. Shehabi Y, Chan L, Kadiman S, Alias A, Ismail WN, et al. (2013) Sedation depth and long-term mortality in mechanically ventilated critically ill adults: a prospective longitudinal multicentre cohort study. Intensive Care Med 39: 910–8.
7. Pang PSK, Suen LKP (2008) Stressors in the icu: a comparison of patients' and nurses' perceptions. J Clin Nurs 17: 2681–9.
8. Battle CE, Lovett S, Hutchings H (2013) Chronic pain in survivors of critical illness: a retrospective analysis of incidence and risk factors. Crit Care 17: R101.
9. Payen JF, Bosson JL, Chanques G, Mantz J, Labarere J, et al. (2009) Pain assessment is associated with decreased duration of mechanical ventilation in the intensive care unit: a post hoc analysis of the dolorea study. Anesthesiology 111: 1308–16.
10. Martin J, Heymann A, Bäsell K, Baron R, Biniek R, et al. (2010) Evidence and consensus-based german guidelines for the management of analgesia, sedation and delirium in intensive care–short version. Ger Med Sci 8: Doc02.
11. Young J, Murthy L, Westby M, Akunne A, O'Mahony R, et al. (2010) Diagnosis, prevention, and management of delirium: summary of nice guidance. BMJ 341: c3704.
12. Barr J, Fraser GL, Puntillo K, Ely EW, Gélinas C, et al. (2013) Clinical practice guidelines for the management of pain, agitation, and delirium in adult patients in the intensive care unit. Crit Care Med 41: 263–306.
13. Patel RP, Gambrell M, Speroff T, Scott TA, Pun BT, et al. (2009) Delirium and sedation in the intensive care unit: survey of behaviors and attitudes of 1384 healthcare professionals. Crit Care Med 37: 825–32.
14. Devlin JW, Bhat S, Roberts RJ, Skrobik Y (2011) Current perceptions and practices surrounding the recognition and treatment of delirium in the intensive care unit: a survey of 250 critical care pharmacists from eight states. Ann Pharmacother 45: 1217–29.
15. Trupkovic T, Kinn M, Kleinschmidt S (2011) Analgesia and sedation in the intensive care of burn patients: results of a european survey. J Intensive Care Med 26: 397–407.
16. Forsgren LM, Eriksson M (2010) Delirium–awareness, observation and interventions in intensive care units: a national survey of swedish icu head nurses. Intensive Crit Care Nurs 26: 296–303.
17. Van Eijk MMJ, Kesecioglu J, Slooter AJC (2008) Intensive care delirium monitoring and standardised treatment: a complete survey of dutch intensive care units. Intensive Crit Care Nurs 24: 218–21.
18. Luetz A, Heymann A, Radtke FM, Chenitir C, Neuhaus U, et al. (2010) Different assessment tools for intensive care unit delirium: which score to use? Crit Care Med 38: 409–18.
19. Gonçalves F, Cordero A, Almeida A, Cruz A, Rocha C, et al. (2012) A survey of the sedation practice of portuguese palliative care teams. Support Care Cancer 20: 3123–7.
20. Pandharipande P, Cotton BA, Shintani A, Thompson J, Pun BT, et al. (2008) Prevalence and risk factors for development of delirium in surgical and trauma intensive care unit patients. J Trauma 65: 34–41.
21. Martin J, Parsch A, Franck M, Wernecke KD, Fischer M, et al. (2005) Practice of sedation and analgesia in german intensive care units: results of a national survey. Crit Care 9: R117–23.
22. Radtke FM, Heymann A, Franck M, Maechler F, Drews T, et al. (2012) How to implement monitoring tools for sedation, pain and delirium in the intensive care unit: an experimental cohort study. Intensive Care Med 38: 1974–81.
23. Girard TD, Kress JP, Fuchs BD, Thomason JWW, Schweickert WD, et al. (2008) Efficacy and safety of a paired sedation and ventilator weaning protocol for mechanically ventilated patients in intensive care (awakening and breathing controlled trial): a randomised controlled trial. Lancet 371: 126–34.
24. Novaes MA, Knobel E, Bork AM, Pavão OF, Nogueira-Martins LA, et al. (1999) Stressors in icu: perception of the patient, relatives and health care team. Intensive Care Med 25: 1421–6.
25. Chanques G, Jaber S, Barbotte E, Violet S, Sebbane M, et al. (2006) Impact of systematic evaluation of pain and agitation in an intensive care unit. Crit Care Med 34: 1691–9.
26. Martin J, Franck M, Sigel S, Weiss M, Spies C (2007) Changes in sedation management in german intensive care units between 2002 and 2006: a national follow-up survey. Crit Care 11: R124.
27. Shehabi Y, Botha JA, Boyle MS, Ernest D, Freebairn RC, et al. (2008) Sedation and delirium in the intensive care unit: an australian and new zealand perspective. Anaesth Intensive Care 36: 570–8.

Is Early Oral Feeding after Gastric Cancer Surgery Feasible? A Systematic Review and Meta-Analysis of Randomized Controlled Trials

Xiaoping Liu[1,2¶], Da Wang[1¶], Liansheng Zheng[1], Tingyu Mou[1], Hao Liu[1*], Guoxin Li[1*]

1 Department of General Surgery, Nanfang Hospital, Southern Medical University, Guangzhou, Guangdong, P.R. China, 2 Department of Gastrointestinal Surgery, The first affiliated hospital of Gannan medical university, Gannan medical university, Ganzhou, Jiangxi, P.R. China

Abstract

Aim: To assess the feasibility and safety of early oral feeding (EOF) after gastrectomy for gastric cancer through a systematic review and meta-analysis based on randomized controlled trials.

Methods: A literature search in PubMed, Embase, Web of Science and Cochrane library databases was performed for eligible studies published between January 1995 and March 2014. Systematic review was carried out to identify randomized controlled trials comparing EOF and traditional postoperative oral feeding after gastric cancer surgery. Meta-analyses were performed by either a fixed effects model or a random effects model according to the heterogeneity using RevMan 5.2 software.

Results: Six studies remained for final analysis. Included studies were published between 2005 and 2013 reporting on a total of 454 patients. No significant differences were observed for postoperative complication (RR = 0.95; 95%CI, 0.70 to 1.29; $P = 0.75$), the tolerability of oral feeding (RR = 0.98; 95%CI, 0.91 to 1.06; $P = 0.61$), readmission rate (RR = 1; 95%CI, 0.30 to 3.31; $P = 1.00$) and incidence of anastomotic leakage (RR = 0.31; 95%CI, 0.01 to 7.30; $P = 0.47$) between two groups. EOF after gastrectomy for gastric cancer was associated with significant shorter duration of the hospital stay (WMD = −2.36; 95%CI, −3.37 to −1.34; $P<0.0001$) and time to first flatus (WMD = −19.94; 95%CI, −32.03 to −7.84; $P = 0.001$). There were no significant differences in postoperative complication, tolerability of oral feeding, readmission rates, duration of hospital stay and time to first flatus among subgroups stratified by the time to start EOF or by partial and total gastrectomy or by laparoscopic and open surgery.

Conclusions: The result of this meta-analysis showed that EOF after gastric cancer surgery seems feasible and safe, even started at the day of surgery irrespective of the extent of the gastric resection and the type of surgery. However, more prospective, well-designed multicenter RCTs with more clinical outcomes are needed for further validation.

Editor: Helge Bruns, University Hospital Oldenburg, Germany

Funding: This study was supported by The National Key Technology R&D Program (No. 2013BAI05B00), the Major Program of Science and Technology Program of Guangzhou (No. 201300000087), Research Fund of Public welfare in Health Industry of Health (No. 201402015), Ministry of Health of PR China, and The program of the national key clinical medical specialty. The funders had no role in study design, data collection and analysis, decision to publish, or preparation of the manuscript.

Competing Interests: The authors have declared that no competing interests exist.

* Email: liuhaofbi@163.com (HL); gzliguoxin@163.com (GXL)

These authors contributed equally to this work.

¶ These authors are co-first authors on this work.

Introduction

Recently, the concept of fast-track surgery is drawing increasing attention, which requires multidisciplinary team work to accelerate recovery during perioperative care [1]. Early oral feeding (EOF) is one of the most important parts of fast-track surgery elements. The advantages of early enteral nutrition after colorectal surgery have been demonstrated in several reports, such as a shorter length of hospital stay and less postoperative morbidity and mortality compared with traditional postoperative oral feeding (TOF) [2–4].

Gastric cancer is the second most common cause of cancer-related death worldwide, of which the global incidence is declining. However, there remains quite higher morbidity rate in Asia compared to that in western countries [5]. Gastric cancer can be cured successfully with surgical resection and the operative technique and anastomotic type for gastric cancer has been gradually standardized [6–8]. Then, surgeons should pay more attention to how to enhance recovery, reduce complications and improve quality of life of patients undergoing gastrectomy for gastric cancer [9–11]. To date, the introduction of fast-track surgery following gastrectomy has been demonstrated for nearly one decade [12–14]. However, as a key element of fast track surgery pathway, the significance of EOF after gastric cancer surgery is still controversial.

The purpose of this study was to assess the feasibility and safety of EOF in patients after gastric cancer surgery through a systematic review based on randomized controlled trials.

Materials and Methods

Search strategy

The relevant literature was searched from PubMed, Embase, Web of Science and Cochrane library databases published between January 1995 and March 2014. The following search terms was used: gastric cancer, gastrectomy, early oral feeding, early oral intake, enhanced recovery and fast-track surgery. Reference lists within selected studies and abstracts published at major international conferences were also searched for potentially eligible studies.

Study inclusion criteria

The studies were limited to be described as the design type of randomized controlled trials (RCTs) with or without blinding method, comparing EOF with TOF following gastrectomy for gastric cancers. Oral feeding was following a stepwise plan from water to other liquids to semi-fluids to normal food. EOF was defined as oral feeding of water or glucose saline initiated before flatus as tolerated; TOF was defined as oral feeding initiated certainly after flatus. Comparative studies that included patients undergoing EOF after gastric cancer surgery through nasogastric enteral nutrition were excluded. We applied restrictions with respect to language in English.

Quality Assessment

The quality of included RCTs was assessed by two reviewers (XP Liu and D Wang) independently according to the Cochrane Collaboration's tool for assessing risk of bias, which addressed seven items: random sequence generation, allocation concealment, blinding of participants and personnel, blinding of outcome assessment, incomplete outcome data, freedom from selective reporting, and freedom from other bias [15]. Disagreement was resolved by consensus and discussion.

Outcomes

The primary outcomes were postoperative complication, tolerability of oral feeding and readmission rates. The secondary outcomes were the duration of hospital stay expressed as hospitalization days after surgery, time of first flatus and incidence of anastomotic leakage. Patients failed to tolerate EOF presented as recurrent nausea, vomiting, abdominal distension without intestinal sound or nasogastric tube was reinserted.

Statistical analysis

Statistical analysis was performed with Cochrane Collaboration's RevMan5.2 software (Cochrane Collaboration, Oxford, UK). For continuous data, results from each study were expressed as a weighted mean difference (WMD) with 95% confidence intervals (CI) and combined for meta-analysis. Data were summarized graphically in forest plots. For dichotomous data, results for each study were performed by using the relative risk (RR). The Mantel–Haenszel method was used to combine the RRs for the outcomes of interest. A funnel plot for postoperative complication was constructed to evaluate publication and other biases [16].

Heterogeneity was measured through X^2 and I^2 test. If between-study heterogeneity existed (I^2>50%), random-effect model was used; otherwise, meta-analysis was done with fixed effect model. $P<0.05$ in two-sided test was considered statistically significant.

Results

Selected studies

A flow chart detailing the process of study identification and selection following the PRISMA statement (see Checklist S1) is shown in Fig.1. Six studies finally remained for further analysis. Included studies were published between 2005 and 2013 and reported on a total of 454 patients [17–22]. In the study by Chen *et al.*, they carried out subgrourp analysis stratified by laparoscopic and open surgery, so L and O were used to tell them apart in the present meta-analysis [17]. The characteristics of these six studies are summarized in Table 1.

Methodological quality of the studies

Risk of bias was assessed by the Cochrane Collaboration's tool. As concerns for early oral feeding being compared, blinding was inherent defect for such studies. Generally, the included studies had a moderate risk of bias (Fig.2).

Primary outcome parameters

Postoperative complication. Primary outcome for this systematic review was postoperative complication. All six studies provided information on postoperative complication. The pooled results indicated no evidence of a significant difference in the number of complications between two groups (RR = 0.97; 95% CI, 0.71 to 1.33; P = 0.85), and there was no remarkable heterogeneity among studies (P = 0.06, I^2 = 50%) (Fig.3A).

The tolerability of oral feeding. Six studies were all included with 224 and 230 cases in each group respectively. Among them, 209 patients tolerated EOF while 15 failed. Using a random effects model, the pooled results showed that there was no significant difference between two groups about tolerability of oral feeding after gastrectomy (RR = 0.99; 95%CI, 0.91 to 1.07; P = 0.72), with obvious heterogeneity (P = 0.03, I^2 = 58%) (Fig.3B).

Readmission rate. In the five studies [18–22] reporting on readmission rate after gastric cancer surgery with 372 patients, the pooled readmission rate was similar between both groups based on fix effects model analysis (RR = 1; 95%CI, 0.30 to 3.31; P = 1.00), without significant heterogeneity (P = 0.55, I^2 = 0%) (Fig.3C).

Secondary outcome parameters

The duration of hospital stay. All included studies reported information on the duration of hospital stay, however, two studies, Chen *et al.* [17] and Wang *et al.* [22] only described the median postoperative hospital stay. So, we excluded them out of this meta-analysis. The duration of hospital stay was significantly shorter with EOF than TOF in all included studies (WMD = −2.19; 95%CI, −3.22 to −1.17; P<0.001). Pooled analysis of the duration of hospital stay showed obvious heterogeneity between studies (P = 0.005, I^2 = 77%) (Fig.4A).

Time to first flatus. Four studies [18–21] provided the complete information on time to first flatus. Time to first flatus was significantly shorter for EOF group than TOF group after gastric cancer surgery (WMD = −19.94; 95% CI, −32.03 to −7.84; P = 0.001). Because of significant heterogeneity (P = 0.0005, I^2 = 83%), a random effects model was used (Fig.4B).

Incidence of anastomotic leakage. Anastomotic leakage is one of the major postoperative complications. We observed that the incidence of anastomotic leakage was comparable for two

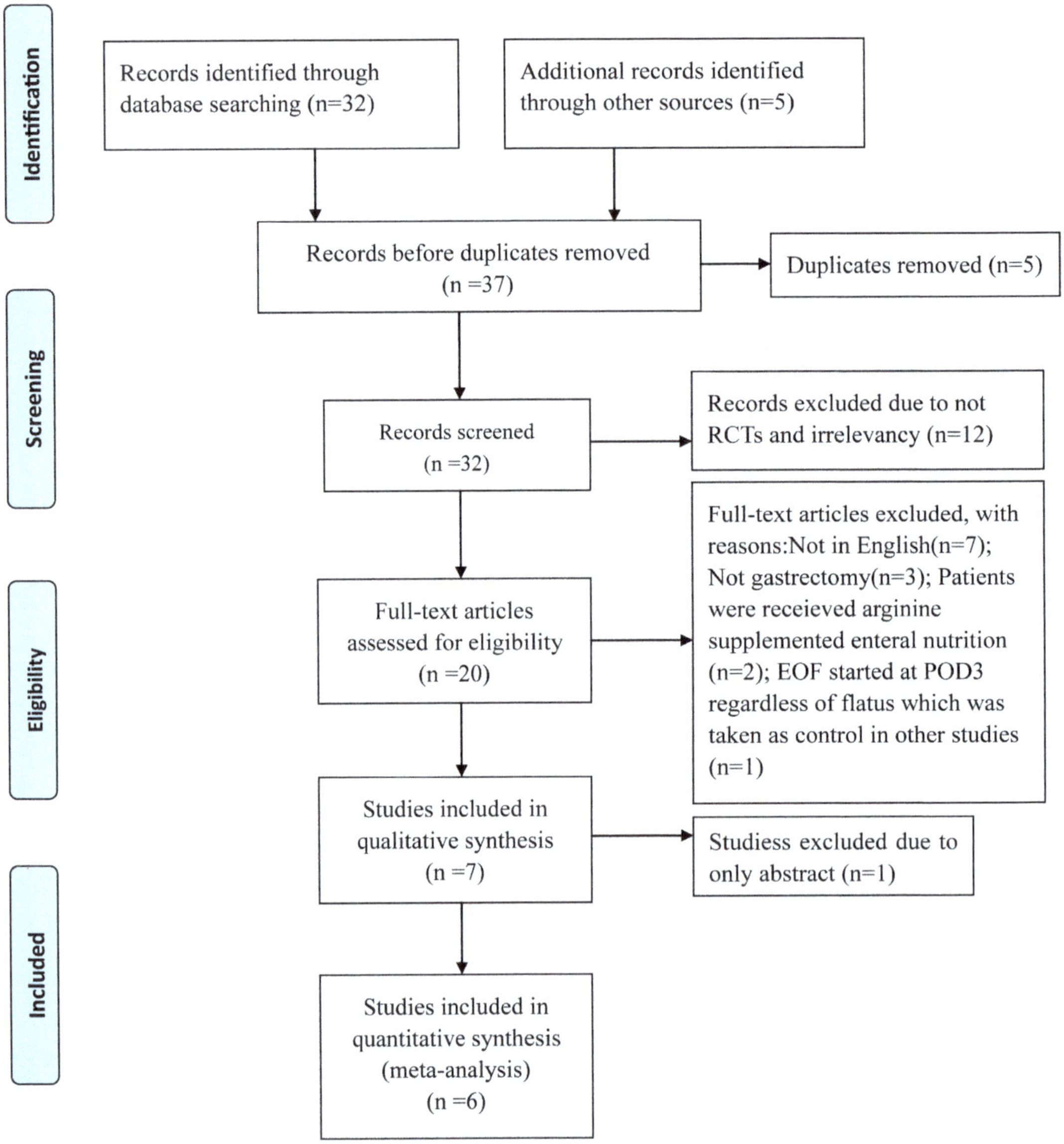

Figure 1. Flow chart of studies identified, included and excluded following PRISMA statement.

groups among all patients as similar in all included studies (RR = 0.31; 95%CI, 0.01 to 7.30; $P = 0.47$) (Fig.4C). There was only one patient suffered anastomotic leakage in Hur *et al.*'s study [19]. So the heterogeneity was not applicable.

Sensitivity analysis. We reanalyzed the primary outcome parameters by including only studies with total sample size no smaller than 50 in order to perform sensitivity analysis. The results were not substantially influenced by sensitivity analysis as shown in Table 2. The results of sensitivity analysis supported the credibility of the evidence in this meta-analysis.

Subgroup analysis. Subgroup analysis according to the time of starting EOF, extent of gastrectomy and type of surgery, were also performed to assess potential effect modification of these variables on outcomes. Tables 3–5 show the results of subgroup analysis. The similar outcomes could be observed in the stratified groups irrespective of the time to start EOF, the extent of gastric resection and the type of surgery.

Publication bias. Publication bias was evaluated by performing a funnel plot of postoperative complication (Fig.5). All included studies reported on this outcome, which were equally distributed on the vertical axis, the result showed no evidence of obvious publication bias.

Discussion

The present meta-analysis showed that early oral feeding (EOF) did not increase postoperative complication, readmission rate and the incidence of anastomotic leakage, either. We found no significant difference in tolerability of oral feeding after gastrectomy between both groups. Furthermore, EOF following gastric surgery was associated with a significant reduction in duration of postoperative hospital stay and time to first flatus compared with TOF.

Though emerging evidence for the advantages of EOF has been demonstrated, many surgeons are still reluctant to administer EOF

Table 1. Characteristics of the studies included in meta-analysis.

Author	Country	Year	Time of oral feeding	Extent of gastrectomy	Group	Number	Age	Gender	BMI	ASA	TNM stage
							(years)	(m/f)	(kg/m^2)	(0/1/2)	(I+II)/(III+IV)
Liu[21]	China	2010	day of surgery	TG, PG, DG	EOF	30	60.7±9.7	18/15	21.84±2.65	2[c]	8/25
					TOF	33	61.9±8.3	15/14	21.28±2.54	2 [c]	7/23
Wang[22]	China	2010	day of surgery	PG, DG	EOF	45	58.76±9.66	32/13	23.85±2.40	NR	NR
					TOF	47	56.87±9.16	29/18	23.25±2.79		
Hur[19]	Korea	2011	POD1	TG, SG	EOF	28	24/4 [a]	20/8	21/7 [b]	10/18[d]	NR
					TOF	26	21/5[a]	13/13	19/7[b]	4/22[d]	
Chen(L)[17]	China	2012	6–8*h* after surgery	DG	EOF	19	59(49–71)	10/9	22.94±2.23	NR	11/8
					TOF	22	62.5(45–72)	10/12	22.99±2.24		11/11
Chen(O)[17]	China	2012	6–8*h* after surgery	DG	EOF	21	64(40–71)	9/12	23.54±2.59	NR	9/12
					TOF	20	64.5(49–75)	12/8	23.47±2.62		7/13
Kim[20]	Korea	2012	POD2	DG	EOF	22	52.64±11.57	13/9	23.40±3.17	0/14/8	21/1
					TOF	22	57.45±14.54	15/7	23.77±3.54	0/14/8	22/0
Feng[18]	China	2013	day of surgery	TG	EOF	59	54.98±11.35	41/18	22.44±3.51	0/3/56	26/33
					TOF	60	55.79±10.06	44/16	21.01±1.78	0/1/59	39/21

BMI: body mass index; ASA: American Society of Anesthesiology; TNM: tumor, node, metastasis; NR: not reported; POD: postoperative day; TG: total gastrectomy; DG: distal gastrectomy; PG: proximal gastrectomy; SG: subtotal gastrectomy;

[a]: Age grouped by <65/≥65;

[b]: BMI grouped by <25 kg/m^2/≥25 kg/m^2;

[c]: median;

[d]: ASA score grouped by 0/(1 and 2).

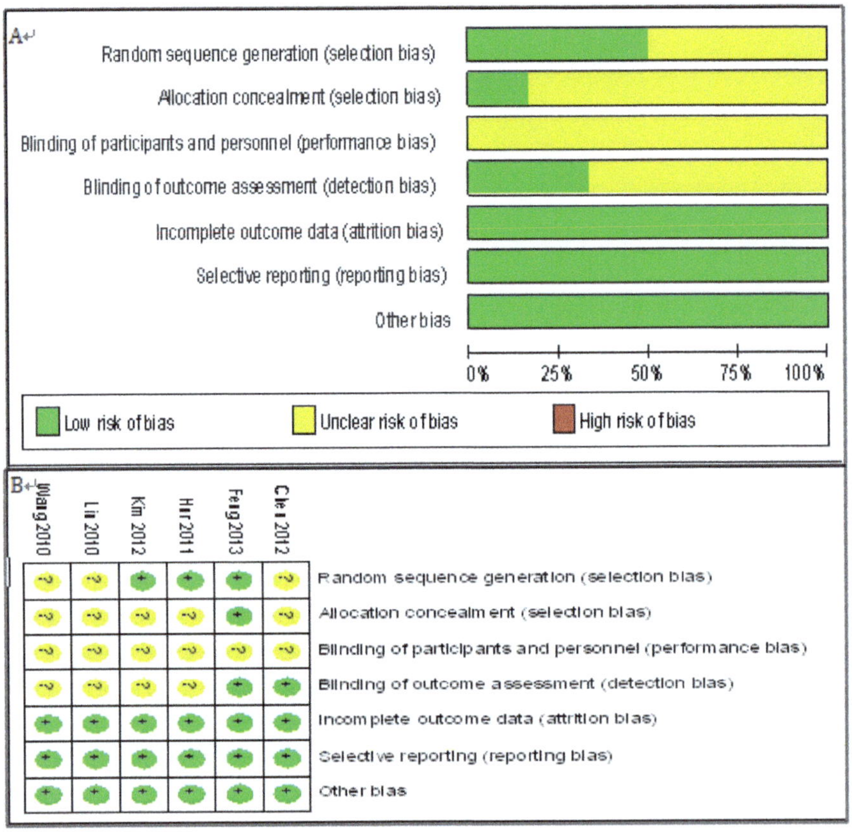

Figure 2. Risk of bias graph. Judgements about each risk of bias item presented in all include RCTs(A) and for each included RCT(B).

to patients after gastrectomy. One reason is fearing an increase of postoperative complications, such as gastric retention and anastomosis dehiscence[23,24]. Regarding the safety of EOF, previous evidence from a systematic review in patients undergoing colonic surgery has shown that EOF is safe without any significant increase in complications [25,26]. What's more, in a meta-analysis of studies comparing early enteral feeding versus "nil by mouth", those patients receiving enteral nutrition had a lower incidence of infection complications undergoing gastrointestinal surgery [27]. The major factor used to justify the traditional practice of oral intake restriction and EOF after gastrectomy is concern for anastomosis leakage [28]. However, restricting EOF is not evidence-based. On the contrary, EOF after upper gastrointestinal surgery was found to promote anastomotic healing and anastomotic strength in intestines and somatic tissues of a rat model [29]. Early postoperative oral diet is easily absorbed, which may accelerate recovery of peristalsis, protect gut mucosal barrier function, and strengthen immune response [30]. Traditional nutritional routes still adhere to the first flatus with postoperative fasting, decompression of nasogastric tube and the supply of a large number of intravenous fluids for several days after gastrectomy. Thus, some pulmonary complications such as atelectasis, pneumonia, gastroesophageal reflux in patients may be induced [31]. In the present meta-analysis, we observed no significant differences between two groups concerning postoperative complications, including the presence of anastomotic leakage.

Inducing gastrointestinal symptoms is another concern to justify EOF restriction after gastrectomy [32,33]. It was supposed that EOF might result in the risk of increasing postoperative nausea and vomiting [4,34,35]. Thus, the patients would not only suffer from intolerance of EOF, but also encounter severe adverse events. Traditionally, the time to resume diet depends on the passage of flatus. However, such an approach was considered extremely conservative through the physiology research of postoperative ileus [36]. Difronzo *et al.* [37] showed that over 80% of patients tolerated EOF after colonic surgery by analyzed 200 patients during a five-year period. From all included studies of this meta-analysis, in spite that nausea, vomiting or abdominal distension occurred in some patients receiving EOF, the symptoms mostly happened in the initial stage of oral diet and did not develop into severe complications. The pooled data showed that there was no significant difference between two groups about tolerability of oral feeding after gastrectomy, and EOF didn't increase the risk of postoperative morbidity and mortality. Therefore, removing a nasogastric tube and early oral intake after gastrectomy as soon as possible is a considerable strategy for postoperative patients [38,39]. Moreover, on the basis of safety and tolerability of EOF, we also see from this meta-analysis, EOF might further shorten the hospital stays, lessen first flatus time and didn't increase the patient's readmission to the hospital. It was considered that EOF following gastrectomy could benefit patients.

From the studies included in this meta-analysis, various time of EOF after surgery between studies was found such an 6 to 8 hours after surgery, the first postoperative day and the third postoperative day et al. Jeong *et al.* [40] reported EOF was safe and feasible on the first postoperative day after gastrectomy, however, an old age (≥70 years) required careful monitoring when applying EOF after surgery. Lewis *et al.* [41] compared early enteral nutrition within 24 *h* of gastrointestinal surgery versus later commencement

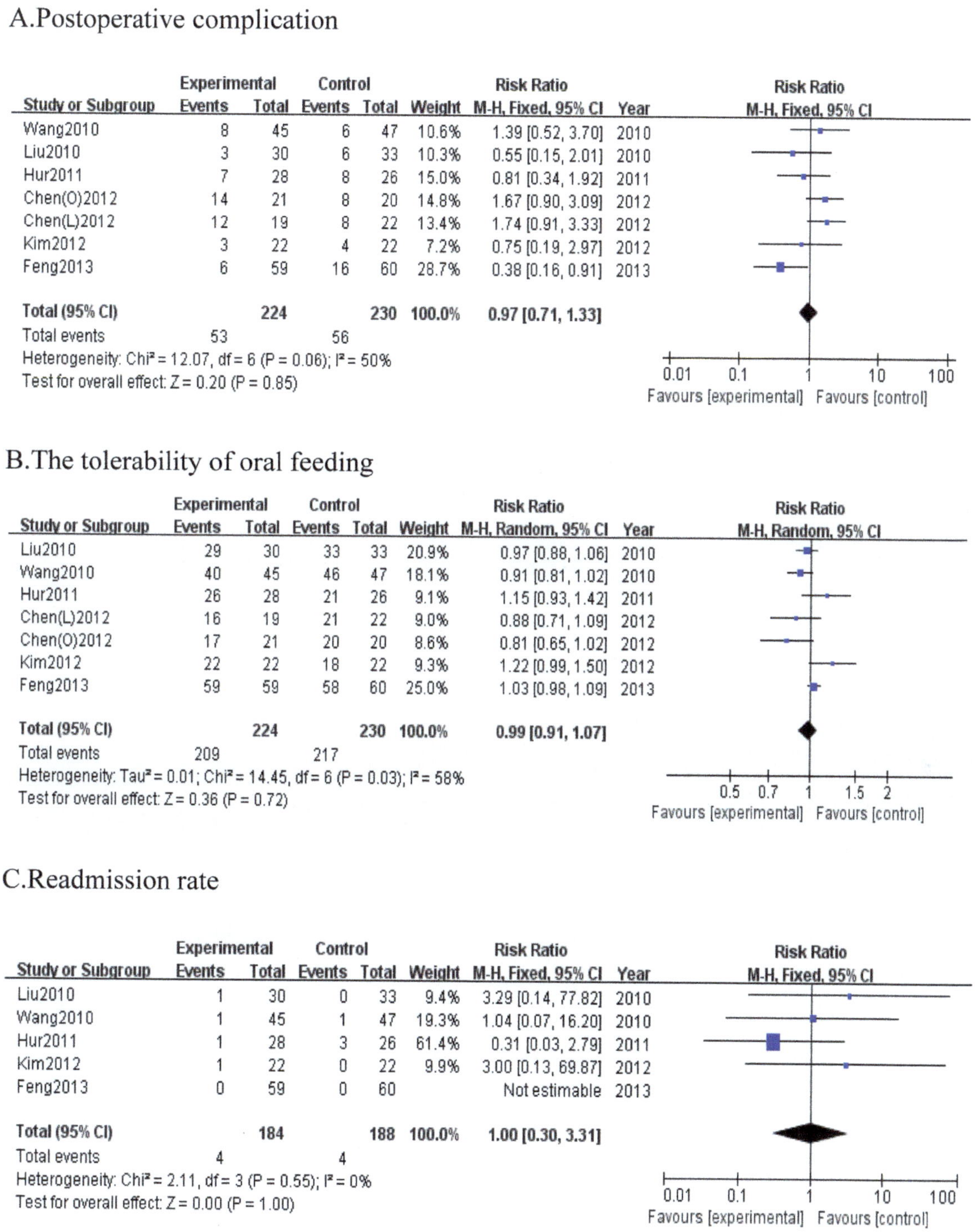

Figure 3. Forest plot displaying the results of the meta-analysis. A. postoperative complication; B. the tolerability of oral feeding; C. readmission rate. RR: Risk ratio; WMD: Weighted mean difference. CI: confidence intervals.

of feeding, it was found that mortality was reduced with early postoperative feeding even though increased vomiting. Thus, the given time of EOF after surgery is still controversial. In our included studies, time of EOF after gastrectomy was mostly based on an accelerated rehabilitation protocol designed for colorectal resection surgery. According to the time of EOF, we divided the included studies into two subgroup, day of surgery subgroup [17,18,21,22] and day after surgery subgroup [19,20]. Most outcomes in EOF were found similar with TOF in the stratified subgroups consistent with the pooled analysis, which somewhat suggested that to start EOF at 6 or 8 hours after surgery might be safe, in spite of small sample studies contributing to it.

Simultaneously, we also analyzed the outcomes stratified into total gastrectomy (TG) subgroup [18] and subtotal gastrectomy (SG) subgroup [17,20,22]. Similar findings were found in both TG and SG group with regard to tolerability of oral feeding, duration

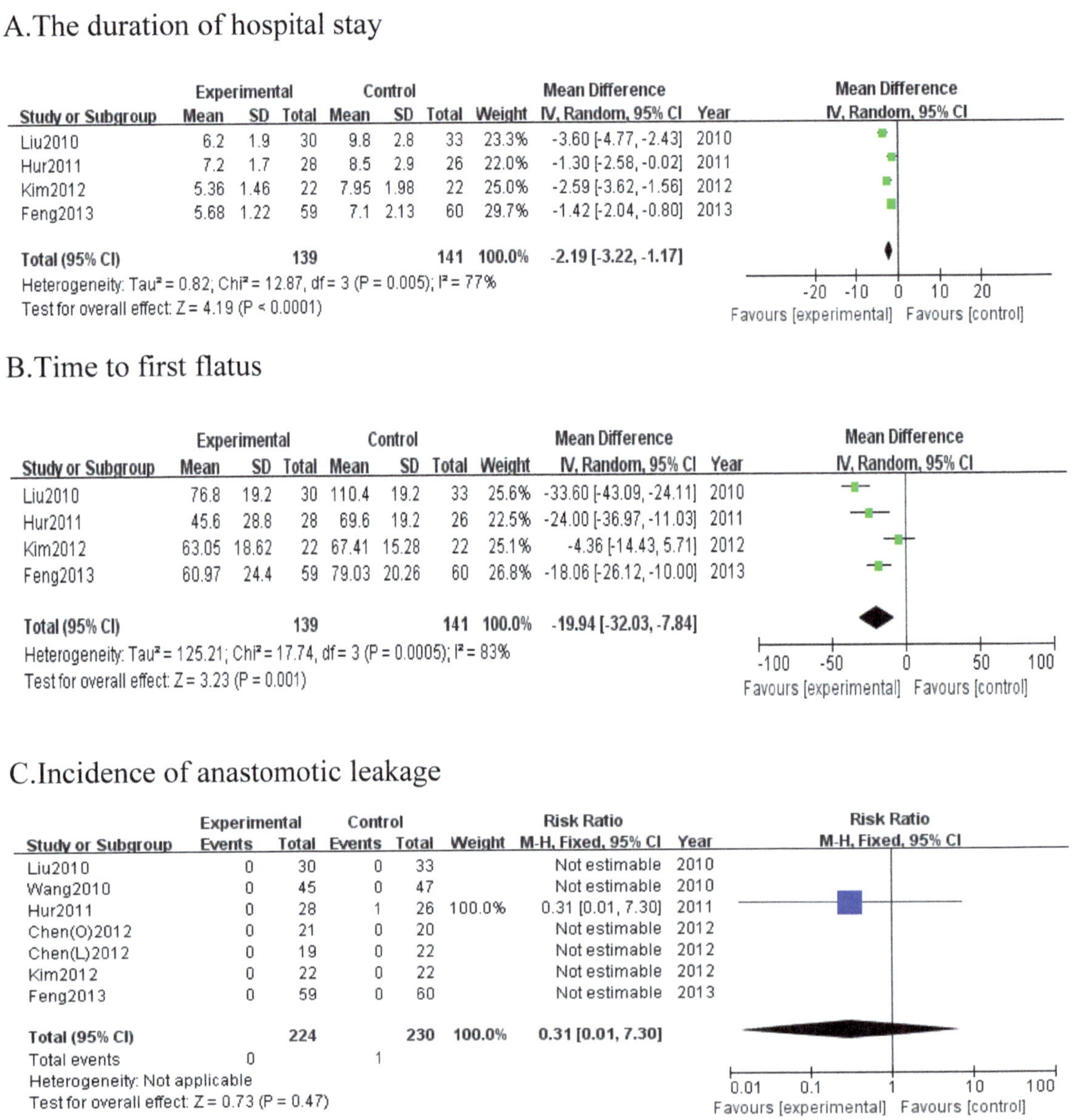

Figure 4. Forest plot displaying the results of the meta-analysis. A. the duration of hospital stay; B. time of first flatus; C. incidence of anastomotic leakage. RR: Risk ratio; WMD: Weighted mean difference. CI: confidence intervals.

of hospital stay and time of first flatus except postoperative complication. For TG, the incidence of postoperative complications seemed lower in EOF group than that in TOF group, which turned out to be opposite for SG. The possible reasons underlying the distinctions between TG and SG might be that the extent of the gastric resection decided types of digestive tract reconstruction, which led to different effects on postoperative physiological functions, like gut motility and metabolism. Thus, some minor gastrointestinal symptoms such as abdominal cramps, colic, nausea and vomiting would be induced, especially in SG which preserved the function of gastric acid secretion, resulting in increased overall postoperative complications. However, no major complications like anastomotic leakage were observed in most studies that had reported on this issue. Besides, it was too difficult to reach a conclusive outcome based on pooled analysis including only two studies with quite small sample sizes. On the whole, no obvious change was observed regarding the primary outcomes of the present meta-analysis. It might still be feasible under careful assessment for both TG and SG. And similar findings were also observed in the subgroup analyses stratified by laparoscopic and open surgery. It is believed that postoperative recovery of bowel motion could be affected by abdominal incision size. Patients in laparoscopy group are supposed to have a better recovery for the intrinsic advantages of minimally invasive surgery over conventional one. Unfortunately, due to limited sample size, such conclusions could not be draw out of the given data. So a large-scale well-designed RCT is warranted to clarify this difference more conclusively. However, in this meta-analysis EOF seemed acceptable for patients in both laparoscopic and open surgery group.

Several limitations were associated with included randomized studies deserving consideration in the interpretation of this meta-analysis. First, small sample size, single-center experience and moderate quality of included studies might decrease the reliability

Table 2. Sensitivity analysis results of primary outcomes by included studies of no less than 50 patients in each group.

Primary outcomes	Number of studies	Patients	WMD/RR	95%CI	Analysis model	*P*	heterogeneity	
		(EOF/TOF)					I^2	*P*
postoperative complication	5	202/208	0.90	0.47, 1.70	Random	0.73	66%	0.02
Tolerability of oral feeding	5	202/208	0.97	0.89, 1.05	Random	0.47	67%	0.02
Readmission rates	4	162/166	0.78	0.20, 3.00	Fixed	0.72	0%	0.47

RR: Risk ratio; WMD: Weighted mean difference. CI: confidence intervals.

Table 3. Results of subgroup analysis comparing the time of EOF after gastrectomy.

Outcomes	Subgroup	Number of studies	Patients	WMD/RR	95%CI	*P*	Heterogeneity	
			(EOF/TOF)				I^2	*P*
Postoperative complication	Day of surgery	5	174/182	1.02	0.72, 1.45	0.91	64%	0.02
	Day after surgery	2	50/48	0.79	0.38, 1.65	0.53	0%	0.92
Tolerability of oral feeding	Day of surgery	5	174/182	0.94	0.86, 1.03	0.21	67%	0.02
	Day after surgery	2	50/48	1.18	1.02, 1.37	0.03	0%	0.71
Readmission rates	Day of surgery	3	134/140	1.78	0.24, 13.09	0.57	0%	0.59
	Day after surgery	2	50/48	0.68	0.14, 3.28	0.63	26%	0.25
Duration of hospital stay	Day of surgery	2	89/93	−2.45	−4.58, −0.32	0.02	90%	0.001
	Day after surgery	2	50/48	−2.00	−3.26, −0.74	0.002	58%	0.12
Time to first flatus	Day of surgery	2	89/93	−25.62	−40.84, −10.40	0.001	83%	0.01
	Day after surgery	2	50/48	−13.74	−32.96, 5.49	0.16	82%	0.02

RR: Risk ratio; WMD: Weighted mean difference. CI: confidence intervals.
Day of surgery: 6 h$\leq$ time to start EOF$\leq$ 24 h after gastrectomy;
Day after surgery: time to start EOF>24 h after gastrectomy.

Table 4. Results of subgroup analysis comparing EOF in TG and SG for gastric cancer.

Outcomes	Subgroup	Number of studies	Patients (EOF/TOF)	WMD/RR	95%CI	*P*	Heterogeneity I^2	Heterogeneity *P*
Postoperative complication	TG	1	59/60	0.38	0.16, 0.91	0.03	Not applicable	
	SG	4	107/111	1.54	1.04, 2.28	0.03	0%	0.72
Tolerability of oral feeding	TG	1	59/60	1.03	0.98, 1.09	0.25	Not applicable	
	SG	4	107/111	0.94	0.81, 1.09	0.44	63%	0.05
Duration of hospital stay	TG	1	59/60	−1.42	−2.04,−0.80	<0.00001	Not applicable	
	SG	1	22/22	−2.59	−3.62,−1.56	<0.00001	Not applicable	
Time of first flatus	TG	11	59/60	−18.06	−26.12,−10.00	<0.0001	Not applicable	
	SG	1	22/22	−4.36	−14.43, 5.71	0.40	Not applicable	

TG: total gastrectomy; SG: subtotal gastrectomy; RR: Risk ratio; WMD: Weighted mean difference. CI: confidence intervals.

Table 5. Results of subgroup analysis comparing EOF in Laparoscopy and open surgery for gastric cancer.

Outcomes	Subgroup	Number of studies	Patients (EOF/TOF)	WMD/RR	95%CI	*P*	Heterogeneity I^2	Heterogeneity *P*
Postoperative complication	Laparoscopy	2	41/44	1.39	0.77, 2.51	0.27	18%	0.27
	Open	5	183/186	0.86	0.59, 1.25	0.43	57%	0.06
Tolerability of oral feeding	Laparoscopy	2	41/44	1.04	0.76, 1.42	0.82	77%	77%
	Open	5	183/186	0.97	0.90, 1.06	0.54	61%	0.04
Readmission rates	Laparoscopy	1	22/22	3.00	0.13, 69.87	0.49	Not applicable	
	Open	4	162/166	0.78	0.20, 3.00	0.72	0%	0.47
Duration of hospital stay	Laparoscopy	1	22/22	−2.59	−3.62,−1.56	<0.001	Not applicable	
	Open	3	117/119	−2.07	−3.45, −0.70	0.003	82%	0.004
Time of first flatus	Laparoscopy	1	22/22	−4.36	−14.43, 5.71	0.40	Not applicable	
	Open	3	117/119	−25.07	−35.05, −15.09	<0.001	67%	0.05

RR: Risk ratio; WMD: Weighted mean difference. CI: confidence intervals.

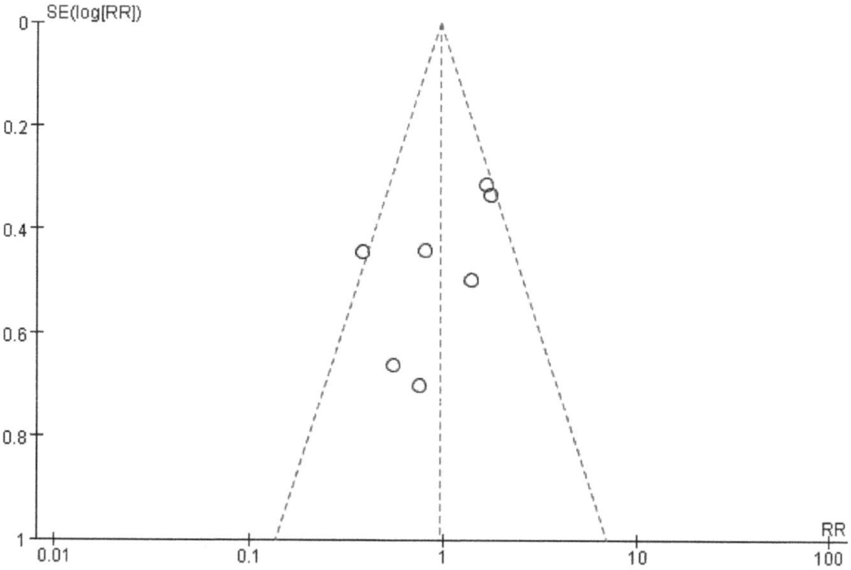

Figure 5. Funnel plot of the studies reporting on postoperative complication. RR: risk ratio; SE: standard error.

of the results. Second, insufficient background of clinical information, differences in operating technique, perioperative nursing system and outcomes examined were discovered in our included studies. Third, obvious bias in population was found. Most of the studies were done in East Asian countries. However, the studies of white and black population were lacked. As widely known, factors such as dietary history, preoperative obesity could also influence the EOF on patients after gastric cancer surgery. Thus, given the above defects, different strategies were used to eliminate bias. Then, subgroup analysis was performed to detect potential bias sources, stratifying the time to start EOF, the extent of the gastric resection and the type of surgery to acquire robust evidence for the conclusions. All these attempts supported the credibility of the evidence in this meta-analysis.

In conclusion, this meta-analysis supported that EOF after gastric cancer surgery seemed feasible and safe, even started at the day of surgery irrespective of the extent of the gastric resection and the type of surgery. However, more prospective, well-designed multicenter RCTs with more clinical outcomes are needed for further validation.

Author Contributions

Conceived and designed the experiments: XPL DW GXL. Performed the experiments: XPL DW LSZ TYM. Analyzed the data: HL DW XPL. Contributed reagents/materials/analysis tools: DW XPL LSZ TYM. Wrote the paper: DW XPL.

References

1. Kehlet H, Wilmore DW (2008) Evidence-based surgical care and the evolution of fast-track surgery. Ann Surg 248: 189–198.
2. Feo CV, Romanini B, Sortini D, Ragazzi R, Zamboni P, et al. (2004) Early oral feeding after colorectal resection: a randomized controlled study. ANZ J Surg 74: 298–301.
3. Zhuang CL, Ye XZ, Zhang CJ, Dong QT, Chen BC, et al. (2013) Early versus traditional postoperative oral feeding in patients undergoing elective colorectal surgery: a meta-analysis of randomized clinical trials. Dig Surg 30: 225–232.
4. Gianotti L, Nespoli L, Torselli L, Panelli M, Nespoli A (2011) Safety, feasibility, and tolerance of early oral feeding after colorectal resection outside an enhanced recovery after surgery (ERAS) program. Int J Colorectal Dis 26: 747–753.
5. de Martel C, Forman D, Plummer M (2013) Gastric cancer: epidemiology and risk factors. Gastroenterol Clin North Am 42: 219–240.
6. Hanna GB, Amygdalos I, Ni M, Boshier PR, Mikhail S, et al. (2013) Improving the standard of lymph node retrieval after gastric cancer surgery. Histopathology 63: 316–324.
7. Lee HJ, Shiraishi N, Kim HH, Hiki N, Uyama I, et al. (2012) Standard of practice on laparoscopic gastric cancer surgery in Korea and Japan: experts' survey. Asian J Endosc Surg 5: 5–11.
8. Koeda K, Nishizuka S, Wakabayashi G (2011) Minimally invasive surgery for gastric cancer: the future standard of care. World J Surg 35: 1469–1477.
9. Chen ZX, Liu AH, Cen Y (2014) Fast-track program vs traditional care in surgery for gastric cancer. World J Gastroenterol 20: 578–583.
10. Yu Z, Zhuang CL, Ye XZ, Zhang CJ, Dong QT, et al. (2014) Fast-track surgery in gastrectomy for gastric cancer: a systematic review and meta-analysis. Langenbecks Arch Surg 399: 85–92.
11. Zhao H, Zhao H, Wang Y, Jing H, Ding Q, et al. (2013) Randomized clinical trial of arginine-supplemented enteral nutrition versus standard enteral nutrition in patients undergoing gastric cancer surgery. J Cancer Res Clin Oncol 139: 1465–1470.
12. Yamada T, Hayashi T, Cho H, Yoshikawa T, Taniguchi H, et al. (2012) Usefulness of enhanced recovery after surgery protocol as compared with conventional perioperative care in gastric surgery. Gastric Cancer 15: 34–41.
13. Grantcharov TP, Kehlet H (2010) Laparoscopic gastric surgery in an enhanced recovery programme. Br J Surg 97: 1547–1551.
14. Hayakawa T, Kaneko H, Konagaya T, Shinozaki K, Kasahara A, et al. (2003) Enhanced somatostatin secretion into the gastric juice with recovery of basal acid output after Helicobacter pylori eradication in gastric ulcers. J Gastroenterol Hepatol 18: 505–511.
15. Armijo-Olivo S, Stiles CR, Hagen NA, Biondo PD, Cummings GG (2012) Assessment of study quality for systematic reviews: a comparison of the Cochrane Collaboration Risk of Bias Tool and the Effective Public Health Practice Project Quality Assessment Tool: methodological research. J Eval Clin Pract 18: 12–18.
16. Liao G, Chen J, Ren C, Li R, Du S, et al. (2013) Robotic versus open gastrectomy for gastric cancer: a meta-analysis. PLoS One 8: e81946.
17. Chen Hu J, Xin Jiang L, Cai L, Tao Zheng H, Yuan Hu S, et al. (2012) Preliminary experience of fast-track surgery combined with laparoscopy-assisted radical distal gastrectomy for gastric cancer. J Gastrointest Surg 16: 1830-1839.
18. Feng F, Ji G, Li JP, Li XH, Shi H, et al. (2013) Fast-track surgery could improve postoperative recovery in radical total gastrectomy patients. World J Gastroenterol 19: 3642–3648.

19. Hur H, Kim SG, Shim JH, Song KY, Kim W, et al. (2011) Effect of early oral feeding after gastric cancer surgery: a result of randomized clinical trial. Surgery 149: 561–568.
20. Kim JW, Kim WS, Cheong JH, Hyung WJ, Choi SH, et al. (2012) Safety and efficacy of fast-track surgery in laparoscopic distal gastrectomy for gastric cancer: a randomized clinical trial. World J Surg 36: 2879–2887.
21. Liu XX, Jiang ZW, Wang ZM, Li JS (2010) Multimodal optimization of surgical care shows beneficial outcome in gastrectomy surgery. JPEN J Parenter Enteral Nutr 34: 313–321.
22. Wang D, Kong Y, Zhong B, Zhou X, Zhou Y (2010) Fast-track surgery improves postoperative recovery in patients with gastric cancer: a randomized comparison with conventional postoperative care. J Gastrointest Surg 14: 620–627.
23. Bisgaard T, Kehlet H (2002) Early oral feeding after elective abdominal surgery—what are the issues? Nutrition 18: 944–948.
24. Csendes A, Diaz JC, Burdiles P, Braghetto I, Maluenda F, et al. (1990) Classification and treatment of anastomotic leakage after extended total gastrectomy in gastric carcinoma. Hepatogastroenterology 37 Suppl 2: 174–177.
25. Vlug MS, Wind J, van der Zaag E, Ubbink DT, Cense HA, et al. (2009) Systematic review of laparoscopic vs open colonic surgery within an enhanced recovery programme. Colorectal Dis 11: 335–343.
26. Minig L, Biffi R, Zanagnolo V, Attanasio A, Beltrami C, et al. (2009) Reduction of postoperative complication rate with the use of early oral feeding in gynecologic oncologic patients undergoing a major surgery: a randomized controlled trial. Ann Surg Oncol 16: 3101–3110.
27. Lewis SJ, Egger M, Sylvester PA, Thomas S, (2001) Early enteral feeding versus "nil by mouth" after gastrointestinal surgery: systematic review and meta-analysis of controlled trials. BMJ 323: 773–776.
28. Sierzega M, Kolodziejczyk P, Kulig J, Polish Gastric Cancer Study G (2010) Impact of anastomotic leakage on long-term survival after total gastrectomy for carcinoma of the stomach. Br J Surg 97: 1035–1042.
29. Fukuzawa J, Terashima H, Ohkohchi N (2007) Early postoperative oral feeding accelerates upper gastrointestinal anastomotic healing in the rat model. World J Surg 31: 1234–1239.
30. Minig L, Biffi R, Zanagnolo V, Attanasio A, Beltrami C, et al. (2009) Early oral versus "traditional" postoperative feeding in gynecologic oncology patients undergoing intestinal resection: a randomized controlled trial. Ann Surg Oncol 16: 1660–1668.
31. Schuchert MJ, Pettiford BL, Landreneau JP, Waxman J, Kilic A, et al. (2008) Transcervical gastric tube drainage facilitates patient mobility and reduces the risk of pulmonary complications after esophagectomy. J Gastrointest Surg 12: 1479–1484.
32. Dag A, Colak T, Turkmenoglu O, Gundogdu R, Aydin S (2011) A randomized controlled trial evaluating early versus traditional oral feeding after colorectal surgery. Clinics (Sao Paulo) 66: 2001–2005.
33. El Nakeeb A, Fikry A, El Metwally T, Fouda E, Youssef M, et al. (2009) Early oral feeding in patients undergoing elective colonic anastomosis. Int J Surg 7: 206–209.
34. Palmer DJ, Prescott SL (2012) Does early feeding promote development of oral tolerance? Curr Allergy Asthma Rep 12: 321–331.
35. Prescott SL, Smith P, Tang M, Palmer DJ, Sinn J, et al. (2008) The importance of early complementary feeding in the development of oral tolerance: concerns and controversies. Pediatr Allergy Immunol 19: 375–380.
36. Klappenbach RF, Yazyi FJ, Alonso Quintas F, Horna ME, Alvarez Rodriguez J, et al. (2013) Early oral feeding versus traditional postoperative care after abdominal emergency surgery: a randomized controlled trial. World J Surg 37: 2293–2299.
37. Di Fronzo LA, Cymerman J, O'Connell TX (1999) Factors affecting early postoperative feeding following elective open colon resection. Arch Surg 134: 941–946.
38. Wu B, Chen XZ, Wen L, Chen XL, Yang K, et al. (2013) The feasibility and safety of early removal of nasogastric tube after total gastrectomy for gastric cancer. Hepatogastroenterology 60: 387–389.
39. Zhou T, Wu XT, Zhou YJ, Huang X, Fan W, et al. (2006) Early removing gastrointestinal decompression and early oral feeding improve patients' rehabilitation after colorectostomy. World J Gastroenterol 12: 2459–2463.
40. Jeong O, Ryu SY, Jung MR, Choi WW, Park YK (2014) The safety and feasibility of early postoperative oral nutrition on the first postoperative day after gastrectomy for gastric carcinoma. Gastric Cancer 17: 324–331.
41. Lewis SJ, Andersen HK, Thomas S (2009) Early enteral nutrition within 24 h of intestinal surgery versus later commencement of feeding: a systematic review and meta-analysis. J Gastrointest Surg 13: 569–575.

Permissions

All chapters in this book were first published in PLOS ONE, by The Public Library of Science; hereby published with permission under the Creative Commons Attribution License or equivalent. Every chapter published in this book has been scrutinized by our experts. Their significance has been extensively debated. The topics covered herein carry significant findings which will fuel the growth of the discipline. They may even be implemented as practical applications or may be referred to as a beginning point for another development.

The contributors of this book come from diverse backgrounds, making this book a truly international effort. This book will bring forth new frontiers with its revolutionizing research information and detailed analysis of the nascent developments around the world.

We would like to thank all the contributing authors for lending their expertise to make the book truly unique. They have played a crucial role in the development of this book. Without their invaluable contributions this book wouldn't have been possible. They have made vital efforts to compile up to date information on the varied aspects of this subject to make this book a valuable addition to the collection of many professionals and students.

This book was conceptualized with the vision of imparting up-to-date information and advanced data in this field. To ensure the same, a matchless editorial board was set up. Every individual on the board went through rigorous rounds of assessment to prove their worth. After which they invested a large part of their time researching and compiling the most relevant data for our readers.

The editorial board has been involved in producing this book since its inception. They have spent rigorous hours researching and exploring the diverse topics which have resulted in the successful publishing of this book. They have passed on their knowledge of decades through this book. To expedite this challenging task, the publisher supported the team at every step. A small team of assistant editors was also appointed to further simplify the editing procedure and attain best results for the readers.

Apart from the editorial board, the designing team has also invested a significant amount of their time in understanding the subject and creating the most relevant covers. They scrutinized every image to scout for the most suitable representation of the subject and create an appropriate cover for the book.

The publishing team has been an ardent support to the editorial, designing and production team. Their endless efforts to recruit the best for this project, has resulted in the accomplishment of this book. They are a veteran in the field of academics and their pool of knowledge is as vast as their experience in printing. Their expertise and guidance has proved useful at every step. Their uncompromising quality standards have made this book an exceptional effort. Their encouragement from time to time has been an inspiration for everyone.

The publisher and the editorial board hope that this book will prove to be a valuable piece of knowledge for researchers, students, practitioners and scholars across the globe.

List of Contributors

Stefan Schilling
Department for Internal Medicine, Staedtische Kliniken Moenchengladbach, Moenchengladbach, Germany

Francesco Maria Fusco, Vincenzo Puro and Giuseppe Ippolito
Department for Infectious Diseases, National Institute for Infectious Diseases "Lazarro Spallanzani", Rome, Italy

Giuseppina De Iaco
Department for Internal Medicine, Azienda Ospedaliero, Universitaria Ospedali Riuniti delle Marche, Torrette, Italy

Barbara Bannister
Department for Infectious Diseases, The Royal Free Hospital, London, United Kingdom

Helena C. Maltezou
Department for Interventions in Health-Care Facilities, Hellenic Center for Disease Control and Prevention, Athens, Greece

Gail Carson
Department of Rare and Imported Pathogens, Health Protection Agency, Porton, United Kingdom

Rene Gottschalk
Department for Infectious Diseases, Port Health Authorities, Frankfurt am Main, Germany

Hans-Reinhard Brodt
Department for Infectious Diseases, Goethe University Frankfurt, Frankfurt am Main, Germany

Philippe Brouqui
Department for Infectious Diseases and Tropical Medicine, Marseilles University, Marseille, France

Lixin Ou, Jack Chen, Kenneth Hillman and Stephanie J Hollis
Simpson Centre for Health Services Research, Australian Institute of Health Innovation & South Western Sydney Clinical School, University of New South Wales, Sydney, New South Wales, Australia

Hassan Assareh
Simpson Centre for Health Services Research, Australian Institute of Health Innovation & South Western Sydney Clinical School, University of New South Wales, Sydney, New South Wales, Australia
Epidemiology, Western Sydney Local Health District, Sydney, New South Wales, Australia

Arthas Flabouris
Intensive Care Unit, Royal Adelaide Hospital, Adelaide, South Australia, Australia

Takahisa Kawano
Department of Emergency Medicine, University of Fukui Hospital, Fukui, Japan

Kei Nishiyama
Department of Primary Care and Emergency Medicine, Kyoto University Graduate School of Medicine, Kyoto city, Japan

Hiroyuki Hayashi
Department of General Medicine, University of Fukui Hospital, Fukui, Japan

Mohsen Bayati
Stanford University, Stanford, California, United States of America

Mark Braverman
Princeton University, Princeton, New Jersey, United States of America

Michael Gillam, Karen M. Mack, George Ruiz and Mark S. Smith
MedStar Health and Washington Hospital Center, Washington, D. C., United States of America

Eric Horvitz
Microsoft Research and University of Washington School of Medicine, Redmond, Washington United States of America

Chih-Hsiang Chang, Pei-Chun Fan, Ming-Yang Chang, Ya-Chung Tian, Cheng-Chieh Hung, Ji-Tseng Fang, Chih-Wei Yang and Yung-Chang Chen
Kidney Research Center, Department of Nephrology, Chang Gung Memorial Hospital, Taipei, Taiwan
Chang Gung University College of Medicine, Taoyuan, Taiwan

Chang Gung University College of Medicine, Taoyuan, Taiwan

Tjeerd-Pieter van Staa
Health eResearch Centre, Farr Institute for Health Informatics Research, University of Manchester, Manchester, United Kingdom
Utrecht Institute for Pharmaceutical Sciences, Utrecht University, Utrecht, the Netherlands

Edmond S.-W. Ng, Ben Goldacre and Liam Smeeth
Department of non-communicable diseases, London School of Hygiene & Tropical Medicine, London, United Kingdom

Martin Gulliford
Primary Care and Public Health Sciences, King's College, London, United Kingdom

Karen S. Palmer
Faculty of Science Simon Fraser University, Burnaby, British Columbia, Canada

Taryn Scott, Sohail M. Mulla, Arnav Agarwal, Afeez Abiola Hazzan, John J. You and Gordon H. Guyatt
Department of Clinical Epidemiology and Biostatistics, Faculty of Health Sciences, McMaster University, Hamilton, Ontario, Canada

Thomas Agoritsas
Department of Clinical Epidemiology and Biostatistics, Faculty of Health Sciences, McMaster University, Hamilton, Ontario, Canada
Divisions of General Internal Medicine and Clinical Epidemiology, University Hospitals of Geneva and Faculty of Medicine, University of Geneva, Geneva, Switzerland

Danielle Martin
Department of Family and Community Medicine, Department of Health Policy Management and Evaluation, University of Toronto and Medical Affairs and Health Systems Solutions at Women's College Hospital, Toronto, Ontario, Canada

Ashley P. Miller
Memorial University of Newfoundland, St. John's, Newfoundland, Canad

Andrew Bresnahan
Michael G. DeGroote School of Medicine, McMaster University, Hamilton, Ontario, Canada

Rebecca A. Jeffery
Faculty of Medicine, Dalhousie University, Halifax, Nova Scotia, Canada

Arnaud Merglen
Paediatric Outcome Research Team, The Hospital for Sick Children, Toronto, Ontario, Canada and Division of General Pediatrics, University Hospitals of Geneva and Faculty of Medicine, University of Geneva, Geneva, Switzerland

Ahmed Negm
Rehabilitation School, McMaster University, Hamilton, Ontario, Canada

Reed A. Siemieniuk
Department of General Internal Medicine, Sunnybrook Health Sciences Centre, Toronto, Ontario, Canada

Neera Bhatnagar
Health Sciences Library, McMaster University, Hamilton, Ontario, Canada

Irfan A. Dhalla
St. Michael's Hospital, Department of Medicine and Institute of Health Policy Management and Evaluation, University of Toronto, Toronto, Ontario, Canada

John N. Lavis
Department of Clinical Epidemiology and Biostatistics, Faculty of Health Sciences, McMaster University, Hamilton, Ontario, Canada
McMaster Health Forum, Centre for Health Economics and Policy Analysis, Department of Political Science, McMaster University, Hamilton, Ontario, Canada and Department of Global Health and Population, Harvard School of Public Health, Boston, Massachusetts, United States of America

Stephen J. Duckett
Grattan Institute, Carlton, Victoria, Australia

Maliwan Hongsuwan, Nantasit Luangasanatip and Anchalee Jatapai
Mahidol-Oxford Tropical Medicine Research Unit, Faculty of Tropical Medicine, Mahidol University, Bangkok, Thailand

Pramot Srisamang
Department of pediatrics, Sappasithiprasong Hospital, Ubon Ratchathani, Thailand

Manas Kanoksil
Department of pediatrics, Udon Thani Hospital, Udon Thani, Thailand

Nicholas P. Day and Ben S. Cooper
Mahidol-Oxford Tropical Medicine Research Unit, Faculty of Tropical Medicine, Mahidol University, Bangkok, Thailand
Center for Tropical Medicine, Nuffield Department of Clinical Medicine, University of Oxford, Oxford, United Kingdom

Sharon J. Peacock
Mahidol-Oxford Tropical Medicine Research Unit, Faculty of Tropical Medicine, Mahidol University, Bangkok, Thailand
Department of Microbiology and Immunology, Faculty of Tropical Medicine, Mahidol University, Bangkok, Thailand
Department of Medicine, Cambridge University, Addenbrooke's Hospital, Cambridge, United Kingdom

Direk Limmathurotsakul
Mahidol-Oxford Tropical Medicine Research Unit, Faculty of Tropical Medicine, Mahidol University, Bangkok, Thailand
Department of Tropical Hygiene, Faculty of Tropical Medicine, Mahidol University, Bangkok, Thailand

Cyrille P. Launay and Anastasiia Kabeshova
Department of Neuroscience, Division of Geriatric Medicine, UPRES EA 4638, UNAM, Angers University Hospital, Angers, France

Laure de Decker
Department of Geriatrics, EA 1156-12, Nantes University Hospital, Nantes, France

Cédric Annweiler
Department of Neuroscience, Division of Geriatric Medicine, UPRES EA 4638, UNAM, Angers University Hospital, Angers, France
Robarts Research Institute, Schulich School of Medicine and Dentistry, the University of Western Ontario, London, Ontario, Canada

Olivier Beauchet
Department of Neuroscience, Division of Geriatric Medicine, UPRES EA 4638, UNAM, Angers University Hospital, Angers, France
Biomathics, Paris, France

Dionne S. Kringos and Niek S. Klazinga
Department of Public Health, Academic Medical Center (AMC)/University of Amsterdam, Amsterdam, the Netherlands

Asgar Aghaei Hashjin
Department of Public Health, Academic Medical Center (AMC)/University of Amsterdam, Amsterdam, the Netherlands

Department of Health Services Management, School of Health Services Management and Information Sciences, Iran University of Medical Sciences, Tehran, Iran

Hamid Ravaghi
Department of Health Services Management, School of Health Services Management and Information Sciences, Iran University of Medical Sciences, Tehran, Iran

Jila Manoochehri
Department of Quality Improvement, Tehran Heart Center Hospital, Tehran University of Medical Sciences, Tehran, Iran

Paula K. O. Yokota, Alexandre R. Marra, Marcelino S. Durão and Oscar F. P. dos Santos
Division of Medical Practice, Hospital Israelita Albert Einstein, São Paulo, Brazil

Marines D. V. Martino
Laboratory of Microbiology, Hospital Israelita Albert Einstein, São Paulo, Brazil

Elivane S. Victor
Statistics Department, Instituto Israelita de Ensino e Pesquisa (IIEP), Hospital Israelita Albert Einstein, São Paulo, Brazil

Michael B. Edmond
Department of Internal Medicine, Virginia Commonwealth University School of Medicine, Richmond, Virginia, United States of America

Charles Grégoire, Cédric Bruel, Sandie Brochon, Franc¸ois Philippar and Adeline Max
Medical-Surgical ICU, Saint Joseph Hospital Network, Paris, France

MaiéGarrouste-Orgeas
Medical-Surgical ICU, Saint Joseph Hospital Network, Paris, France

IAME, UMR 1137, Paris Diderot University, Sorbonne Paris Cité, Paris, France

Antoine Périe
Maison des Adolescents, University Hospital Cochin, Paris, France
INSERM U-669, University Paris Sud and University Paris Descartes, UMR-S0669, Paris, France

Philippe Mouricou
Management department, ESSCA School of Management PRES UNAM, Boulogne- Billancourt, France

Benoit Misset
Medical-Surgical ICU, Saint Joseph Hospital Network, Paris, France
University Paris Descartes, Paris, France

Nguyen Hanh Nguyen
Institute of Population, Health and Development, Ha Noi, Viet Nam

Hoa L. Nguyen
Institute of Population, Health and Development, Ha Noi, Viet Nam
Oxford University Clinical Research Unit, Ho Chi Minh City, Viet Nam

Quang Ngoc Nguyen and Dat Tuan Phan
Viet Nam National Heart Institute, Ha Noi, Viet Nam

Duc Anh Ha
Ministry of Health, Ha Noi, Viet Nam

Robert J. Goldberg
Department of Quantitative Health Sciences, University of Massachusetts Medical School, Worcester Massachusetts, United States of America

Calpurnia Jayakumar and Urszula Oldakowska-Ganesan Ramesh
Vascular Biology Center, Georgia Regents University, Augusta, GA, United States of America

Lidia Lewandowska and Joanna Matuszkiewicz-Rowińska
Department of Nephrology, Dialysis & Internal Diseases, Medical University of Warsaw, Warsaw, Poland

Jedynak, Michalina Galas and Marek Krawczyk
Department of General, Transplant and Liver Surgery, Medical University of Warsaw, Warsaw, Poland

Stephen Looney
Department of Biostatistics and Epidemiology, Georgia Regents University, Augusta, GA, United States of America

Małgorzata Dutkiewicz
Department of General and Nutritional Biochemistry, Medical University of Warsaw, Poland

Ilona W. M. Verburg and Nicolette F. de Keizer
Department of Medical Informatics, Academic Medical Center, University of Amsterdam, Amsterdam, the Netherlands

Evert de Jonge
Department of Intensive Care, Leiden University Medical Center, Leiden, the Netherlands

Niels Peek
Department of Medical Informatics, Academic Medical Center, University of Amsterdam, Amsterdam, the Netherlands
Health eResearch Centre, Centre for Health Informatics, University of Manchester, Manchester, United Kingdom

Wenming Wu, Xiafei Hong, Lilan Fu, Shanglong Liu, Lei You, Li Zhou and Yupei Zhao
Department of General Surgery, Peking Union Medical College Hospital, Chinese Academy of Medical Sciences and Peking Union Medical College, Beijing, China

Alexandra Farag, Michael Nartey, Jamie L. Fleet and Sachin Shah
Division of Nephrology, Department of Medicine, Western University, London, Ontario, Canada

Amit X. Garg and Arsh K. Jain
Division of Nephrology, Department of Medicine, Western University, London, Ontario, Canada
Department of Epidemiology and Biostatistics, Western University, London, Ontario, Canada

Eric McArthur
Institute for Clinical Evaluative Sciences, London, Ontario, Canada

Greg A. Knoll
Division of Nephrology, Kidney Research Centre, Ottawa Hospital Research Institute, University of Ottawa, Ottawa, Ontario, Canada

S. Joseph Kim
Division of Nephrology, Toronto General Hospital, University Health Network, University of Toronto, Toronto, Ontario, Canada

Janneke Horn
Department of Intensive Care Medicine, Academic Medical Center, Amsterdam, the Netherlands

Camiel Verhamme and Ivo N. van Schaik
Department of Neurology, Academic Medical Center, Amsterdam, the Netherlands

Luuk Wieske
Department of Intensive Care Medicine, Academic Medical Center, Amsterdam, the Netherlands
Department of Neurology, Academic Medical Center, Amsterdam, the Netherlands
Laboratory of Experimental Anesthesiology and Intensive Care (LNENINCNA), Academic Medical Center, Amsterdam, the Netherlands

Esther Witteveen and Marcus J. Schultz
Department of Intensive Care Medicine, Academic Medical Center, Amsterdam, the Netherlands
Laboratory of Experimental Anesthesiology and Intensive Care (LNENINCNA), Academic Medical Center, Amsterdam, the Netherlands

Daniela S. Dettling-Ihnenfeldt and Marike van der Schaaf
Department of Rehabilitation, Academic Medical Center, Amsterdam, the Netherlands

Laura Marije Hofstra, Arjen J. Stam, Monique Nijhuis and Annemarie M. J. Wensing
Department of Medical Microbiology, Virology, University Medical Center Utrecht, Utrecht, the Netherlands

Tania Mudrikova
Department of Internal Medicine and Infectious Diseases, University Medical Center Utrecht, Utrecht, the Netherlands

Sigrid Otto and Kiki Tesselaar
Laboratory of Translational Immunology, University Medical Center Utrecht, Utrecht, the Netherlands

Lisa M. Vallely
Sexual and Reproductive Health Unit, Papua New Guinea Institute of Medical Research, Alotau, Milne Bay Province, Papua New Guinea

Primrose Homiehombo
Sexual and Reproductive Health Unit, Papua New Guinea Institute of Medical Research, Goroka, Eastern Highlands Province, Papua New Guinea

Angela Kelly-Hanku
Sexual and Reproductive Health Unit, Papua New Guinea Institute of Medical Research, Goroka, Eastern Highlands Province, Papua New Guinea
International HIV Research Group, School of Public Health and Community Medicine, University of New South Wales, Sydney, Australia

Antonia Kumbia
Division of Obstetrics and Gynaecology, Eastern Highlands Provincial Hospital, Goroka, Eastern Highlands Province, Papua New Guinea

Glen D. L. Mola
School of Medicine and Health Sciences, University of Papua New Guinea, Port Moresby, Papua New Guinea

Andrea Whittaker
School of Social Sciences, Monash University, Victoria, Australia

Nathan N. O'Hara and Gerard P. Slobogean
Department of Orthopaedics, University of British Columbia, Vancouver, British Columbia, Canada

Rodney Mugarura
Department of Orthopaedics, Makerere University, Kampala, Uganda

Maryse Bouchard
Department of Orthopaedics, Seattle Children's Hospital, Seattle, Washington, United States of America

M. Isabel Asensio-Cruz
Unidad Médico-Quirúrgica de Enfermedades Respiratorias, Instituto de Biomedicina de Sevilla (IBiS), Hospital Universitario Virgen del Rocio/ Universidad de Sevilla, Sevilla, Spain

Jose Luis Lopez-Campos and Carmen Calero
Unidad Médico-Quirúrgica de Enfermedades Respiratorias, Instituto de Biomedicina de Sevilla (IBiS), Hospital Universitario Virgen del Rocio/ Universidad de Sevilla, Sevilla, Spain
Centro de Investigación Biomédica en Red de Enfermedades Respiratorias (CIBERES), Instituto de Salud Carlos III, Madrid, Spain

Ady Castro-Acosta and Francisco Pozo-Rodriguez
Centro de Investigación Biomédica en Red de Enfermedades Respiratorias (CIBERES), Instituto de Salud Carlos III, Madrid, Spain
Hospital 12 de Octubre, Instituto de Investigación i+12, Madrid, Spain

Xiaohui Wang and Rujia Yu
Center of Infectious Diseases, West China Hospital, Sichuan University, Chengdu, China
Division of Infectious Diseases, State Key Laboratory of Biotherapy, Chengdu, China

Lin Cai
Department of Intensive Care Unit, West China Hospital, Sichuan University, Chengdu, China

Wenzhi Huang
Department of Infection Control, West China Hospital, Sichuan\ University, Chengdu, China

Zhiyong Zong
Center of Infectious Diseases, West China Hospital, Sichuan University, Chengdu, China
Division of Infectious Diseases, State Key Laboratory of Biotherapy, Chengdu, China
Department of Infection Control, West China Hospital, Sichuan\ University, Chengdu, China

Alawi Luetz, Felix Balzer, Finn M. Radtke, Bjoern Weiss and Claudia Spies
Department of Anesthesiology and Intensive Care Medicine, Campus Charité Mitte and Campus Virchow-Klinikum, Charité - Universitätsmedizin Berlin, Berlin, Germany

Christina Jones
Whiston Hospital, Critical Care Unit, Prescot, Liverpool, United Kingdom

Giuseppe Citerio
Hospital San Gerardo, Department of Emergency Medicine, Monza, Italy

Bernhard Walder
Service d'Anesthesiologie, Hôpitaux Universitaires de Genève, Geneva, Switzerland

Klaus-Dieter Wernecke
Sostana GmbH, Berlin, Germany

Da Wang, Liansheng Zheng, Tingyu Mou, Hao Liu and Guoxin Li
Department of General Surgery, Nanfang Hospital, Southern Medical University, Guangzhou, Guangdong, P.R. China

Xiaoping Liu
Department of Gastrointestinal Surgery, The first affiliated hospital of Gannan medical university, Gannan medical university, Ganzhou, Jiangxi, P.R. China

Index